The Chiropractic Theories

Principles and Clinical Applications

Third Edition

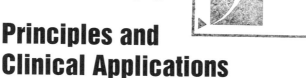
Robert A. Leach, AA, DC, FICC

Chairman, Mississippi Associated Chiropractors Committee on Research
Postgraduate Faculty, National College of Chiropractic, Logan College of Chiropractic, Life Chiropractic College West
Private general practice of chiropractic, Starkville, Mississippi

with contributions from
Reed B. Phillips, DC, PhD
President, Los Angeles College of Chiropractic

Charles A. Lantz, DC, PhD
Director of Research, Life Chiropractic College West

illustrated by Robert S. Fritzius, BS and
 Joseph A. MacGown

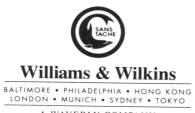

Williams & Wilkins

BALTIMORE • PHILADELPHIA • HONG KONG
LONDON • MUNICH • SYDNEY • TOKYO

A WAVERLY COMPANY

Editor: John Butler.
Managing Editor: Linda Napora
Copy Editor: Anne K. Schwartz
Designer: Dan Pfisterer
Illustration Planner: Ray Lowman
Production Coordinator: Anne Stewart Seitz

Copyright ©, 1994
Williams & Wilkins
428 East Preston Street
Baltimore, MD 21202, U.S.A.

Printed in the United States of America

First Edition, 1980
Second edition, 1986

Library of Congress Cataloging in Publication Data

Leach, Robert A.
   The chiropractic theories : a synopsis of scientific research /
  Robert A. Leach, with contributions from Reed B. Phillips, Charles
  A. Lantz : illustrated by Robert S. Fritzius. -- 3rd ed.
      p. cm.
      Includes bibliographical references and index.
      ISBN 0-683-04904-6
      1. Chiropractic--Philosophy. 2. Dislocations. I. Title.
      [DNLM: 1. Chiropractic. 2. Phillips, Reed B. 3. Lantz, Charles
  A.   WB 905 L434c 1994]
  RZ242.L42 1994
  615.5'34--dc20
  DNLM/DLC   93-17891
  for Library of Congress   CIP

97
4 5 6 7 8 9 10

To Vicki, Robbie, Zach, and Amber.
Thank you for your patience and love.
I will always appreciate your
support of "Daddy's book."

Foreword

According to one old proverb, leisure is a time to do something useful. Not everyone handles leisure in that proverbial way, of course. Rare individuals put their leisure to serious and demanding tasks, even as youthful students. Robert A. Leach as a young student of chiropractic was that kind of person. The first edition of *The Chiropractic Theories* was motivated by the desire to bring together scientific findings relating to the practice of chiropractic and then to share that knowledge with the chiropractic profession.

Five years passed, and Dr. Leach took on the task of writing a second edition while fully occupied in the private practice of chiropractic. Leisure for him remained a time to do something useful. That half-decade was a time of rapid increase in research relating to the profession. The task of summarizing and synthesizing was more difficult than it had been earlier, but the second edition also met with success. My own copy, within easy reach, is well thumbed; its worn pages are a testimony to its usefulness as a handy reference of advances in chiropractic research.

Seven years have passed. Research productivity relating to chiropractic has increased exponentially in the number of published studies. It took a quantum leap in the rigor of methodological and statistical standards. This Third Edition will continue to serve as a guide for chiropractors and students. With our commitment to research, we affirm our service to humankind.

ROBERT ANDERSON, M.D., PH.D., D.C.
Professor of Anthropology
Mills College
Oakland, California

Preface

This is a book about a hope, a fear, and a future. Quite simply, the hope is in the development of science-minded practitioners who will explore the horizons of chiropractic practice in the 21st century. Even as Galileo first peered into the universe to discover that his own world was not flat, chiropractic scientist/practitioners and researchers must look beyond preconceived notions and antiquated theories to discover the true nature of the chiropractic lesion and the true effectiveness of the chiropractic adjustment. Will the paradigm of chiropractic adjustment contributing to wellness be established? Will its effectiveness be limited to musculoskeletal conditions? Or will stress-related or even infectious and malignant processes be shown to improve after chiropractic care? Is bone-out-of-place a rational hypothesis and metaphor to explain chiropractic effectiveness? Can we operationally define a chiropractic lesion, or do we instead explain what happens after adjustment as a *biological effect*? Dare we even ask such questions, let alone seek answers to them? Certainly, just as Galileo was scourged for asking and answering provocative questions in his day, modern chiropractic scientist/practitioners and researchers will be ostracized in direct proportion to the depth of their questioning. The hope then, is that the questions posed in the coming decades will be piercing.

The fear within the pages of this text is unstated but lurks within each chapter nonetheless. It is a fear on the one hand that hypothesis will be taken as fact and thus make further inquiry unnecessary, or alternatively, that since this is all so much speculation and without basis (i.e., without harder randomized prospective trials directed to each question raised in this text), then we can dismiss the whole subject out of hand and exclusively relegate chiropractic to the "safer" domain of acute lower back pain. *The fear then is that we will take for granted that with which we have been given charge, and fail to pursue our hope in scientific inquiry.*

The future is embodied by the final chapters of this text, which embrace the new research mindset: *the methodology, protocol and terminology that chiropractors simply must embrace if indeed we want any role in health care in the 21st century.* Inter- and intraexaminer reliability, outcomes assessment, dependent and independent variables, the role for the scientist/practitioner in development of a scientific database for chiropractic practice—

these and other topics and issues raise questions around which the very existence of chiropractic will turn in the future.

Just as our past was defined by the war with medicine (perhaps stayed somewhat by the decision of the U.S. Supreme Court in December 1991 to uphold Judge Susan Getzendanner's permanent injunction against the AMA for conspiracy to illegally boycott the chiropractic profession [*Wilk et al. v. AMA et al.* U.S. no. 76 c 3777. September 25, 1987]), I believe the future will be defined by our ability to wage war against ignorance of the methods and practices of science within our own ranks. To that end this third edition is humbly brought forth.

New chapters reflecting the new research terminology have been included in this text: *Segmental Dysfunction Hypothesis, Soft Outcome Measures of Dysfunction, Hard Outcome Measures of Dysfunction, Facilitation Hypothesis,* and *Developing Chiropractic Scientist/Practitioners*. Moreover, nearly all chapters that appeared in the second edition have been extensively revamped and/or completely rewritten. One new chapter in particular, *Clinical Aspects of Dysfunction*, is a brief yet thorough review of all the clinical outcome research regarding chiropractic adjustment—for a wide array of human health problems—that has been published in peer-reviewed bioscientific journals (occasionally research that has not appeared in appropriate science journals is presented—albeit not without risk—due to its provocative nature; such "alternative" data are identified appropriately).

In the end, however, this text should be viewed as a beginning, as a starting point for students of chiropractic, for chiropractic clinicians in the field who dare to question the how and why of their practice, for scientist/practitioners who are actively engaged in clinical research and practice, and for full-time chiropractic researchers. This third edition has a slant that is decidedly different from prior editions, with clinical applications aimed at the practitioner in private practice. The theme remains unchanged: *we must have testable hypotheses systemized in some manner that can be used as a platform for scientific inquiry.*

Truly from humble beginnings—originally begun in 1975 as a response to *Consumer Reports'* articles on chiropractic (Consumer Reports 1975;40: 542–547 and 1975; 40:606–610)—this work has now been read by nearly one in five chiropractors world-wide. If those who read this edition would but assertedly embrace development of the science of chiropractic, then the fear within these pages can be exchanged instead for a hope and a future.

ROBERT A. LEACH, AA, DC, FICC

Acknowledgments

A number of individuals were involved with the production of this manuscript; their help and inspiration will not be forgotten. Thanks must begin with those who helped with prior editions, as their effort is still reflected in the current work.

To those whose constructive criticism made the first edition possible, Thomas D. S. Key, Ed.D., Sc.D., Mario Vitelli, Ph.D., D.C., M.D., and R. J. Watkins, D.C., D.A.B.C.R., I again extend my heartfelt thanks. Your efforts continue to bear fruit.

To Thomas Blackshear, B.S., M.S. (proofreading), and Robert Fritzius, B.S. (illustrations), my thanks again for your contributions to the second edition.

The current (third) edition similarly benefitted from many individuals. Thanks go to Joseph F. Unger, Jr., D.C., and to Frank Pederick, D.C., for providing information regarding craniosacral research and to Irvin Korr, Ph.D., for guidance regarding questions pertaining to osteopathic scientific investigations. Thanks also to Joseph MacGown who contributed most of the new illustrations. Especially I would like to thank Michael Patterson, Ph.D., at the Kansas College of Osteopathic Medicine and Surgery, for information and critical assessment regarding portions of Chapter 8; Dana Lawrence, D.C., at the National College of Chiropractic, for criticism of Chapter 9; and Walter Wardwell, Ph.D., for inspiration and criticism as well.

Joseph Keating, Jr., Ph.D., provided not merely some criticism of this work, but much more importantly, he has been an inspiration and mentor since we first met. For caring about chiropractic and our patients, Joe, words will never adequately express my thanks.

Finally, Vicki, thank you again for your help with manuscripts of prior editions, for allowing me to rant and rave about issues and ideas, and for caring as you do.

It were not best that we should
all think alike; it is difference
of opinion that makes horseraces.

Samuel Langhorne Clemens
(Mark Twain)

Contents

Section 2
Pathophysiology of Segmental Dysfunction

Chapter 5   Segmental Dysfunction Hypothesis 43
  Early Evidence 44
  Experimental Evidence 45
    Normal Anatomy and Physiology 45
    Mechanisms of Zygapophyseal Pathophysiology 47
    Physiology of Joint Manipulation 49
  Discussion 51
  Summary 52
Chapter 6   Soft Outcome Measures of Dysfunction 55
  Range of Motion 55
    Motion Palpation 56
    Regional Motion Testing 57
    Algometry 60
    Validity and Reliability 60
    Studies of Algometry in Physical Medicine and Dentistry 61
    Studies of Algometry and Chiropractic Manipulation 63
  Pain and Functional Status Questionnaires 63
    Reliability and Validity 64
  Leg Length Tests 65
  Discussion 67
  Summary 68
Chapter 7   Hard Outcome Measures of Dysfunction 73
  Surface Electromyography 73
    Normal Paraspinal EMG Findings 74
    Abnormal Paraspinal EMG Findings 74
    EMG Changes after Manipulation/CMT 76
  Thermography 76
    Normal Paraspinal Thermographic Findings 77
    Abnormal Paraspinal Thermographic Findings 78
    Thermographic Findings After CMT 78
  Motion Studies of the Spine 78
    Cineroentgenography and Videofluoroscopy 79
    Stress X-Rays 79
    Motion Studies after CMT 80
  Measures of Physical Performance 80
    Normal Spinal Muscle Strength 80
    Abnormal Spinal Muscle Strength 82
    Spinal Muscle Strength after Manipulation/CMT 83
  Discussion 83
  Summary 84
Chapter 8   Facilitation Hypothesis 89
  Neurobiology of Kinesthetic Receptors 89

Section 3
Pathophysiology of
Vertebral Subluxation Complex

Section 4
Spinal Pathophysiology
and Neurodystrophy

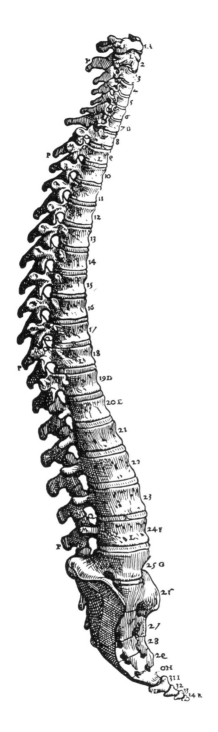

Introduction

Men occasionally stumble over
the truth, but most of them
pick themselves up and hurry
off as if nothing had happened.

Sir Winston Leonard Spencer Churchill

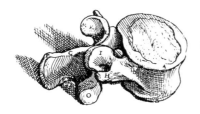

Chapter 1

General Introduction

*H*ugh Hefner got married. Nintendos replaced Cabbage Patch Kids. The Berlin Wall came tumbling down. Hospitals started cooperating with chiropractors. Perhaps just as unbelievable, the 1980s saw the bone-out-of-place hypothesis questioned by chiropractic researchers.

Bone-out-of-place, a concept rooted in 19th century medical thought (see Chapter 4), has been a primary component of chiropractic theory since the inception of the profession (1). Now, however, the predominate thinking seems to be that segmental dysfunction (SDF—see Section 2), and not intervertebral subluxation (see Section 3), is the primary lesion that chiropractors treat.

Whether SDF is actually a stage in subluxation pathophysiology (see "Subluxation Hypothesis," Chapter 10, and Appendix B, "Integrated Biochemical Model for VSC") or is a separate clinical entity often leads to animated debate among some researchers.

Others in research, thwarted by a failure to find validity or reliability in chiropractic analytic methodology, are advocating research on the effects of chiropractic (2). Their question: does chiropractic manipulation exert an affect on pathophysiology, just as would, for example, massage?

As we approach our profession's centennial and the 21st century, chiropractors and chiropractic researchers appear to be scrambling for answers to these and other age-old questions regarding manipulation science and theory.

This text has been written to provide the student, practitioner, and researcher with a comprehensive synopsis of scientific and medical literature relevant either directly or indirectly to chiropractic theories.

The need for this review and discussion is underscored by the fact that these questions have a direct bearing on chiropractic practice and, hence, legislative, educational, practice scope, ethical, and other issues.

Developing Hypotheses

Many hypotheses have been developed regarding causes and effects of segmental dysfunction and intervertebral subluxation. Most of them have been stated by one or more practitioners who then devised or patterned a technique after the hypothesis (Table 1.1). Certainly it is beyond the scope of this book to investigate them all; an attempt has been made to present hypotheses when (*a*) there is a substantial amount of scientific and/or medical literature in which the idea is explored and (*b*) based on these studies, there is a reasonable probability that the hypothesis is correct to some degree and therefore should be investigated further.

An understanding of the development of theory is necessary so that the reader can

Table 1.1
Principal Chiropractic Techniques[a]

Technique	Inventor
Activator methods	W. C. Lee and A. W. Fuhr
Ajustment of the spastic muscle	Spastic Muscle Research Bureau, Inc.
Applied kinesiology	G. Goodheart
Atlas subluxation complex and correction	R. Gregory
Basic technique (Logan basic)	H. B. Logan
Bioenergetic synchronization	M. T. Morter
Chiroenergetics	E. H. Kimmel
Chiro-Manis treatment	J. M. Cox
Chiropractic neurobiochemical analysis	W. K. Ehmann
Concept therapy	H. Dill
Craniopathy	C. Cottam
Directional nonforce technique	R. Van Rumpt
Endonasal and allied techniques	D. D. Gibbons
Fixation analysis-movement palpation	H. Gillet and M. Liekens
Gonstead technique	C. S. Gonstead
Gonstead cervical chair technique	C. S. Gonstead
Grostic procedure	J. Grostic
Kinesiology	F. Stoner
Life cervical technique	D. Jones
Mears technique	D. B. Mears
Palmer upper cervical	B. J. Palmer
Perianal postural reflex	R. J. Watkins
Pettibon method	B. E. Pettibon
Pierce-Stillwagon	W. V. Pierce
Polarity therapy	E. E. Jarvis
Receptor-tonus method	R. L. Nimmo
Reinert's disc move	O. C. Reinert
Rolfing	I. P. Rolf
Sacrooccipital technique	M. B. DeJarnette
Spears painless system	L. Spears and D. Spears
Spinal touch treatment	W. Lamar Rosquist
Thompson terminal point technique	J. C. Thompson
Toftness system	I. N. Toftness
Von Fox combination technique	R. Von Fox

[a]Information from Kfoury P. H. Catalog of Chiropractic Techniques. St. Louis: Logan College of Chiropractic, 1977

study the text and keep the data in proper perspective (see Chapter 2, written by Reed Phillips). Review of differences in terminology between the various health professions is the purpose of Chapter 3, "Manipulation Terminology"; and the history of the various chiropractic hypotheses is explored briefly in Chapter 4.

Central Axioms

The axiom common to all chiropractic theories has traditionally been that an intervertebral subluxation (subluxation is defined in Chapter 3) somehow alters the normal neurophysiological balance found in a healthy individual.

As previously mentioned, that axiom has been challenged by a shift in the thinking of chiropractic researchers in the past decades away from the static concept of subluxation and toward a dynamic concept of segmental dysfunction.

Accordingly, edition three of this text reviews the medical and chiropractic concepts of intervertebral subluxation with related hypotheses in Section 3, while a new Section 2 reviews the concept of SDF with its related hypotheses. Section 2 begins with the chiropractic and osteopathic concept of segmental dysfunction, leading to the secondary concept of facilitation. Tertiary hypotheses are that facilitation of spinal segments create aberrant somatoautonomic as well as somatosomatic reflexes. A chapter on clinical aspects of SDF is a major feature of this section.

Section 3 includes chapters on hypotheses relevant primarily to the medical model for intervertebral subluxation, including neuropathy, myelopathy, and vertebrobasilar insufficiency. From the aspect of the research data presented, the medical model for subluxation describes a more severe clinical picture. Clinical aspects of intervertebral subluxation as a phase of VSC are presented in this section

These hypotheses clearly overlap (Fig. 1.1), and traditional thinking has the intervertebral subluxation model including the concept of aberrant motion (see Appendix B on the vertebral subluxation complex, by Charles Lantz).

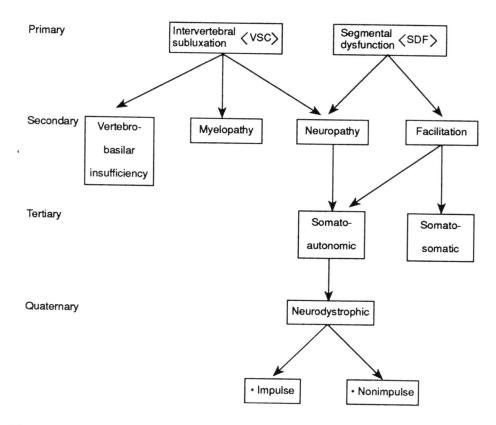

Figure 1.1. Hypothesized effects of segmental dysfunction and intervertebral subluxation.

A new Section 4 is concerned with hypotheses regarding the relationship of spinal lesions to neurodystrophy. A final quaternary hypothesis is that by a variety of mechanisms, neurodystrophy can be created involving both impulse and nonimpulse mechanisms. Again, clinical considerations and implications are reviewed.

An updated and expanded Section 5 includes chiropractic research issues, including diagnosis, effectiveness, and theory. Based on the available scientific literature, this author has further developed these hypotheses. Working definitions have been adapted from the original authors' contributions (Table 1.2), and references from the medical and scientific literature are used to lend objectivity to the discussion. Chiropractic references are given weight when published in peer-reviewed journals. Many of the references contained herein have not been readily available to the chiropractic profession, as years of dust have all but hidden them in the stacks at various medical and osteopathic college libraries. Unveiling these old data and comparing them with modern findings will, it is hoped, provide a clear overview of facts relevant to the various chiropractic theories.

Need for Synthesis

More than ever before, a clear presentation of chiropractic theories is necessary. Probably more than 150 case presentations and clinical investigations of chiropractic have been reported in the *Journal of Manipulative and Physiological Therapeutics* alone since the first edition of this textbook was published in 1980. In addition, legitimate chiropractic research efforts have appeared in *Spine*, *Manual Medicine*, and other peer-reviewed science and medical journals. This monograph attempts to synthesize these data to update the student and practitioner, with a new emphasis on clinical applications, while providing some literature review helpful for the researcher as well.

Efforts to synthesize chiropractic research data are further justified by the need to accurately dispense this information to the academic community, as well as the public at large. Federal inclusion of chiropractic in Medicare and Medicaid programs, recent advances in chiropractic service utilization by some hospitals, licensing of chiropractors by all 50 states, federal recognition of chiropractic education, and steadily increased

Table 1.2
Hypotheses Relating to Chiropractic Theory

Segmental dysfunction—common spinal lesion recognized by lessened or otherwise altered mobility, altered pressure threshold to pain, and signs of neuromuscular dysfunction

Facilitation—chronic neural dysfunction associated with persistent segmental dysfunction, including lowered skin resistance, aberrant sudomotor responses; high vasomotor and sudomotor activity, and may result in abnormal somatoautonomic reflex activity

Vertebral subluxation complex—SDF commonly progresses to intervertebral subluxation and spinal degeneration

Nerve compression—intervertebral subluxations may interfere with the normal transmission of nerve energy by irritating or compressing the spinal nerve roots

Compressive myelopathy—intervertebral subluxation may, in some severe cases (even in the absence of fracture/dislocation) irritate, compress, or destroy the spinal cord

Vertebrobasilar arterial insufficiency—cervical intervertebral subluxations that may cause deflection or compression of the vertebral arteries, thereby altering cerebral circulation

Neurodystrophy—Neural dysfunction is stressful to the visceral and other body structures, and this "lowered tissue resistance" can modify the nonspecific and specific immune responses and alter the trophic function of the involved nerves

Axoplasmic aberration—axoplasmic transport may be altered in certain cases in which the spinal nerve roots or spinal nerves are compressed or irritated by intervertebral subluxation or facilitation

---

use by the public all point to a need for increased awareness of chiropractic research and theory (3–5). As our nation contemplates inclusion of chiropractic in federal health insurance, this synthesis of data gains added importance.

In any given year, probably 15 million Americans see a chiropractor (6), and based on ACA members' 1989 median gross incomes ($174,500.00)(7) and given 30,000 U.S. practitioners, they spend more than 5 billion for their care. Probably 1 in 4 Americans has been to a chiropractor at one time or another (8, 9), and roughly 80% believe chiropractic is effective (7). Moreover, so many Americans now believe chiropractic is effective for back pain, that 31% will see a chiropractor if the back pain persists longer than 2 weeks (10).

Perhaps as impressive as these gains in the public eye, chiropractic has won its day in court against the American Medical Association and others who conspired to eliminate the profession (11). In 1987, U.S. District Court Judge Susan Getzendanner issued a permanent injunction, citing lawless behavior on the part of the AMA (11). In 1990, that decision was upheld by the Court of Appeals (12), and the Supreme Court refused to hear an appeal by the AMA. All this has permitted referrals between doctors of medicine and chiropractic to increase, along with increased cooperation in education and research as well.

This progress in education and public relations, and in political and social arenas, begs the question, what advances are being made in chiropractic research? In addition to addressing this question, the purpose of this text is to provide a review of literature necessary for research, education, and practice.

The presentation of data in this book follows standard journal style. Following Chapter 4, chapters begin with a review of older literature (chiropractic, medical, and/or scientific) dealing with the subject matter at hand. Review of current clinical, experimental, and in some cases, postmortem studies are also accomplished. A general discussion precedes the chapter summary, which acts to highlight important concepts. This format is designed to simplify the presentation of these studies, which might otherwise appear to be too complex for quick comprehension.

Summary

Chiropractic researchers are questioning some of the basic tenets of chiropractic theory. Researchers are no longer focusing exclusively on subluxation and segmental dysfunction, but on the effects of chiropractic manipulation as well. Hypotheses reviewed in this text include those related to subluxation, segmental dysfunction, neurodystrophy, and chiropractic research issues. The need for systemization and synthesis of chiropractic research data is underscored by advances in utilization of chiropractic services. It is within the scope of this book to review and synthesize these data to provide a basis for understanding chiropractic theory, as well as provide the researcher, practitioner, and student with a model for research, debate, and study.

REFERENCES

1. Gibbons RW. The evolution of chiropractic: medical and social protest in America. In: Haldeman S, ed. Modern developments in the principles and practice of chiropractic. New York: Appleton-Century-Crofts, 1980: 3–24.

2. Keating JC Jr. Science and politics and the subluxation. Am J Chiro Med 1988;1: 107–110.

3. Howie LJ. Utilization of selected medical practitioners: United States, 1974. Int Rev Chiro 1978;32:41–47.

4. Davidson GM, ed. U.S. Dept of HEW issues approval, Council on Chiropractic Education is now the official accrediting agency for all colleges. Dig Chiro Econ 1974;17:6.

5. Carmichael JP. Chiropractic residency at Lindell Hospital: a program description. J Manipulative Physiol Ther 1988;11:177–180.

6. Berk ML, Schur CL. Nonphysician health care providers: use of ambulatory services, expenditures, and sources of payment. Data preview #22. Natl Health Care Expenditures Study. DHHS Publication, No. 86-3394. Rockville, MD, 1985.

7. Anonymous. ACA annual statistical survey. Washington D.C.: American Chiropractic Association, 1990.

8. Wardwell WI. The Connecticut Survey of Public Attitudes toward Chiropractic. J Manipulative Physiol Ther 1989;12:167–173.

9. Brooks R. Attitudes toward chiropractic health care in Oklahoma. Oklahoma City; Chiropractic Association of Oklahoma, 1984.

10. Deyo RA. Descriptive epidemiology of low back pain and its related medical care in the United States. Spine 1987;12:264–268.

11. Goodley PH. Chiropractic and Judge Getzendanner's injunction. [Letter] JAMA 1988; 260:1717.

12. Associated Press. Ruling against AMA upheld in chiropractors' lawsuit. Des Moines Register; Feb 9, 1990:3A.

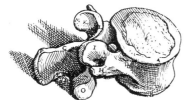

Chapter 2

Philosophy and Theory

If we indoctrinate the young person in an elaborate set of fixed beliefs, we are insuring early obsolescence. The alternative is to develop skills, attitudes, habits of mind and the kinds of knowledge and understanding that will be instruments of continuous change and growth on the part of the young person. Then we will have fashioned a system that provides for its own continuous renewal.

John Gardner

*T*he diabolical debate over philosophy continues to divide the chiropractic profession. "Straights" and "super-straights" challenge the "mixers" and "medipractors," all in the name of chiropractic. Yet in the midst of this tribal divisiveness, scientific verification of the effectiveness of chiropractic care continues to bolster social acceptance of the profession. Recognition of chiropractic as an acceptable health care alternative is being broadcast over the airways and in the printed media. Externally, the profession moves strongly toward legitimacy; internally, it languishes in the mire of mediocre thought.

Chiropractic extends from the extremes of the rampant empiricist (anything is acceptable) to the dogmatic devotee of fundamentalism (strict adherence to a very limited perspective). There should be a common thread that can bind this profession together, however loose that binding may be. The fundamentals of philosophy and theory may provide this thread of continuity. This chapter attempts to coalesce the common philosophical foundations that lead to critical thought and productive theoretical development.

Definitions of Philosophy

There are numerous definitions of philosophy. In the December 1991 issue (vol. 21, no. 4) of the *Chiropractic Journal of Australia* (an issue totally dedicated to philosophy), there are no less than six different definitions of the term *philosophy*, without referring to a particular branch of philosophy or to philosophy and chiropractic. Durant offers an interesting perspective, "Philosophy is harmonized knowledge making a harmonious life; it is the self-discipline which lifts us to serenity and freedom"(1). Can philosophy bring harmony, serenity, and freedom to chiropractic? or is philosophical conflict healthy to the future development of the chiropractic construct?

These traditional definitions provide a foundation:

Philosophy—
1. Pursuit of wisdom
2. A search for a general understanding of values and reality by chiefly speculative rather than observational means
3. An analysis of the grounds of and concepts expressing fundamental beliefs (2).

If philosophy is defined as the pursuit of wisdom, understanding, and the analysis of beliefs, then harmony, serenity, and freedom are within our professional grasp. Harmony implies the absence of debate and dialogue, which to some suggests stagnation and decline.

Divisions of Philosophy

Philosophy is divided into a variety of branches:

Metaphysics—study of the fundamental nature of reality and existence and of the essences of things; often subdivided into *ontogeny*—study of being and *cosmology*—study of the physical universe;

Epistemology—study of the nature, basis, and extent of knowledge (a priori and empirical);

Logic—study of the principles and methods of reasoning (inductive and deductive);

Ethics—study of human conduct, character, and values (relativism, objectivism, and subjectivism);

Aesthetics—study of the creation and principles of art and beauty, and of thoughts, feelings, and attitudes (3).

This categorization is designed to enhance and clarify the science of philosophy. Essentially, philosophical thought is an inescapable part of human existence and can be directed to any subject. But the philosophical thoughts directed to a subject, i.e., the study of ———, do not in turn become the subjects' philosophy. For example, the pursuit of wisdom, the understanding of values, and the analysis of beliefs (Webster's definition of philosophy) of a religion are part of the philosophy of religion but are not the "religious philosophy" or "tenets" of that religion. The pursuit of wisdom, the understanding of values, and the analysis of beliefs regarding chiropractic are the components of the philosophy of chiropractic but not "chiropractic philosophy" or "tenets" of chiropractic. By definition, there is no "chiropractic philosophy," only a philosophy of chiropractic (4).

This statement is not intended to inflame adherents of "chiropractic philosophy" terminology; it is an attempt to clarify meaning, according to definitions acceptable to the academic community and to society in general. "Disrespect for the position of the academic community itself, is an expression of ignorance" (4).

Philosophy and Chiropractic: Divisions in the Profession

Discussions of the philosophy of chiropractic tend to center in the metaphysical branch of philosophy, or the study of the fundamental nature of things. It is within this branch of philosophical thought that concepts of materialism, mechanism, vitalism, and holism reside. The mechanistic and vitalistic concepts associated with D. D. and B. J. Palmer are chronicled elsewhere in this text (see Chapter 4). The reader should be aware that there is variety of thought in the fundamental belief systems associated with chiropractic, which in large measure contributes to confusion in the profession's philosophical debate.

Coulter (5) claims that contemporary philosophy of chiropractic is actually a philosophy of health that can be viewed as the offspring of five distinct philosophies: (*a*) vitalism, (*b*) holism, (*c*) naturalism, (*d*) conservatism (therapeutic), and (*e*) critical rationalism. He speaks of three interrelated principles in this chiropractic philosophy of health: (*a*) the innate tendency of the body to restore and maintain health through homeostatic mechanisms; (*b*) health as an expression of biological, psychological, social, and spiritual factors, with disease or illness being multicausal; and (*c*) the belief that healthful living contributes significantly to health and the patient is responsible for active participation in obtaining improved health. The doctor facilitates this process.

An alternative perspective is repeated by Rondberg (6) in *The Philosophy of Chiropractic*, which attributes chiropractic the status of a branch of philosophy. Quoting from Rondberg's work, "In chiropractic, the basic underlying precepts remain unchanged and unchangeable. These beliefs—this philosophy—is the WHY of chiropractic. Chiropractic doesn't *HAVE* a philosophy . . . Chiropractic *IS* a philosophy." Rondberg also refers to underlying principles, listing the key ones as (*a*) the existence of a *Universal Intelligence*, (*b*) the presence of an inborn *Innate Intelligence* in all living things, (*c*) that health is the expression of the Innate Intelligence through *Innate Matter*, via *Innate Energy*, and (*d*) that *Dis-ease* is the result of the interference with the transmission of Innate Energy causing a decrease in the expression of Innate Intelligence. According to Rondberg, these assumed unchanging principles form the basis of the "super" straight chiropractic approach to health care which consists solely in the detection of the subluxation (the cause of nerve interference) and its removal through the specific chiropractic adjustment.

The irony in the dichotomy presented above is that many adherents at both ends of the spectrum exemplified by Coulter and Rondberg believe in a universal intelligence, an innate intelligence, and the expression of life as the combination of matter and energy. Some may vary in their descriptions of the governance of that expression of life; recognizing, however, that an external or unexplainable force or entity may exist. Both perspectives give central focus to the neuromusculoskeletal system and speak of the homeostatic mechanisms of the body or the body's ability to heal. This irony is more significant when one realizes that medicine adheres to similar concepts of an unexplainable life force, homeostasis, and the body's ability to heal itself (7).

So why the debate between chiropractic and medicine and between elements within the chiropractic profession? Fundamental beliefs seem to be comparable but not compatible. One major difference is the apparent self-appointment of straight chiropractic to an independent branch of philosophy and its unchanging character (see also Chapter 16). The remaining issues dividing the groups reside in the role assigned to the philosophy (i.e., the ability to pursue wisdom, seek understanding of values, and analyze fundamental beliefs and concepts).

Pseudoscience versus Science

If philosophy leads to wisdom and understanding, there must be a method by which this occurs. *Knowledge*, the foundation of wisdom and understanding, is obtained in a variety of ways. Intuition, authority, experience, and logic are all methods of obtaining knowledge. Intuition lacks objectivity and cannot be measured in a mechanistic paradigm. Authority is subject to bias and misinterpretation. Experience through the senses may be subject to interpretive errors. Through deductive reasoning based on a predetermined set of laws or inductive reasoning based on empirical observation, logic may also prove a potentially fallible source of knowledge.

To eliminate error from our knowledge base, a method called science has come into existence. In a very defined manner, knowledge is scrutinized to determine validity and reliability. The scientific method, formidable in its power, is a time-proven way to evaluate knowledge. Using such tools as controls, randomization, masking, repeated measures, and statistical tests, science attempts to refute hypotheses by exposing error. The detection of error nulls the hypothesis and calls the theory into question. If error is not found, the theory is strengthened, and the pursuit of wisdom and understanding is enhanced. The essence of the scientific method is the testable hypothesis. (Whoso loveth correction loveth knowledge, but he that hateth reproof is brutish. Proverbs 12:1) The inability to test the hypothesis moves the hypothesis from the realm of science to the realm of pseudoscience, from objective rational thinking to metaphysical mysticism.

This is not to deny the role of discovery in the field of science; many concepts and ideas have come into existence prior to being subjected to the scientific method. Science is discussed here to emphasize its role in exposing error, as opposed to opening the door to new discoveries.

Theory Development

What is a theory? *Theory*, as a systematic abstraction, implies an organization of words or other labels that represent objects, properties, or events in the real world (8). In experiencing life, we often strive to understand the many injustices or the unexplainable beauty that we see or feel. Organizing these sensations or feelings brings order to the myriad of stimuli that inundate life. Through this organizational process, one systematically abstracts reality and attempts to explain the meaning or the purpose or the reason why life exists as it does. A theory is formed.

Causal explanations are expressed in theory. The value of a theory is related to its ability to provide an explanation of why something exists or why something happens. A theory is thus strengthened when it generates multiple hypotheses that can withstand the rigors of the scientific method. (*Falsification* is the process of refining knowledge by finding error with testable hypotheses.) As theory develops, knowledge expands, and paradigm clarification ensues. Paradigms determine how we interpret the world around us. They help create the road map to our reality. They form the network upon which our theories hang and are tested. Our *paradigm* is the aggregation of our fundamental beliefs, our philosophy.

Theories that fail to produce testable hypotheses are of little value in the pursuit of wisdom and knowledge, for they allow no opportunity to eliminate error. Nontestable hypotheses lead to poorly substantiated theories, and they in turn fail to provide a paradigm that will lead to productive research. Our fundamental beliefs are suscep-tible to gross error with no means of detection. Reality can become dogmatic, irrational, even incomprehensible, and subject to whims of thought and unrealistic perceptions. There is a Flat Earth Society in existence today (9).

Theory to Philosophy

Where does theory fit and what is its usefulness? Testable hypotheses subjected to scientific scrutiny lead to the reduction of error and the clarification of our theoretical explanation of our existence within the confines of our paradigm. This approach is very mechanistic and leads to reductionism; the whole is equal to the sum of its parts. This is counter to the holistic or vitalistic concept of a life force that makes the whole greater than the sum of its parts.

Thus another dilemma. Can the scientific method lead us back to our philosophical roots from which original theories have been postulated? Can science prove philosophy? The answer is No, given the current state of science. Science proves nothing. Science eliminates error by disproving the testable hypothesis. If done properly and frequently, theories are questioned, paradigms are altered, and fundamental beliefs may be subject to reinterpretation.

Hence the relationship of science and philosophy. Through the methods of science with all its limitations, wisdom is pursued, values are challenged, and fundamental beliefs are analyzed. When fundamental beliefs and reality are in conflict, either paradigms change or new ones are created, as described by Kuhn (10).

Philosophy remains speculative; it is not rigorously objectively tested but is rigorously argued. When objective testing and argumentation bring fundamental beliefs into question, our interpretations of reality may need reevaluation. Einstein's theory of relativity did not negate Newton's laws, but it did add to our understanding of reality; it changed our paradigm and perhaps our philosophy.

Agenda for Chiropractic

What is the significance of all this to chiropractic? There is a philosophy related to chiropractic that has many common elements throughout the varied factions within the profession; some factions elevate these tenets to a transcendent level. The commonality of our philosophical tenets should bring harmony to chiropractic, according to Durant (1).

The factionalism appears to occur when one descends from philosophical tenets to practical application of fundamental beliefs; when one moves from philosophy to theory, from nontestable to testable explanations.

To state that an innate intelligence manages the health of the body is an unmeasurable philosophical tenet common to chiropractic and medicine. To state that a subluxation (however defined) interferes with the ability of this innate intelligence is also untestable, since there are no objective means of measuring innate intelligence. (The Keating Innatometer is yet to be validated scientifically (11).) But, when a subluxation is operationally defined, it becomes measurable, which removes a statement about the role of the subluxation from the category of philosophical tenet to that of theory or hypothesis (see also Chapters 16 and 17).

The subluxation theory, to be of value, must produce testable hypotheses that are subject to scientific scrutiny. Only by this process can the theory be refuted and abandoned or validated to contribute to the pursuit of wisdom and understanding and support our philosophical tenets.

The dichotomy in chiropractic is that some in the profession seek scientific validation of the theories related to subluxation while others continue to revere subluxation as a philosophical construct not subject to question. The latter position is dogmatic, antiscientific, and akin to blind faith in a theology rather than a philosophy. Such a position invites cultist, antiscientific, and anti-intellectual labeling. Moreover, this closed-mindedness can be construed to support irrationality and irresponsibility when practitioners limit their clinical responsibility to the detection and removal of an unmeasurable philosophical tenet (the subluxation).

On the other hand, when theories are used to derive testable hypotheses and the scientific method is used to conduct the tests, new knowledge and deeper understanding contribute to the pursuit of wisdom. This process is rational, responsible, and frightful. Frightful in the sense that fundamental beliefs may be brought into question, challenged, and even changed. Adoption of this approach opens the mind and the profession to growth and expansion but carries the threat of change to fundamental rituals and traditions.

The chiropractic profession appears to be approaching the same sort of crossroad that homeopathy faced at the turn of the century, as described by Starr (12). With one foot in science and one foot in prescientific mysticism, homeopaths failed to produce evidence to support the value of their existence and essentially disappeared from the health care delivery scene. If chiropractic adopts the philosophical justification approach to their existence, the role of scientific investigation will be devalued and evidence supporting the worth of chiropractic will be lacking. If the profession adopts the merits of scientific investigation stimulated by theoretical development derived from a proper understanding of the role of philosophy, there is hope for continuance.

Chiropractic Theories

This book is designed to present a brief historical and philosophical review, thorough review of relevant chiropractic and medical research, and a theoretical basis for the profession. It represents a monumental effort in a very small domain. Chiropractic needs critical thinkers who can draw upon our philosophical tenets to develop new theories as well as test the hypotheses of the old ones. Stagnation of thought is a symptom of a dis-ease referred to as hardening of the categories (13). Where are the Einsteins of chiropractic? On the lecture circuit? In the colleges? As comprehensive as this text is, there should be additional volumes of critical thought attesting to the maturity of this profession (see Chapter 16).

The future of chiropractic is in the hands of the profession. Our philosophy need not be abandoned. Our theories need testing. New theories are to be derived. Critical thinking must supplant stagnation of thought. With all that chiropractic has to offer society, it is shameful that it stands at a crossroad that could lead to its demise if wrong choices are made. Wise choices usually result from the pursuit of wisdom rather than from intellectual arrogance or ignorance.

Summary

Philosophy includes the branches of metaphysics, ontology, cosmology, epistemology, logic, ethics, and aesthetics.

The interconnections of philosophy and science are complex. This parsimonious presentation of those interconnections is intended to provide an infrastructure for the remainder of this text. Some argue the philosophy of chiropractic is the result of five distinct philosophies: vitalism, holism, naturalism, conservatism (therapeutic), and critical rationalism. Theories of chiropractic are in their infancy.

Science is the method used to scrutinize knowledge through a process termed falsification. Knowledge can only be examined if it is first expressed as a testable hypothesis. While science cannot "prove" philosophy, it can refute theories and eliminate error by disproving testable hypotheses. Scientific discovery and philosophical debate are essential to future growth and development of the profession. It is argued that closing our minds to new thoughts and new ideas or reinterpretation of old ideas in new settings is professional suicide. Finally, the search for wisdom and understanding through critical analysis of our fundamental beliefs is advocated.

REFERENCES

1. Durant W. The pleasures of philosophy. New York: Simon & Schuster, 1953:xii.

2. Webster's new collegiate dictionary. Springfield, Mass.: G & C Merriam, 1979.

3. The world book encyclopedia, vol 15. Chicago: World Book, 1988:383–385.

4. Coulter I. Chiropractic philosophy has no future. Chiro J Aust 1991;21(4):129–131.

5. Coulter I. An institutional philosophy of chiropractic. Chiro J Aust 1991;21(4):129–131.

6. Rondberg T. The philosophy of chiropractic. Chandler, Ariz.: Terry A. Rondberg, 1989.

7. Ledermann E. Philosophy and medicine. Philadelphia: JB Lippincott, 1970:24.

8. Chinn P, Jacobs M. Theory and nursing. St Louis: CV Mosby, 1987:18.

9. Radner D, Radner M. Science and unreason. Belmont, Calif.: Wadsworth, 1982:1.

10. Kuhn T. The structure of scientific revolutions. 2nd ed. Chicago: University of Chicago Press, 1970.

11. Keating J. Interexaminer reliability of the innatometer. J Manipulative Physiol Ther 1990;13(4):229–233.

12. Starr D. The social transformation of American medicine. New York: Basic Books, 1982:107–108.

13. Adams A. personal communication.

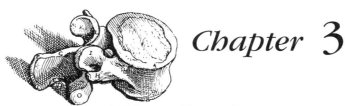

Chapter 3

Manipulation Terminology

*T*here are significant barriers to interprofessional and even intraprofessional communication about chiropractic adjustment (i.e., chiropractic manipulative therapy, (CMT)) and osteopathic and physiotherapeutic procedures. Variations between the professions and within the chiropractic profession in diagnostic and treatment procedures and criteria complicate communications, largely because of terminological differences.

This chapter broadly reviews the traditional approaches to defining the manipulative lesion, the current definitions used by the professions, and medical versus chiropractic subluxation and segmental dysfunction, in an attempt to clarify this material and expedite comprehension of issues that will arise in subsequent chapters. Certainly progress in chiropractic and manipulation research and attempts to clarify manipulation terminology will provide a more satisfactory foundation for dialog in the 21st century than now exists.

Traditional Definitions of the Manipulable Lesion

Historically, the medical definition of the manipulable lesion centered around use of the term "subluxation." In fact, the medical author Hieronymus as early as 1746 stated

Subluxation of joints is recognized by lessened motion of the joints, by slight change in the position of the articulating bones and by pain . . . most displacements of vertebrae are subluxations rather than luxations (1).

Of course the earliest "manipulable lesions" might have included posterior curvatures caused by falls as opposed to incurable humpback associated with disease (2).

In the 19th century, manipulation was a fashionable medical treatment of spinal curvatures and weaknesses. Perhaps the most classic concept of the century was that of "spinal irritation" of the marrow, easily diagnosed by eliciting tenderness on pressure over the offending vertebral spine (2). Hence, early medical concepts of the manipulable lesion centered around use of the term subluxation to describe a slightly misaligned vertebra, and involved spinal curvatures and spinal irritations producing a wide variety of illnesses. Loss of proper joint motion and point tenderness are described as aspects of the lesion. Early osteopathic criteria for the manipulable lesion included palpation of bony maladjustment, when marked, and of localized tension. Muscular contraction associated with the lesion was recognized by "generally increased tone of the spinal muscles, or by the occurrence of localized "knots" or "strings" in the irregularly contracted muscles of the deeper spinal layers" (3).

Localized sensitivity to palpation (i.e., point tenderness) is described and x-ray is used to verify the lesion routinely by 1917. Rigidity and less reliable findings, including skin and hair changes in the affected area, are noted as well as antalgia, as indicating the manipulable lesion (3). In contrast, early chiropractic definitions of the manipulable lesion (i.e., subluxation) were given by D. D. Palmer (4): "a partial or incomplete separation; one in which the articulating surfaces remain in partial contact" and by B. J. Palmer (5):

1. Misalignment with co-respondents above and below wherein three different abnormal directions from its normal position are in permanent misalignment
2. Occlusion of a foramen through which nerves pass
3. Pressure upon nerves
4. Interference to transmission of mental impulse supply.

Although neither of the Palmers consider joint motion as a factor in subluxation, several early chiropractic authors discuss the concept (see Chapter 4), and Henry J. Gillet may have popularized the notion with the publication of his *Belgian Notes on Fixation* in 1951 (6):

> A vertebral articulation can become fixed in any of the positions it normally takes in spinal movement. Vertebrae do not 'slip out of place,' they are not 'displaced' out of their physiological boundaries, they have not gone out of their limits of motion. When we adjust subluxations we do not 'replace' vertebrae.

Clearly, traditional medical, osteopathic, and chiropractic attempts to identify and define the manipulable lesion included concepts of misalignment, point tenderness, restricted motion, muscular contraction, and other phenomena. While lacking quantification and specific qualification, these concepts have set the stage for redefinition of the lesion(s) in light of contemporary understanding.

Defining the Methods of Manipulation

Spinal manipulative therapy (SMT) describes generally the use of any of a variety of manipulative procedures by the various practitioners of the healing arts (7). Three major healing professions, as well as other minor healing arts, use SMT.

Under the auspices of orthodox medicine, physical therapists and some medical doctors practice manipulation, "the forceful passive movement of a joint beyond its active limit of motion" (8). This technique involves the use of long levers and slow, passive articular movements (9). When a joint is passively mobilized to the end of its passive range of motion, the resistance encountered is thought to be due to tensing of the joint capsule. The joint undergoing mobilization is passively moved, back and forth, up to the point where resistance is met (10).

In contrast, osteopathic manipulative therapy (OMT) often involves active participation of the patient; the osteopathic profession uses a wide variety of manipulative and mobilization techniques (11). The chiropractic profession is the largest health profession in the world in which SMT is the central method of treatment. Chiropractic manipulative therapy (CMT) is unique in many aspects, however. CMT is also termed "adjustment" and involves the use of short-lever, specific, high-velocity, controlled forceful thrusts by hand or instrument, which are directed at specific articulations (12). CMT is intended to force the joint surfaces beyond the initial barrier of resistance and to the anatomical limit of "safe" joint play.

Roston and Haines (13) and Meal and Scott (14) have provided evidence that the "crack" associated with CMT suggests that the range of motion of a joint has been extended into the so-called paraphysiological space (Fig. 3.1). This key component of most methods of CMT is based on the concept developed by Roston and Haines (13) and modified by Sandoz (16) that initially joints behave elastically until the joint surfaces suddenly separate. At that point,

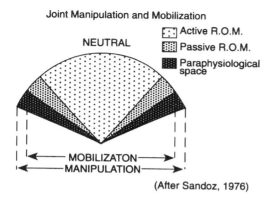

Joint Manipulation and Mobilization

NEUTRAL

[∷] Active R.O.M.
[▦] Passive R.O.M.
[■] Paraphysiological space

←— MOBILIZATON —→
←—— MANIPULATION ——→

(After Sandoz, 1976)

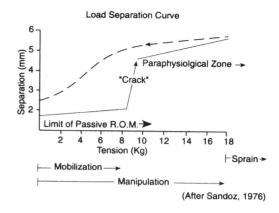

Load Separation Curve

Separation (mm)

← Paraphysiolgical Zone →

"Crack"

Limit of Passive R.O.M. →

Tension (Kg)

├— Mobilization —→

├———— Manipulation ————→

├Sprain→

(After Sandoz, 1976)

Figure 3.1. Mobilization is said to differ from manipulation in that in the former, a joint is passively moved back and forth up to its barrier of initial resistance, while in the latter, a thrust forces the joint beyond its initial barrier of resistance and into its so-called paraphysiological space (13, 16).

Figure 3.2. In a classic study by Roston and Haines (13), it was determined that at a certain point, distraction of a joint (8.3 kg of tension in the metacarpophalangeal joint) produces rapid separation of joint surfaces (2 to 4.7 mm in their study) along with a cracking noise. Other studies suggest that this is due to liberation of gases from the synovial fluid, a process termed cavitation. (Adapted from Sandoz R. Some physical mechanisms and effects of spinal adjustments. Ann Swiss Chiro Assoc 1976;6:91–141.)

where the "crack" is heard, the normal subatmospheric pressure in the joint space is altered dramatically as gases are liberated from the synovial fluid (evidenced by a radiolucent cavity seen on x-ray)(13, 15). This process is known as *cavitation* (Fig. 3.2).

After manipulation, the gases are gradually resorbed back into the synovial fluid. During this refractory period, which lasts approximately 20 minutes in the metacarpophalangeal joint, a second crack cannot be produced. Haldeman's (17) suggestion that types of manipulation should be distinguished in research on SMT is underscored by evidence that mobilization techniques cannot mimic the effects of a local anesthetic injection in relieving spontaneous myoelectrical activity associated with spinal joint dysfunction, whereas the manipulative thrust (i.e., CMT, OMT) can (18).

To further complicate matters, a variety of manipulative thrust maneuvers are used by chiropractors, osteopaths, and medical doctors. One must carefully compare the results of various trials of manipulation accordingly, considering that the differences between the various methods of manipulation may have a significant impact on clinical outcomes.

Defining Subluxation—Medical versus Chiropractic Perspectives

Current medical and chiropractic attempts to define intervertebral subluxation have generally centered around the use of radiographic criteria. In general terms, medical subluxation often refers to an operable spinal lesion that is considered unstable:

Semiluxation; an incomplete luxation or dislocation; though a relationship is altered, contact between joint surfaces remains (19).

For example, spondylolisthesis is graded by degrees of slippage (viz., Meyerding grades I, II, or III (20)), and surgery is considered when progressive slippage (i.e. instability) is demonstrated radiographically in conjunction with back and/or leg pain, despite conservative therapeutic intervention (21).

That mild or moderate trauma affecting the cervical spine in adolescents and children can result in rotary subluxation of the atlas is recognized by Birney and Hanley

(22). In their series of 84 cases of injury, 23 resulted in this type of subluxation and responded well to traction or a soft collar.

Hyperanteflexion sprain is the term preferred by Braakman and Penning (23) to describe anterior subluxation of C2-C3. While advocating Minerva jacket or collar and bed rest for the child with this lesion, they consider it potentially a surgical lesion in an adult:

> In adults [,] surgical fusion may be indicated in cases of recurrent or severe angulation. In minor angulation a policy of 'wait and see' is adopted. Fusion is effected by bone grafting either by the posterior [approach] or [by the] anterior approach. Wiring may help in establishing reduction of the angulation during the operation (23).

Translation of a vertebra in the cervical spine when it is flexed or extended is not considered significant unless it is beyond a 3.5-mm slip (24). Similarly, radiographic criteria for subluxation in the lumbar spine defining segmental instability as occurring whenever there is 3 mm of slippage have been described in the literature but are challenged by evidence that on lumbar flexion/extension, 20% of 59 asymptomatic individuals have 4 mm or more of translational motion (25).

Similarly, atlantoaxial translation can be severe and even life threatening and has been associated with Reiter's disease and rheumatoid arthritis, even without trauma. This type of subluxation is considered unstable when the atlantodental interval increases to 9 mm on cervical flexion (26).

Traditionally, chiropractic radiographic criteria for subluxation have been much broader than medical criteria. For example, a 1–2 mm lateral deviation of atlas on axis would have been labeled a subluxation by some types of chiropractic analyses, while medical radiographers would label the same finding a normal variant. Moreover, chiropractic radiographic technique researchers have had mixed results determining reliability of some of these measures (27, 28).

Another area of disagreement between chiropractic and medical use of the term subluxation pertains to scoliosis and angular deformities such as cervical kyphosis (Fig. 3.3). This appears to be a semantic difference, with medical authors referring to these lesions as "abnormal curvatures," and chiropractors referring to them as vertebral subluxation complex (VSC) (see also Chapter 10) (29–31). Since initial studies indicate that at least one chiropractic manipulative technique has a beneficial corrective effect on cervical hypolordosis and kyphosis, and given that at least some spinal curvatures can be corrected with heel-lift therapy, there is merit to use of the term VSC (31, 32).

From this cursory review of the professions' use of the term subluxation, we can see that confusion might arise from two primary sources: (a) differing radiographic criteria between the chiropractic and medical professions, and (b) semantic differences in labeling spinal disorders. By careful reporting and quantitatively describing spinal lesions, the professions can enjoy improved inter- and intraprofessional communications and research in the future.

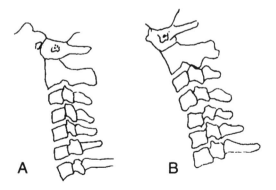

Figure 3.3. Disagreement over use of the term subluxation by medical and chiropractic authors is exemplified by cervical hypolordosis (*A*) and cervical kyphosis (*B*). Medical authors refer to these radiographic findings as abnormal curvatures, while chiropractic authors prefer the terms subluxation or vertebral subluxation complex (From 32, used by permission.) (30, 31).

Defining Segmental Dysfunction

While a more thorough study of segmental dysfunction (SDF) is presented in Chapter 5, a cursory review here will serve to clarify clinical differences between SDF and VSC. Researchers and clinicians use terms such as somatic dysfunction (osteopathy), spinal joint dysfunction (manual medicine), and spinal fixation (chiropractic), to describe the manipulable lesion that current investigators are still in the process of defining operationally. For purposes of symmetry, this text will use the term segmental dysfunction to describe this spinal lesion.

Segmental dysfunction refers to a localized spinal lesion that exhibits asymmetry or reduction in motion, associated with disturbed muscular activity, sensitivity to percussion, and sensitivity to deep pressure (33–36).

As previously stated, VSC relies largely on radiographic criteria for the diagnosis to be established. By contrast, researchers are using inclinometers and goniometers to measure motion derangements, pressure threshold devices to measure point tenderness, and more sophisticated electromyography (EMG) to measure aberrant myoelectric activity associated with SDF (37–39).

Indeed, classic osteopathic research indicates that electrical skin resistance, myoelectrical activity, and sudomotor reflexes are altered by SDF (40). Recent investigations indicate that manipulation may be effective in changing abnormal electrodermal activity and EMG activity associated with SDF as well (18, 38).

Clinically, when the practitioner locates the tender spinous, "taut" erector spinae muscles and isolates the restriction in joint motion, the diagnosis of SDF is established. Qualitatively and quantitatively, however, the operational definition of this lesion has yet to be established (see also Chapter 9).

Perhaps most importantly, a unifying model of VSC-SDF has yet to be established. Although there have been considerable attempts to create such a model (see Chapter 10; see also Appendix B), clinically operational definitions of stages of degenerative and inflammatory changes associated with SDF and VSC have yet to be devised and tested. Further, even within the chiropractic profession, a standardized nomenclature to define radiographic aspects of the VSC is unavailable (41). Efforts to remedy these issues through research should have a profound impact on chiropractic practice in the 21st century. In the interim, uniform definitions such as those recently endorsed by the American Chiropractic Association Advisory Panel on Technique (M. Gatterman, personal communication) will aid greatly in using these terms (Table 3.1).

Summary

There are significant barriers to interprofessional and intraprofessional communication regarding CMT, diagnostic and treatment procedures, and criteria for the application of SMT. Early and contemporary concepts of the manipulable lesion (SDF) suggest an area exhibiting tenderness, loss of proper joint motion, and abnormal muscular contraction.

Some physiological aspects of chiropractic and osteopathic manipulation have been compared with physiotherapeutic mobilization techniques. Differing aspects of medical subluxation and VSC have been discussed. Confusion between the professions arises because of differing radiographic criteria regarding diagnosis of the lesion and differences in semantics as well.

SDF is defined and discussed briefly in light of current research activity. However, research has yet to provide operational definitions of SDF and VSC, and efforts to do so may be expected to profoundly affect chiropractic practice in the 21st century.

Table 3.1
ACA Advisory Panel on Technique Adopted Terminology (1993)

Motion segment—A functional unit made up of the two adjacent articulating surfaces and the connecting tissues binding them to each other.
Spinal motion segment—Two adjacent vertebrae and the connecting tissues binding them to each other.
Subluxation—A motion segment, in which alignment, movement integrity, and/or physiological function are altered although contact between joint surfaces remains intact.
Manipulable subluxation—A subluxation in which altered alignment, movement, and/or function can be improved by manual thrust procedures.
Subluxation complex—A theoretical model of motion segment dysfunction (subluxation) that incorporates the complex interaction of pathological changes in nerve, muscle, ligamentous, vascular, and connective tissues.
Subluxation syndrome—An aggregate of signs and symptoms that relate to pathophysiology or dysfunction of spinal and pelvic motion segments or to peripheral joints.
Manual therapy—Procedures by which the hands directly contact the body to treat the articulations and/or soft tissues.
Manipulation—A manual procedure that involves a directed thrust to move a joint past the physiological range of motion, without exceeding the anatomical limit.
Mobilization—Movement applied singularly or repetitively within or at the physiological range of joint motion, without imparting a thrust or impulse, with the goal of restoring joint mobility.
Adjustment—Any chiropractic therapeutic procedure that utilizes controlled force, leverage, direction, amplitude, and velocity, which is directed at specific joints or anatomical regions. Chiropractors commonly use such procedures to influence joint and neurophysiological function.

REFERENCES

1. Watkins RJ. Subluxation terminology since 1746. ACA J Chiro 1968;Sept:65–70.

2. Lomax E. Manipulative therapy: a historical perspective from ancient times to the modern era. In: Goldstein M, ed. The research status of spinal manipulative therapy. Washington, D.C.: GPO, 1975:11–17.

3. Burns L. The effects of lumbar lesions (bulletin #5). Chicago: AT Still Research Institute, 1917:14–15.

4. Palmer DD. The science, art and philosophy of chiropractic. Portland, Ore.: Portland Printing House, 1910:490.

5. Palmer BJ. The subluxation specific—the adjustment specific. Davenport, Ia.: Palmer School of Chiropractic, 1934:329.

6. Gillet H. Belgian notes on fixation. Privately published, 1951.

7. Wardwell WI. Discussion: the impact of spinal manipulative therapy on the health care system. In: Goldstein M, ed. The research status of spinal manipulative therapy. Washington, D.C.: GPO, 1975:11–17.

8. Friel JP, ed. Dorland's illustrated medical dictionary. 25th ed. Philadelphia: WB Saunders, 1974:909.

9. DeHesse P. Chirotherapy. Prescott, Ariz., published privately, 1946:13–26.

10. Cassidy JD, Kirkaldy-Willis WH, McGregor M. Spinal manipulation for the treatment of chronic low back and leg pain: an observational study. In: Buerger AA, Greenman PE, eds. Empirical approaches to the validation of spinal manipulation. Springfield, Ill.: Charles C Thomas, 1985:119–148.

11. Greenman PE. Manipulative therapy in relation to total health care. In: Korr IM, ed. The neurobiologic mechanisms in manipulative therapy. New York: Plenum, 1978:43–53.

12. Janse J. History of the development of chiropractic concepts; chiropractic terminology. In: Goldstein M, ed. The research status of spinal manipulative therapy. Washington, D.C.: GPO, 1975:25–42.

13. Roston JB, Haines RW. Cracking in the metacarpo-phalangeal joint. J Anat 1947;81: 165–173.

14. Meal GM, Scott RA. Analysis of the joint crack by simultaneous recording of sound and tension. J Manipulative Physiol Ther 1986;9:189–196.

15. Unsworth A, Dowson D, Wright V. Cracking joints: a bioengineering study of cavitation in the metacarpophalangeal joint. Ann Rheum Dis 1971;30:348–358.

16. Sandoz R. Some physical mechanisms and effects of spinal adjustments. Ann Swiss Chiro Assoc 1976;6:91–141.

17. Haldeman S. What is meant by manipulation? In: Buerger AA, Tobis JS, eds. Approaches to the validation of manipulation therapy. Springfield, Ill.: Charles C Thomas, 1977:299–302.

18. Thabe H. Electromyography as a tool to document diagnostic findings and therapeutic results associated with somatic dysfunctions in the upper cervical spinal joints and sacroiliac joints. Manual Med 1986;2:53–58.

19. Hensyl WR, ed. Stedman's medical dictionary. 24th ed. Baltimore: Williams & Wilkins, 1982:1356.

20. Meyerding HW. Spondylolisthesis: surgical treatment and results. Surg Gyn Obstet 1932;54:371–377.

21. Hanley EN, Levy JA. Surgical treatment of isthmic lumbosacral spondylolisthesis. Spine 1989;14:48–50.

22. Birney TJ, Hanley EN. Traumatic cervical spine injuries in childhood and adolescence. Spine 1989;1277–1282.

23. Braakman R, Penning L: Injuries to the cervical spine. In: Vinken PJ, Bruyn GW, eds. Handbook of clinical neurology. Injuries to the spinal cord part 1. Vol. 25. New York: Elsevier, 1976:242.

24. White AA, et al. Biomechanical analysis of clinical stability in the cervical spine. Clin Orthop 1975;109:85–96.

25. Hayes MA, Howard TC, Gruel CR, Kopta JA. Roentgenographic evaluation of lumbar spine flexion-extension in asymptomatic individuals. Spine 1989;14:327–331.

26. Hotta Y, et al. Non-osseous dural compression in rheumatoid atlanto-axial subluxation. Spine 1989;14:236–241.

27. Sigler DC, Howe JW. Inter- and intra- examiner reliability of the upper cervical x-ray marking system. J Manipulative Physiol Ther 1985;8:75–80.

28. Jackson BL, Barker WF, Gambale AG. Reliability of the upper cervical x-ray marking system: a replication study. Chiropractic 1988;1:10–13.

29. Norris SH, Watt I. The prognosis of neck injuries resulting from rear-end vehicle collisions. J Bone Joint Surg 1983;65-B:608–611.

30. Lantz CA. The vertebral subluxation complex part 1: an introduction to the model and the kinesiological component. Chiro Res J 1989;1:23–36.

31. Owens E, Leach RA. Changes in cervical curvature determined radiographically following chiropractic adjustment. In: Proceedings of the 1990 International Conference on Spinal Manipulation. Washington, D.C.: Foundation Chiroprac Educ Res, 1990: 165–169.

32. Leach RA. An evaluation of the effects of chiropractic manipulative therapy on hypolordosis of the cervical spine. J Manipulative Physiol Ther 1983;6:17–23.

33. Johnston WL. Inter- rater reliability in the selection of manipulable patients. In: Buerger AA, Greenman PE, eds. Empirical approaches to the validation of spinal manipulation. Springfield: Charles C Thomas, 1985: 106–118.

34. Nansel DD, Cremata E, Carlson J, Szlazak M. Effect of unilateral spinal adjustment on goniometrically assessed cervical lateral flexion end-range assymetries in otherwise asymptomatic subjects. J Manipulative Physiol Ther 1989;12:419–427.

35. Eder M, Tilscher H. Chiropractic therapy, diagnosis and treatment. (Gengenbach MS, English language ed). Rockville, Md.: Aspen, 1990:23–30.

36. Dvorak J, Dvorak V. Manual medicine, diagnostics. New York, Thieme-Stratton, 1984: 47–49.

37. Patterson MM, Steinmetz JE. Long-lasting alterations of spinal reflexes: a potential basis for somatic dysfunction. Manual Med 1986;2:38–42.

38. Ellestad SM, Nagle RV, Boesler DR, Kilmore MA. Electromyographic and skin resistance responses to osteopathic manipulative treatment for low-back pain. JAOA 1988;88: 991–997.

39. Waldorf V, Devlin L, Nansel D. The assessment of normal paraspinal musculature on
50 female and 50 male subjects in the prone
and standing positions. In: Proceedings of
the 1990 International Conference on Spinal
Manipulation. Washington, D.C.: Foundation
Chiropr Educ Res, 1990:255–262.

40. Korr IM. Sustained sympathicotonia as a factor in disease. In: Korr IM, ed. The neurobiologic mechanisms in manipulative therapy.
New York: Plenum, 1978:229–268.

41. Cashman SJ. Nomenclatures of anatomical
distortions of the spine: a comparison. J Manipulative Physiol Ther 1988;11:31–35.

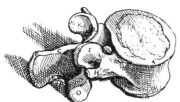

Chapter 4

History of the Chiropractic Theories

"When we circle the wagons we shoot inwards!" declared Ian Coulter, Ph.D., past president of the Canadian Memorial Chiropractic College at a conference recently (1). It is a sad commentary that we chiropractors are often our own worst enemy. Throughout our first century of existence, since the first Palmer father-son disputes, a divided profession has hampered clinical, public relations, legislative, and research endeavors (2–4). By focusing on dogma and disputes about personalities, untested hypotheses, and treatments rather than concentrating on scientific research into clinical questions and rational philosophy, the profession was doomed to irrational development (5). Despite these turbid beginnings, the last two decades have seen a remarkable transition toward more scientific education and toward the application of scientific method to chiropractic research.

This chapter briefly explores the prechiropractic 19th century medical use of manipulation and turn-of-the-century metaphysical beliefs, and traces chiropractic from these roots to the present experience.

Spinal Irritation

While we do not know much about the ancient (viz., around 2700 BC) Chinese uses of manipulation, we do know of them through the writings of Kong-Fou (6). In contrast, Hippocrates was quite descriptive in recording his manipulative technique, succussion (i.e., shaking up violently), by hand, by foot, using wood as a lever, and even by sitting on the hump to reduce it forcibly (7). The Greek physician used extension and pressure "taking into consideration whether the reduction should naturally be made straight downwards, or towards the head, or towards the hip" (8).

However, it was the 19th century before discoveries such as the Bell-Megendie law and Marshall Hall's theory of reflex action again placed the spinal cord in the medical limelight. "Spinal irritation" became a clinical entity following coinage of the term by Thomas Brown in 1828 in the *Glasgow Medical Journal* (7). In 1832, the *American Journal of Medical Sciences* began carrying news from Europe about spinal irritation, and eminent physicians reported diagnostic progress. Tenderness of the appropriate vertebra, corresponding to the diseased organ in question, clinched the diagnosis (7).

J. Evans Riadore, who wrote *Irritation of the Spinal Nerves* in 1843, is probably the contemporary father of the nerve compression hypothesis, according to Donald Tower (9). Tower quotes Riadore as saying, "if any organ is deficiently supplied with nervous energy or of blood, its functions immediately, and sooner or later its structure, become deranged." Riadore concluded that irritation of nerve roots resulted in disease and advocated manipulation to treat this disorder. It is noteworthy that Riadore made these conclusions two years before D. D. Palmer (Fig. 4.1), the founder of chiropractic, was even born. In 1894, Sir William Gowers, a prominent physician in the London Hospital, said, "function depends upon the release of force—nerve force" (10).

Thus, the stage was set for Andrew Taylor Still (the founder of osteopathy) and D. D. Palmer. Still and Palmer were probably outraged at the late nineteenth century medical treatment for spinal irritation, which included cauterization and application of leeches to the tender dorsal area (7). Probably the hypothesis adopted by Palmer resulted largely from this nineteenth-century contemporary medical thought, and manipulation was adopted as a more conservative mode of treatment than the aforementioned remedies. However, Palmer's theories developed from more than a refined mechanistic viewpoint (i.e., using mechanical and physical principles to treat spinal mechanical disorders). Palmer's theories apparently evolved from nineteenth-century spiritual and vitalistic beliefs as well.

Vitalism: Metaphysical Roots of Innate

American spiritualism is said to date to 1848. Modern spiritualists still hold to traditional spiritualistic principles including the belief "that the phenomena of nature, both physical and spiritual, are the expression of infinite intelligence" (11). Spiritualists of the late 19th century commonly held colorful seances to contact spirits.

In 1875, Theosophy was founded by spiritualist Helena Blavatsky, with one of its objectives being to investigate, "unexplained laws of nature and the psychical powers latent in man" (11). One of the beliefs of Theosophy is that ultimately spiritual and natural laws are the same.

Donahue (12), in a thorough investigation of the subject, concludes that D. D. Palmer was probably a student of metaphysics from about 1870, became a student of science while practicing magnetic healing about 1890, and after "discovering" chiropractic in 1895 (or 1896; J. Keating, Jr., personal communication), attempted to merge science with metaphysics. Starting the Palmer School and Cure in 1897, Palmer's first graduates included a significant number who already held degrees in medicine or osteopathy. Initially Palmer must have taught a mechanistic philosophy in line with contemporary medical thinking at the turn of the century, as it is believed the founder was well read in current medical literature. Indeed perhaps the first known Palmer writing, according to Gibbons (13), was published in 1899 and was called "Luxation on Bones Cause Disease." Reprinted by son B. J. Palmer in Davenport newspaper advertisements in 1902 and unearthed after investigation by Cyrus Lerner, D. D. Palmer states:

> All diseases are prolonged until the pressure upon the nerves leading to the parts affected are freed from the pressure. The manner of removing the pressure is done by the use of the hands of the operator. The muscles, nerves and bones of the patient are manipulated in such a manner as to adjust the system properly to itself . . . This pressure is caused by the luxation or displacement (partial or complete) of the bones or by contraction of the muscles drawing on or across the nerves . . . (13)

Not only is the above passage of interest because of the absence of any mention of metaphysical concepts, but it is also interesting that D. D. Palmer's first writings refer

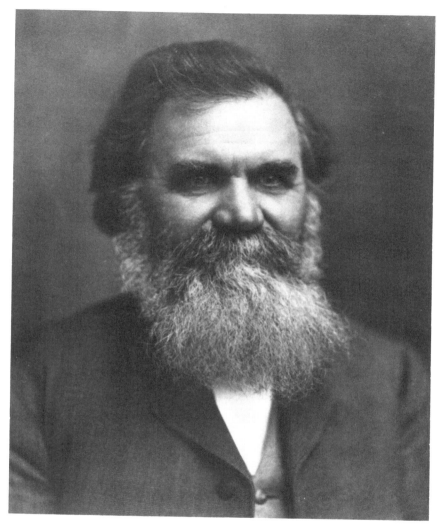

Figure 4.1. D. D. Palmer founded chiropractic in 1895. His writings were apparently based on turn-of-the-century scientific knowledge, but were influenced by spiritualistic and vitalistic beliefs as well. (From Palmer College of Chiropractic Archives.)

to nerve pressure caused by contracted muscles. That concept was lost in Palmer's text, yet perhaps was more correct than his "bone out of place" concept, in light of today's understanding of neurophysiology.

However, known theosophical influences, what he read, his close association with the famous theosophical writer and lecturer W.J. Colville, and the timing and character of his first ideas on "innate philosophy" suggest a strong metaphysical influ-

ence (12). Hence, in his 1910 text, Palmer states

To express the **individualized** intelligence which runs all the functions of our bodies during our wakeful and sleeping hours, I chose the name Innate. Innate—born with. And so far I would not change it except to replace it with the name of that individualized entity which really is a part or portion of that All Wise, Almighty, Universal Intelligence, the Great Spirit, the Greek's Theos, the Christian's

God, the Hebrew's Helohim, the Mahometan's Allah, Hahneman's Vital Force, New thot's Divine Spark, the Indian's Great Spirit, Hudson's Subconscious Mind, the Christian Scientist's All Goodness, the Allopath's Vis Medicatrix Naturae—the healing power of nature (14).

Rejecting or unaware of contemporary mechanistic theory and a 1905 paper by Albert Einstein on special relativity, Palmer chose to adopt vibratory theory—that nerves vibrated normally at approximately 200 vibrations per minute, representing "tone" of the nervous system (12, 15). According to Donahue (12), Palmer was aligned with turn-of-the-century Theosophists in adopting a more modern version of the centuries-old universal ether theory (i.e., that natural forces work through an invisible medium). Palmer apparently believed (like other occultists) that thoughts were also explainable by vibratory theory and could be sent telepathically. Palmer may have been pushed into combining a questionable scientific theory with metaphysical beliefs by other influences as well.

Morikubo Trial: Chiropractic Philosophy Unique

In 1906, in Scott County, Iowa, D. D. Palmer was sentenced to serve three months in jail for practicing medicine without a license, but he paid a fine and was released early (J. Keating, Jr., personal communication). Understanding that religious and spiritual healing were judiciously considered in many health statutes at the time, he might have considered his system as meeting both scientific and religious criteria necessary for the legal survival of chiropractic. This assumption is based upon his direct statement (15) and on the influence he and his son B. J. (Fig. 4.2) must have felt by the outcome of the trial of Dr. Shegataro Morikubo in La Crosse County, Wisconsin, in 1907.

Morikubo, a Palmer-educated chiropractor, was charged with practicing medicine, surgery, and osteopathy without a license

(16). B. J. Palmer hired a prominent local attorney and state senator, Thomas Morris, to defend the Japanese-American, and he quickly mounted an effective defense. Indeed the Palmer-picked attorney's first successful defense of a chiropractor over the charge of practicing medicine without a license, based upon chiropractic's unique philosophy, may have been the cement for B. J.'s clinging to the metaphysically based Innate philosophy.

Perhaps a better understanding of the Palmers' fears of medical persecution—and hence the need for a strategy to defend against it—can be gleaned from Chittendon Turner's (17) observation that by 1930, at least 30,000 jail terms had been served by chiropractors for practicing medicine without a license (Fig. 4.3). A review of B. J. Palmer's writings suggests that one primary (if not the primary) reason for clinging to Innate philosophy was to provide a defense against medical persecution. Indeed a pamphlet he wrote just before his death, "Shall Chiropractic Survive?," classically warns that straying away from Innate philosophy in the future would spell the very death of the profession through losses in court and the legislatures:

> The above letter shows that THE ONLY COURSE to pursue, is an honest, straight, sincere presentation OF CHIROPRACTIC AS IS, not as it would be what THE NCA has been attempting to enforce down the throats of our profession legislatively.
>
> All thinking and honest chiropractors will see, by evidence contained in the BLUE BOOK, the necessity of getting on, staying on, and sticking closely TO chiropracTIC IF they wish to KEEP CHIROPRACTIC AS A DISTINCT AND SEPARATE PROFESSION. NO OTHER WAY CAN, HAS, OR EVER WILL WIN (18).

In fact, to B. J. Palmer, the necessity for preserving the TIC in chiropractic (TIC refers to principled chiropractic) was akin to preserving chiropractic itself. Loss of this metaphysically based philosophy meant the profession was watered down, and adher-

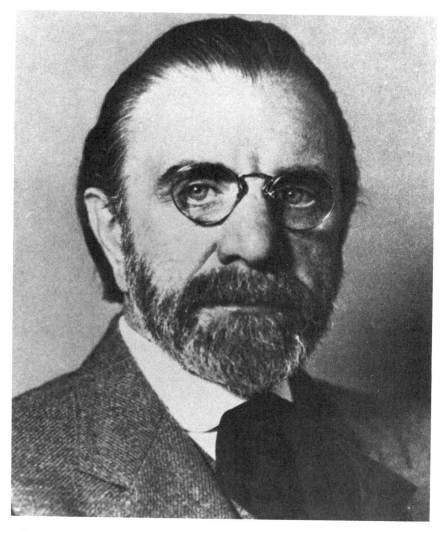

Figure 4.2. B. J. Palmer, son of the founder, is acknowledged as the "developer" of chiropractic. Due to an intense struggle within chiropractic and with organized medicine at about the time of the Morikubo trials, B. J. may have been pressured into adopting a metaphysical philosophy to protect the profession in courts of law. (From Palmer College of Chiropractic Archives.)

ents to any other philosophy were as low as dogs:

MEDI-practic or MEDI-practor.
MEDI, first two syllables of MEDI-cine.
and,
A MEDI-practor, falsely misrepresents MEDI-cine AND chiropractic, is an imposter to both, using subterfuging deceptions to both professions.

A MEDI-practor is a mongrel, belonging to neither species or professions (18).

With this understanding of the influences on D. D. Palmer's and B. J. Palmer's beliefs, we can more fully appreciate their struggle to develop a metaphysical philosophy of chiropractic and their desire to protect that philosophy at any cost.

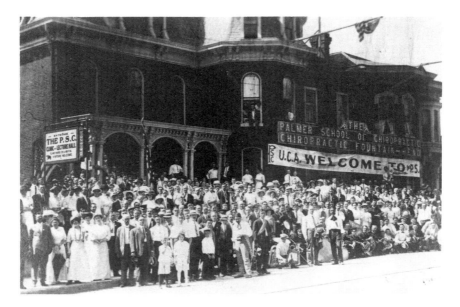

Figure 4.3. Palmer School of Chiropractic as it appeared early in the century. By the 1930s, 30,000 jail terms were served by chiropractors, creating the need for a philosophy to defend the profession in courts of law. (From Palmer College of Chiropractic Archives.)

Palmer's Contribution

Harvey Lillard was a janitor in Davenport, Iowa, who had lost his hearing for 17 years until he met D. D. Palmer. Palmer discovered that Lillard's deafness had begun after a joint in his back had "given away" while he was stooping. Palmer says he reasoned that replacing the bone's alignment would restore the hearing, which it apparently did, and the chiropractic experience began (14).

D. D. Palmer admitted several times that he was not the first to use manipulation to correct human ailments, but he did claim to be the first to use the spinous and transverse processes of vertebrae as levers enabling the doctor to "rack" the bones back to their normal juxtaposition. Palmer (14) also "named the mental act of accumulating knowledge, the cumulative function, corresponding to the physical vegetative function—growth of intellectual and physical—together, with the science, art and philosophy—chiropractic." Palmer's writings are a classic in the profession today. His 1910 textbook, *The Science, Art and Philosophy of Chiropractic*, included some contradictions, verbal assaults against his son and other would-be chiropractic educators of the time, and metaphysically based philosophy, in addition to legitimate turn-of-the-century clinical and scientific information.

Palmer's hypothesis was that a bone out of place in the spine (i.e., subluxation), from accidents or poisons, resulted in nerve impingement, increased or decreased body tonus, and thereby disease. Correction of the spinal subluxation was followed by convalescence and a return to optimum health. Palmer rejected both the germ theory and the older humoral theory of disease causation (i.e., that disease results when the four humors—blood, phlegm, and yellow and black bile—are out of balance)(14).

While Palmer's concept of nerve vibration creating tone has obviously been displaced, his hypothesis that too much or not enough nerve function is disease was a forerunner to later accepted scientific concepts of homeostasis, and was the beginning of what are today known as the nerve compression and neurodystrophic hypotheses (see Chapters 11 and 14).

Palmer's contribution to chiropractic philosophy and theory was to be rejected by some dissenters because of its metaphysical and spiritual components and for other reasons. Nevertheless, it is conceivable that the Palmers' approach to mixing the metaphysical with turn-of-the-century scientific knowledge—to prevent medical persecution from destroying the fledgling profession—did provide the profession with some sense of identity and purpose, in addition to providing a legal defense against the charge of practicing medicine without a license.

To this day, a significant minority of chiropractors continue to accept Innate philosophy, although according to Donahue (2):

> The whole concept of Innate of course rests on accepting on faith the basic premises without hope of any concrete proof. From a strictly scientific viewpoint, Innate must be rejected out of hand because it fails the most fundamental requirement of science, namely testability. From the standpoint of logic, the whole concept of Innate depends on the logical fallacy called word magic. Giving names and definitions to unprovable spiritual entities like Innate and soul cannot guarantee their existence.

Perhaps the tragedy for the chiropractic profession and for chiropractic patients and potential patients was that continuing acceptance of this theosophy and philosophy undermined critical rationalism that when fully applied to chiropractic education, research, and practice, would have promoted the very growth in the profession the Palmers desired most (19).

Setting Palmer's philosophical mistakes aside, his steadfast contribution to the creation and development of our profession—an alternative to drugs and surgery for millions—despite often intense medical persecution, cannot be underemphasized nor easily dismissed.

Dissenters: Other Schools and Leaders

Before the Morikubo trial, other schools of chiropractic had already developed in rejection of perceived flaws in the Palmer educational curriculum. One of D. D. Palmer's first graduates, Solon Massey Langworthy, founded the American School of Chiropractic and Nature Cure by 1903 (13, 20). In 1906, Langworthy, Oakley Smith, and Minora Paxson (Fig. 4.4) published the first textbook on chiropractic, preceding the first Palmer textbook by several weeks. Their two-volume text, *Modernized Chiropractic*, was used by attorney Morris to establish chiropractic's unique philosophy in winning the Morikubo court case. (However, the Langworthian philosophy Morris cited to win the Morikubo case was later changed altogether by B. J. Palmer; J. Donahue, personal communication.)

This classic text presented the theory of motion restriction and joint fixation while rejecting the Palmer hypothesis of "bone out of place" as too simplistic:

> In case of a simple vertebral subluxation, the vertebra is not lodged in a fixed and permanent abnormal position like the displaced brick in the wall; to consider it so is preposterous for it is a moveable bone in a flexible and moveable column. A simple subluxated vertebra differs from a normal vertebra only in its field of motion and the center of its field of motion; because of its being subluxated, its various positions of rest are differently located than when it was a normal vertebra . . . its field of motion may be too great in some directions and too small in others (21).

Smith, Langworthy, and Paxson's theory, however advanced for its era, was rejected at the time, while the Palmer hypothesis was embraced by the profession. Laments Sandoz (21):

> We cannot help regretting that the far more adequate concept of Smith, Langworthy and Paxson did not prevail. But this is history. Let the past be past. The fact is that for generations of chiropractors, basically, a vertebral subluxation consisted in an off-centering of a vertebra . . .

Moreover, Langworthy's theory of chiropractic (that it should be limited to treating spinal subluxations) became the first contro-

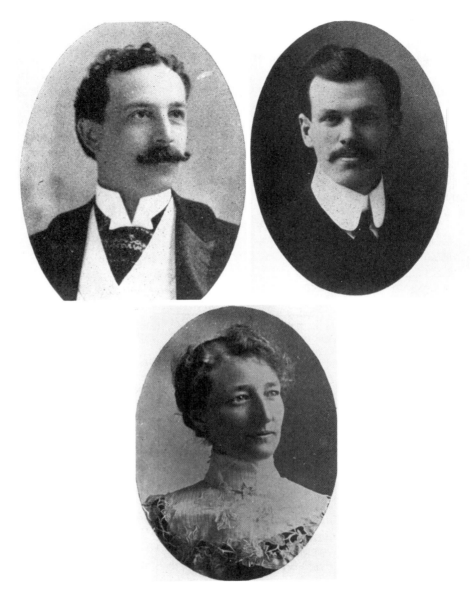

Figure 4.4. Solon Massey Langworthy (*top left*), Oakley Smith (*top right*), and Minora Paxson (*bottom*) as they appeared early in the 20th century. The three wrote the first chiropractic textbook, *Modernized Chiropractic*, in 1906. Langworthy started one of the first dissenting schools in 1903. Smith later founded "Naprapathy," and Paxson was the first licensed chiropractor in the U.S. (Illinois drugless license #438, dated May 24, 1904). (From Palmer College of Chiropractic Archives.)

versy with the Palmers (who at that time emphasized adjusting any subluxation). Yet Langworthy may go down as one of the key figures in early chiropractic history, having accomplished a number of "firsts" in a critical period of development of the profession, 1903–1906, when the Palmers faced staggering debts, medical persecution, and jail terms, and when other leadership was unavailable (Table 4.1)(13). His concepts were the precursor to the segmental dysfunction hypothesis (see Chapters 5 and 9).

Table 4.1.
Solon Massey Langworthy "Firsts" for Chiropractic During "Lost Years" of Chiropractic (1903–1906)[a]

Concepts
   First use of the term subluxation
   First reference to intervertebral foramina
   First anatomical description of intervertebral openings
   First reference to the brain as the source of all nerve force
   First chiropractic reference to erect posture in man as a factor in abnormal spinal mechanics
   First reference to human stature being affected by laws of gravity
   First reference to health/disease and the supremacy of nerves as opposed to the supremacy of
      blood (osteopathy)
   First reference to subluxation as a fixation and to a "field of motion" of a vertebra
Achievements
   Coauthored first chiropractic textbook, *Modernized Chiropractic*
   Was impetus for Swanburg's classic anatomical research on the intervertebral foramen
   Graduates of his school were responsible for first state legislature to enact chiropractic law
      (Minnesota)

[a] Based upon research by Cyrus Lerner as reported in (13).

Minora C. Paxson, meanwhile, accomplished some "firsts" of her own. Coauthor of the first chiropractic textbook, she later was the first chiropractor to receive a state license (Illinois license #438, declaring her drugless practice to be chiropractic, dated May 24, 1904) (22).

Oakley Smith went on to "discover" the art of Naprapathy, or the manipulation of "ligatights" (tight ligaments that irritate nerves and thereby cause various diseases; not unlike D. D. Palmer's early idea that muscles can constrict nerves) (22). He started the Chicago College of Naprapathy in 1905, which is the forerunner to today's Chicago National College of Naprapathy. In northern Illinois, there were reportedly 800 to 1000 naprapaths practicing their art until a recent court ruling that only chiropractors, osteopaths, and physicians can practice Napropathy (22).

Another early Palmer graduate, John Howard (Fig. 4.5), started the National School of Chiropractic in Davenport, Iowa, in 1906 (23). In 1908, hoping to expose the students to a better education in diagnosis, he moved the school to Chicago. Within a few years, two graduates of Rush Medical College, William Schulze and Arthur Forester, joined Howard in assuring high stan-

dards in diagnosis and care from National graduates. Light, heat, water, electricity, and other forces were used with chiropractic and were defined as physiological therapeutics as early as 1915 at National College (23). Schulze expanded the clinical diagnostic opportunities for National students by securing admission privileges to all clinics and autopsies at Cook County Hospital (20).

Still another dissenter was Joy Loban, who objected to B. J. Palmer's introduction of the x-ray to chiropractic. Leaving his philosophy class at Palmer with 50 of his students, he formed the Universal College of Chiropractic down the street from Palmer College in Davenport, Iowa (Fig. 4.5). He developed perhaps the most detailed approach to meric system adjusting in the literature (viz., a system for adjusting specific vertebra to have an affect upon a specific organ or disease process), although largely in line with D. D. and B. J. Palmer's beliefs at the time (20).

Willard Carver opened the Carver-Denny School of Chiropractic in 1906 and developed the structural approach theory, that the spine was a weight-bearing structure that adapted to various stresses; he rejected the concept that individual joints subluxate (24). He named his approach "relatology,"

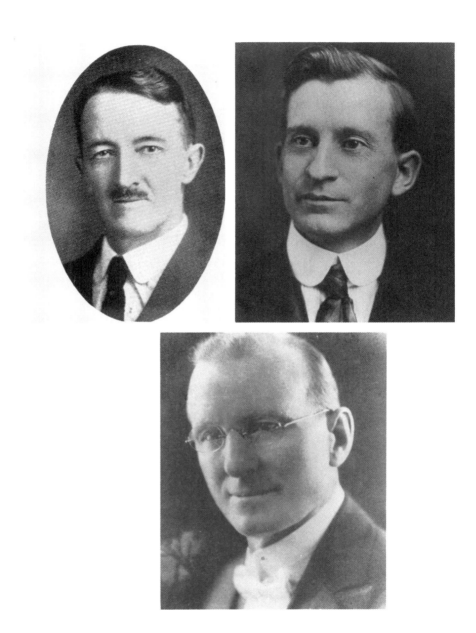

Figure 4.5. John Howard (*top left*), founded the National School of Chiropractic in 1906. Another early dissenter was Joy Loban (*top right*), a philosophy instructor for B. J., who objected to the use of x-ray and formed the Universal College of Chiropractic with 50 ex-Palmer students. In 1906, Willard Carver (*bottom*) opened a chiropractic college that later merged with present-day Logan College. He advocated a structural approach theory, emphasizing that the spine was a weight-bearing structure that adapts to various stresses. (From Palmer College of Chiropractic Archives.)

emphasized the scientific approach to teaching and research, was the first to introduce minor surgery to chiropractic education, and lengthened the chiropractic curriculum to three years. Carver remained influential in chiropractic throughout his life, and in 1921 published the famous *Carver's Chiropractic Analysis* (25). After his death, his school was absorbed by Logan College of Chiropractic.

In 1912, Alva Gregory (10) (Fig. 4.6) reiterated Palmer's hypothesis and explained without metaphysical philosophy:

> The most frequent point of mechanical interference with the normal nerve function is where the nerves make their exit from the neural canal through the foramina formed by notches in the adjacent pedicles of vertebrae.

Gregory, a medical doctor and student of Palmer, published a complex treatise, *Spinal Treatment Science and Technique*, in which he stated that excitability, conductivity, reflexivity, and efferent transmission may all be affected by nerve interference (10).

A Profession Divided

B. J. Palmer apparently followed his father's influence initially in describing chiropractic as the process of adjusting by hand all subluxations of the 300 articulations of the skeleton, with particular emphasis on the 52 articulations of the spine (20). Hence, Palmer was originally a segmentalist, but by 1911 he began to change his viewpoint.

B. J. became one of the first purchasers of x-ray equipment sometime between 1908 and 1911, installing a Sheidel-Western at Palmer School of Chiropractic (26). B. J.'s purpose was apparently to "verify or deny palpation findings and to verify or deny proof of the existence of vertebral subluxations" (26). Ernest A. Thompson headed the first "Spinographic" department at PSC by 1918 for some 20 years, and in 1924, Warren L. Sausser at the Universal Chiropractic College in Pittsburgh, Pa., became the first to make an upright 14 × 36-inch view of the spine (26). Throughout the coming decades,

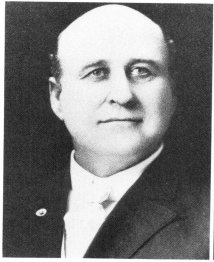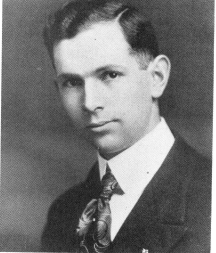

Figure 4.6. Alva Gregory (*left*), a medical doctor and student of D. D. Palmer, emphasized nerve interference from a mechanical vewpoint without metaphysical philosophy in his 1912 text. Ernest A. Thompson (*right*) was a pioneer in x-ray at the Palmer School, heading the first "Spinographic" Department for 20 years, some time after installation of the Sheidel-Western Unit at PSC around 1910. (From Palmer College of Chiropractic Archives.)

B. J. Palmer would attempt to make techno-logical breakthroughs that would advance chiropractic science and art. He commis-sioned a number of projects including de-velopment of the neurocalameter, an instru-ment used to detect heat variance in the skin paraspinally. He combined this instrument with x-ray, in an effort to promote a more accurate method of detecting subluxations that could damage the spinal cord itself:

> . . . subluxations, which would diminish the size of lateral foramina would, by the fact of subluxation of bone on bone, diminish the size of the opening from above downward on that spinal cord [without fracture or death], consequently this opens up a larger and broader viewpoint (27).

B. J. Palmer (28) established four criteria for his definition of "subluxation": misalign-ment of the vertebra in relation to adjacent segments, occlusion of a foramen (including the spinal canal and the intervertebral foramina) that contains nerves, pressure upon nerves, "and interference to transmis-sion of mental impulse supply" (i.e., action potentials; connection of God above with God within). He went on to assert that the only two vertebrae in the spine that could be subluxated were the atlas and the axis (he predicted that it was only at these levels that "occlusion of a foramen" could result in spinal cord or nerve pressure from a sub-luxation; he incorrectly predicted that spinal nerve root compression could occur also at these levels but nowhere else in the spine). This hypothesis resulted in his formation of a chiropractic adjustive technique in which only the first or second cervical vertebrae were adjusted. Because this was the so-called major subluxation, Palmer's method of correction was called the "hole in one" (HIO) technique.

It was Palmer's assertion that "no chiro-practor can practice chiropractic without an NCM" (neurocalometer—after developing this instrument Palmer then marketed it) and that any chiropractor not using the NCM with the HIO technique was incapable of practicing honestly. Such comments and re-action to them led to the great division in the chiropractic profession (3). After he de-livered his talk "The Hour Has Struck" at the lyceum (homecoming) of the Palmer School of Chiropractic in 1924, only a small seg-ment of the chiropractic profession would hold to his rigid beliefs (3). In fact, some may have been upset that Palmer had a fiduciary interest in the use of the neu-rocalometer and was "demanding" its imme-diate profession-wide use through lease ar-rangements.

Part of the backlash against the NCM and HIO technique included the creation of Lin-coln Chiropractic College by four of Palmer School of Chiropractic's leading instructors, in 1926. Outraged by the PSC emphasis on HIO, the NCM, and restrictions on academic freedom, the four created the first chiroprac-tic institution to require four academic years of instruction (20). The importance of diag-nosis was emphasized, and the assertion that only a neurocalometer could verify sub-luxation was rejected.

In 1935, Hugh B. Logan's new theory that subluxations of the spine were secondary to subluxations of the sacrum resulted in the formation of Logan Basic College of Chiro-practic, a four-year institution. Other sublux-ations in the spine should be left alone, ac-cording to Logan's theory, later published in a textbook with the assistance of his son, Vinton (20). The dissenters continued to voice concerns regarding educational and research reforms. By the mid-thirties, the Langworthy concept (stimulated perhaps by osteopathic influences; J. Keating, Jr., per-sonal communication) was beginning to be taken seriously, gaining new allies in the profession.

Fixation Concept

Marcel and Henri Gillet, Belgian chiro-practors, and Fred Illi, a Swiss chiropractor, revitalized the Smith-Langworthy-Paxson concept with a number of papers and inves-tigations on lack of proper joint motion (20). Rather than "bone out of place," an injured joint becomes fixed as fluid edema develops about the strained capsule and tissues, concluded Illi, after years of research (from 1932 to 1975) and gross anatomy dissections with Joseph Janse at National College of Chiropractic (29). In addition, Illi reviewed more than 800 cineroentgenographic studies of spinal and pelvic mechanics, rejected the bone-out-of-place hypothesis, and hypothesized instead:

> One cannot put a vertebra back into place the way one does a fracture or a dislocation. What one really does is: to restore the function of a vertebra (29).

Instead, this early chiropractic scientist/practitioner (S/P) redefined chiropractic:

> The art and science concerned with the study and treatment of the mechanics, statics and dynamics of the human body, particularly of the vertebral column and pelvis, for the primary purpose of eliminating neuropathological reflexes and their consequences (29).

His research rejected the wisdom of mid-1930s anatomists, including the orthodox thinking of the era that the sacroiliac joint was diarthrodial. Instead, Illi is credited with demonstrating an intraarticular sacroiliac ligament in dissections at National College of Chiropractic (Illi's ligament), and he correctly described sacroiliac motion based upon his cineroentgenographic studies (29). Moreover, his research regarding pelvic dynamics during gait, the dampening effect of the iliolumbar ligament on L5 and spinal motion, and pathological gait and mechanics was an excellent improvement upon Carver's principles of spinal mechanics and Langworthy's concept of motion restriction.

Research and Education Reform

By the 50th year of chiropractic, 35 years after Abraham Flexner's stinging indictment of medical education in America, chiropractic education and research reformers were beginning to voice their concerns more aggressively. Two primary camps had already formed in chiropractic, the one led by B. J. Palmer, promoting the HIO major subluxation philosophy, and the other, led by a number of individuals who advocated lengthening chiropractic education and holding to the application of scientific method in chiropractic research and practice (20, 30).

One primary advocate of the latter group was C. O. Watkins, at one time chairman of the board of the National Chiropractic Association (NCA; founded in 1930 and forerunner to the present-day American Chiropractic Association). Watkins' views on chiropractic education and research were revolutionary for the 1940s, and according to Keating (30), in 18 papers, Watkins advocated the application of scientific method to chiropractic practice, research, and education. He believed that the practitioner's role included the generation and publication of clinical data. Watkins believed that public relations activity should be modest and accurate in the portrayal of research findings and that public relations masquerading as science should be rejected (see Chapters 16 and 17).

Perhaps the most revolutionary of all Watkins' concepts, however, was his view of professional unity. He suggested that "natural unity" would occur only as a by-product of organized, systematized, chiropractic research. Scientific data, rather than personalities, beliefs, or hypotheses, would become the source of authority to guide and direct chiropractic practice. Chiropractors with different theories would be united by studying their differences and sharing growth by investigation (30). Some of Watkins' writings provided the impetus for the later development of the NCA/ACA committees on research, accreditation, and education, forerunners to the present-day Council on Chiropractic Education and Foundation for Chiropractic Education and Research.

Scientific Revolution: Defining a New Chiropractic Paradigm

If chiropractic can be defined as a paradigm by how chiropractors act and what they say they believe, then surely some paradigm shift began with the dissenters and continues to this day. Certainly B. J. Palmer's unwillingness or inability to perform and publish accepted scientific research (see also Chapter 9: "CMT and Type O Disorders") in the face of a medical profession that was becoming increasingly scientific (or at least that had the appearance of being scientific) didn't fare well with many chiropractors or with the general public (3, 4).

By the 1950s, B. J. Palmer was summarizing the research developed since the 1930s at the B. J. Palmer Research Clinic. While the title of the book was impressive, *Chiropractic Clinical Controlled Research*, unfortunately the contents were less than satisfactory (4, 31). Palmer was a prolific writer, but his motive for conducting research appears to have been his desire to see proof that "chiropractic works" rather than to find out whether and for what chiropractic works (30). Accordingly, an array of technological diagnostic equipment was developed and/or used at the PSC to "prove" that HIO philosophy was right. The Ellis Micro-Dynameter (developed independently but used by Palmer), the neurocalometer, neurotempometer, and the electroencephaloneuromentimpograph (forerunner to the electroencephalograph) were but a few of the Palmer-led developments used to document subluxation detection and correction and its clinical correlates (31). However, apparently no research statistician was employed during those decades at PSC to control or collect the clinic's data. As a result of the lack of sufficient statistic expertise, design, and analysis, uncontrolled statistical measures and unpublished and unpublishable data are all that remains.

Probably B. J. Palmer's primary research mission was to show that chiropractic was more than a cure for a specific condition or disease, but instead was a cure for "the cause of dis-ease" (30, 31). However, the lack of controlled clinical studies from the PSC outpatient clinic dealt a blow to chiropractic's development as a form of "wellness" care.

For chiropractic theories, Verner's *The Science and Logic of Chiropractic* was refreshing; at last a chiropractor was beginning to accept the role that germs play in disease, while at the same time redefining the role of the nervous system, which not only fights disease processes but also influences the chemical and environmental control necessary for health:

> It should not be assumed that because the nervous system occupies such a supremely powerful or influential position . . . the body can meet every emergency. It cannot. However, neural mechanisms are always involved in infection and immunity, just as they are in everything else. Very frequently they dominate the situation; they hold the balance of power. It is in such cases that Chiropractic operating through such neural mechanisms, may be employed to advantage (32).

By 1953, Verner teamed up with C. W. Weiant and R. J. Watkins to write *Rational Bacteriology*. This book summarizes the problem of dogmatic adherence to one theory or another and admonishes the profession to try to understand bacteriology rather than disregard its study (33).

By the late 1960s, legitimate chiropractic basic science research was funded at the University of Colorado. Annual conferences reported progress and have continued from 1970 to the present, under the direction of C. H. Suh. Meanwhile, osteopathic researcher Irvin Hoff's pioneering work (see Chapter 15) on the concept of damage to axoplasmic transport as a result of nerve compression or irritation was further studied by Suh's colleagues (34, 35). While initial hopes were that a computer model would be developed for more accurate radiographic interpretation of biomechanical spinal dysfunction or subluxation, the programs have apparently never been perfected. At least they have not been distributed or used. The University of Colorado research may not have led to clinically useful information; however, important basic science research relevant to chiropractic hypotheses was published in a variety of biomedical journals and is reported throughout this text (e.g., see Luttges and Triano's work in Chapter 11).

While a number of impressive joint chiropractic-osteopathic-medical conferences were held throughout the 1970s and 1980s that probably sparked the renaissance of legitimate chiropractic clinical research efforts seen in the 1980s, the real chiropractic research renaissance may be only now beginning (36–40).

Coulter (41) concludes that chiropractic is a paradigm, based on a number of observations: most chiropractors choose the profession through a conversion experience, a gestalt transformation, after care given to them and their families (i.e., many chiropractors decided to go to chiropractic school after first benefitting from adjustments), and chiropractic has adopted extremely dogmatic positions both internally and externally throughout its history. In addition, chiropractors have tended to ignore or rationalize information that would challenge their basic tenets. Finally, chiropractic is used consciously to solve health puzzles that have been unresolved by other health care disciplines. Coulter states, however, that chiropractic is not like other health care paradigms in that usually health care paradigms give rise to distinct research traditions during which the paradigm is tested over a wide range of health care puzzles (41). Coulter argues that instead, chiropractic has attempted to substantiate its fundamental principles with the research of outside professions. As an alternative, Coulter (42) would have the profession begin to adopt a philosophy of "wellness" care without metaphysical beliefs. In this way, chiropractic research would be guided by efforts to establish effectiveness of chiropractic in restoring homeostatic mechanisms in the body and in determining to what extent and under what circumstances the body is a self-healing mechanism.

Beginning the 1990s with a research conference entitled Bridging the Gap Between Research and Clinical Practice, the Foundation for Chiropractic Education and Research received 128 scientific papers and accepted only 73 for presentation (43). That chiropractic has matured enough to produce 128 legitimate research projects in one year, of sufficient quality to be submitted to the International Conference on Spinal Manipulation is impressive by itself. That chiropractic is becoming selective in what it describes as "research" or as "clinical research" is perhaps much more important. In fact, development of a cadre of legitimate chiropractic researchers meeting regularly and publishing their work in legitimate indexed biomedical journals may be evidence of a paradigm shift away from antiscientific epistemology and theosophy in chiropractic. Further evidence for a paradigm shift may be found in the number of chiropractors subscribing to the only medically indexed chiropractic science journal, the *Journal of Manipulative and Physiological Therapeutics*, and in the proliferation of refereed science journals pertaining to chiropractic, and in increasing debate of once dogmatic chiropractic philosophy (see also Chapters 16 and 17).

As the profession faces the 21st century, it appears that the long awaited "scientific revolution" in chiropractic is indeed in progress. It is currently being led by a number of researchers at a host of chiropractic colleges and by an equal number of private general practitioners. Keating (30) points out that the process of scientific development is critical to the development and perhaps to the very survival of the profession, especially as cost effectiveness and inclusion in federally mandated programs become issues to be reckoned with. Indeed, while the profession can perhaps thank B. J. Palmer's philosophy for its survival despite often intense medical persecution, it appears that it must now shed that philosophy and replace it with one that is testable, to promote patient welfare and insure its future survival (19).

Summary

Chiropractic evolved from a mix of 19th century medical knowledge regarding spinal irritation and theosophical and metaphysical beliefs commonly held in the early 1900s. While D. D. Palmer's observation that a deaf man regained his hearing following manipulation sparked the chiropractic experience, metaphysical concepts like Innate intelligence were initially deemed necessary to preserve chiropractic in the face of intense medical persecution, including 30,000 jail terms meted out to chiropractors by 1930 for practicing medicine without a license.

Dissenters to the Palmer "bone out of place," Innate intelligence philosophy developed other schools that finally produced a shift in the chiropractic paradigm. Although B. J. Palmer continued to exert a strong influence over a core of followers that exists to this day, education and research reformers like C. O. Watkins, Fred Illi, Joseph Janse, Scott Haldeman, and a host of others began to gradually shift the thinking of the profession toward adopting the principles and methods of science in chiropractic philosophy, education, research, and practice. There is evidence that a paradigm shift is occurring in chiropractic, being led by a host of researchers at chiropractic colleges, a few scientist practitioners, and an increasing number of practitioners interested in acquiring new scientific knowledge regarding chiropractic practice.

REFERENCES

1. Coulter ID. Of clouds, clocks and chiropractors: towards a theory of irrationality. Presentation at the Canadian Memorial Chiropractic College Homecoming Conference: Philosophy of chiropractic into the 21st century. Toronto, April 27, 1990.

2. Donahue J. D. D. Palmer and innate intelligence: development, division and derision. Chiro Hist 1986;6:31–36.

3. Gibbons RW. The evolution of chiropractic: medical and social protest in America. In: Haldeman S, ed. Modern developments in the principles and practice of chiropractic. New York: Appleton-Century-Crofts, 1980: 3–24.

4. Leach RA. Chiropractic research: an author's perspective. Chiropractic research: attitudes that hinder. Chiropractic 1988;1:14–17.

5. Donahue JH. A proposal for the development of a contemporary philosophy of chiropractic. Am J Chiro Med 1989;2:51–53.

6. Dintenfass J. Chiropractic: a modern way to health. New York: Pyramid, 1970.

7. Lomax E. Manipulative therapy: a historical perspective from ancient times to the modern era. In: Goldstein M, ed. The research status of spinal manipulative therapy. Washington, D.C.: Government Printing Office, 1975:11–17.

8. Hippocrates. Hippocrates, with an English translation by Dr. E. T. Withington, volume III. Cambridge: Harvard University Press, 1959:299.

9. Tower D. Chairman's summary: evolution and development of the concepts of manipulative therapy. In: Goldstein M, ed. The research status of spinal manipulative therapy. Washington, D.C.: Government Printing Office, 1975:59.

10. Gregory A. Spinal treatment science and technique. Oklahoma City: Palmer-Gregory College, 1912.

11. Judah JS. The history and philosophy of the metaphysical movements in America. Philadelphia: Westminister Press, [n.d.]:64–65, 93.

12. Donahue JH. D.D. Palmer and the metaphysical movement in the 19th century. Chiro Hist 1987;7:23–27.

13. Gibbons RW. Solon Massey Langworthy: keeper of the flame during the "lost years" of chiropractic. Chiro Hist 1981;1:15–21.

14. Palmer DD. Text-book of the science, art and philosophy of chiropractic. Portland: Portland Printing House, 1910.

15. Palmer DD. The chiropractor. Los Angeles: Beacon Light Printing, 1914:1.

16. Rehm WS. Legally defensible: chiropractic in the courtroom and after, 1907. Chiro Hist 1986;6:51–55.

17. Turner C. The rise of chiropractic. Los Angeles: Powell, 1931.

18. Palmer BJ. Shall chiropractic survive? Davenport, Ia.: Palmer School of Chiropractic, 1959;16:105–106.

19. Leach RA. In pursuit of valid chiropractic theory: demanding excellence in the 21st century. Presentation at the Canadian Memorial Chiropractic College Homecoming: Philosophy of chiropractic into the 21st century, Toronto, April 27, 1990.

20. Montgomery DP, Nelson JM. Evolution of chiropractic theories of practice and spinal adjustment, 1900–1950. Chiro Hist 1985;5: 71–76.

21. Sandoz R. Some critical reflections on subluxations and adjustments. Ann Swiss Chiro Assoc 1989;9:7–29.

22. Zarbuck MV. A profession for 'Bohemian chiropractic': Oakley Smith and the evolution of naprapathy. Chiro Hist 1986;6:77–82.

23. Ransom JF. The origins of chiropractic physiological therapeutics: Howard, Forester and Schulze. Chiro Hist 1985;4:47–52.

24. Rosenthal MJ. The structural approach to chiropractic: from Willard Carver to present practice. Chiro Hist 1981;1:25–28.

25. Carver W. Carver's chiropractic analysis. Oklahoma City: Carver Chiropractic College, 1921.

26. Canterbury R, Krakos G. Thirteen years after Roentgen: the origins of chiropractic radiology. Chiro Hist 1986;6:25–29.

27. Palmer BJ. The science of chiropractic. Davenport, Ia.: Palmer School of Chiropractic, 1911.

Palmer BJ. The subluxation specific—the adjustment specific. Davenport, Ia.: Palmer School of Chiropractic, 1934.

[...]aker WJ. A clinical reformation in chiropractic: the research of Dr. Fred Illi. Chiro [...]t 1985;5:59–62.

30. Keating JC, Mootz RD. Commentary: the influence of political medicine on chiropractic dogma: implications for scientific development. J Manipulative Physiol Ther 1989; 5:393–398.

31. Palmer BJ. Chiropractic clinical controlled research. Davenport, Ia: Palmer School of Chiropractic, 1951.

32. Verner JR. The science and logic of chiropractic. Brooklyn: Cerasoli, 1941:220.

33. Verner JR, Weiant CW, Watkins RJ. Rational Bacteriology. New York: Wolf, 1953:204.

34. Suh CH. Researching the fundamentals of chiropractic. In: Suh CH, ed. Proceedings of the 5th Annual Biomechanics Conference on the Spine. Boulder: University of Colorado, 1974:1–52.

35. Triano JJ, Luttges MW. Nerve irritation: a possible model of sciatic neuritis. Spine 1982;7:129–136.

36. Goldstein M, ed. The research status of spinal manipulative therapy. Washington, D.C.: Government Printing Office, 1975.

37. Buerger AA, Tobis JS, eds. Approaches to the validation of manipulation therapy. Springfield, Ill.: Charles C Thomas, 1977.

38. Korr I, ed. Neurobiologic mechanisms in manipulative therapy. New York, Plenum, 1978.

39. Haldeman S, ed. Modern developments in the principles and practice of chiropractic. New York: Appleton-Century-Crofts, 1980.

40. Buerger AA, Greenman PE, eds. Empirical approaches to the validation of spinal manipulation. Springfield, Ill.: Charles C Thomas, 1985.

41. Coulter ID. The chiropractic paradigm. J Manipulative Physiol Ther 1990;13:279–287.

42. Coulter ID. The patient, the practitioner and wellness: paradigm lost, paradigm gained. J Manipulative Physiol Ther 1990;13:107–111.

43. Wolk S, ed. Proceedings of the 1990 International Conference on Spinal Manipulation. Arlington, Va.: Foundation for Chiropractic Education and Research, 1990.

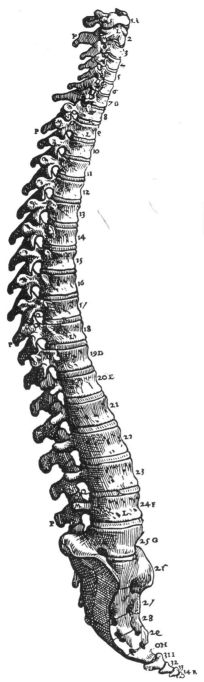

Section 2

Pathophysiology
of Segmental
Dysfunction

Subjectivity and objectivity commit
a series of assaults on each other
during a human life out of which the
first one suffers the worse beating.

André Breton

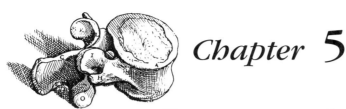

Chapter **5**

Segmental Dysfunction Hypothesis

*I*s there a manipulable lesion? Indeed, is there a specific, identifiable lesion that responds favorably to spinal manipulative therapy (SMT) or to chiropractic manipulative therapy (CMT; also referred to as "adjustment")? Or are there physiological and clinical effects of CMT that can be reliably and reproducibly measured whether or not a lesion is detected? Research into these questions has caused considerable debate within the profession. Tireless efforts to quantify and qualify the lesion and to find a suitable outcome measure or measures capable of predicting manipulative effectiveness have met with mixed and often disappointing results.

Several emerging trends should lend hope to researchers and practitioners of CMT that a discriminable lesion does exist. This section (Section 2) focuses on what is known of that lesion and its effects. This chapter focuses on the *segmental dysfunction* (SDF) hypothesis, discussing historical and experimental aspects of the lesion, as well as the physiology of joint manipulation. SDF refers to abnormal spinal function that is limited to a single motion unit (e.g., C5-C6; see also Chapter 3). Subsequent chapters detail research on the so-called hard and soft outcome measures being tested as

monitors of manipulative effects and effectiveness. *Regional dysfunction* (RDF) is discussed in light of current research in those chapters as well. A relatively new concept in chiropractic, termed "somatic dysfunction" in the osteopathic literature, RDF refers to abnormal spinal function that is limited to a specific spinal region (e.g., thoracolumbar, cervical). Recent chiropractic research suggests that RDF may be more reliably detected and associated with manipulative effectiveness than SDF. Chapter 8 details purported neurological correlates of the lesion, including such concepts as facilitation and somatoautonomic phenomena. Finally, Chapter 9 reviews clinical studies of manipulative correction of the lesion (by use of CMT unless otherwise noted) and discusses clinical aspects of the lesion. This section addresses the questions posed earlier and attempts to lay the groundwork for further study and investigation of SDF and RDF, while providing the clinician with information critical to the practice of chiropractic.

A triad of signs has been classically accepted as evidence for existence of a manipulable lesion, or SDF. These include point tenderness or altered pain threshhold to pressure in the adjacent paraspinal musculature or over the spinous process. Loss of normal motion in one or more planes and abnormal contraction or tension within the adjacent paraspinal musculature complete the triad. Hence, for purposes of discussion, the *segmental dysfunction hypothesis* is defined here as

> a common spinal lesion recognized by lessened or otherwise altered mobility, altered pressure threshhold to pain, and signs of neuromuscular dysfunction.

From this basic definition, this chapter lays the groundwork for the initial working or operational definitions of SDF and RDF presented in Chapter 9, which can be used in the clinic setting.

Early Evidence

Perhaps the first author to discuss "subluxation" in terms of loss of joint motion was Hieronymus (see also Chapter 3). In 1746, he identified lessened motion in the joints, pain, and slight change in joint alignment as indicators of the lesion (1). One of D. D. Palmer's (founder of chiropractic, 1895; see also Chapter 4) first descriptions of the manipulable lesion in 1899 included the concept that "contraction of the muscles drawing on or across the nerves . . ." causes nerve pressure that must be manipulated to be restored (2). Certainly the first chiropractic textbook, *Modernized Chiropractic*, in 1906 succinctly rejected "bone-out-of-place" as too simplistic an explanation for chiropractic subluxation. Adopting instead the concept that vertebral subluxation involves a vertebra that has an altered field of motion, Langworthy, Smith, and Paxson were clearly the first chiropractic proponents of SDF (See also Chapter 4)(3, 4). Chiropractor Fred Illi reviewed more than 800 cineroentgenographic studies from 1932 to 1975 and concluded that CMT restores function and motion and does not merely replace a misaligned vertebra (5). Henri Gillet's notes on spinal fixation (a term for the hypomobile type of SDF), written in 1951, are a classic within the profession to this day; indeed,

Sandoz (6) argues that the profession is shifting toward the concept of a dynamic lesion, largely because of the work of these chiropractic pioneers.

Meanwhile, early osteopathic evidence of the lesion was reported in 1917 by Louisa Burns (7). Burns' description of increased paraspinal muscle tone, with "knots" or "strings" in irregularly contracted muscles, was a forerunner to the work of J. S. Denslow, Irvin Korr, and other osteopathic researchers to follow.

Denslow and Hassett (8) studied *muscle spasm* (i.e., skeletal muscle that displays some degree of rigidity, is tender, and is resistant to pressure deformation) in individuals with postural abnormalities. Electromyographic (EMG) recordings were made of the spinal extensors in subjects lying prone with the head in the midline. Sometimes, when electrodes were placed for 1 to 45 minutes, no activity would be recorded; it was suggested that these muscles were in the normal resting state, as confirmed in other EMG studies. In other muscles, spontaneous myoelectric activity was demonstrated without apparent cause; they labeled these "lesions." Using a pin prick, pressure, needle scratching, and ice as noxious stimuli, spontaneous activity was evoked 72.7% of the time (based on 55 applications) in "lesioned" areas and only 0.9% of the time in control muscles. When activity was evoked in control muscles (glutei, tibialis anterior, and extensor digitorum longus), it was always transient; in contrast, "lesioned" muscles' activity persisted up to 10 minutes. Similar findings were demonstrated in nonpain (as opposed to back pain) patients. The authors reasoned that additional activity evoked from "lesioned" muscles could be an indirect indicator of afferent bombardment to the spinal cord (see also Chapter 8) and evidence of an osteopathic spinal lesion (SDF)(8).

Denslow (9) examined this phenomena by applying pressure stimuli to the spinous process of human subjects, with EMG analysis of paraspinal musculature. He demonstrated areas of altered threshold for reflex muscle contraction that stayed constant in repeat measures of the same individual on different days. He reasoned that the different areas could be explained by changes in the environment of deep pressure receptors, stretch receptors, and free nerve endings. In addition, he hypothesized an imbalance in excitor-inhibitor influences (see also Chapter 8).

Based upon these and other investigations, the initial definition of RDF included the concepts of:

1. Asymmetry and structural and functional disrelationships, including postural deviations (11, 12);
2. Increased, decreased, or otherwise abnormal joint motion (11–13);
3. Neurologic phenomena, which include tissue texture abnormalities as evidenced visually and by light and deep palpation (i.e., changes in color, temperature, and consistency).

These initial investigations and observations are the basis for the current efforts in chiropractic to find suitable criteria for the detection and correction of SDF. But before discussing the current clinical evidence regarding SDF, a brief discussion of experimental evidence including a review of normal anatomy and physiology of the motion segment is in order.

Experimental Evidence

NORMAL ANATOMY AND PHYSIOLOGY

The motion segment in the spine may be thought of as the functional unit (Fig. 5.1), composed of an anterior segment, which consists of any two vertebral bodies separated by an intervertebral disc, and a posterior segment, which consists of the articular facets (14). In addition, the ligaments, muscles, tendons, and other soft tissues that play a role in movement must be considered.

To better appreciate the role of SDF in influencing the nervous system—and hence the need for a variety of outcome measures

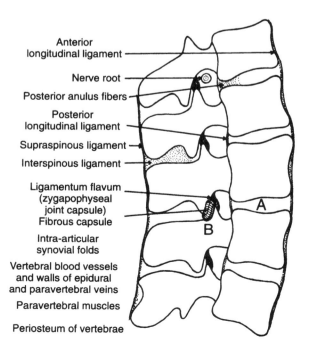

Anterior longitudinal ligament
Nerve root
Posterior anulus fibers
Posterior longitudinal ligament
Supraspinous ligament
Interspinous ligament
Ligamentum flavum (zygapophyseal joint capsule)
Fibrous capsule
Intra-articular synovial folds
Vertebral blood vessels and walls of epidural and paravertebral veins
Paravertebral muscles
Periosteum of vertebrae

Figure 5.1. Schematic illustration of pain sensitive aspects of the lumbar spine. The concept of a motion segment of the spine is derived from Junghann's (14) study of the functional unit. Consisting of the articular triad of one intervertebral joint (A) anteriorly (viz., the intervertebral disc—fibrocartilaginous material responsible for mobility and load transmission) and two synovial zygapophyseal joints (B) posteriorly (viz. the facets—guide vertebrae while restraining them from excessive shear, flexion, and axial rotational forces that could injure the discs). (Adapted from Giles LGF. Anatomical basis of low back pain. Baltimore: Williams & Wilkins, 1989:3.)

to detect the lesion and its effects—requires an understanding of articular neurology. Haldeman (16) reviews the literature on a number of high-threshold sensory receptors in animals and man that give rise to the perception of pain. Wyke (17, 18) has pioneered the field of articular neurology, defining a number of mechanoreceptors and nociceptive-free nerve endings (nociceptors) in greater detail than was previously known. Our current understanding of articular neurology, as well as the Korr model of spinal fixation, are presented in Chapter 8.

Here our focus is on the anatomy of the zygapophyseal joints themselves, since they are thought to play a primary role in SDF and hypomobility. (The posterior segment of the functional unit has also been referred to as "posterior elements.") These are true diarthrodial joints, having a posterolateral fibrous capsule with reinforcing strands from the interspinous ligament, a synovial lining, and a medial capsule formed by the ligamentum flavum. The articular cartilage (Fig. 5.2) is arranged in bundles of hyaline, and when loaded, it interacts with proteoglycans and extracellular fluids to give it the property of shock absorption. The fibrous capsule is said to have a relatively poor blood supply, which makes it understandably slow to heal once damaged (15).

Apparently, spinal joint cavities normally contain only a small volume of synovial fluid. The zygapophyseal joint synovial folds in the lumbar spine project into the joint cavity. A synovial membrane lines the folds (Fig. 5.3) and secretes synovial fluid (viz., hyaluronate), clears away waste materials

Figure 5.2. Adult articular cartilage as found in the zygapophyseal joints, is composed of collagen bundles arranged horizontally in the gliding zone. This orientation becomes vertical in the radial zone. Load bearing is said to arise from an interplay between collagen fibers and hydrated proteoglycan complexes. (Adapted from Giles LGF. Anatomical basis of low back pain. Baltimore: Williams & Wilkins, 1989:16.)

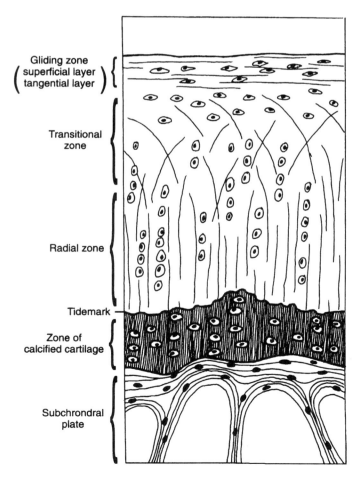

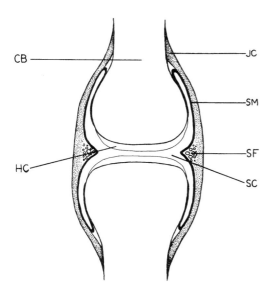

Figure 5.3. A typical synovial joint. *CB*, cancellous bone; *HC*, hyaline cartilage; *JC*, fibrous joint capsule; *SC*, synovial cavity; *SF*, synovial fold with synovial membrane and subsynovial tissue; *SM*, synovial lining membrane. (Adapted from Giles LGF. Anatomical basis of low back pain. Baltimore: Williams & Wilkins, 1989:18.)

(viz., phagocytic "A" cells), and regulates the movement of chemicals necessary for maintenance of the joint (solutes, electrolytes, and proteins)(15).

The anterior element of the functional unit, the intervertebral disc, certainly a critical factor in spinal pain and dysfunction, is discussed in some detail in Chapter 10.

MECHANISMS OF ZYGAPOPHYSEAL PATHOPHYSIOLOGY

A number of mechanisms have been suggested to explain pain originating in the zygapophyseal joints. Hadley (19) cites joint derangement due to ligamentous and capsular instability, including capsular tension, encroachment of the intervertebral foramen (IVF), intraarticular synovial fold inclusions, and impingement of the superior articular process against the pedicle above and the lamina below. Schmorl and Junghanns' (20) studies suggested degenerative changes

within the joint, and meniscal "incarceration" as key sources of back pain. Jackson (21) cites joint effusion with capsular distension as a cause of capsular pain. Haldeman (22) cites joint effusion with direct diffusion as a cause of nerve root pain as well. Farfan (23) suggests that joint capsule adhesions may be a primary factor in causing low back pain.

Giles (15, 24, 25) has extensively investigated the lumbar apophyseal joints and appears to favor release of a trapped intraarticular synovial fold and stretching of the joint capsule (which may have fibrotic scarring) as likely explanations for beneficial effects of spinal manipulative therapy.

A recent review of the literature, as well as their own investigation of histological variations, prompted Jones et al. (26) to discuss possible consequences of mechanically pathological zygapophyseal meniscoids. They studied all lumbar zygapophyses in 10 fresh cadaveric specimens at Logan Chiropractic College. Some meniscoids were found in all lumbar spines; they were usually bilateral in distribution and varied in size and morphology. Histological evaluation revealed variations in fibroadipose tissue, calcification, synovium, fibrocartilage, vascularity, ossifications, and osteoid matrix. The predominant finding was vascular fibroadipose tissue. In four of five meniscoids studied microscopically, calcified hyaline cartilage with chondrocytes, and fibrocartilage in the process of becoming calcified was observed.

In contrast with the findings of prior researchers, Jones et al. (26) documented the presence of fibrocartilage within some meniscoids, some sites of endochondral ossification within meniscoid tissues, and the occasional presence of vascular tissue within fibrocartilaginous tissue (Fig. 5.4). Their other findings were in accord with previous research. Based upon these findings, the researchers predict that chronic intersegmental hypomobility (CIH; viz. SDF) may result from meniscoid entrapment, with subsequent development of fibrocartilaginous tissue. Hence, their findings support and

Figure 5.4. In contrast with prior research, Jones and co-workers (26) demonstrated fibrocartilage within some meniscoids, some sites of endochondral ossification within meniscoid tissues, and occasional vascular tissue within fibrocartilaginous tissues. **A**, A crescent-shaped fibrocartilaginous meniscoid from a lumbar zygapophyseal joint (at tip of scalpel; *LSp*, lumbar spinous process). **B**, A rather large representative fibroadipose meniscoid body is jutting superiorly into the right L2/L3 zygapophyseal joint (at tip of forceps). (Photographs courtesy of J. Paul Ellis, Assistant Professor, Logan College of Chiropractic).

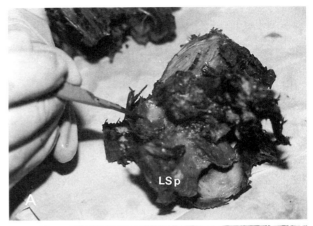

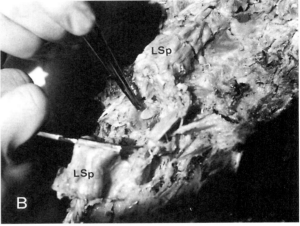

expand Kos and Wolf's (27) theory of joint fixation. Kos and Wolf (27) held that acute locked-back syndrome results from the entrapment of a joint meniscoid between the superior and inferior articular processes, typically after a patient bends forward while twisting the trunk. A "catch" is felt upon returning to the upright position, along with sharp pain that gradually worsens within the next 24 to 48 hours. Soon the patient is unable to fully extend the lumbar spine. As the entrapped apex creates a dent in the articular cartilage of the facet, range of motion is increasingly restricted. Jones et al. (26) detailed the effects of the pathological meniscoid in terms of mechanical and chemical changes that would create CIH or SDF (Table 5.1).

These findings are indirectly supported clinically by research suggesting that the relief in discogenic and facet syndromes (viz. the posterior elements of the spinal column) is not due to release of opioids. Indeed, Zusman and co-workers (28) were able to demonstrate significant relief in patients receiving high-velocity manipulation, but pain returned after subsequent intravenous injection with naloxone or a saline solution. Although interesting, their study still could not rule out cerebrospinal fluid–mediated, or other centrally acting, "nonopioid" pain control mechanisms.

Helbig and Lee (29), in attempting to clinically define facet syndrome, reviewed 22 consecutive cases of lumbar facet syndrome treated with facet joint injection. Retrospec-

Table 5.1.
Some Hypothesized Pathophysiological Effects of an Entrapped Joint Meniscoid[a]

Concept	Statement of Hypothesis
Joint capsule tension	Increased joint capsule tension results in increased mechanoreceptor activity; subsequent increase in nociception lowers pain threshold and creates hypertonic paraspinal musculature; pain-spasm-pain cycle begins
Capsular adhesions	Extra- and intracapsular adhesions form secondary to the joint hypomobility; these progressive contractures of the capsule and fibroadipose connective tissue growths across the joint space can obliterate the joint cavity
Biochemical alterations	Glycosaminoglycan is lost from cartilaginous and ligamentous structures related to the joint, including the endplates
Degenerative changes	Premature degeneration ensues as normal stresses are applied to the dysfunctioning joint; bone minerals are lost with increasing hypomobility as a consequence of the piezoelectric effect (i.e., electric current produced by pressure that is placed on a crystal such as calcium)

[a] Adapted from Jones TR, James JE, Adams JW, Garcia J, Walker SL, Ellis JP. Lumbar zygapophyseal joint meniscoids: evidence of their role in chronic intersegmental hypomobility. J Manipulative Physiol Ther 1989;12:374–385.

tively, 100% prolonged relief was obtained in patients meeting certain diagnostic criteria (see also Chapter 9, "Clinical Aspects of Segmental Dysfunction"). These findings suggest some biochemical role (e.g., reduction of inflammation within the facet) for pain relief.

In contrast, Lewit (13) demonstrated that cervical range of motion does not increase significantly even with the use of myorelaxants in patients under narcosis. He advocates manipulation of the "entrapped meniscus."

Finally, percutaneous block of the dorsal rami of C3, C4, and C5 was accomplished by denervation using thermocouple needles heated to 80°C for 90 seconds in a study by Hildebrandt and Argyrakis (30). Using this method to block nociception and afferent activity from free nerve endings associated with the cervical apophyseal joints, improvement or total relief was obtained in 23 of 35 patients with chronic headache and neck pain, even after an average follow-up of 14 months. The authors speculated that even greater success might have been possible with block of the C2 dorsal rami, which was not attempted because of variable innervation and difficulty of the procedure at that level. These studies and others suggest that some mechanism of pathophysiology involving the zygapophyses may play a primary role in the production of pain, dysfunction, and disability arising from mechanical spinal disorders. From the clinical viewpoint, conservative intervention must be shown to have a physiological effect on the facets, to achieve improvement in SDF. In this regard, a review of the physiology of joint manipulation is in order.

PHYSIOLOGY OF JOINT MANIPULATION

After the initial investigations of Roston and Haines (31) and Unsworth, Dowson, and Wright (32), Sandoz (33) proposed a mechanism for the effects of adjustment on a joint. Three zones of physiological movement are recognized when adjusting a joint, according to Sandoz (33) (see Fig. 3.1):

1. Zone of physiological movement— passive range of motion, active range of motion, and mobilization procedures operate within this zone. Low-force and so-called nonforce adjustive

procedures operate within this zone as well.

2. Paraphysiological zone of movement—the zone of joint play where the high-velocity thrust suddenly separates the articular surfaces (i.e., coaptation), overcoming an elastic barrier of resistance and producing an audible release (viz. "cracking" or "popping" sound), as well as the appearance of a radiolucent cavity in the joint space (i.e., vacuum phenomenon). The gas content of synovium in the metacarpophalangeal (MCP) joint was found to be 80% carbon dioxide—the audible release was said to occur as a result of cavitation in the synovial fluid (32). It has been demonstrated that for 15–20 minutes after MCP manipulation, while the radiolucent cavity is still present, a second attempt to manipulate the joint will be unsuccessful and painful. This time period has been referred to as the refractory period (32). Typical chiropractic diversified adjustive procedures operate within this zone of movement.

3. Pathological zone of movement— once the barrier of normal anatomical integrity has been reached, further movement in a joint results in sprain, medical (surgical) subluxation, or luxation. Sprain can involve simple elongation to complete rupture of the joint capsule.

Meal and Scott (34), in an effort to determine when joint separation occurs in relation to the audible release, measured sound waves—produced by manipulation of the MCP joints—recorded in conjunction with joint tension. Tensions needed to induce an audible release varied from 3 kg in habitual "knuckle crackers" to 23 kg in "non–knuckle crackers." The duration of the audible varied from 0.025 to 0.075 second. A characteristic double-peak wave form was observed, with reduction in tension occurring between the two peaks. This wave form was identical to those produced by cervical spine adjusting. They also observed that joints that were easier to manipulate produced audible releases of lower amplitude. In addition, when a low pressure weather system was occurring, MCP joints appeared to give an audible release under less tension and with a lowered amplitude. There was no evidence of those changes, including changes in coaptation, for the mobilized joints. They concluded that researchers should clearly distinguish the effects of mobilization versus manipulation.

Haas (36) suggests that successful synovial joint cavitation, or manipulation, depends upon seven parameters: joint and patient stiffness, joint and patient elasticities, the proportion of energy received into the joint and patient by the thrust, and joint distraction at the point of cavitation.

In a classic initial clinical investigation of force measurements during chiropractic manipulative therapy (CMT), Herzog et al. (37) measured the preload force, the duration of the treatment, and the point of contact at the instant peak force was applied. Two chiropractors each gave three sacroiliac adjustments using "Thompson technique" to a single patient. While the duration of the manipulative thrust was similar for both doctors, there was a considerable difference between them in mean preload force, in mean peak force, and in the depth of the manipulative thrust. The exact point of contact varied between the practitioners as well.

Conway and co-workers (38) of the University of Calgary, in conjunction with the College of Chiropractors of Alberta and the Canadian Memorial Chiropractic College, further delineated mechanical factors involved in synovial joint manipulation by studying CMT applied at the T4 spinal level. One chiropractor made a light thrust, followed two seconds later by a cavitation-producing manipulation (adjustment) on one patient. The same chiropractor also made a cavitation-producing manipulation on nine additional subjects. Initial findings suggest that force at cavitation (as measured by a thin (2 mm) pressure mat fixed at T4, and electronically synchronized with two accelerometers mounted on the skin at T3 and T5) reached 580 newtons (N). When the thrust did not produce cavitation, peak force measured 460 N. Other differences were noted as well, suggesting that the difference between preload and peak force, and the average increase in thrust force might be responsible for cavitation. Further research to isolate which of those three variables—or which combination of those variables—may be responsible for cavitation is under way.

Discussion

Synovial joint manipulation has been shown in initial investigations to have significant physiological effects not seen after joint mobilization or simple range-of-motion procedures. The phenomena of coaptation of joint surfaces with concomitant audible release, radiographic appearance of a vacuum within the joint associated with cavitation, and the observation that a refractory period exists following manipulation in which a second manipulation is unsuccessful, are seen after manipulation of the MCP but are not observed with mobilization (Table 5.2). Further evidence that there are physiological effects of manipulation that are distinct is found in studies suggesting improvement in paraspinal myoelectric activity and in radiographic appearance of bone alignment following OMT and CMT, respectively, but not following mobilization of spinal joints (see also Chapter 10).

Besides the purely mechanical impact of CMT on joint dynamics and on potentially pathological meniscoids, the greatest clinical effects of CMT may be due to increasing circulation within the joint itself. Poorly understood biochemical processes, including cavitation and the movement of CO_2 within the synovium, and inflammatory changes secondary to trauma must also be considered (see also Chapter 8). Experimentally induced deep somatic inflammatory lesions in anesthetized rats (viz., injection of mustard oil as an inflammatory agent versus mineral oil as a control substance into the trapezius, suboccipital, and masseter muscles) have been recently demonstrated to evoke abnormal myoelectric responses similar to those seen in mechanical spinal pain (47). Hence, one role for CMT in reducing such abnormal myoelectric activity might be associated

Table 5.2.
Physiological and Mechanical Aspects of Manipulative versus Nonmanipulative Joint Procedures

Aspect	Active ROM	Mobilization	Manipulation[a]	OMT[b]	CMT[c]
Movement within paraphysiological zone	Yes (33)	Yes	Yes	Yes	Yes
Increased joint range-of-motion	No	Yes[d]	Yes (35)	Yes	Yes
Coaptation[e]	No	No	Yes (31–34)	Yes	Yes
Vacuum phenomenon	No	No	Yes (31, 32, 35, 39)	Yes	Yes
Audible release	No	No	Yes (31–35)	Yes	Yes
Refractory period	No	No	Yes (32)	Yes	Yes
Reduction in abnormal myoelectric activity	?	No	?	Yes (41, 42)	Yes (40)
Radiographic appearance of improved joint alignment[f]	?	?	?	?	Yes (43–46)

[a] Nonspecific manipulation.
[b] Osteopathic manipulative therapy.
[c] Chiropractic manipulative therapy (adjustment).
[d] Range of motion improves significantly more after manipulation than after mobilization (35).
[e] Coaptation—sudden separation of joint surfaces.
[f] In cases of cervical hypolordosis and retrolisthesis.

with increased circulation in an area of deep somatic dysfunction (SDF or RDF). Thus CMT would interrupt the so-called pain-spasm-pain cycle. Realization of the forces necessary to cause cavitation might also help to understand the clinical and physiological correlates of manipulation or CMT as opposed to "nonforce" or "low-force" adjusting techniques. Certainly experimental research to more fully elucidate these mechanisms is needed.

Relevant to material reviewed in this chapter is the debate over what might be the central component of SDF or RDF. Is the central component of SDF or RDF typically (a) a locked joint capsule or pathological meniscoid? (b) abnormal muscle function? or (c) abnormal biochemical processes within the synovial joint? This chapter has addressed items a and c in some detail. Indeed, there is good evidence to suggest that they go hand in hand, and that they are related to SDF. However, at least some evidence suggests an important role for abnormal muscle function with regard to RDF (see Chapter 7). Certainly, given the body's penchant for inflammatory changes as the initial response to stressors of any sort, some role for all three components seems likely (see also Chapter 14).

Summary

This chapter reviews early evidence for segmental dysfunction (SDF) and regional dysfunction (RDF), including the classic triad of clinically accepted signs: point tenderness (diminished pressure-pain threshold), loss of normal joint motion in one or more planes, and abnormal contraction or tension within the adjacent paraspinal musculature (1–7, 11–13).

Experimental evidence for the lesion is reviewed, including evidence for mechanisms of zygapophyseal pathophysiology based on postmortem examinations (15, 19–26). These findings are discussed in light of clinical studies of patients with specific posterior joint syndromes (28–30). Hypothesized pathophysiological effects of entrapped joint meniscoids are reviewed (26). An overview of normal joint manipulation physiology is presented, with an explanation of the zone of physiological movement, the paraphysiological zone of movement (in which coaptation of the joint surfaces by an adjustment results in cavitation, the audible release, appearance of a radiolucent cavity, the vacuum phenomenon, and a refractory period in which no further cavitation is possible), and the pathological zone of movement (31–35). Experiments to determine forces necessary to achieve cavitation are reviewed as well (37,38). Discussion of these concepts concludes with three components of SDF or RDF that may be central to the lesion: (a) a locked joint or entrapped or pathological meniscus, (b) abnormal muscle function, and (c) abnormal biochemical processes within the synovial joint.

REFERENCES

1. Watkins RJ. Subluxation terminology since 1746. ACA J Chiro 1968;5:65–70.

2. Gibbons RW. The evolution of chiropractic: medical and social protest in America. In: Haldeman S, ed. Modern developments in the principles and practice of chiropractic. New York: Appleton-Century-Crofts, 1980: 3–24.

3. Gibbons RW. Solon Massey Langworthy: keeper of the flame during the "lost years" of chiropractic. Chiro Hist 1981;1:15–21.

4. Montgomery DP, Nelson JM. Evolution of chiropractic theories of practice and spinal adjustment, 1900–1950. Chiro Hist 1985;5: 71–76.

5. Baker WJ. A clinical reformation in chiropractic: the research of Dr. Fred Illi. Chiro Hist 1985;5:59–62.

6. Sandoz R. Some critical reflections on subluxations and adjustments. Ann Swiss Chiro Assoc 1989;9:7–29.

7. Burns L. Evidence of the existence of lesions. Still Res Inst Bull 1917;5:14–15.

8. Denslow JS, Hassett CC. The central excitatory state associated with postural abnormalities. J Neurophysiol 1942;5:393–402.

9. Denslow JS. An analysis of the variability of spinal reflex thresholds. J Neurophysiol 1944;7:207–215.

10. Denslow JS, Korr IM, Krems AD. Quantitative studies of chronic facilitation in human motoneuron pools. Am J Physiol 1947;150:229–238.

11. Greenman PE. Manipulative therapy in relation to total health care. In: Korr IM, ed. The neurobiologic mechanisms in manipulative therapy. New York: Plenum, 1978:43–52.

12. Drum D. The vertebral motor unit and intervertebral foramen. In: Goldstein M, ed. The research status of spinal manipulative therapy. Washington, D.C.: Government Printing Office, 1975:63–75.

13. Lewit K. The contribution of clinical observation to neurobiological mechanisms in manipulative therapy. In: Korr IM, ed. The neurobiologic mechanisms in manipulative therapy. New York: Plenum, 1978:3–25.

14. Schmorl G, Junghanns H. The human spine in health and disease. New York: Grune & Stratton, 1971:35–39.

15. Giles LGF. Anatomical basis of low back pain. Baltimore: Williams & Wilkins, 1989: 15–17.

16. Haldeman S. The neurophysiology of spinal pain syndromes. In: Haldeman S, ed. Modern developments in the principles and practice of chiropractic. New York: Appleton-Century-Crofts, 1980:119–141.

17. Wyke BD. The neurology of joints: a review of general principles. Clin Rheum Dis 1981;7:223–239.

18. Wyke BD. Articular neurology: a review. Physiotherapy 1972;58:94–99.

19. Hadley LA. Anatomico-roentgenographic studies of the spine. Springfield, Ill.: Charles C Thomas, 1964:125–130,375,378.

20. Schmorl G, Junghanns H. The human spine in health and disease. 2nd ed. New York: Grune & Stratton, 1971:21–24, 35–39, 142–150, 221–223.

21. Jackson R. The cervical syndrome. Springfield, Ill.: Charles C Thomas, 1978: 143–146.

22. Haldeman S. Why one cause of back pain? In: Buerger AA, Tobis TS, eds. Approaches to the validation of manipulation therapy. Springfield, Ill.: Charles C Thomas, 1977: 187–197.

23. Farfan HF: The scientific basis of manipulative procedures. Clin Rheum Dis 1980; 6:159–78.

24. Giles LGF. Anatomical basis of low back pain. Baltimore: Williams & Wilkins, 1989: 166–168.

25. Giles LGF. Innervation of zygapophyseal joint synovial folds in low-back pain. Lancet 1987;2:692.

26. Jones TR, James JE, Adams JW, Garcia J, Walker SL, Ellis JP. Lumbar zygapophyseal joint meniscoids: evidence of their role in chronic intersegmental hypomobility. J Manipulative Physiol Ther 1989;12:374–385.

27. Kos J, Wolf J. The intervertebral meniscus and its possible role in intervertebral joint blockage. J Orthop Sports Phys Ther 1972; 1:8–9.

28. Zusman M, Edwards BC, Donaghy A. Investigation of a proposed mechanism for the relief of spinal pain with passive joint movement. J Manual Med 1989;4:58–61.

29. Helbig T, Lee CK. The lumbar facet syndrome. Spine 1988;13:61–64.

30. Hildebrandt J, Argyrakis A. Percutaneous nerve block of the cervical facets—a relatively new method in the treatment of chronic headache and neck pain. Manual Med 1986;2:48–52.

31. Roston JB, Haines RW. Cracking in the metacarpo-phalangeal joint. J Anat 1947;81: 165–173.

32. Unsworth A, Dowson D, Wright V. Cracking joints. A bioengineering study of cavitation in the metacarpophalangeal joint. Ann Rheum Dis 1971;30:348–358.

33. Sandoz R. Some physical mechanisms and effects of spinal adjustments. Ann Swiss Chiro Assoc 1976;6:91–141.

34. Meal GM, Scott RA. Analysis of the joint crack by simultaneous recording of sound and tension. J Manipulative Physiol Ther 1986; 9:189–195.

35. Mierau D, Cassidy JD, Bowen V, Dupuis P, Noftall F. Manipulation and mobilization of the third metacarpophalangeal joint. A quantitative radiographic and range of motion study. Manual Med 1988;3:135–140.

36. Haas M. The physics of spinal manipulation. Part IV. A theoretical consideration of the physician impact force and energy requirements needed to produce synovial joint cavitation. J Manipulative Physiol Ther 1990; 13:378–383.

37. Herzog W, Hessel BW, Conway PJW, McEwen MC. Force measurements during spinal manipulative therapy. Foundation for Chiropractic Education and Research: Proceedings of the 1990 International Conference on Spinal Manipulation, 1990:292–295.

38. Conway P, Herzog W, Zhang Y, Hasler E, Ladly K. Identification of mechanical factors that may cause cavitation during spinal manipulative treatments. Foundation for Chiropractic Education and Research: Proceedings of the 1991 International Conference on Spinal Manipulation, 1991:281–284.

39. Fuiks DM, Greyson CE. Vacuum pneumoarthrography and spontaneous occurrence of gas in joint spaces. J Bone Joint Surg 1950; 32A:933–938.

40. Humphreys CR, Triano JJ, Brandl MJ. Sensitivity of H-reflex alterations in idiopathic low back pain patients vs. a healthy population. J Manipulative Physiol Ther 1989;12:71–78.

41. Thabe H. Electromyography as tool to document diagnostic findings and therapeutic results associated with somatic dysfunctions in the upper cervical spinal joints and sacroiliac joints. Manual Med 1986;2:53–58.

42. Ellestad SM, Nagle RV, Boesler DR, Kilmore MA. Electromyographic and skin resistance responses to osteopathic manipulative treatment for low-back pain. J Am Osteopath Assoc 1988;88:991–997.

43. Leach RA. An evaluation of the effects of chiropractic manipulative therapy on hypolordosis of the cervical spine. J Manipulative Physiol Ther 1983;6:17–23.

44. Owens EF, Leach RA. Changes in cervical curvature determined radiographically following chiropractic adjustment. Foundation for Chiropractic Education and Research: Proceedings of the 1990 International Conference on Spinal Manipulation, 1990:165–169.

45. Plaugher G, Cremata EE, Phillips RB. A retrospective consecutive case analysis of pretreatment and comparative static radiological parameters following chiropractic adjustments. J Manipulative Physiol Ther 1990;13:498–506.

46. Lopes M, Plaugher G, Ray S. Closed reduction of lumbar retrolisthesis: a report of two cases. Foundation for Chiropractic Education and Research: Proceedings of the 1991 International Conference on Spinal Manipulation, 1991:110–114.

47. Yu XM, Hu JW, Vernon HT. Electromyographic responses of neck muscles to an inflammatory agent in anesthetized rats. Foundation for Chiropractic Education and Research: Proceedings of the 1991 International Conference on Spinal Manipulation, 1991:30–34.

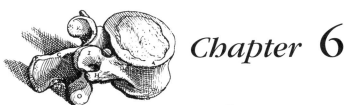

Chapter **6**

Soft Outcome Measures of Dysfunction

A number of outcome measures have been used to identify effects of chiropractic manipulative therapy (CMT) (and osteopathic manipulative therapy; OMT) on segmental dysfunction (SDF) and regional dysfunction (RDF). It is hoped that obtaining and quantifying measures of our patients' conditions will lead to more accurate assessment of SDF and/or RDF, more efficacious care, and ultimately to enhanced communication with governmental and third-party payers, who are demanding more accountability from all practitioners of health care as we approach an era of national health insurance (1). The so-called soft outcome measures associated with SDF and RDF will be discussed here.

In this text we refer to outcome measure as a synonym for any dependent variable that might vary as a result of chiropractic or other intervention. Keating (1) states that dependent variables include clinical outcome assessments—which he alternatively defines as any patient complaint (e.g., visual analog pain score, Oswestry Low Back Pain Disability Questionnaire) or measure of performance (e.g., time lost from work)—and mediating factors (such as muscle spasm detected by electromyography, radiographically identifiable intervertebral subluxation, or movement restriction based on passive range of motion testing).

Typically, measures that are considered "hard" include physical findings that often require more sophisticated technology to obtain. These comprise the focus of Chapter 7. Softer measures may be easier to collect in the clinic setting and are often less obtrusive. These measures, including patient self-reports of symptoms or behavior, have been traditionally regarded as subjective and unreliable. However, mounting evidence suggests the softer measures may be more reliable and more applicable to research and detection of SDF as well as RDF.

Range of Motion

Fixation or hypomobility has long been considered the key component of SDF in chiropractic clinical practice. Range-of-motion testing to clinically validate lost or excessive mobility is generally conducted on a regional (e.g., cervical rotation; lateral cervical flexion) or on an intersegmental (e.g., lateral flexion of L4 on L5) basis. While inter- and intraobserver reliability studies have somewhat validated the use of passive and active gross or regional motion procedures, testing of intersegmental motion has resulted in contradictory findings. The following is a review of these studies.

MOTION PALPATION

In a literature review, Keating (2) concludes that studies of motion palpation of the lumbar motion segments (viz. intersegmental motion) have not provided strong evidence of interexaminer reliability. Nansel and co-workers (3) found poor interexaminer reliability with respect to detection of side of greatest fixation in the cervical spines of 270 asymptomatic students. These chiropractic efforts are at odds with osteopathic research by Johnston (4, 5) and physiotherapy research by Jull and Bullock (6) suggesting good agreement between examiners when testing for intersegmental motion.

More recently, Jull, Bogduk, and Marsland (7) demonstrated excellent sensitivity and specificity in manual detection of cervical zygapophyseal joint dysfunction. They operationally defined symptomatic joints by three findings on palpation involving posteroanterior glides centrally over the spinous processes and performed unilaterally over the zygapophyses of the cervical spine:

1. Abnormal "end feel" (resistance at the extreme end of range of motion);
2. Abnormal resistance to motion;
3. Reproduction of pain with passive movement.

Passive intervertebral cervical movements in flexion, extension, lateral flexion, and rotation were assessed as well. When all three findings were present, as assessed by the blinded manipulative therapist, independent diagnosis by means of medial-branch nerve blocks in 14 cases and by additional fluoroscopically controlled intraarticular zygapophyseal joint blocks in an additional 6 cases confirmed the manipulator's observations. The manipulator correctly predicted 17 true symptomatic joints and found four cases of asymptomatic joints only; local anesthetics (1.5 ml of 0.5% bupivacaine in the case of medial branch blocks, and 1 ml of 1% lignocaine in the case of intraarticular zygapophyseal blocks) brought the expected total

relief of symptoms for at least 3 and 1 hour(s), respectively, at the sites predicted by the manual palpatory procedure (7).

In a novel approach to the problem of reliability of motion palpation, Byfield (8) created a mechanical model, equipped with intersegmental fixators—which acted as universal joints—and covered with a chamois leather, which was blindly palpated by eight chiropractors and 19 chiropractic students. Based on 300 tests of palpation of known preset fixations, there were 25 true-positive and 218 true-negative observations, and 24 false-negative and 33 false-positive observations. The findings suggested high specificity despite a high expected rate of chance agreement (K = 0.35; observed agreement, 81.0%; expected chance agreement, 70.6%; specificity, 86.8%; sensitivity, 51.0%).

If the Byfield model is clinically relevant, it suggests that chiropractors may be able to differentiate SDF when given patients with more prominent pain-related hypomobility (i.e., patients in moderate or severe pain as opposed to asymptomatic students (2, 3). Evidence of that may have been provided by a recent study by Vernon and co-workers (9). Moderate agreement (79%; K = 0.63; P <.05) between examiners checking intersegmental motion and sensitivity to pressure (see "Algometry," later in this chapter) was found in the lumbar spine in patients with acute low back pain (9).

Moreover, Herzog and co-workers (10) have demonstrated good intraexaminer agreement (68% agreement on positive findings, 79% agreement on negative findings, and 72% agreement on the correct side; P = .01) as well as good interexaminer agreement (54–78%; average of three sessions, P = .01) between 10 chiropractors and 11 patients, using motion palpation of the sacroiliac joints. In these patients, severity of the sacroiliac joint syndrome (SIJS) did not seem to influence agreement scores. However, chiropractor expertise did correlate negatively with intraexaminer reliability. The authors suggested that retraining in the motion palpation technique (viz., observation of normal posterior, inferior ilium motion and normal anterior, inferior sacral motion while the patient is raising the knee as high as possible while standing) may be indicated for older practitioners if this sample is representative.

In view of these mixed findings, motion palpation, a promising technique that is widely used in the profession to test for intersegmental motion asymmetry, will continue to be a controversial diagnostic test pending the outcome of further research (2–10).

REGIONAL MOTION TESTING

In contrast with the lack of concordance sometimes seen between examiners (and between researchers) regarding testing for intersegmental motion, tests of gross motion have been found to be reliable indicators of spinal motion asymmetry, and good reliability has been documented between examiners.

For example, Johnston et al. (11) studied 161 subjects, using one osteopathic physician and two osteopathic students to check passive gross motion in six planes. Examiners checked passive range of motion in the spine, noted whether they felt a palpable sense of symmetry, and recorded the side of greatest resistance when asymmetry of motion was detected. To reduce error, each examiner made three repeat observations on each subject and later repeated the process a second time. Records were first examined for interexaminer agreement within each set of three tests and then for agreement between the two sets of tests. Finally, disagreements between examiners were evaluated to determine the extent to which inconsistent results were due to system error. Using this protocol these researchers demonstrated high confidence levels for cervical lateral flexion (expected agreement = 5; observed = 12; z = 2.5; P = .03), extremely high confidence levels for cervical rotation (expected agreement = 8.3; observed agreement = 18; z = 3.64; P = .0005), but unsatisfactory confidence levels for tests of dorsal and lumbar rotation, and only random agreement for tests of dorsal lateral flexion and lateral shifting of the hips.

Gill and colleagues (12) demonstrated excellent repeatability for detection of lumbar flexion and extension, using the modified Schober method. This method requires that the subject be standing; a line is drawn on the skin between the posterior superior iliac crests, representing the top of the sacrum. Marks are placed 10 cm above and 5 cm below the first line in the midline. The distance between the two marks is recorded in centimeters in each posture in this technique of mensuration. This method was determined to be more reliable than three other systems, including the two-inclinometer method now accepted as the profession-wide standard by the AMA *Guides to the Evaluation of Permanent Impairment* (13). The two inclinometer method was determined to be reliable in tests of lumbar extension but not flexion (12).

However, the AMA guidelines call for repeat flexion tests correlated with straight leg raising as a check for patient effort (13), a procedure not tested by Gill et al. (12). It is felt that the additional checks for patient effort and aids such as automated inclinometers capable of calculating compound joint motion permit increased clinical efficiency and speed of testing (Fig. 6.1). Indeed, recent joint chiropractic and medical research by Dillard and co-workers (14) demonstrated that expensive computer-aided inclinometry such as the Isotechnologies B-200 is not as reliable as the two inclinometer method. In their study, the two inclinometer method endorsed by the AMA resulted in reliability coefficients approaching 0.8 in lumbar flexion. Combined dorsal-lumbar flexion/extension and right rotation were also significantly repeatable measures, in contrast with the findings of Gill et al. (12).

In a classic set of experiments, Nansel et al. (15) were the first to demonstrate not only the reliability of goniometrically established cervical lateral flexion measurements but also the side-specificity of CMT in correction of asymmetry in lateral cervical motion. Although it had long been held that

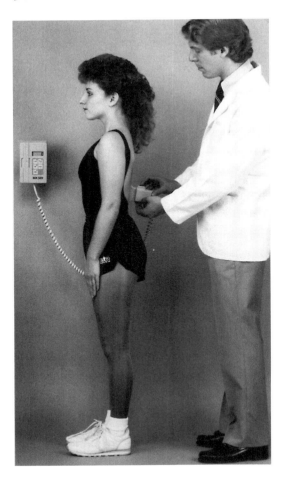

of less than 5° did not always meet minimum confidence levels. Hence, retest 30 minutes later yielded very high correlation coefficients when the larger end-range differences were documented (r = 0.94; n = 66). Based upon the criterion of only accepting subjects exhibiting more than 8° of left/right asymmetry, sitting adjustments (high-velocity thrust) to the least restricted side (n = 11), sitting adjustments to the most restricted side (n = 14), set-up without thrust (n = 9), and nonintervention control groups were used. While the two control groups exhibited no posttreatment changes in asymmetries, there was significant (P <.025) improvement when adjusting the least restricted side. In contrast, when adjusting the side of greatest restriction, there was highly significant improvement (P <.001) in motion on the side of restriction only.

In further work, Nansel and co-workers (16) have established that correction of cervical lateral flexion asymmetries by a single adjustment is short-lived (viz. return to pretreatment asymmetry within 48 hours) in patients with significant histories of neck pain and trauma. Conversely, subjects without pain appear to have more lasting correction of their asymmetry with a single adjustment (16).

Finally, Nansel, Peneff, and Quitoriano (17) studied the effects of adjusting upper versus lower cervical segments in asymptomatic chiropractic students with lateral flexion asymmetries (n = 43), rotational asymmetries (n = 40), and both lateral flexion and rotational asymmetries (n = 15). Blinded goniometric recordings were made with the patients' eyes closed (prior work had established increased reliability on retest when patients close their eyes during goniometric assessment). More than 350 asymptomatic subjects were screened to obtain 98 with end-range asymmetries of more than 10°. Results strongly demonstrated that lateral flexion asymmetries are corrected most efficiently with sitting bilateral lower cervical adjustments (P <.001), although sitting upper cervical bilateral adjustments were somewhat effective as well (P <.05).

Figure 6.1. The use of digital inclinometry and repeat testing has improved the reliability of range-of-motion examinations. Cybex's EDI 320 is the only automated inclinometer on the market and is capable of calculating compound joint motions (e.g., dorsal flexion measured at the dorsolumbar transition minus sacral flexion measured over the sacrum equals true lumbar flexion angle). (Photo courtesy of Cybex, a division of Lumex, Inc. Photographer, Barry Axelrod.)

adjustments were most effective when delivered on the side of greatest restriction of motion, these researchers were the first to document this phenomenon, an important concept in clinical correction of SDF. In their initial blinded experiments it was found that left versus right lateral flexion end-range differences of 8° or more were always highly significant (P <.001); however, asymmetries

Conversely, rotational asymmetries responded significantly to sitting upper cervical bilateral adjustments (P <.001), but not to bilateral lower cervical adjustments. The findings were further corroborated by results of adjusting the students with both rotational and lateral bending asymmetries. Hence, of the eight who received bilateral upper cervical (C2–C3 segments) adjustments, rotational asymmetries were significantly ameliorated within 30 minutes (P <.001), while there was no significant change in lateral flexion asymmetry. Moreover, the seven who received bilateral lower cervical (C6–C7 segments) adjustments showed significant improvement in lateral flexion (P <.01) but not in rotational asymmetry (Fig. 6.2).

The authors concluded that their work offered strong evidence for the regional independence of rotational versus lateral flexion asymmetries. Of more than 350 students tested, only 15 had both lateral flexion and rotational asymmetries simultaneously. Within the larger group of 83 subjects and the smaller group of 15 subjects, adjustments were axis-specific (upper cervical adjustments ameliorating rotational asymmetries, and lower cervical adjustments ameliorating lateral flexion asymmetries). The authors felt that the segmental level at which adjustments were delivered (rather than the manner in which they were performed) was the most important factor responsible for the axis or level-specific effects (17).

In summary, while motion palpation to detect intersegmental motion restrictions and fixations has not consistently been shown to be a reliable indicator of SDF, tests of passive gross motion in spinal regions have been shown to be reliable. Correction of asymmetries detected using these techniques by side-specific as well as level-specific

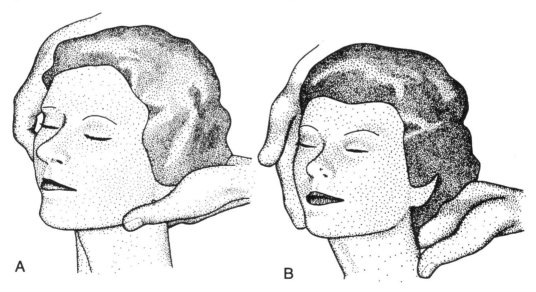

A   B

Figure 6.2. Nansel and co-workers (15–17) in a series of classic experiments, confirmed that side-specific and level-specific chiropractic adjustments resulted in significant amelioration of rotational and side-bending cervical motion asymmetries. These researchers at Palmer West University determined that adjustments delivered to the side of rotational or side-bending restriction were significantly more effective than adjustments delivered to the contralateral side. **A**, When rotational asymmetries were present, adjustments to the upper cervical spine were more effective. **B**, When side-bending asymmetries were present, adjustments to the lower cervical spine were significantly more effective in reducing the asymmetry and restoring normal motion.

adjustments suggests that passive gross motion may be a reliable indicator of RDF.

Algometry

Algometry refers to measurement of pain. Since initial investigations were reported in 1953, a number of research efforts have contributed to assessment of pain perception utilizing force gauges, including most recently several studies by Fischer (18–22). Fischer distinguishes dolimetry and algometry from measurement of *pressure tolerance* (PTo, the maximum force a person can tolerate) and measurement of *pressure-pain threshold* (PPT, the minimum force that causes discomfort or pain). Fischer prefers measurement of PPT for a number of reasons: (*a*) PPT is the minimum level of pain or discomfort that is felt by the patient and recorded by the examiner, and is therefore less traumatic to the patient; (*b*) measurement of pressure tolerance may be intrusive enough to actually alter the excitability of the underlying tissues, making repeat measures less indicative of the norm for that patient (viz., less reproducibility); and (*c*) the point of measurement is defined more precisely (18–22).

The rationale for current use of algometry in chiropractic practice and research and its potential application for determination of SDF can be gleaned from a review of current uses of algometry in physical medicine. Certainly initial investigations of CMT using PPT as an outcome measure and clinical reliability studies of algometry have been promising and will be discussed. These studies, taken collectively, offer good evidence that the point tenderness classically associated with SDF may be more precisely quantified using this instrumentation.

VALIDITY AND RELIABILITY

In Fischer's experiences with algometry, the use of a force gauge fitted with a rubber disk having a surface of 1 cm^2 was the method of choice, rather than earlier force gauges having a smaller 0.5-cm plunger surface diameter. He concluded that forces could be transmitted more deeply into the tissues with the larger plunger diameter and a gauge with a range of 0 to 11 kg (Fig. 6.3)(20).

A study of validity and reproducibility of the pressure threshold meter (PTM) in establishing PPT was conducted by Fischer (19) on 24 male and 26 female normal volunteers at 9 sites. Normative values were obtained based upon these evaluations (for normative values see Table 9.2). In that investigation the rate of delivery of pressure was constant, at approximately 1 kg/sec. Reliability was established by comparing left/right values in the same patient. Over nine sites in the 50 patients, there were no significant left/right differences with the exception of the m. infraspinatus in females (P <.05).

In a separate study of pressure tolerance over bone and muscle, Fischer (18) examined the maximum amount of pressure that could be tolerated without excessive effort. Hence, 30 female and 20 male pain-free volunteers were examined at four sites and were told to "say stop when you cannot stand the pressure any longer." He found that use of algometry (1 kg/sec) to measure the patient's tolerance for pain is best conducted at two of the sites over the deltoid muscle 2 cm below the acromion at the lateral aspect of the arm; and over the chin, with the knees flexed to 60° and the algometer at a 90° angle to the tibial shaft and 6 cm distal to the tibial tubercle. Normal values were established, and there were no significant left/right differences, suggesting good reproducibility and reliability. Based upon these findings and his clinical experiences, Fischer (20) established the following criteria for determination of abnormal PPT findings:

1. Left/right asymmetries in PPT >2 kg/cm^2;
2. PPT < 3 kg at all muscle and bone sites;
3. PPT values below established normals (see Chapter 9).

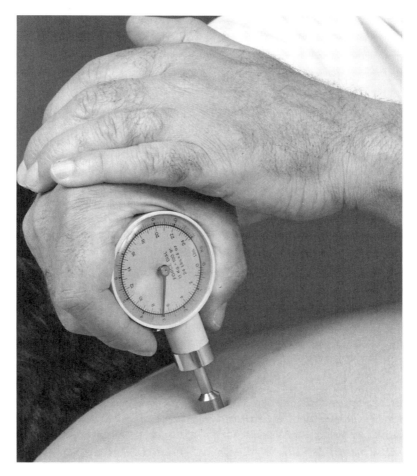

Figure 6.3. The use of algometry in chiropractic research and practice is increasing rapidly. Fischer (18–22) has helped pioneer its use in physical medicine for quantification of myofascial trigger points. He uses a force gauge with a 0–11 kg range and a surface of 1 cm² and advocates application of constantly increasing pressure at the rate of 1 kg per second. Chiropractic researchers have subsequently used the pressure threshold meter (PTM) to identify segmental dysfunction associated with a manipulable spinal lesion (32). Its further use as an outcome measure for assessment of improvement after chiropractic adjustment is being investigated (30, 31, 33). (Photograph courtesy of Andrew A. Fischer, M.D., Ph.D.)

General considerations based upon his work and reviews of the literature suggest that both PPT and PTo are reduced in females more than in males. However, age has not been statistically correlated with PTo. Clinical considerations and implications of abnormal PPT and PTo examinations, including determination of excessive sensitivity, evidence of myofascial trigger points, and chronic pain syndrome are discussed in more detail in Chapter 9.

The reliability, validity, and reproducibility of the PTM have been the subjects of a number of investigations in physical medicine, psychology, and even dentistry. They are discussed below.

STUDIES OF ALGOMETRY IN PHYSICAL MEDICINE AND DENTISTRY

List, Helkimo, and Falk (23) assessed 25 healthy volunteers and 20 patients with craniomandibular dysfunction in an inter- and intraobserver reliability study of algometry using the PTM. Six sites along the masseter muscle, the anterior temporal muscle, and the zygomatic arch were evaluated by one examiner with the PTM, by repeat recordings at each marked point. High reliability coefficients (r = 0.79–0.94) were demonstrated at all of the sites, and even movement of the instrument up to 3 mm off the marked sites resulted in reliability coefficients of the same magnitude. Comparison of PTM data with a finger palpation score obtained by a second examiner resulted in good correlation between the examiners at all sites (p <.05). The authors concluded that PTM is useful for evaluation of PPT in the masticatory system in clinical and experimental research. Certainly temporomandibular joint dysfunction has been the focus of some chiropractic attention and treatment, and the PTM could be an important outcome measure in any future chiropractic studies of this lesion.

Gerecz-Simon and co-workers (24) evaluated PPT with a pressure algometer in 54 female and 72 male subjects with rheumatoid arthritis (36 subjects), osteoarthritis (36 subjects), ankylosing spondylitis (18 male subjects), or no symptoms (36 healthy control volunteers). Six sites were evaluated (three sites over bone and three sites over muscle) at points not corresponding to "trigger points" associated with fibromyalgia. Results revealed significantly higher PPT in patients with ankylosing spondylitis than in those with osteoarthritis. PPT in osteoarthritis patients was significantly higher than that in normal subjects. Patients with rheumatoid arthritis had significantly lower PPT than controls. Females had lower PPT than males.

Takala (25) demonstrated intraobserver reliability coefficients ranging from 0.71 to 0.92, using algometry to detect PPT over upper trapezius and levator scapulae muscles in 70 women. Day-to-day repeatability was measured in 10 women and proved to be acceptable. Interobserver reliability coefficients based on two examiners checking PPT in 93 men at the same two sites varied from 0.68 to 0.79. Women had lower PPT than men, but values varied widely, even among asymptomatic individuals. Accordingly, Takala recommended that the device be used as an outcome measure in therapeutic trials but not as a primary diagnostic or screening tool.

Ohrbach and Gale (26) studied validity and reliability of the PTM for detecting PPT in 45 patients with myogenous temporomandibular disorder. There was strong validity in PPT measures between patients and matched controls. The PPT was significantly reduced at the site of pain as opposed to control sites in contralateral nonpainful muscles. Moreover, PPT was significantly lower at sites producing referred pain than at sites producing only localized pain on palpation. They concluded that reliability of PPT was better than reliability of the signs and site-specific symptoms, and recommended use of the procedure in clinical trials of temporomandibular disorders.

Decreased PPT was demonstrated in 50 chronic muscle tension-type headache sufferers by Langemark and co-workers (27). There was a negative correlation between headache severity and PPT in the temporal region, compared with 24 healthy controls. There was a positive correlation between PPT in the temporal and occipital regions, and a correlation was found between PPT and cold pain thresholds as well.

These studies seem to confirm initial osteopathic investigations that demonstrated reliability of determining deep tissue tension manually (28). Johnston et al. (29) found agreements ranging from 79 to 86%, using manual palpation alone, among five student palpators.

More recently, chiropractic researchers have demonstrated correction of trigger points and improvement in PPT in the cervical spine and lumbosacral region after CMT, using the PTM.

STUDIES OF ALGOMETRY AND CHIROPRACTIC MANIPULATION

Vernon and co-workers (30) at the Canadian Memorial Chiropractic College demonstrated significant improvement (increase) in PPT from 40 to 56% in patients with chronic cervical pain receiving a single chiropractic rotational adjustment, but not in a control group receiving oscillatory mobilization only (p <.0001). The blinded pilot study was carried out on nine subjects.

Similarly, Hsieh and Hong (31), in a pilot study, found evidence of increased PFT in myofascial trigger points in the trapezius and rhomboid muscles after diversified chiropractic adjusting. Pretreatment mean PPT was 1.28 ± 0.36 kg/cm^2/sec, and the posttreatment mean PPT was 2.05 ± 0.47 kg/cm^2/sec. A single session of cervical and/or upper thoracic high-velocity, low-amplitude diversified adjustments was administered to areas of palpable fixation in the five patients.

Vernon and co-workers (32), in a blinded evaluation, also provided initial evidence that palpable spinal fixations correlate well with lumbar trigger points, as assessed by the PTM (agreement was 79%; K 0.63; p <.05). In their study, the sacroiliac motion palpation test of Gillet and the AP glide dynamic joint play test of Gillet, Grice, Cassidy, and Faye were used by one blinded assessor to document specific restrictions in joint motion in the lumbosacral region, while a second examiner documented the location of subjective pain and maximal tender points. A third blinded assessor used the PTM to assess lumbar paraspinal PPT. The moderately high correlations between reduced PPT and joint movement fixation offered perhaps the first good chiropractic evidence for reliability of these techniques for the determination of a specific SDF.

To determine manipulative effectiveness in cases of chronic sacroiliac joint syndrome (SIJS), Osterbauer and co-workers (33) studied the Activator chiropractic technique and used the PTM and a pain scale and functional disability questionnaire (see the discussion on the Visual Analog Scale and Oswestry Modified Low Back Pain Questionnaire below) as outcome measures. In nine subjects with confirmed SIJS (viz., positive Yeoman's test, sacral pressure, and the supported Adam's test), after Activator adjusting for five weeks (three sessions per week), there was significant improvement in the baseline Visual Analog Score (p <.05), in pain threshold over bone (p <.05); (value in kg/cm^2/sec) and in the Oswestry score (p <.05) but not in pain threshold over muscle, although this improved as well. Similarly, the number of positive SIJS orthopaedic test findings at posttest improved significantly over the 1-week baseline in these chronic (more than 6 months duration) cases (Fisher's exact probability test; one-tailed p <.05).

Thus, algometry using a PTM and a constant rate of delivery of force (e.g., 1 kg/cm^2/sec) reliably monitors PPT, myofascial trigger points, and excessive sensitivity, and correlates well with spinal fixations and trigger points that respond well to CMT. Its use as an outcome measure in further research and practice has been widely advocated, despite some variance between asymptomatic individuals.

Pain and Functional Status Questionnaires

Both practitioners and researchers often prefer "hard" measures of clinical improvement (e.g., straight leg raising, paraspinal EMG activity, and motion x-rays of the spine) to the so-called soft measures. Indeed, third-party payers and courts are widely seen to prefer such documentation. Unfortunately, the boundary between soft and hard measures of spinal function is often vague. For example, while interobserver agreement on assessment of functional x-rays of the spine is often poor, test-retest reliability of a number of pain and function questionnaires and patient self-reports is actually quite acceptable (34, 35). Moreover, using the same example, functional A-P and lateral lumbar spine films offer little practical information toward the detection of SDF (although obviously necessary to rule out pathology and identify congenital or developmental defects), while self-reports and visual analog scales yield quantified data regarding the direct impact of the lesion upon the patient's symptoms, functional ability, and psychological status.

Some of the criteria used to assess the value of pain and functional status indices include the following:

1. Practicality—can the test be self-administered quickly?
2. Comprehensiveness—is a wide range of function and behavior included?
3. Reproducibility—what is the test-retest reliability (for self-administered questionnaires) and the interobserver reliability (for questionnaires administered by an interviewer)?
4. Validity—does the instrument correlate well with other physical measures of function?
5. Responsivity—can the questionnaire detect subtle yet clinically relevant changes in the patient's functional status?

RELIABILITY AND VALIDITY

A number of instruments have been tested for reliability and validity of assessment of pain and function, primarily of the lower back region. While a descriptive presentation of these instruments is beyond the scope of this chapter, a few select indices include:

Visual analog scale (VAS)—The scale consists of a 100-mm continuous line. Patients place a mark to indicate their pain level, somewhere between "No Pain" and "Unbearable Pain." The VAS is scored by placing a metric ruler against the line. Good correlations

with the McGill pain questionnaire ($r = 0.63$) have been reported (36).

McGill pain questionnaire (MPQ)—Melzack (37) introduced this instrument in 1975, which has since become a standard in pain assessment. Twenty scales of verbal descriptors are arranged into four subscales. Validity has been established by correlation with other instruments.

Oswestry low back pain questionnaire—This 10-question self-report describes a variety of daily activities from walking, sitting, and lifting to sex life, and is scored with ordinal responses. Validity is suggested by correlations with trunk mobility and muscle function in patients with lower back pain (38, 39).

Neck disability index (NDI)—The index, a modification of the Oswestry questionnaire, was developed by researchers at the Canadian Memorial Chiropractic College to rate the effect of cervical spine disability on activities of daily living. The NDI correlates with MPQ ($r = 0.73$) and with VAS ($r = 0.60$); test-retest reliability is 0.80 (34).

Finally, use of these measures as tests of the manipulable lesion (SDF) is validated throughout the chiropractic literature. For example, the visual analog scale reveals significantly less pain in patients with acute mechanical lower back pain after CMT, despite the absence of any significant change in plasma β-endorphin concentrations (40). The Oswestry LBP questionnaire was used in the exhaustive British randomized trial of chiropractic versus hospital outpatient treatment for patients with mechanical LBP; Oswestry scores were 7% more improved in the chiropractic-treated LBP patients, which correlated well with increased improvement in straight leg raising and lumbar flexion in the group receiving CMT (41). Leach, Owens, and Giesen (39) recently found significant loss of normal lumbar flexion-relaxation on EMG (see Chapter 8), significant reduction in lumbar paraspinal PPT, and elevated Oswestry and VAS scores in patients with acute LBP, but not in control patients. Results of these and similar studies in the chiropractic literature suggest the validity of using these intruments as outcome measures for SDF treatment by CMT.

Leg Length Tests

Perhaps the oldest of the soft outcome measures of subluxation complex or SDF has until recently received little attention from the research community. Despite wide-spread regular use throughout the profession, physical measurements of leg length inequality, specifically the Derefield pelvic leg check (DPLC), have been poorly understood and remain to be validated.

The DPLC is not to be confused with medical radiographic procedures to determine an anatomically short leg. Instead, the chiropractic test is considered a functional test of lumbopelvic mechanics. The test involves assessing the prone patient's sole-heel interfaces bilaterally for a short leg, then flexing the knees to 90° to see if the short leg stays short or appears shorter (viz., negative Derefield; D−), evens, or becomes the long leg (viz., positive Derefield; D+)(42).

Cooperstein (42) created a kinesiological model to study the DPLC, which involves either: (*a*) hypertonic/futile thigh extensors (long leg D+ test); and (*b*) hypertonic/futile thigh flexors (short leg D+ test) with increased tonicity, so that as the knees are flexed to 90°, there is the appearance of a short leg that becomes long; or (*c*) hypertonic/effective thigh flexors (long leg D− test) with increased tonicity such that as the knees are flexed to 90° the long leg stays long; and (*d*) hypertonic/effective thigh extensors (short leg D− test) with thigh flexors that remain unchanged as the knees are flexed to 90° (Fig. 6.4).

DeBoer and co-workers (43) made a preliminary investigation of the DPLC on 40 students, with three different examining doctors rechecking each student two times. While interexaminer reliability was fair between two examiners, it was poor for the third. However, the study was an attempt to replicate the test as it is conducted in the field, so no training program was attempted prior to the research to enhance the reliability of the test. Furthermore, intraexaminer reliability was more acceptable, with interclass correlation coefficients ranging from .52 to .77.

Danelius (44) took issue with the conclusions reached by DeBoer and co-workers (43), suggesting instead that high correlations between examiners checking straight versus knee-flexed leg lengths was probably due to transference by the examiner of leg shortness or longness from the straight- to the flexed-knee position. He calculates that trunk muscles would have to pull the hip joint cephalward fully three inches to record a 0.25-inch difference in heel heights.

Shambaugh, Sclafani, and Fanselow (45) tested a variant of the Derefield test (the Derefield-Thompson test for leg length inequality) for reliability, using 26 subjects with five different examiners. This chiropractic test purportedly determines if there is a cervical subluxation or SDF; if the Derefield test is negative, the patient is instructed to turn the head to the left and right—a change in leg length indicates a cervical lesion. After each subject had been sequentially examined for leg length inequality by five examiners in five different rooms, using the aforementioned procedure, they were randomly given no treatment, cervical adjusting, or gluteal massage. The entire cycle was repeated five times. Results suggested that clinicians could reliably detect leg length inequalities to less than 3 mm (both interexaminer and intraexaminer reliability were acceptable) and a change in leg length inequality when the head was rotated. Pierce-Stillwagon cervical adjustments were administered on either the first, second, third, or fourth visit to the treatment room to 16 students who had never or rarely been adjusted prior to the research. The level of adjustment was based upon cervical x-ray

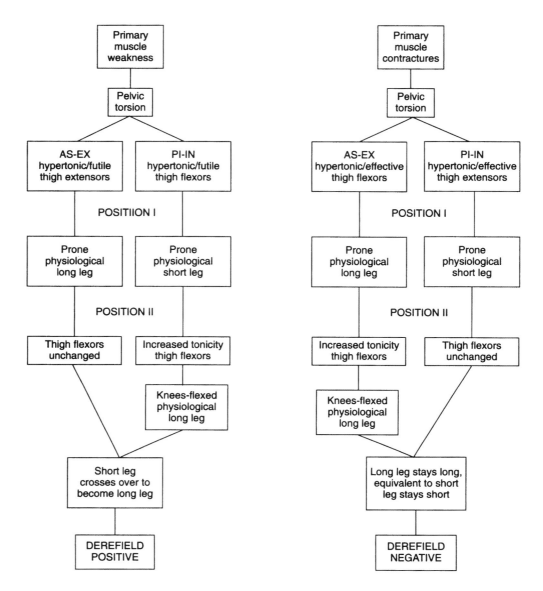

Figure 6.4. The Derefield pelvic leg check (DPLC) remains an enigma despite some evidence of good interexaminer reliability. Cooperstein (42) created a model for study of the still widely used chiropractic test for putative lumbopelvic dysfunction or subluxation. The Cooperstein model predicts that either the long or short leg anterior thigh may exhibit relative hypertonicity and that the asymmetry seen in the DPLC may result from guarding responses instituted by stretch reflexes (viz., hypertonic/futile thigh flexors in one case, and hypertonic/effective thigh flexors in the other). (Adapted from Cooperstein R. The Derefield pelvic leg check: a kinesiological interpretation. Chiro Technique 1991;3:60–65.)

listings and a Derma-Therma-Gram heat reading. Neither cervical adjusting nor gluteal massage produced a significant change in observed leg length inequalities. However, this study was criticized for purported errors in statistical evaluation (46, 47). Specifically, Shambaugh and co-workers used the t-test instead of K or the interclass correlation coefficient for comparisons between examiners. In reply, Shambaugh (48) presented raw data and calculated coefficients using the SAS system, revealing excellent rater agreements (P = .984 when head in center; P = 0.98 when head turned right or left).

Youngquist, Fuhr, and Osterbauer (49) used a novel approach to determine the interexaminer reliability of an isolation test used by Activator technique to determine the presence of cervical subluxation or SDF. Of 72 subjects from a practice that used Activator adjusting technique exclusively, one group (n = 34) had received regular manipulation to the C1 vertebra using the Activator mechanical adjusting device, while a second group (n = 38) had no history of C1 adjusting. Two blinded assessors used the isolation test (patient tucks chin in while lying prone as the examiner flexes knees to 90°), and reliability between examiners was good on two separate occasions (group 1, 24 subjects: K = 0.52, P <.01; group 2, remaining 48 subjects tested one week later: K = 0.55, P <.001). Highly significant concordance was 79% overall for the presence or absence of C1 subluxation or SDF.

Fuhr and Osterbauer (50) have advocated using a ruler to further quantify relative leg length inequalities. Using a second assistant to record the inequality at the heel-sole interface with 30 prone subjects checked by 4 examiners, interexaminer reliability was fair to good (K = 0.31–0.75).

Falltrick and Pierson (51) found good interrater agreement (R^2 = 0.638, K = 0.799) between two subjects measured six times alternately by two examiners using a new apparatus to determine leg length inequality in the prone position. They found no correlation between prone leg length and head rotation, type of table, galvanic stimulation (viz., ipsilateral application at the middorsal and midlumbar levels producing tetanic contractions) or presence or absence of purported cervical subluxation or SDF, based on clinical criteria, in tests on 36 other subjects. The lack of correlation between head rotation and leg length inequality changes contradicted the findings of Shambaugh and co-workers (45, 48).

Improvements in future trials may be expected if examiners test for the paper sign (i.e., it is easier to withdraw paper placed under the flexed knee when the subject isometrically extends the flexed knee against resistance; easier removal suggests increased thigh stiffness) after first creating an artificial Derefield (viz. confirm that the state of contraction of the quadriceps altered the flexed-knee leg length inequality by asking the subject to extend one of the flexed knees mildly against the examiner's resistance; the examiner observes leg length inequality at the level of the medial maleoli) (42). Having first tested for a Derefield response using isometric contraction, then confirming with a paper test that the mechanism relates to pressure of the distal thigh against the table, Cooperstein (42) suggests that the paper sign will be more often seen on the short leg side in D+ patients and more often seen on the long leg side in D− patients. Until more research is done, the Derefield phenomenon will remain an enigma, although its use in clinical practice continues.

Discussion

The use of functional status and pain questionnaires yields important information to the clinician and researcher about physical, social, and psychological aspects of the patient's condition. These indices have shown test-retest and interobserver reliability that often exceeds that of other so-called hard outcome measures, and validity has been established by correlations between the instruments. Their use is advocated for practice and research, whether the underlying lesion is an SDF, another mechanical or pathological disorder, or unknown.

Moreover, as previously discussed, algometry and regional range of motion, especially when controlled carefully (e.g., using the two-inclinometer method with repeat testing, and algometry for the detection of PPT) has been correlated with fixation and shown to respond favorably to side-specific adjustments. This suggests the validity of using these techniques to detect SDF, and further quantification of clinical effects of the lesion can be obtained by using the functional and pain questionnaires just reviewed.

Nansel and co-worker's (16) finding that patients with long-standing complaints of pain and trauma gain only short-term amelioration of motion restriction is in line with experimental evidence on spinal learning and facilitation. In such patients with chronic complaints, a series of adjustments would predictably be necessary to effect more lasting improvement, based on the findings of these researchers (see also Chapter 8).

If Feinstein (52) is correct, "hardness" is more appropriately applied to measures that demonstrate good reliability and reproducibility. If this approach is correct and preliminary chiropractic research findings are validated, future editions of this text may have to include regional gross motion palpation, algometry, and functional indices under the heading of "hard outcome measures," and report radiographic, electromyographic, and some other physiological measures under the heading of "soft outcome measures."

Certainly the continuing use of the Derefield test for leg length inequality must remain suspect, perhaps more because of questions of validity than questions of reliability. Indeed, a number of authors have demonstrated good reliability for the Derefield and other chiropractic functional leg length tests, but these tests have not correlated well with clinical findings in most cases. Furthermore, flexing the knees 90° creates confounding biomechanical problems regarding interpretation: according to Dane-

lius (44), if the actual prone leg inequality was in the commonly found 5 ± 2 mm range, according to the quadratic formula, the leg length inequality in the flexed knee position would fall between 0.009 and 0.59 mm, or not be observable. In reply, DeBoer (53) cites hip rotation secondary to putative pelvic subluxation or SDF, forcing one knee to dig into the table cushion while the other rises slightly off the table, and femoral-tibial joint rotation displacing the knee both laterally and cephalad as examples of biomechanical changes during knee flexion that could create the discrepancies in leg length inequality observed in some of these studies.

Summary

There is good reliability and reproducibility for assessments of regional spinal motion (e.g., cervical lateral flexion) but there are mixed findings with regard to manual palpatory tests of intersegmental motion (e.g., L1/L2 motion restriction in lateral flexion). Regional motion restrictions have been shown to improve significantly with side-specific and level-specific CMT in blinded chiropractic investigations.

Another outcome measure traditionally considered soft is palpation for taut muscle bands or tender paraspinal muscles indicating the level of an SDF. However, development of the PTM provides the practitioner with a method of detecting taut muscles that has acceptable reliability and validity. A novel chiropractic investigation that positively correlated low PPT (trigger points) with joint fixations and pain in a blinded trial demonstrated the clinical utility for this approach. Clearly, algometry holds promise as an outcome measure for one aspect of SDF.

Functional status and pain questionnaires have a high degree of test-retest reproducibility and good correlations with other indices, and examiner-assisted tools have shown good interobserver reliability as well. Moreover, these instruments are perhaps more clinically effective in qualitatively and quantitatively assessing the patient's pain and function than are other tests and methods (e.g., functional x-rays) traditionally thought to be clinically important.

Finally, while various chiropractic tests of leg length inequality have generally demonstrated good interexaminer reliability, their validity is questioned by a lack of concordance with clinical findings. Specifically, the Derefield test has promising reliability, but biomechanical problems confound the interpretation when the knees are flexed to 90°, and exact implications of the phenomenon remain unknown.

REFERENCES

1. Keating JC Jr. Toward a philosophy of the science of chiropractic: a primer for clinicians. Stockton, Calif.: Stockton Foundation for Chiropractic Research. 1992:104.

2. Keating JC. Inter-examiner reliability of motion palpation of the lumbar spine: a review of quantitative literature. Am J Chiro Med 1989;2:107–110.

3. Nansel DD, Peneff AL, Jansen RD, Cooperstein R. Interexaminer concordance in detecting joint-play asymmetries in the cervical spines of otherwise asymptomatic subjects. J Manipulative Physiol Ther 1989;12:428–433.

4. Johnston WL. Segmental definition: part I. A focal point for diagnosis of somatic dysfunction. J Am Osteopath Assoc 1988;88:99–105.

5. Johnston WL. Segmental definition: part II. Application of an indirect method in osteopathic manipulative treatment. J Am Osteopath Assoc 1988;88:211–217.

6. Jull G, Bullock M. A motion profile of the lumbar spine in an aging population assessed by manual examination. Physiother Pract 1987;3:70–81.

7. Jull G, Bogduk N, Marsland A. The accuracy of manual diagnosis for cervical zygapophyseal joint pain syndromes. Med J Aust 1988;148:233–236.

8. Byfield D. Preliminary studies with a mechanical model for the evaluation of spinal motion palpation in the lumbar spine. Proceedings of the 1990 International Conference on Spinal Manipulation, Washington, D.C., May 11–12, 1990:215–219.

9. Vernon H, Cote P, Beauchemin, Bonnoyer B. A correlative study of myofascial tender points and joint fixations in the lumbopelvic spine in low back pain. Proceedings of the 1990 International Conference on Spinal Manipulation, Washington, D.C., May 11–12, 1990:236–240.

10. Herzog W, Read LJ, Conway PJW, Shaw LD, McEwen MC. Reliability of motion palpation procedures to detect sacroiliac joint fixations. J Manipulative Physiol Ther 1989;12:86–92.

11. Johnston WL, Elkiss ML, Marino RV, Blum GA. Passive gross motion testing: part II. A study of interexaminer agreement. J Am Osteopath Assoc 1982;81:304–308.

12. Gill K, Krag MH, Johnson GB, Haugh LD, Pope MH. Repeatability of four clinical methods for assessment of lumbar spinal motion. Spine 1988;13:50–53.

13. Editors. Guides to the evaluation of permanent impairment. 3rd ed. Chicago: American Medical Association, 1988:75–95.

14. Dillard J, Trafimow J, Andersson GBJ, Cronin K. Motion of the lumbar spine: reliability of two measurement techniques. Spine 1991;16:321–324.

15. Nansel DD, Cremata E, Carlson J, Szlazak M. Effect of unilateral spinal adjustments on goniometrically-assessed cervical lateral-flexion end-range asymmetries in otherwise asymptomatic subjects. J Manipulative Physiol Ther 1989;12:419–427.

16. Nansel D, Peneff A, Jansen R, Cremata E, Carlson J, et al. Time course considerations for the effect of lower cervical adjustments with respect to the amelioration of cervical lateral flexion passive end-range asymmetries, and on blood pressure, heart rate, and plasma catecholamine levels. Proceedings 1990 International Conference on Spinal Manipulation, Washington, D.C., May 11–12, 1990:345–351.

17. Nansel D, Peneff A, Quitoriano J. Effectiveness of upper vs. lower cervical adjustments with respect to the amelioration of passive rotational vs. lateral-flexion end-range asymmetries in otherwise asymptomatic subjects.

Proceedings 1991 International Conference Spinal Manipulation, April 12–13, 1991: 21–25.

18. Fischer AA. Pressure tolerance over muscles and bones in normal subjects. Arch Phys Med Rehabil 1986;67:406–409.

19. Fischer AA. Pressure threshold meter: its use for quantification of tender spots. Arch Phys Med Rehabil 1986;67:836–838.

20. Fischer AA. Pressure algometry over normal muscles. Standard values, validity and reproducibility of pressure threshold. Pain 1987; 30:115–126.

21. Fischer AA. Pressure threshold measurement for diagnosis of myofascial pain and evaluation of treatment results. Clin J Pain 1987; 2:207–214.

22. Fischer AA. Documentation of myofascial trigger points. Arch Phys Med Rehabil 1988;69:286–291.

23. List T, Helkimo M, Falk G. Reliability and validity of a pressure threshold meter in recording tenderness in the masseter muscle and the anterior temporalis muscle. Cranio 1989;7:223–229.

24. Gerecz-Simon EM, Tunks ER, Heale J-A, Kean WF, Buchanan WW. Measurement of pain threshold in patients with rheumatoid arthritis, osteoarthritis, ankylosing spondylitis, and healthy controls. Clin Rheumatol 1989;8:467–474.

25. Takala E-P. Pressure pain threshold on upper trapezius and levator scapulae muscles. Scand J Rehabil Med 1990;22:63–68.

26. Ohrbach R, Gale EN. Pressure pain thresholds, clinical assessment, and differential diagnosis: reliability and validity in patients with myogenic pain. Pain 1989;39:157–169.

27. Langemark M, Jensen K, Jensen TS, Olesen J. Pressure pain thresholds and thermal nociceptive thresholds in chronic tension-type headache. Pain 1989;38:203–210.

28. Johnston WL. Interexaminer reliability studies: spanning a gap in medical research—Louisa Burns Memorial Lecture. J Am Osteopath Assoc 1982;81:819–829.

29. Johnston WL, Allan BR, Hendra JL, Neff DR, Rosen ME, et al. Interexaminer study of palpation in detecting location of spinal segmental dysfunction. J Am Osteopath Assoc 1983;82:839–845.

30. Vernon HT, Aker P, Burns S, Viljakaanen S, Short L. Pressure pain threshold evaluation of the effect of spinal manipulation in the treatment of chronic neck pain: a pilot study. J Manipulative Physiol Therap 1990;13: 13–16.

31. Hsieh J, Hong C. Effect of chiropractic manipulation on the pain threshold of myofascial trigger point: a pilot study. Proceedings 1990 International Conference on Spinal Manipulation, Washington, D.C., May 11–12, 1990:359–363.

32. Vernon H, Cote P, Beauchemin D, Bonnoyer B. A correlative study of myofascial tender points and joint fixations in the lumbo-pelvic spine in low back pain. Proceedings 1990 International Conference on Spinal Manipulation, Washington, D.C., May 11–12, 1990: 236–240.

33. Osterbauer P, Fuhr A, Widmaier R, Petermann E, DeBoer K. Preliminary clinical and biomechanical assessment of patients with chronic sacroiliac syndrome. Proceedings 1990 International Conference on Spinal Manipulation, Washington, D.C., May 11–12, 1990:403–404.

34. Vernon HT. Applying research-based assessments of pain and loss of function to the issue of developing standards of care in chiropractic. Chiro Technique 1990;2:121–126.

35. Triano JJ. The subluxation complex: outcome measure of chiropractic diagnosis and treatment. Chiro Technique 1990;2:114–120.

36. Huskisson EC. Measurement of pain. Lancet 1974;2:1127–1131.

37. Melzack R. The McGill pain questionnaire: major properties and scoring methods. Pain 1975;1:277–299.

38. Fairbank J, Couper J, Davies J, O'Brien J. The Oswestry low back pain questionnaire. Physiotherapy 1980;66:271–273.

39. Leach R, Owens E, Giesen J. Thoraco-lumbar asymmetry detected in low back pain patients with hand held post style surface electromyography. Proceedings 1991 International Conference on Spinal Manipulation, Washington, D.C., April 12–13, 1991: 325–332.

40. Sanders GE, Reinert O, Tepe R, Maloney P. Chiropractic adjustive manipulation on subjects with acute low back pain: visual analog

pain scores and plasma β-endorphin levels. 1990;13:391–395.

41. Meade TW, Dyer S, Browne W, Townsend J, Frank AO. Low back pain of mechanical origin: randomised comparison of chiropractic and hospital outpatient treatment. Br Med J 1990;300:1431–1437.

42. Cooperstein R. The Derefield pelvic leg check: a kinesiological interpretation. Chiro Technique 1991;3:60–65.

43. DeBoer K, Harmon RO, Savoie S, Tuttle CD. Inter- and intra-examiner reliability of leg-length differential measurement: a preliminary study. J Manipulative Physiol Therap 1983;6:61–66.

44. Danelius BD. Letter to the editor. J Manipulative Physiol Ther 1987;10:132–133.

45. Shambaugh P, Sclafani L, Fanselow D. Reliability of the Derifield-Thompson test for leg length inequality, and use of the test to demonstrate cervical adjusting efficacy. J Manipulative Physiol Ther 1988;11:396–399.

46. DeBoer KF, Wagnon RJ. Letter to the editor. J Manipulative Physiol Ther 1989;12:151.

47. Haas M, Nyiendo J. Letter to the editor. J Manipulative Physiol Ther 1989;12:316–317.

48. Shambaugh JP. In reply. J Manipulative Physiol Ther 1989;12:317–320.

49. Youngquist MW, Fuhr AW, Osterbauer PJ. Interexaminer reliability of an isolation test for the identification of upper cervical subluxation. J Manipulative Physiol Ther 1989;12:93–97.

50. Fuhr AW, Osterbauer PJ. Interexaminer reliability of relative leg-length evaluations in the prone, extended position. Chiro Technique 1989;1:13–18.

51. Falltrick DR, Pierson SD. Precise measurement of functional leg length inequality and changes due to cervical spine rotation in pain-free students. J Manipulative Physiol Ther 1989;12:364–368.

52. Feinstein AR. Clinical biostatistics XLI. Hard science, soft data, and challenges of choosing clinical variables in research. Clin Pharmacol Ther 1977;22:485–498.

53. DeBoer K. Letter to the editor: in reply. J Manipulative Physiol Ther 1987;10:133.

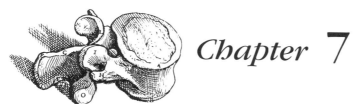

Chapter 7

Hard Outcome Measures of Dysfunction

*T*here are a number of outcome measures that employ a variety of technologies to assess spinal function, with the hope of defining more precisely the diagnosis and status of spinal disorders. Certainly these technologies, considered to be objective and "harder" than palpation and other more observer dependent measures, have received considerable attention from chiropractic researchers recently. Of these so-called hard outcome measures, perhaps the most widely studied and advocated include electromyography (particularly with regard to surface scanning of the erector spinae muscles), infrared and liquid crystal thermography, videofluoroscopy, motion radiography, and physical performance evaluation including muscle strength testing. This chapter reviews the current status of these measures and the advantages and disadvantages of collecting hard outcome measures in chiropractic practice. These dependent variables are reviewed with relation to segmental dysfunction (SDF) and/or regional dysfunction (RDF) and with relation to adjustment or chiropractic manipulative therapy (CMT).

Surface Electromyography

Electromyography (EMG) has been used extensively to monitor myoelectric paraspinal activity in research of neck and low back pain (LBP) and dysfunction. Surface EMG electrodes placed on the belly of paraspinal muscles 3 cm bilateral to the spinous process at L4/L5, for example, measure erector spinae m. and multifidus m. myoelectric activity (viz., depolarizations). Altered nerve activity to a muscle may be associated with altered nerve activity to the segmentally related spinal joints (*Hilton's law*).

Both needle (fine wire) and surface electrodes have been used to differentiate normal from dysfunctional muscle activity in the spine. A wide variety of band-widths, methodologies, and skin preparations have been used. Dynamic examinations such as having the patient perform a task, or bend at the waist and return to the upright position, have been compared with examinations of EMG activity during maximal voluntary trunk contractions against resistance. While there is some confusion regarding outcomes, seeming contradictions between researchers, and increasing evidence that information gained from needle-EMG differs from that gleaned from surface EMG examination, there is also good evidence that both techniques can be useful in characterizing spinal pain and muscle syndromes. The role of fine-wire EMG in assessing radicular lesions is well documented but beyond the scope of this discussion, which focuses instead on surface EMG.

NORMAL PARASPINAL EMG FINDINGS

Allen (1) first suggested that normal and abnormal backs could be more precisely characterized by use of EMG. He hypothesized that EMG could be useful in preemployment physical assessment. After 30 tests on 20 subjects, with a gain as high as 50 microvolts, using a 3-channel electroencephalograph, metal surface electrodes with resistance from 15,000 to 20,000 ohms, and dynamic examinations including trunk flexion and reextension (viz., both standing and sitting postures), side bending, and other activities, he was the first to observe normal lumbar paraspinal activity during motion. He found that with full trunk flexion, the sacrospinalis muscles are quiescent, although they are active during flexing and extending, both before and after the silent phase. During this phase, the rectus abdominis muscles are silent as well; in fact, rectus activity was not seen during normal trunk flexion or extension in hundreds of tests for this activity (except when the subject was trying to force beyond full flexion). Allen concluded that during full flexion, the weight of the torso appears to be supported on the posterior ligaments and fascia while the sacrospinalis m. falls silent, a phenomenon since termed the *flexion/relaxation* (F/R) response.

Allen (1) also determined that the erector spinae muscles were inactive during trunk extension past the upright position, except when extension was forced or contraction was made against resistance. While considerable effort has been made to validate the F/R response, there has been comparatively little mention in subsequent literature of his findings of extension-relaxation.

Flexion-relaxation was recently confirmed in tests comparing fine-wire needle electrodes with surface electrodes in 10 female subjects with no recent or prior history of back pain. Wolf et al. (2), while finding some differences between the two types of EMG, did confirm an F/R response past 60° of forward bending. During return to the neutral position from lumbar side-bending, there was increased contralateral paraspinal EMG activity. Sihvonen et al. (3) documented F/R in 16 pain-free males and females and concluded that functional rectified electrical patterns were essentially the same during flexion and reextension, using either intramuscular or surface electrodes. Kippers and Parker (4) confirmed in the lumbar spine that F/R occurs at 80° ± 13°. F/R has been confirmed recently in the cervical spine by chiropractic researchers Meyer and co-workers (5) in 10 asymptomatic subjects.

Hence, F/R has been well documented in various studies of neck and back flexion in asymptomatic subjects. Contralateral paraspinal EMG activity is elevated in side bending, and the erectors are progressively less active during trunk flexion to approximately 80°, where they fall silent (viz., F/R). Their activity increases again during reextension to the neutral position, where they again become relatively silent. Unless extension is forced, the erectors again fall silent with full extension of the trunk (1–5).

ABNORMAL PARASPINAL EMG FINDINGS

A number of researchers have used more complicated EMG procedures, including assessment of spinal loading, H/M ratios, median frequency (MF), and measures of paraspinal EMG during a series of tasks, to successfully differentiate patients with chronic or acute LBP from asymptomatic controls (6–9). Unfortunately, these procedures generally do not lend themselves well to clinical settings, where assessment must be faster yet discriminatory.

Others have used dynamic examinations of trunk flexion and reextension to document F/R in normal control subjects but not in acute or chronic LBP patients (10–12). While Ahern et al. (13) and Sherman (14) were unable to document F/R differences between control and LBP patients, they did not test their patients past 50° and 30° of flexion, respectively.

Osteopathic researchers using dynamic examinations of cervical side-bending (lateral flexion) have been able to associate abnormal EMG activity with goniometrically established lateral flexion motion restrictions (15, 16).

Generally, researchers have been unable to detect left/right paraspinal asymmetries in surface EMG examinations between control and acute or chronic LBP patients, either prone, sitting, or standing. Meeker et al. (17) used hand-held post-style surface EMG and could not detect left/right paraspinal asymmetries between acute, chronic, and asymptomatic subjects, either sitting or prone. The hand-held devices have been advocated as a faster method of assessing paraspinal EMG activity, appropriate for clinicians.

However, Hoyt et al. (18) did confirm significant left/right lumbar paraspinal asymmetries in patients with chronic LBP by continuously sampling surface EMG activity during 10 minutes of quiet standing; although others have suggested that they may have been measuring muscle fatigue (19).

Leach, Owens, and Giesen (20) documented left/right paraspinal asymmetry during full flexion (as well as by averaging left and right activity during neutral, flexed, and extended postures), loss of F/R (Fig. 7.1), and thoracolumbar asymmetry (a novel measure not previously reported: T10 paraspinal activity less L3 paraspinal activity) in acute LBP patients but not in controls, using hand-held post-style surface EMG (i.e., paraspinal surface scanning). They emphasized repeat measures, appropriate 80–200 Hz band width, and strict protocol and skin preparation and used a variety of outcome measures to define the level of back pain experienced by their subjects (Fig. 7.1). Blinded pressure-pain threshold was significantly lower in the back pain group (p <.05, left side L3; p <.01, right side L3). Oswestry low back pain questionnaires indicated 23.2% activities of daily living disability in the back pain group, and visual analog scales revealed an average level of pain of 3.9 at the time of examination. They emphasized that previous investigators had not described the intensity of back pain in their studies using more than one or two outcome measures to compare with the EMG findings. Some studies make no reference to outcome measures, and chronic back pain patients may have no or little pain at the time of EMG examination. These researchers found that loss of F/R correlated significantly with the presence of myofascial trigger points and disability and correlated negatively with diminished straight leg raising (as expected). They predicted that since these outcome measures respond to manipulative therapy and specifically to CMT, loss of F/R could become part of a "global" assessment for RDF or VSC (20) (see also Chapter 9).

Leach et al. (20) were in accord with the findings of Triano and Schultz (12), who demonstrated a significant relationship between Oswestry disability and presence or loss of F/R in the erector muscles of 48 males and females. Triano and Schultz noted significant loss of F/R in the back pain subjects, associated with significantly less lumbar flexion/extension. In their series, F/R was absent in all but one LBP patient with an Oswestry score of more than 24% disability.

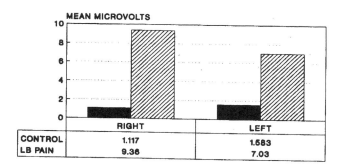

Figure 7.1. F/R response at L3. A significant loss in F/R was seen in patients having LBP, but not in controls. ■, Control; ▨, LBP. Right, p = .011; left, p = .026.

	RIGHT	LEFT
CONTROL	1.117	1.583
LB PAIN	9.36	7.03

EMG CHANGES AFTER MANIPULATION/CMT

While discriminability of surface EMG in detecting LBP has been questioned, studies have confirmed high test/retest (intrasubject) reliability (21, 22), and a number of studies have suggested reduced lumbar paraspinal myoelectric activity after both osteopathic manipulative therapy (OMT) and CMT. Denslow, Korr, and Krems (23) made early observations that spinal lesions were associated with long-lasting alterations in EMG and electrodermal activity (EDA) (see also Chapters 5 and 9).

Shambaugh (24) found reduced lumbar paraspinal surface EMG activity after CMT, and reductions in left/right EMG asymmetry in adjusted subjects (but not in control subjects) lying prone. More recently, Cramer et al. (25) found evidence of reduction in the H/M ratio after CMT (viz., side-lying manipulation to the painful level) but not after control procedures (viz., ice, sham ultrasound, and brief, gentle soft tissue massage). An earlier chiropractic investigation by Humphreys, Triano, and Brandl (8) found significant (P <.001) reduction in H/Mmax ratios in 12 LBP patients after CMT (viz., three adjustments at 2- or 3-day intervals; side-lying high-velocity thrusts), which improved toward values seen in an untreated control group of 39 subjects. Charbonneau and Boucher (26) provided initial evidence that the Hmax/Mmax ratio is not as sensitive to manipulation as is the Tmax/Mmax ratio, which decreased 39% after CMT in six subjects with sacroiliac joint dysfunction.

Ellestad et al. (27) documented significant reductions in paraspinal surface EMG activity in both control-manipulated and LBP-manipulated subjects; however, there was a greater reduction in activity in the LBP group after OMT. Nonmanipulated control and LBP groups had no significant changes in EMG activity. In a separate analysis of arousal levels, they confirmed significant reduction in EDA in the LBP-manipulated group only after OMT, while control-manip-

ulated and nonmanipulated control and LBP groups remained unchanged in this measure of autonomic activity. Conversely, in a small case series study of cervical trauma cases, osteopathic researchers noted paradoxical evidence that cervical paraspinal surface EMG activity increases after OMT (28).

Others have continued to confirm reduction in EMG activity after manipulation (29, 30). Thabe (29) found that in cases of cervical and sacroiliac dysfunction, manipulation resulted in an instantaneous cessation of abnormal spontaneous multifidus m. activity as assessed by needle EMG. This effect was more robust than the effect seen after either intramuscular injection, intraarticular injection, or mobilization procedures.

These studies taken collectively, seem to support the reflex-spasm model of LBP suggested by some researchers, but downplayed due to lack of agreement between researchers looking for left-right asymmetry associated with LBP (19). Certainly it appears that EMG examinations at end-ranges of motion averaged together or during full flexion (20), those made during prolonged quiet standing (to assess fatigue associated with LBP?)(18), and those using various stressful postures or loading (to assess patterns of EMG activity associated with LBP?) (12, 25) are possible techniques for assessing muscle dysfunction related to LBP (and regional dysfunction) and for monitoring clinical improvement after CMT.

Thermography

Thermography was introduced into the profession as a method of detecting vertebral subluxation by B. J. Palmer (31) in 1924. Since that early use of the Neurocalometer, much has been written about the use of heat-sensing equipment to detect not only spinal and other musculoskeletal lesions but also metastatic lesions of the breast, and other applications as well. The discussion here focuses on current efforts to validate thermography as an outcome measure of segmental dysfunction (SDF; perhaps the initial stage of vertebral subluxation) (see also Chapter 10).

A variety of methods are in use to qualify and quantify body surface temperature. Thermocouples, thermistors, and crystals, in direct contact with the skin, cause a reaction that increases skin temperature beneath the sensor; thermopiles and radiometers detect temperature beneath the skin as well. These properties must be taken into consideration both when reviewing the literature on this technology and when applying these measures clinically. Surface temperature is thought to be a measure of vasomotor tone within the peripheral arterioles and precapillary sphincters, which regulate heat loss form the body's core temperature by controlling constriction of these surface vessels. Hence, thermography is thought to measure the sympathetic-mediated tone of these vessels. With increased sympathetic function, vasospasm associated with vessel constriction and decreased thermal emission is expected at the cutaneous region. Conversely, increased thermal emission might be associated with decreased postganglionic function (i.e., denervation) or α-receptor blockade (e.g., due to release of vasoactive substance such as substance P) (32).

NORMAL PARASPINAL THERMOGRAPHIC FINDINGS

A number of investigators have developed normative values for paraspinal thermographic evaluation. Feldman and Nickoloff (33) evaluated the cervical spines of asymptomatic factory workers and found strong bilateral paraspinal thermographic symmetry.

Kelso et al. (34) found a normal variation in skin temperature of 2–3.5°C in the backs of 35 subjects with no symptoms or history of major surgery or major illness. Eight thermograms were made with a GE Thermoscan after the patients were gowned with only the back exposed and allowed to acclimate to a room maintained at 30°C. Subjects were standing, seated, or prone. Analysis of variance revealed that the variation was too large to allow any conclusions regarding a pattern of normal thermographic symmetry for all subjects. Large variance was also observed in any one subject. The authors concluded that small continuous changes in thermographic patterns must be considered normal in future research on thermography and that discontinuities represent a nonuniform source of heat delivered to or lost from the skin.

In a more recent and more controlled and comprehensive 5- year study of infrared thermography (IRT), Uematsu and co-workers (35) determined that normal bilateral variation in the spine was minimal (2 SD, 98% confidence: cervical, 0.33 C; thoracic, 0.33 C; lumbar, 0.65 C) in 90 healthy volunteers without pain. Short- and long-term reproducibility was excellent.

Hand-held temperature scanners have been used in the chiropractic profession since Palmer (31) and have been under scrutiny recently. Plaugher et al. (36) found that a "break" (i.e., a positive finding using the typical hand-held scanners: meter needle moving briskly from side to side at one segmental level indicating a wide temperature variation and, purportedly, evidence of a spinal subluxation) could be only fairly agreed upon between examiners in the lumbar (kappa coefficient [K] = .35) and cervical spines (K = .41), although agreement was somewhat better in the thoracic spines (K = .64) of 19 normal females without pain. On test-retest, examiner one had marginal agreement (K = .44), while examiner two was more likely to reproduce his results with good reliability (K = .64). Overall, reliability of the Nervoscope instrument method of assessing abnormal temperature patterns theoretically associated with chiropractic subluxation was only marginal to fair in this study.

Hence, reliability of computerized IRT and liquid crystal thermography appears to have promise, but reliability of hand-held thermographic scanners is marginal to fair, according to initial investigations (see also Chapter 9 for normative thermographic values).

ABNORMAL PARASPINAL THERMOGRAPHIC FINDINGS

While a complete discussion of issues relating to infrared thermography (IRT) is beyond the scope of this chapter, an overview of examination differences between IRT and other types of imaging (viz., magnetic resonance imaging (MRI) and computerized tomography (CT)), as well as between IRT and other types of diagnostic tests (e.g., fine-wire EMG), is in order.

In determining root level spinal lesions and disc lesions, IRT appears to have excellent predictive value (94.7%) and specificity (87.5%) where left/right asymmetry >1°C is the cutoff for normal (35). When compared with MRI and CT for detecting chronic low back pain, IRT actually exceeded the predictive values of the other imaging techniques (IRT, 92%; MRI, 89%; CT, 87%; myelography, 80%) (37). Using IRT, Thomas and co-workers (37) found significant (>1°C asymmetry) leg abnormalities in 21 of 22 MRI-positive disc cases.

So et al. (38) compared thermography with fine-wire EMG studies in 27 normal patients and 30 patients with LBP. They concluded that while the tests agreed positively or negatively 71% of the time, EMG was more successful in localizing the lesion and indeed in determining the side of involvement. While relative limb warming was seen in patients with acute denervation, and limb cooling in more chronic cases, the authors argued that thermographic findings did not correlate well with dermatomal distribution. Extensive review of the literature on IRT shows that these reservations are echoed by Handelsman (39), at the National Center for Health Services Research and Health Care Technology Assessment, and others as well (40).

THERMOGRAPHIC FINDINGS AFTER CMT

In contrast, a chiropractic researcher in a classic initial investigation demonstrated the value of IRT as an outcome measure for pa-tients with lumbar disc herniation treated by chiropractic. Ben Eliyahu (41) used liquid crystal IRT before, during, and after up to 6 months of either physical therapy and flexion-distraction (11 patients) or physical therapy and chiropractic side-lying manipulation (12 patients) for CT- or MRI-confirmed lumbar disc herniation. Both groups had significant reductions in anatomical areas of thermal asymmetry, but significantly more symmetry was achieved in the group receiving side-lying manipulation (P <.05, T = 7.74). Ben Eliyahu (32) and others argue that thermograms reveal sympathetic-mediated dermatomal distributions of asymmetry that cannot be detected by other methods. (These differ from dermatomes; researchers suggest "autonomes" or "*thermatomes*" to describe thermographic patterns that may overlap several neurological levels). Hence, IRT can measure somatoautonomic reflexes not otherwise measurable.

Diakow (42) and Kelso and Grant (34), among others, have correlated thermography with myofascial trigger points thought to be associated with SDF (43). These trigger points and thermographic asymmetries improved with chiropractic and osteopathic manipulative care.

These studies offer hope that IRT can become a meaningful outcome measure for the detection and monitoring of sympathetic activity associated with SDF. Indeed, recent experimental research by chiropractic investigators demonstrated that after sciatic transection, a 5.1°C rise in temperature is seen in the affected rat hind paw by IRT (44). This significant change persists for 42 days but returns to the sham-operated group level after 63 days. Clinically, IRT may be less invasive and more appropriate for monitoring such changes than other imaging techniques.

Motion Studies of the Spine

Dynamic imaging of the spine is generally accomplished by use of videofluoroscopy, cineroentgenography, and *motion roentgenography* (viz., "stress views" of the spine; x-rays made at the end-ranges of spinal motion).

CINEROENTGENOGRAPHY AND VIDEOFLUOROSCOPY

Cineroentgenography of the spine, pioneered by chiropractic investigators (see Chapter 4, "History of the Chiropractic Theories"), has now largely been replaced in chiropractic by videofluoroscopy. The technique has not been shown to be helpful for measurement of segmental or total range of motion in the cervical spine (because of intraindividual variation) in a recent test/retest trial (45). However, cineradiography is recommended with prolonged spinal pain (>7 weeks) and radicular pain to assess compression and spinal stenosis, as well as for postsurgical pain (>6 months) (46).

Indeed, cineroentgenography and videofluoroscopy have been advocated in medicine and chiropractic for detection and evaluation of spinal motion disorders (47, 48). Recently, Antos et al. (48) investigated the reliability of the technique for detection of fixation defined as:

> failure on forward flexion to increase the distance between the spinolaminar junctions by more than 50% of the distance noted in the neutral position (48).

There was strong (K = .80) and statistically significant (P <.0001) agreement between two blinded chiropractors reviewing 48 videotapes of cervical flexion occurring at the C4/C5 interspace, using this fixation criterion.

STRESS X-RAYS

Motion x-rays (x-rays made at the end-range of a spinal motion) have been widely advocated in chiropractic and medical settings as an entry-level test for abnormal spine motion or segmental dysfunction (SDF). Unfortunately, motion x-rays, or so-called stress views, suffer from some of the same limitations that other movement-related outcome measures have. For example, Grice and Tschumi (49) found improvement in lateral bending x-rays and reduction in multifidus and quadratus lumborum EMG activity after CMT. However, Phillips et al. (50) found no significant differences in demographic, historical, and/or clinical data in patients having abnormal versus normal intersegmental motion on flexion, extension, and lateral-bending lumbar x-rays. Perhaps that should be expected, since according to Haas and colleagues (51), three doctors could not agree convincingly on when a lateral-bending SDF existed, from blinded examination of x-ray films. Reliability between examiners was good only for lumbar rotation, and only for upper lumbar analysis.

In contrast with these criticisms raised by chiropractic researchers for lumbar motion studies, medical radiologists and orthopedists studying cervical flexion/extension found good agreement between examiners using Penning's method of measurement, but poor agreement using Buetti-Bauml's method. They found that passive examination yielded significantly more hypo- and hypermobile segments than the otherwise routine active x-ray examination. (In a passive x-ray examination, the patient's head is moved to the end-range of a motion and held in place during exposure (52).)

More recently, in a computer-assisted follow-up study using flexion/extension radiographic assessment, Dvorak and co-workers (53) found significantly more hypomobile segments in four different groups of LBP patients than in normal controls. Patients with lytic spondylolisthesis, radicular syndromes, degenerative joint disease, and undifferentiated LBP all had more hypomobile segments, while young athletes with LBP had significantly more hypermobile segments than normal control subjects. Instead of deeming this finding useful, however, the authors felt that since the hypomobility was spread between the various segments in these four groups equally, the technique was unnecessary, especially with regard to indicating a need for surgical intervention.

Medical researchers continue to investigate the lumbar spine for abnormal segmental motion and translations (e.g., retrolisthesis or anterolisthesis is defined as at least 3 mm of slip), with flexion/extension films as well, advocating loaded procedures that stress and magnify the motion disorders (54, 55). For example, patients with lumbar spondylolisthesis were placed in axial traction and compression; translatory instability of 5–15 mm was found in about half the patients after normal flexion/extension films had been negative.

Perhaps the critical issue regarding chiropractic detection of motion disorders (specifically, SDF) by use of motion radiography concerns the radiation exposure to the patient, especially with repeat examinations (56). As an initial screening and detection procedure, few argue the indispensability of a radiographic series. However, until more is known about the validity of using these examinations as an indicator for manipulative intervention, their use will continue to be advocated by some (48, 49) and questioned by others (50, 51).

MOTION STUDIES AFTER CMT

A review of the literature cited in the Chiropractic Library Consortium's *Index to Chiropractic Literature 1985–1989* and the 1990 index yields no current studies using videofluoroscopy, cineroentgenography, or flexion/extension x-ray to document the effectiveness of CMT in correcting motion disorders of the spine.

However, in a prospective study of 25 patients with LBP, Grice and Tschumi (49) found evidence of improvement in lateral-bending asymmetry in the lumbar spine after CMT. They sampled surface EMG activity and noted reduction in muscular hyperactivity (multifidus and quadratus lumborum) after CMT as well. They found that the range of lateral lumbar flexion was increased after CMT in 24 of 25 patients and that 19 of 25 had improvement in lumbar spine mechanics, according to preset criteria. None of

eight normal subjects showed abnormal myoelectric activity on the concave side of the lumbar curve during lateral bending, but EMG activity was elevated on the concave side during side-bending in LBP patients (49). (During side-bending, paraspinal EMG activity is normally higher on the side of convexity.) These improved EMG findings associated with improved radiographic motion studies after CMT generally confirm the earlier observations of osteopathic researchers (27–29).

Measures of Physical Performance

Recently, much attention has been focused on tests of endurance and physical performance as a potential outcome measure for the determination of functional spine problems and as a potential monitor of effectiveness of chiropractic manipulative therapy (CMT). Initial observations suggest that, for example, good upper body strength contributes to reduction in injuries related to materials handling. Conversely, when maximum isometric effort is less than the load requirements of the job, injuries increase threefold. Further, when conservative intervention has reached maximum effectiveness, rehabilitation focusing on enhanced performance results in continuing improvement in functional spinal pain syndromes (57).

Hence, the evaluation of chronic and recurrent pain patients has been enhanced by use of tests of physical performance. Reciprocal strength ratios (e.g., for the spine, an extensor/flexor trunk strength ratio of 1.3 is the normal mean), flexibility, and endurance levels have known validity for setting treatment goals. For optimal measurement, patient motivation must be assessed, and the testing procedure should closely simulate the job activity performed by the patient (57).

NORMAL SPINAL MUSCLE STRENGTH

At 72° trunk flexion, average lumbar erector spinae m. strength (trunk extension strength) has been established using Medx (a computerized muscle testing apparatus) at >100–200+ ft/lb in females and >200–450+ ft/lb in males (averages: females, 175; males, nearly 350, ±1 SD) (58).

Vernon et al. (59) tested 40 asymptomatic young adults in six ranges of neck movement with a modified sphygmomanometer-dynamometer (MSD) in paired trials. There were high correlation coefficients (.79–.97) for all ranges of motion. Left/right symmetry in cervical rotation and in lateral bending was within 6–8%. Tests confirmed the relative weakness of the cervical flexors, compared with the cervical extensors, and the flexion/extension ratio was determined to be .57/1 (i.e., in normal subjects, cervical flexors are approximately 40% weaker than the cervical extensors). Moreover, lower cutoffs (1 SD) were established: 2.5 for flexion, 4.5 for extension, 4.0 for rotation, and 4.5 for lateral flexion (units in mm Hg/sec). Similarly, Triano and Schultz (60) demonstrated a full trunk extension to flexion ratio of 1.35 in pain-free controls.

In the National Institute of Occupational Safety and Health (NIOSH) standardized lift tasks test, the patient assumes several postures: lifting with the legs and back, using the legs and standing erect, and using the arms, as well as in push/pull tasks (57).

Jerome and co-workers (61) attempted to establish normative data for flexion and extension of the trunk, using peak torque and best work repetition, two commonly reported isokinetic measurements, and a new composite muscle performance index (MPI). Collecting data on 160 subjects using the Cybex II TEF Unit, they found a significant decrease in peak torque of extension in females as velocity of contraction increased. They also determined that significant variance between six measures of isokinetic strength across the subjects was explained by patient height, weight, and age. Of the variables, body weight had the largest quantitative effect on isokinetic measurements in their sample. They defined *strength testing* as that carried out at velocities less than or

equal to 60°/second; *power testing* is carried out at more functional speeds faster than 60°/second. They concluded that protocols involving slower velocities test both fast- and slow-twitch fibers, while high-velocity protocols test only faster twitch muscle fibers. Because these protocols test various aspects of muscle performance, they chose a muscle performance index that incorporated both peak torque at lower velocities and average power at higher velocities. Unfortunately, they were unable to provide "normative" data for their MPI that would be clinically applicable.

Delitto, Rose, Crandell, and Strube (62) found good-to-excellent intraexaminer reliability for isokinetic trunk strength testing using the LIDOBACK dynamometer. In 29 men and 32 women without LBP, at speeds of 60, 120, and 180°/second, 10 tests of flexion and extension were repeated 1 and 3 weeks later. Peak torque/body-weight ratios, E/F ratios, and average work per repetition were calculated for flexion and extension at each speed. Intraclass correlation coefficients were .74–.88 for peak torque and .88–.93 for average work per repetition, with the exception of .69 for men at 180°s/second. The authors did suggest that increased practice for women and longer rest periods for men enhanced reliability of the technique.

Recent tests have demonstrated good interexaminer reliability for manual muscle testing with such devices as a computerized dynamometer (e.g., supine iliopsoas m. strength averaged 12.48–14.48 kg by three different examiners on 13 males, using maximal isometric contraction followed by a phase of "break")(58). In the "break" test, at the point of maximum isometric contraction, the examiner applies slightly more pressure until a "break" in contraction occurs or no further motion is possible. Using the "break" test, intratester Pearson coefficients for repeat testing on the same day ranged from 0.84 to 0.98, and from 0.86 to 0.96 for iliopsoas tests made 1 week apart on normal subjects (63).

Testing with hand-held dynamometer-type muscle-testing devices such as the ISMAT correlate well with manual "break" testing (64). The breaking force necessary on the normal side for hip flexion (testing iliopsoas m. strength in the seated position) was 36.7 kg (mean; range, 17.2–62.1 kg). Hip abduction and hip flexion were weaker in the pathologic limb in 87% of the tests on 128 patients (64).

A novel study comparing isometric trunk strength and myoelectric responses of the erector spinae m. in elite wrestlers and tennis players was done by Sward and co-workers (65). Ten male wrestlers had more symmetrical trunk strength values than normative data published in any previous study (flexion, 852 newtons (N); extension, 951 N; right and left side-bending, 759 N and 744 N, respectively). Nine male tennis players, in contrast, were stronger in left side-bending than in right side-bending (643 N left; 557 N right; $p < .01$) and stronger in extension than in flexion (835 N extension; 638 N flexion; $p < .01$). Both groups developed fatigue bilaterally in the lumbar erector spinae m., as assessed by EMG, although to a greater degree in the tennis players (65).

ABNORMAL SPINAL MUSCLE STRENGTH

A variety of measures of physical performance are used to differentiate LBP and CLBP patients from normals.

Triano and Schultz (60) demonstrated a trunk extension to flexion ratio of 1.08 in LBP patients with raw Oswestry scores of less than 8.5, and of 0.84 when raw Oswestry scores exceeded 10.5. Conversely, they found trunk extensors in normal subjects were stronger than trunk flexors (1.35 ratio). They also found significant correlations between loss of flexion-relaxation (F/R) in the lumbar spine (surface EMG electrodes placed 3 cm bilateral to midline at L3) and increasing ratings of Oswestry disability ($p < .001$) and trunk strength ratios ($p < .05$; hence, as trunk extensor/flexor ratio drops, there is a loss of F/R), and in loss of

trunk range of motion in flexion and extension ($p < .01$; although pain subjects could still flex 71°s on average, enough to normally elicit a F/R response).

Improvement in the trunk flexion to extension strength ratio can be accomplished using Medx (58). In addition to reducing the frequency of future back injuries and enhancing treatment efficacy, use of such technology may help to offset the effects of aging and disabling pathological changes in the lumbar spine (58).

Evidence suggests that patients who perform one dynamic exercise per week improve their lumbar extension strength as much as those using Medx two and three times per week (66). Predominance of muscle fiber type helps determine the type of exercise regimen necessary (66). (Type I fibers are slow twitch and require low ATPase activity; type II fibers are fast twitch and require high ATPase activity.)

Triano et al. (67) used real-time feedback during exertion to determine whether patients were using maximal voluntary contraction. Using a visual feedback system, 20 LBP patients improved extension 19% and improved flexion 9%, compared with verbal coaching. While both systems had strong test-retest reliability ($r = .95–.99$), and the methods correlated well with each other ($r = .96$, flexion; $r = .97$, extension), visual feedback consistently resulted in stronger effort ($p < .15$, flexion; $p < .001$, extension) (67).

Inconsistencies between researchers in establishing normal agonist/antagonist ratios was emphasized by Hondras et al. (68). Comparing the Isostation B200 with the Daytronic Uniaxial Load Cell mounted in an upright static testing frame (STF), they found essentially no correlation between the two in terms of the 2-second values and peak force values (while testing E/F ratios). Indeed, as patients' perception of LBP increased (as assessed by Oswestry questionnaire), STF values decreased and B200 values increased. They made eight recommendations for improving the use of these instruments to measure E/F ratios. Without such improvements, according to these chiropractic researchers, doctors using these two instruments would reach opposite conclusions and exercise recommendations (68).

In summary, good reliability is found in functional strength assessment when appropriate protocols are used, and abnormal E/F ratios and other abnormal findings can lead to strengthening programs beneficial in pain control and prevention.

SPINAL MUSCLE STRENGTH AFTER MANIPULATION/CMT

While it has been clearly demonstrated that lumbar extensor muscles (and trunk flexors/extensors) can be strengthened using full-range-of-motion variable-resistance exercises, functional capacity tests of muscle strength have not been used as outcome measures of CMT per se until recently (57, 66–68). Pelvic stabilization, one session per week training regimens, and other recommendations have been made regarding the use of these instruments to aid in erector spinae muscle evaluation and strengthening; however, assessments after CMT without weight training, to evaluate the effectiveness of CMT in improving muscle function, have been only rarely reported in the chiropractic literature (57, 65, 66–68).

Recent reports by Bonci and colleagues (69, 70) regarding improvement in biceps and trunk erector strength immediately following cervical and dorsolumbar CMT, respectively, give some of the first evidence that functional strength testing has the potential of becoming a valid clinical tool for assessing improvement after CMT.

Discussion

After reliability, perhaps the critical test of an outcome measure is its suitability or validity in the chiropractic clinical setting. The ability of the four measures discussed in this chapter to predict the presence or absence of SDF, RDF, or VSC is a primary consideration in determining their value in a chiropractic setting. Inasmuch as we are still in the process of operationally defining these primarily chiropractic lesions, outcome measures that reveal improvement in neuromusculoskeletal or other function after CMT are of equal importance. To varying degrees, the so-called hard outcome measures discussed in this chapter do reveal significant changes after CMT.

Surface EMG appears to be useful as a quick clinical test for pain-related muscle dysfunction. Using the newer hand-held post-style electrodes, for example, an examiner can efficiently and quickly test for absence of the flexion/relaxation phenomenon, which correlates clinically with diminished straight leg raising, Oswestry disability, a poor E/F ratio, and myofascial trigger points as assessed by algometry (12, 20). Straight leg raising, Oswestry disability, and myofascial trigger points (diminished pressure-pain threshold, see Chapter 6) respond well to CMT. Functional strength testing, specifically the trunk E/F ratio, has been tested and found to be a reliable indicator of abnormal muscle function related to LBP. However, determination of the E/F ratio after CMT alone has been only rarely reported to date (57, 65, 66–68).

Thermographic evaluation in chiropractic has been historically a primary test for presence of VSC (31). While the hand-held thermographic scanners traditionally have been a classic test of the presence of a chiropractic lesion, more recent research indicates only marginal-to-fair intraexaminer reliability using this method; the computerized and liquid crystal infrared thermographic systems are far more reliable (and more expensive).

Motion studies have been boosted by recent research indicating strong agreement between examiners reviewing videofluoroscopic studies of flexion and extension in the cervical spine (48). Some medical and chiropractic researchers advocate motion x-ray films at the end-ranges of spinal movement and indicate good reliability for the detection of motion disorders, under certain conditions (49, 52–55). These studies show promise that an operational definition of an identifiable motion disorder relating to pain and dysfunction can be developed, which would be sensitive to corrective changes after CMT. Discussion of these measures with regard to clinical assessment is found in Chapter 9.

At least one criticism of all these measures has revolved around clinical value. What use is there to knowing that the E/F ratio is abnormal, that the F/R phenomenon is lost, and that the thermographic and radiographic criteria for a lesion have been met? Aside from the very practical aspect of quantifying the patient's disorder to gauge the length and type of intervention, these outcome measures are useful when malingering or hysteria is suspected. Certainly if these measures become part of a global measure of SDF, RDF and/or VSC, their status will be enhanced further.

Summary

Of the so-called hard outcome measures reviewed in this chapter, only two, electromyography and thermography, have been tested before and after CMT in a number of studies (23–30, 32, 38–40). Little information is available regarding changes in radiographic motion studies or in functional strength assessment after CMT (47–49, 54, 62, 64–67).

For example, surface EMG scanning (specifically, loss of lumbar flexion-relaxation), correlates well with other known and reliable measures of LBP used in manipulation research (viz., visual analog scale, Oswestry LBP disability questionnaire, straight leg raising, and algometry) (12, 20). Moreover, surface EMG examinations after CMT or osteopathic manipulation reveal significant reductions in hyperactive responses and a return to normal myoelectric patterns (23–30, 49).

Thermography is gaining acceptance, based upon reliability studies of liquid crystal, infrared, and paraspinal scans using hand-held thermocouples (32–35). Thermography seems to correlate well with MRI and CT examinations in determining the presence of disc disorders,(33, 35), and thermographic paraspinal asymmetries appear to improve after CMT (41–43).

While there is less information regarding motion studies and functional strength assessment after CMT, the initial studies reveal good reliability for the techniques and good improvement after CMT. Certainly, these assessments (specifically the trunk flexor/extensor ratio and the use of stress x-rays and videofluoroscopy) hold promise, and further research is indicated.

REFERENCES

1. Allen CEL. Muscle action potentials used in the study of dynamic anatomy. Br J Phys Med 1948;11:66–73.
2. Wolf LB, Segal RL, Wolf SL, Nyberg R. Quantitative analysis of surface and percutaneous electromyographic activity in lumbar erector spinae of normal young women. Spine 1991;16:155–161.
3. Sihvonen T, Partanen J, Hanninen O. Averaged (rms) surface EMG in testing back function. Electromyogr Clin Neurophysiol 1988;28:335–339.
4. Kippers V, Parker AW. Posture related to myoelectric silence of erectores spinae during trunk flexion. Spine 1984;9:740–745.
5. Meyer J, Anderson A, Berk R. The flexion-relaxation phenomenon: does it exist in the

cervical spine? Proceedings of the 1990 International Conference on Spinal Manipulation, Foundation for Chiropractic Education and Research, Washington, D.C., 1990: 157–159.
6. Triano JJ, Luttges M. Myoelectric paraspinal response to spinal loads: potential for monitoring low back pain. J Manipulative Physiol Ther 1985;8:137–145.
7. Roy SH, DeLuca CJ, Casavant DA. Lumbar muscle fatigue and chronic lower back pain. Spine 1989;14:992–1001.
8. Humphreys CR, Triano JJ, Brandl MJ. Sensitivity study of H-reflex alterations in idiopathic low back pain patients vs. a healthy population. J Manipulative Physiol Ther 1989;12:71–78.

9. Triano JJ. Condensations/commentaries. DC Tracts 1989;1:133–137.

10. Nouwen A, Van Akkerveeken PF, Versloot JM. Patterns of muscular activity during movement in patients with chronic low back pain. Spine 1987;12:777–892.

11. Sihvonen T, Partanen J. Segmental hypermobility in lumbar spine and entrapment of dorsal rami. Electromyogr Clin Neurophysiol 1990;30:175–180.

12. Triano JJ, Schultz AB. Correlation of objective measure of trunk motion and muscle function with low-back disability ratings. Spine 1987;12:561–565.

13. Ahern DK, Follick MJ, Council JR, Laser-Wolston N, Litchman H. Comparison of lumbar paravertebral EMG patterns in chronic low back pain patients and non-patient controls. Pain 1988;34:153–160.

14. Sherman A. Relationships between strength of low-back muscle contraction and reported intensity of chronic low-back pain. Am J Phys Med 1985;64:190–200.

15. Johnston WL, Vorro J. Biomechanical measurements of changes in cervical muscle function following osteopathic manipulative treatment. J Am Osteopath Assoc 1983; 83:131.

16. Vorro J, Johnston WL, Hubbard R. Biomechanical analysis of symmetric and asymmetric cervical function. J Am Osteopath Assoc 1982;82:140–141.

17. Meeker W, Matheson D, Milus T, Wong A. Lack of correlation between scanning EMG asymmetries and history and presence of low back pain: analysis of pilot data. Proceedings of the 1990 International Conference on Spinal Manipulation, Foundation for Chiropractic Education and Research, Washington, D.C., 1990:230–235.

18. Hoyt WH, Hunt HH, DePauw MA, et al. Electromyographic assessment of chronic low-back pain syndrome. J Am Osteopath Assoc 1981;81:728–730.

19. Nouwen A, Bush C. The relationship between paraspinal EMG and chronic low back pain. Pain 1984;20:109–123.

20. Leach RA, Owens EF, Giesen JM. Correlates of myoelectric asymmetry detected in low back pain patients using hand held post-style surface electromyography. J Manipulative Physiol Ther 1993;16:140–149.

21. Cram JR. Clinical EMG for surface recordings: vol 2. Seattle: Clinical Resources, 1990.

22. Sheres BM, Freely K, Egyed E. Are surface electrode EMG data reliable? Today's Chiropractic 1991;20:22–24, 25.

23. Denslow JS, Korr IM, Krems AD. Quantitative studies of chronic facilitation in human motoneuron pools. Am J Physiol 1947; 105:229–238.

24. Shambaugh P. Changes in electrical activity in muscles resulting from chiropractic adjustment: a pilot study. J Manipulative Physiol Ther 1987;10:300–304.

25. Cramer G, Hondras M, Humphreys R, Triano J. The H/M ratio as an outcome measure of chiropractic treatment efficacy in acute low back pain. Proceedings of the 1990 International Conference on Spinal Manipulation, Foundation for Chiropractic Education and Research, Washington, D.C., 1990:71–73.

26. Charbonneau M, Boucher J. Segmental modulation of T and H reflexes and M wave following a chiropractic adjustment: a pilot study. Proceedings of the 1990 International Conference on Spinal Manipulation, Foundation for Chiropractic Education and Research, Washington, D.C., 1990:393–398.

27. Ellestad SM, Nagle RV, Boesler DR, Kilmore MA. Electromyographic and skin resistance responses to osteopathic manipulative treatment for low-back pain. J Am Osteopath Assoc 1988;88:991–997.

28. Beal MC, Vorro J, Johnston WL. Chronic cervical dysfunction: correlation of myoelectric findings with clinical progress. J Am Osteopath Assoc 1989;89:891–900.

29. Thabe H. Electromyography as tool to document diagnostic findings and therapeutic results associated with somatic dysfunctions in the upper cervical spinal joints and sacroiliac joints. Manual Med 1986;2:53–58.

30. Gatto R, Bargero V, Robere G. Computerized electromyographic biofeedback in valuation of "myialgy" caused by "minor intervertebral derangement". Abstracts of the 9th International Congress of the Federation Internationale de Medecine Manuelle, London, Sept 18–22, 1989:99.

31. Palmer BJ. The subluxation specific—the adjustment specific. Davenport, Ia.: Palmer School of Chiropractic, 1934:13.

32. Ben Eliyahu DJ. Infrared thermography in

the diagnosis and management of sports injuries: a clinical study and literature review. Chiro Sports Med 1990;4:46–53.

33. Feldman F, Nickoloff E. Normal thermographic standards in the cervical spine and upper extremities. Skeletal Radiol 1984; 12:235–249.

34. Kelso AF, Grant RG, Johnston WL. Use of thermograms to support assessment of somatic dysfunction or effects of osteopathic manipulative treatment: preliminary report. J Am Osteopath Assoc 1982;82:182–188.

35. Uematsu S, Edwin DH, Jankel WR, Kozikowski J, Trattner M. Quantification of thermal asymmetry. Part I. Normal values and reproducibility. J Neurosurg 1988;69:552–555.

36. Plaugher G, Lopes MA, Melch P, Cremata EE. The inter- and intraexaminer reliability of a paraspinal skin temperature differential instrument. J Manipulative Physiol Ther 1991; 14:361–367.

37. Thomas D, Cullum D, Siahamis G, Langlois S. Infrared thermographic imaging, magnetic resonance imaging, CT scan and myelography in low back pain. Br J Rheumatol 1990; 29:268–273.

38. So YT, Aminoff MJ, Olney RK. The role of thermography in the evaluation of lumbosacral radiculopathy. Neurology 1989;39: 1154–1158.

39. Handelsman H. Thermography for indications other than breast lesions. Health Technol Assess Rep 1989;(2):1–32.

40. Hoffman RM, Kent DL, Deyo RA. Diagnostic accuracy and clinical utility of thermography for lumbar radiculopathy: a meta analysis. Spine 1991;16:623–628.

41. Ben Eliyahu D. Infra-red thermographic assessment of chiropractic treatment in patients with lumbar disc herniations—a clinical study. Proceedings of the 1990 International Conference on Spinal Manipulation, Foundation for Chiropractic Education and Research, Washington, D.C., 1990:405–411.

42. Diakow PRP. Thermographic imaging of myofascial trigger points. J Manipulative Physiol Ther 1988;11:114–117.

43. Fischer AA, Chang C. Temperature and pressure threshold measurements in trigger points. Thermology 1986;1:212–215.

44. Gerow G, Callton M, Meyer JJ, Demchak JJ, Christiansen J. Thermographic evaluation of rats with complete sciatic nerve transection. J Manipulative Physiol Ther 1990;13: 257–261.

45. Van Mameren H, Drukker J, Sanches H, Beursgens J. Cervical spine motion in the sagittal plane (I) range of motion of actually performed movements, an x-ray cinematographic study. Eur J Morphol 1990;28:47–68.

46. Quebec Task Force on Spinal Disorders. Scientific approach to the assessment and management of activity-related spinal disorders: a monograph for clinicians. Spine 1987; 12:S3–59.

47. Bell GD. Skeletal applications of videofluoroscopy. J Manipulative Physiol Ther 1990; 13:396–405.

48. Antos JC, Robinson GK, Keating JC Jr, Jacobs GE. Interrater reliability of fluoroscopic detection of fixation in the mid-cervical spine. Chiro Technique 1990;2:53–55.

49. Grice AS, Tschumi PC. Pre and post manipulation lateral bending radiographic study and relation to muscle function of the low back. Ann Swiss Chiro Assoc 1985;8: 149–165.

50. Phillips RB, Howe JW, Bustin G, Mick TJ, Rosenfeld I, Mills T. Stress x-rays and the low back pain patient. J Manipulative Physiol Ther 1990;13:127–133.

51. Haas M, Nyiendo J, Peterson C, Thiel H, Sellers T, Cassidy D, Yong-Hing K. Interrater reliability of roentgenological evaluation of the lumbar spine in lateral bending. J Manipulative Physiol Ther 1990;13:179–189.

52. Dvorak J, Froehlich D, Penning L, Baumgartner H, Panjabi MM. Functional radiographic diagnosis of the cervical spine: flexion/extension. Spine 1988;13:748–755.

53. Dvorak J, Panjabi MM, Chang DG, Theiler R, Grob D. Functional radiographic diagnosis of the lumbar spine: flexion/extension and lateral bending. Spine 1991;16:562–571.

54. Paaganen H, Erkintalo M, Dahlstrom S, Kuusela T, et al. Disc degeneration and lumbar instability. Magnetic resonance examination of 16 patients. Acta Orthop Scand 1989;60: 375–378.

55. Friberg O. Functional radiography of the lumbar spine. Ann Med 1989;21:341–346.

56. Goldstein M. Introduction, summary and analysis. In: Goldstein M, ed. The research status of spinal manipulative therapy. Washington, D.C.: Government Printing Office, 1975:3–7.

57. Triano JJ. The subluxation complex: outcome measure of chiropractic diagnosis and treatment. Chiro Technique 1990;2:114–120.

58. Leggett SH, Pollack ML, Graves JE, et al. Quantitative assessment of full range of motion lumbar extension strength. Med Sci Sports Exerc 1988;20:s87.

59. Vernon H, Aker P, Aramenko M, Battershill D, Alepin A, Penner T. The use of a modified sphygmomanometer dynamometer in isometric strength tests in the neck: reliability and normative data. Proceedings of the 1990 International Conference on Spinal Manipulation, Foundation for Chiropractic Education and Research, Washington, D.C., 1990: 170–173.

60. Triano JJ, Schultz AB. Correlation of objective measure of trunk motion and muscle function with low-back disability ratings. Spine 1987;12:561–565.

61. Jerome JA, Hunter K, Gordon P, McKay N. A new robust index for measuring isokinetic trunk flexion and extension: outcome from a regional study. Spine 1991;16:804–808.

62. Delitto A, Rose SJ, Crandell CE, Strube MJ. Reliability of isokinetic measurements of trunk muscle performance. Spine 1991;16: 800–803.

63. Hsieh C-Y, Phillips RB. Reliability of manual muscle testing with a computerized dynamometer. J Manipulative Physiol Ther 1990;13:72–82.

64. Marino M, Nicholas JA, Gleim GW, Rosenthal P, Nicholas SJ. The efficacy of manual assessment of muscle strength using a new device. Am J Sports Med 1982;10:360–364.

65. Sward L, Svensson M, Zetterberg C. Isometric muscle strength and quantitative electromyography of back muscles in wrestlers and tennis players. Am J Sports Med 1990;18: 382–386.

66. Lanzisera FP, Rowe-Lanzisera L. Medx isometric strength evaluation of the lumbar spine: normal and abnormal findings. Proceedings of the 1990 International Conference on Spinal Manipulation, Foundation for Chiropractic Education and Research, Washington, D.C., 1990:198–211.

67. Triano JJ, Baker JA, McGregor M, Torres B. Optimizing measures of maximum voluntary contraction. Proceedings of the 1990 International Conference on Spinal Manipulation, Foundation for Chiropractic Education and Research, Washington, D.C., 1990:285–287.

68. Hondras MA, Baker JA, Torres BA, McGregor M, Triano JJ. Repeatability of isometric trunk strength testing in the isostation B200 vs. a static upright testing frame. Proceedings of the 1990 International Conference on Spinal Manipulation, Foundation for Chiropractic Education and Research, Washington, D.C., 1990:288–291.

69. Bonci A, Ratliff C. Strength modulation of the biceps brachii muscles immediately following a single manipulation of the C4/C5 intervertebral motor unit in healthy subjects; preliminary report. Am J Chiro Med 1990;3: 14–18.

70. Bonci A, Ratliff C, Adams E, Mirtz T. Strength modulation of the erector muscles immediately following manipulation of the thoracolumbar spine. Chiropractic 1990;6:29–33.

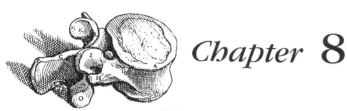

Chapter **8**

Facilitation Hypothesis

*S*egmental dysfunction (SDF), regional dysfunction (RDF), and vertebral subluxation complex may well be defined operationally in the coming decade, as chiropractic scientists and others continue to refine the use of outcome measures for assessment of these lesions (see also Chapters 5–7). Yet how can such mechanical spinal lesions effect the diverse conditions purported to respond to chiropractic manipulative therapy (CMT) or adjustment? How could nature fail to protect the spine from the falls, accidents, and postures said to cause chronic spinal lesions?

This chapter explores these questions and attempts to provide some good answers; however, the reader will probably find even more probing questions to replace them. The hypothesis of segmental facilitation appears to be gaining even more respect from researchers who study manipulative therapy, but much remains to be learned, and several neurobiologic mechanisms have been forwarded to explain the phenomenon. *Segmental facilitation* has been defined as a lowered threshold for firing in a spinal cord segment, as a result of afferent bombardment associated with spinal lesions (1).

Beginning with a review of kinesthetic receptors associated with the effects of a lesion, this chapter reviews recent concepts regarding somatic afferent bombardment of the dorsal horn associated with spinal le-

sions. Nociception appears to be a key component of facilitation, and the concepts of "spinal learning," habituation, and sensitization of reflexes are reviewed.

Spinal pathways and physiology are briefly reviewed to show the role of facilitation in promoting somatoautonomic reflexes. Clinical and experimental evidence of facilitation is reviewed, along with somatoautonomic reflexes and sympathicotonia associated with the lesion.

Since D. D. Palmer's (2) observation that a janitor's hearing was restored after an adjustment, chiropractors have wanted an explanation for some of the "miraculous" cures said to occur after CMT. This chapter explores the concepts of SDF, RDF, and facilitation as precursors to somatoautonomic dysfunction, which might justify the use of CMT for treatment of other than pain syndromes, such as Palmer and other early pioneers reported.

Neurobiology of Kinesthetic Receptors

Several receptors signal the nervous system about the position and inclination of the joints of the spinal column. These joint receptors together with the various muscle receptors, which report the tension of the skeletal muscles, must play an important role in any afferent bombardment accompanying SDF.

JOINT RECEPTORS

The joint receptors include the complex nerve endings, free nerve endings, and Vater-Pacini corpuscles (3–5). Of the complex nerve endings, the spray or Ruffini-type endings are the most common within the joint capsules and nearby ligaments. These endings, which are supplied by type A beta afferents (Table 8.1), are sensitive to stretch and intraarticular pressure changes and indicate movement and position (3–5). Also sensitive to stretch and intraarticular pressure change is the Golgi tendon-type receptor sometimes found in ligaments near the joint. Simple coiled end organs, found in the adventitia of blood vessels, represent the third type of complex nerve endings (3–5).

Free nerve endings are found in articular capsule blood vessels, synovial membrane, and external parts of the collateral ligaments. These nociceptive (pain) receptors are supplied by unmyelinated and small myelinated fibers.

Vater-Pacini corpuscles are not found in synovial membrane but are sometimes seen in the intervertebral joints; they are stimulated by movements that distort their lamellar endings and are highly sensitive, rapidly adapting, receptors (3–5).

Wyke (6) states that all synovial joints have the following types of receptor nerve endings:

Type I—Globular corpuscles in the outer layers of the fibrous capsule; thinly encapsulated mechanoreceptors.

Type II—Conical corpuscles in the deeper layers of the fibrous capsule; thickly encapsulated mechanoreceptors.

Type III—Larger corpuscles on the surface of joint ligaments; thinly encapsulated mechanoreceptors.

Type IV—Unmyelinated nerve fibers that weave throughout the capsule; nociceptors.

Giles (7) used electron microscopy to assess innervation of 50 fresh surgical zygapophyseal specimens (posteromedial fibrous joint capsule of the inferior recess, the adjoining ligamentum flavum, and synovial fold of the inferior joint recess). This chiropractic anatomist used fresh laminectomy specimens instead of older cadaveric material. He demonstrated paravascular myelinated fibers in 5 of 13 synovial folds, using epon/araldite sections, and in 8 of 17 silver-impregnated specimens. No neural structures were seen in the ligamentum flavum using either preparation, but encapsulated nerve fibers were visualized in 3 of 13 epon/araldite and in 3 of 17 zygapophyseal joint inferior recess accessory capsules. In 12 of 17 zygapophyseal joints treated with silver impregnation, nerve fibers were traced to unencapsulated endings in the fibrous portion of the capsule. Using gold chloride impregnation, nerve fibers were clearly demonstrated in 8 of 16 specimens (Fig. 8.1). Immunofluorescent substance P profiles verified that these were nerve fibers. Fiber diameters ranged from 0.5 to 1.2 μm

Table 8.1.
Properties of Various Mammalian Nerve Fibers

Fiber type	Diameter (μm)	Velocity (m sec)	Function
A (α)	13–22	70–120	Motor, proprioception; sensory transmission of nociception
(β)	8–13	30–70	Touch, kinesthesia
(γ)	4–8	15–40	Motor, spindle excitation; touch, pressure
(δ)	1–5	5–30	Nociceptive reflexes, heat, cold, pressure
B	1–3	3–15	Preganglionic autonomic
C	0.2–1.3	0.2–2.3	Pain (possibly heat, cold, pressure), postganglionic autonomic

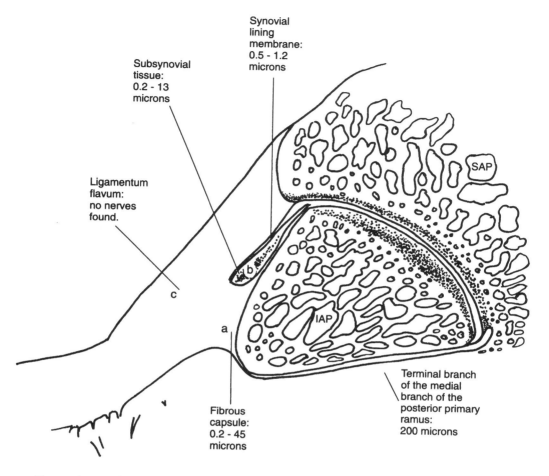

Figure 8.1. Schematic illustration of findings of L. G. F. Giles. A composite of L4/5 and L5/S1 zygapophyseal joints from fresh human surgical laminectomy specimens. Microscopy revealed nerve fibers, fasciculi, and encapsulated endings in both the accessory capsule at L5/S1 and the posteromedial fibrous capsule at L4/5 (*a*); nerve fibers and fasciculi were observed in subsynovial tissue and nerve fibers were located in the synovial membrane (*b*), but no neural elements were found in the ligamentum flavum (*c*). (*SAP*, superior articular process; *IAP*, inferior articular process). (Adapted from Giles LGF. Anatomical basis of low back pain. Baltimore: Williams & Wilkins, 1989:81.)

in the synovial lining membrane, from 0.2 to 13 μm in the subsynovial tissues, and from 0.2 to 45 μm in the accessory fibrous capsule (L5/S1) and/or the posteromedial fibrous capsule (L4/5) (7).

Another type of free nerve ending is the sinuvertebral nerve; its endings provide the fascia, ligaments, periosteum, intervertebral joints, and intervertebral disc with an afferent supply (3–7).

MUSCLE RECEPTORS

The muscle receptors play a central role in the Korr model of SDF (presented below in this chapter). Muscle receptors include the muscle spindle receptors, Golgi tendon organs, pressure receptors, and unmyelinated pain receptors. The function of these receptors is understood in some detail by neurophysiologists (3–5, 8, 9).

The muscle spindle (Fig. 8.2) consists of 3–10 intrafusal muscle fibers that are pointed at their ends and attached to the sheaths of the surrounding extrafusal (skeletal muscle) fibers. The heavily nucleated central region of the intrafusal fiber cannot contract but can be stretched when surrounding muscle is stretched or when the ends of the intrafusal fibers are contracted. Encompassing the central region is the primary (or annulospiral) receptor, which is supplied by a large type A afferent nerve fiber. The flower-spray receptor is a secondary receptor in the muscle spindle; it lies between the annu-

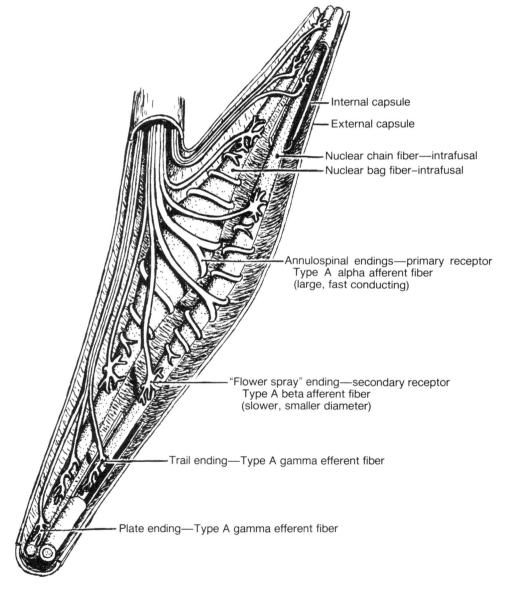

Internal capsule

External capsule

Nuclear chain fiber—intrafusal

Nuclear bag fiber–intrafusal

Annulospinal endings—primary receptor
Type A alpha afferent fiber
(large, fast conducting)

"Flower spray" ending—secondary receptor
Type A beta afferent fiber
(slower, smaller diameter)

Trail ending—Type A gamma efferent fiber

Plate ending—Type A gamma efferent fiber

Figure 8.2. Muscle spindle. Two types of intrafusal fibers as well as the annulospiral and flower spray receptors are shown. An external capsule surrounds the entire muscle spindle. The muscle spindle is an important component of the Korr hypothesis of SF. (Adapted from Warwick R, Williams PL, eds. Gray's Anatomy, 35th ed. Philadelphia: WB Saunders, 1973:800. (5).)

lospiral receptor and the contractile portion of the intrafusal fiber on both sides. The intrafusal fiber itself receives its efferent innervation from type A gamma motoneurons (fusimotor). The surrounding extrafusal muscle fibers are supplied by large type A alpha motoneurons (skeletomotor).

Muscle belly stretching results in intrafusal fiber stretching and activation of the annulospiral endings. The large type A alpha afferent nerve fibers of the annulospiral receptor synapse directly on type A alpha motoneurons in the anterior horn of the spinal column. Hence, when the annulospiral endings are activated, reflex contraction of the extrafusal fibers of the same muscle belly occurs. This contraction, in turn, shortens the intrafusal fibers and stops the annulospiral excitation, which allows the muscle to relax. Because this entire mechanism is mediated at a spinal level, it is a servo mechanism. This mechanism of reflex contraction, called the stretch reflex (i.e., myotatic reflex), protects the muscle from stretch beyond its desired length. The annulospiral receptors also are activated on contraction of the intrafusal muscle fibers that contract the two ends of the spindle while stretching the middle.

The primary and secondary muscle spindle receptors differ importantly in their phasic responses. The annulospiral endings are more sensitive to changes in intrafusal fiber length and respond faster than the secondary flower-spray receptors. At maximum physiologic length, however, the secondary receptors discharge at higher rates than do the primary receptors. During the resting state, the primary receptors maintain a basal level of activity while the flower-spray endings are inactive.

There is some overlap in fusimotor (gamma motoneuron) and skeletomotor (alpha motoneuron) activity. Burke and co-workers (10) suggest that fusimotor activation during skeletomotor activation provides background discharge for the spindle endings so they can detect irregularities in movement and reflexly correct them.

The Golgi tendon organ is another muscle receptor that receives its afferent supply from large type A nerve fibers. This organ consists of receptor endings in a tendon attached to 10–15 extrafusal muscle fibers; it is stimulated by tension produced in these fibers or by passive stretch of the muscle tendon.

Two types of pressure receptors are also found in skeletal muscle. Regular free nerve endings are the most common pressure-sensitive receptors found in extrafusal muscle. These type A delta fibers also convey nociceptive and thermal sensations at relatively low rates of conduction. Perhaps the most familiar pressure receptor located in muscular tissues is the pacinian corpuscle. This organ is located mainly in the fascia surrounding skeletal muscle fibers. The pacinian receptor consists of concentric lamellae with an unmyelinated nerve ending. The myelinated afferent supply to the pacinian corpuscle transmits impulses for rapid mechanical deformation but no stretch.

Unmyelinated pain receptors comprise another category of muscle receptors. These free branching nerve endings are activated by ischemia, pressure, and thermal changes. They are the terminal endings of the perivascular nerves.

Somatic Afferent Input and Nociception

Of the 10 billion cells in the human nervous system, a single segment of the spinal cord—which controls several muscles and receives a rich sensory input—contains thousands of neurons (11). This rich afferent input is composed primarily of nonmyelinated C fibers (nociceptors); the large fibers from the muscle stretch receptors (type A alpha afferents) comprise only a small percentage of the cross-section of the dorsal root. However, the large type A alpha afferents synapse directly with motor neurons in the ventral cord; the nociceptors synapse with interneurons and are thus subject to modification by excitatory and inhibitory influences.

With regard to the sympathetic preganglionic neurons, synaptic influences arise from two primary sources: peripheral input from somatic and visceral afferents to the spinal cord and central input from spinally projecting brainstem neurons (12). Researchers agree that the primary afferent fibers capable of influencing preganglionic cells include the myelinated fibers conducting at below 40 m/sec, the unmyelinated fibers (viz., A, B, and C fibers of cutaneous nerves as well as muscle nerve fibers of groups II, III, and IV), and the small myelinated and unmyelinated afferent fibers of visceral nerves (12).

A brief overview of dorsal horn and spinal neurophysiology pertinent to SDF and VSC is provided after a review of current concepts of sensitization of receptor fields to nociception.

RECEPTOR FIELD SENSITIZATION TO NOCICEPTION

A key factor to any hypothesis regarding facilitation concerns the mechanism by which receptor fields in damaged or traumatized tissues become sensitized to activation from even low-threshold stimuli. Mense (13) recently reviewed the literature and concluded that a number of substances released from pathologically altered tissues influence neurological activity. These endogenous substances in damaged skeletal muscle (and found in other deep tissues affected by a mechanical lesion) apparently enable weak and previously subthreshold stimuli to excite nociceptors and elicit muscle pain. While bradykinin has been shown to be important in this regard, prostaglandin E_2 (PGE_2) may be more important, as it not only sensitizes nociceptors but also enhances the excitatory influence of bradykinin on muscle receptors (13). Another substance capable of enhancing the effects of bradykinin is 5-hydroxytryptamine.

Interactions between these substances are likely as they are released together in pathologically altered muscle, and neuropeptides such as substance P (SP), and calcitonin gene-related peptide (CGRP) may play a role in receptor field sensitization as well (13). The exact role of SP is poorly understood. Kumazawa and Mizumura (14) were able to demonstrate excitation of testicular nociceptors by SP. However, nothing is known of the role of SP on receptor endings in skeletal muscle (the potential role of SP in nociception and in central modulation of neural activity will be discussed in more detail later in this chapter) (13).

Hence, endogenous substances released in the deep and superficial tissues as a result of trauma might be the first insult to the integrity of the nervous system, causing localized tenderness or even muscle pain (13). By lowering the threshold for nociceptor activation, these substances might set the stage for facilitation at the corresponding segmental level of the spinal cord, as well as initiate subsequent pathological processes discussed below in this chapter.

SPINAL PATHWAYS AND NOXIOUS STIMULI

All somatic sensations of a mechanoreceptive, nociceptive, or proprioceptive nature must enter the dorsal horn of the spinal column before proceeding to higher neural centers. It is here that processing begins, and the nervous system must decide which data are important and which can be "ignored." The central nervous system (CNS) may be thought of as a system of literally hundreds of neuronal pools, some of which are very large (e.g., cerebral cortex) (15). Many afferent and efferent fiber tracts as well as interconnecting neurons can be found within any given pool. Apparently, it is this network that allows the nervous system to instantaneously process the billions of pieces of information that it is fed every minute (15).

It has been said that the primary pathway in the spine for nociceptive sensations is the lateral spinothalamic system (neospinothalamic tract)(16). Although other tracts are functional in nociceptive discrimination (e.g., dorsal column system, spinocervicothalamic tract, paleospinothalamic tract, spinoreticular tract, and multisynaptic ascending propriospinal system), the three discriminative ascending pain pathways are the neospinothalamic tract, the dorsal column system, and the spinocervicothalamic tract (16)(Fig. 8.3).

Of these, perhaps the best known is the lateral spinothalamic system. Although these fibers respond best to type A delta fiber stimulation (as well as to type C fiber stimulation), this tract may not be that important in the transfer of noxious stimuli, since few of these fibers actually even reach the thalamus; most terminate in the lower reticular formation (17). Type A and C fiber stimulation affects both wide-dynamic-range and high-threshold spinothalamic tract cells. In addition to pain, this system conveys thermal, crude touch, pressure, tickle, itch, and sexual sensation to the reticular formation (17). Recently Schouenborg and Dickenson (18) demonstrated long-lasting alterations in dorsal horn activity after noxious pinching

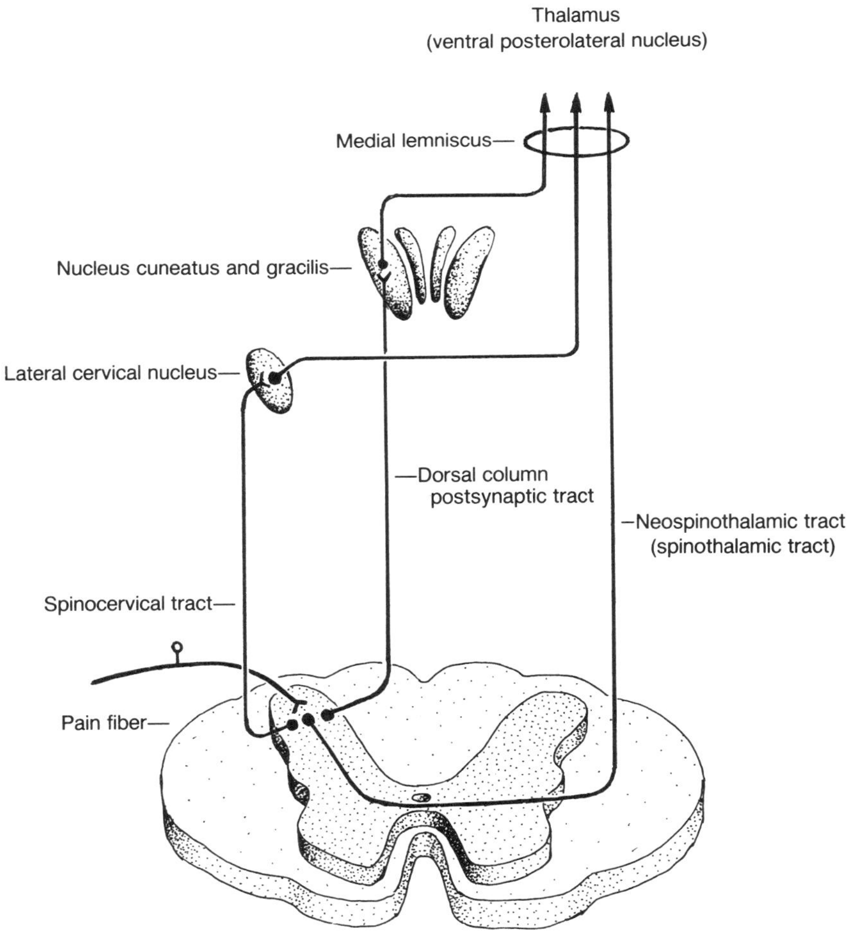

Figure 8.3. Three pathways for pain that are considered discriminative. The spinothalamic tract is considered the oldest known and perhaps the most direct pathway for nociception (pain). (Adapted from Haldeman S. Neurophysiology of spinal pain syndromes. In: Haldeman S, ed. Modern developments in the principles and practice of chiropractic. New York: Appleton Century Crofts. 1980:119–141.)

of the skin, which appeared to cause late discharges in nociceptive C fibers.

If facilitation of a spinal segment can be demonstrated through neurophysiological research (an issue discussed below), the question we are next faced with is, Can segmental afferent bombardment of dorsal horn cells affect normal somatic and autonomic function? Coote (12) describes several pathways by which somatic sensations could affect normal sympathetic reflexes. In addition to synapsing directly in the tract of Lissauer, the small somatic and visceral afferents entering the dorsal horn may synapse in the substantia gelatinosa, where synaptic contacts with Lissauer may occur for up to six segments; this feature involves somatosympathetic and viscerosympathetic reflexes (12). There is no evidence that afferent pathways involved in autonomic reflexes have this type of organization; however, if such organization exists, it would explain one route for afferent bombardment affecting segmental levels up to six segments on either side of the input (19).

Those afferent impulses that reach laminae IV and V or the dorsal horn (which contributes to the dorsolateral system) may ascend via the ventral funiculus, anterolateral fasciculus, and dorsolateral funiculus. This pathway is especially important because it is the main ascending afferent pathway for sympathetic reflexes that have been mediated by medullary or supramedullary regions (12). The lamina V and VI cells are perhaps the most interesting of all the neuronal pools, as they are the only cells of the dorsal horn to receive inputs from both small somatic and small visceral afferent fibers. These cells are largely responsible for the activation of sympathetic reflexes (12).

Gardner (20) delineated the role of the spinocervicothalamic tract in which input to the dorsolateral funiculus ascends to the lateral cervical nucleus, where the impulses synapse before ending in the thalamic region. Kajander and Giesler (21) demonstrated that neurons in the lateral cervical nucleus could be sensitized by sustained thermal stimuli, suggesting that the spinocervicotha-

lamic pathway receives prominent input from A-nociceptors.

Ample evidence suggests that somatic afferent input does indeed affect autonomic and somatic reflexes (22–26). Supramaximal stimulation of forelimb muscle type A delta fibers evoked small early responses in thoracic sympathetic nerves with latencies in the range of 92 to 157 msec (27). Corbett et al. (28) showed that in humans (tetraplegic patients), muscle spasm can stimulate blood pressure and heart rate increases. Indeed, chronic spinal pain with its afferent bombardment may actually result in an increased arousal response, a decrease in the performance of difficult tasks that lead to pain (i.e., a more sedentary lifestyle), and decreased evidence of muscle spasm (29). However, although Collins et al. (29) concluded that chronic low back patients have less muscle spasm than matched controls, others have criticized their study because of the use of an EMG bandpass that may have been too wide (30). In contrast, their findings of increased frontalis EMG and increased electrodermal activity (EDA) in patients with chronic low back pain are corroborated indirectly by evidence of significant reductions in EMG and EDA activity in manipulated patients with LBP, compared with control patients not receiving manipulation (31).

Somatic afferent inputs remote from the level of sympathetic efferent activity may evoke specific sympathetic reflex responses. Nonnoxious stimulation of the skin anywhere in the body, for example, increases sympathetic postganglionic activity to cutaneous vascular beds but decreases it to muscular vascular beds. Noxious stimulation of the skin produces the opposite effects. Burgess and Perl (32) and Bessou and Perl (33) have demonstrated that both myelinated and unmyelinated fibers are necessary for relay of cutaneous noxious and innocuous thermal stimuli.

Coote (19) has established two important principles with regard to somatosympathetic reflexes: (a) a spatial organization is seen in some somatosympathetic reflexes and (b) somatic afferent input can enter the cord at one segment and the relevant sympathetic preganglionic neurons be located at an entirely different segmental level. Beacham and Perl (34) demonstrated that preganglionic units at one spinal level could be activated with a shorter latency by afferent input from an adjacent segment than by afferent input to the same segment.

Hence, a number of pathways appear to be involved in the transmission of somatoautonomic activity. However, somatosympathetic reflexes, for example, can habituate or sensitize (19). Receptor field sensitization (as previously discussed) can play a role in the modulation of these pathological reflexes, as can central processes such as descending inhibition in the dorsal columns (discussed below). Before discussing central modulation of somatic afferent bombardment, we will consider several important neurobiologic models of SDF. These models help explain how SDF can occur and create afferent bombardment that would initiate these reflexes.

Neurobiologic Models of SDF

Several neurobiologic models have been proposed to account for SDF. Some might be categorized as *noninflammatory/neurologic* models, since they rely primarily on electrophysiological research that indicates that afferent input to the spinal pathways can cause sustained alterations in neural excitability.

Other models combine the concepts of long-lasting alterations in spinal reflexes due to afferent bombardment with the factor of inflammatory changes secondary to tissue trauma. We might categorize these as inflammatory/neurological models, since they depend upon both electrophysiological research and known influences of peptides and inflammation on nerve propagation.

These models may help us understand how the clinical findings associated with SDF (e.g., altered pressure-pain thresholds, altered segmental motion, and altered myo-

electric responses; see Chapters 6 and 7) can create a sustained source of altered afferent dorsal horn stimulation and inflammation, which can subsequently alter somatoautonomic and sympathetic reflexes and impair health through segmental facilitation.

NONINFLAMMATORY/ NEUROLOGICAL MODELS

Early observations by a team of osteopathic researchers laid the foundation for our current understanding of human segmental facilitation. Led by J. S. Denslow, these scientists also were the first to publish manipulation research in refereed science journals in the 1940s (see citations and more discussion of this work in Chapter 5). For example, Denslow, Korr, and Krems (35) applied pressure over selected spinous processes and observed changes in erector spinae muscles in 30 young men. They found that in certain subjects, even a small amount of pressure (1– kg) applied to the spinous process at some segments resulted in some degree of hyperexcitability in the spinalis muscles on one or both sides of the spine. Hence, spontaneously evoked spike potentials were seen more often at these sites, and activity was triggered easily, even from pressure applied at more distant segmental levels. They determined that these areas were "facilitated" and had a low threshold for activity (35).

Much greater pressures (3–7+ kg) could be applied to other spinous processes in the same subjects before evoked potentials were seen in the adjacent erector spinae muscles; these were labeled moderate- or high-threshold segments. Indeed, pressure applied over high-threshold spinous processes did not trigger reflex activity at adjacent high-threshold segments but caused activity at distant low-threshold or facilitated segments in the same spine. Procainization of tissues around the spinous processes at facilitated segments did not prevent this reflex activation by pressure over other distant high-threshold areas (35). These facilitated segments remained so for months in the same subjects and corroborated other work demonstrating long-lasting areas of altered galvanic skin response in "lesioned" segments (see discussion in Chapter 5).

Korr Model

Based upon these observations, Korr (36) developed perhaps the first model to explain neurological effects of SDF. According to Korr, in a zone of segmental facilitation (that might be associated with SDF), which includes anterior and lateral horn cells as well as cells of ascending pain pathways, both motor and autonomic function are affected. These neurons become hyperresponsive to input from the brain and the body. Both afferents from the musculoskeletal tissues adjacent to the SDF and visceral afferents may be involved in this facilitation.

Korr (36) discounted the role of joint receptors in his hypothesis, stating that little evidence suggests that joint receptors can influence motor activity. Instead, he focused on the muscle spindle as the coordinator that may increase or decrease muscle contraction according to the direction of motion of the joint. This reflex muscle contraction can then produce joint motion by its action or prevent joint motion in an area of SDF.

The mechanism Korr (36) used to explain such a phenomenon involves the fusimotor background discharge that is seen during type A alpha motoneuron activity. He explained that the CNS adjusts the slack in the muscle spindle that occurs during extrafusal contraction by adjusting the level of background activity in the fusimotor system. Not only is the slack in the spindle taken up by increased gamma motor activity, but the CNS turns the level of background activity up or down, depending on the needs of the muscle. For example, athletes who wish to swing a bat or hockey stick in a wide arc must be able to "preset" the gamma activity in their muscles so that large changes in muscle length may be swiftly and smoothly accomplished. In this example, the CNS would turn down the level of background activity in the fusimotor system of the involved muscles so that as the skeletal mus-

cles contract gradually, there is only a gradual simultaneous contraction of the intrafusal fibers. On the other hand, tennis players who play the net must have this background activity increased, to return the ball with a minimum of muscle motion. In this way, the CNS can set and reset spindle sensitivity through the fusimotor system. Korr called this a type of automatic "gain" that controls the length-regulating mechanism for each skeletal muscle.

Sometimes, cerebral influences may set the spindle sensitivity at the wrong level for correct muscular activity. Tension and stressful situations may result in the "gain" being set too high in the fusimotor system; muscles may be tense and resistant to change in length, and according to the Korr hypothesis, the person is said to be "jumpy" or "irritable."

With the idea of "gain" kept in mind, it is easy to visualize the main points of the Korr hypothesis (Fig. 8.4):

1. The CNS orders skeletal muscle contraction (which carries with it background "low-gain" gamma motoneuron activity).
2. At the same time, vertebral attachments are suddenly approximated (by external forces or by the unexpected withdrawal of a load or force that is opposing strong isometric extrafusal contraction), which results in slackening of the muscle spindles quickly and, thereby, silencing of the annulospiral activity.
3. Without an annulospiral report, the CNS assumes that the gamma motor "gain" is not set high enough for the primary receptor endings to transmit the impulses for the contraction. The CNS then turns up the "gain" to compensate for this discrepancy. Increasing the gamma motor activity likewise results in increased fusimotor activity, and the muscle is contracted further.
4. As the body recoils from the forced motion and the vertebral attachments attempt to return to their normal

position, they are now opposed in this by the now resistant muscle. The joint surfaces are approximated, and increased frictional resistance prevents normal motion.

5. Gravity and postural reflexes tend to stretch the muscle to resting length, and the joint receptors continue to report their true position. The "high-

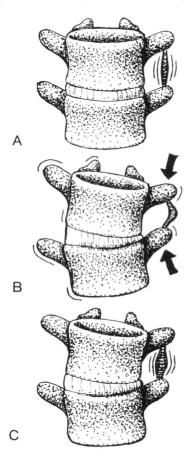

A

B

C

Figure 8.4. Schema of the Korr (11) model of SDF. *A.* CNS orders skeletal muscle contraction. *B.* At the same time, vertebral attachments are approximated by external forces, etc. (this has the effect of silencing annulospiral receptor activity). *C.* CNS turns up the gamma motor neuron "gain," thereby increasing the intensity of the contraction. Due to this contraction, the vertebral attachments cannot return to their normal position; gravity and postural reflexes further stretch the muscle, which causes continued resistance and high "gain" or "spasm" activity.

gain" activity, however, causes the muscle to resist, and the muscle is in "spasm." Afferent input could be expected to create segmental facilitation at this level of SDF.

Korr proposed two mechanisms whereby manipulation would successfully turn down the fusimotor "gain" and thereby relax the muscle spasm. First, stretching the intrafusal fibers by forcefully stretching the muscle against its spindle-maintained resistance would produce a barrage of afferent impulses intense enough to signal the CNS to reduce the gamma motoneuron discharge. Second, the Golgi tendon organs would be stimulated by forced stretch of the skeletal muscle causing both gamma and alpha motoneuron inhibition. Korr predicted that both the slow-range-of-motion, long-lever type of manipulation and the rapid, high-velocity, short-lever type of chiropractic adjustment would be successful in stretching the muscles against their resistance (36).

Later Korr (37) proposed a number of factors that might modify the site, nature, and severity of SDF, with resultant segmental facilitation. Posture and attitude, descending pathways, neuroendocrine mechanisms, and endocoids (viz., the peptides, especially endogenous opioids such as enkephalins and endorphins) were factors he cited that are discussed in detail later in this chapter and elsewhere in this text. Korr (38) more recently argued that this model (as well as another he proposed by which "garbled" collective input from joint proprioceptors triggers facilitation) deserves attention from researchers interested in joint manipulation.

Patterson-Steinmetz Model

Another model relating to the findings of Denslow, Korr, and Krems (35) was forwarded by M. Patterson and J. Steinmetz at the College of Osteopathic Medicine, Ohio University, in 1986. Patterson and Steinmetz (39) based their model on animal research in which a spinal fixation is created experimentally. Previous researchers had known that creating a small lesion in the cerebellum of an anesthetized dog, for example, would cause the limbs on one side to actively flex and remain in that position. If the cord was then severed (provided 3 or 4 hours had elapsed since the lesion was created), the limbs retained the flexed posture (Fig. 8.5). This became the basis for the concept of *spinal learning*, in that although the influence of the instigating lesion in the cerebellum had been removed, the "learned" influence in the spine had remained. From 1976 to 1986, Patterson and Steinmetz (39) determined that:

1. There is a gradient effect of lesions created; partial spinal fixation (limb flexion) occurred in anesthetized rats if cord section occurred after 35 minutes, but by 45 minutes, sectioning

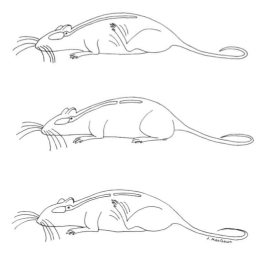

Figure 8.5. Schema of *spinal learning* as determined from experiments that formed the basis for Patterson and Steinmetz's facilitation hypothesis. They and others showed that creating a small lesion in the cerebellum of an anesthetized animal would cause the limbs on one side to actively flex and remain in that position (*top*). Immediate severance of spinal cord at T7 results in paralysis of the hind limb (*middle*). If the hind limb flexion is allowed to remain for even 45 minutes, it becomes "learned" by the spine and remains despite section of the cord (*bottom*).

caused all animals to retain their limb flexion.

2. The cerebral cortex and brainstem are not necessary for observed alterations in spinal reflex excitability; animals with spinal transections at the T12 level (and hence without brainstem or cortex influence) actually had limb flexion established faster (within 30 minutes of cord sectioning).

3. Direct stimulation of the hind limb producing reflex flexion of the limb showed fixation within 35–40 minutes. Thus the effect could be produced by afferent inputs from the limbs themselves and did not necessitate descending influences from the brain.

4. Spinal fixation is not the result of changes in afferent input due to electrical stimulation of the skin; hence, skin areas stimulated to produce flexion and its retention can be completely anesthetized with no loss of hind-limb flexion. Therefore, alterations being studied *are due to changes in spinal reflex circuits* and not due to peripheral inputs alone.

5. Fixation of hind-limb flexion cannot occur without the spinal cord remaining intact; direct stimulation of severed ventral spinal roots controlling hind-limb flexion did not result in retention of flexion following stimulation. Hence, the effect did not occur in the muscle or at the neuromuscular junction but was a result of alterations in the afferent inputs or in the spinal cord reflex excitability.

6. After 45 minutes of stimulation, spinal cord section at T7 induced a reappearance of hind-limb flexion, regardless of the duration of stimulation delivered or the length of recovery allowed after the stimulation (in studies lasting 3 days).

They concluded that spinal fixation can be generated by either central or peripheral inputs to segmental circuits; that the reflex can be created in a short time, given a sufficient stimulus; and that the increased excitability outlasts spinal transection and prolonged periods of otherwise normal activity.

Patterson and Steinmetz (39) concluded that in an area of SDF with accompanying motion disorder and muscle tension, visceral spasm, or other initiating disorder, if the initial stimulus is sufficient or lasts long enough, there may be segmental facilitation even after the instigating stimulus is removed. Once this facilitation occurs, despite the removal of the afferent source of stimulation, the abnormal segmental reflex circuit itself participates in maintaining the symptoms, thus creating a cycle of increased output with any sensory input.

According to this model, manipulation would be highly effective in stopping the cycle, especially soon after the start of an initiating stimulus. However, once the excitability changes were fixated in the cord, a "neural scar" of hyperexcitable but subliminally excited neurons would remain, which would be abnormally responsive to additional stimuli. They further predict that alterations at the segmental level in these spinal reflex circuits may not be easily removed, insuring increased susceptibility to recurrence for at least hours, days, or months after the acute problem is resolved.

More recently, Patterson, Bartelt, and Johnson (40) demonstrated that spinal fixation could be ameliorated somewhat by contralateral hind limb stimulation. This finding suggested a role for the crossed extensor reflex pathway in inhibition of hind-limb flexion after spinal section. Johnson, Bartelt, Johnson, and Patterson (41) demonstrated a dose-response effect of d-amphetamine on persisting hind-limb flexion. Hence, increased spinal fixation with increasing amphetamine administration suggested involvement of catecholamine in long-lasting alterations of spinal reflexes, or facilitation. Bartelt, Johnson, and Patterson (42) have recently demonstrated significantly less hind-limb flexion in spinalized rats in which repeated removal of the flexion is accomplished through repeated measures

(viz., testing the limb numerous times to see how much weight is needed to remove the flexion). They questioned whether this change was associated with a muscular or a neural mechanism (42). Finally, Patterson, Bartelt, Johnson, and Howe (43) recently used animals placed in a restraint box for 30 minutes to demonstrate that stress increases the severity of hind-limb flexion in subsequently hind limb–stimulated and spinalized rats.

Patterson (personal communication) recently confirmed that current research of this phenomenon indicates that a wide variety of stressors (viz., noise and swimming stress) increases spinal fixation in spinalized rats. Hence, spinal reflexes may be altered for long periods of time or permanently by a wide variety of central or peripheral afferent inputs and may be mediated or excited by various stressors. The human facilitated segment, according to this model, becomes an important part of body dysfunction, as it limits the ability of the body to respond to stress, changing internal or external demands, and challenges created by our daily existence (39, 44).

Other Noninflammatory/Neurological Models

Various models hypothesizing the effects of SDF on the nervous system have been forwarded by a number of researchers. Some include the concept of relative hypoxemia as a corollary to the muscle tissue damage seen in an area of chronic SDF (45). Schmidt (46) favors a gamma motoneuron feedback loop triggered by nociception. Animal experiments demonstrate that both acute allogenic stimulation of the muscle nociceptors and chronic stimulation of small type III and IV muscle afferents can lead to a permanent increase in muscle tone (46). This is a variation of the Korr (36) hypothesis (presented above), which was based upon an alteration in background fusimotor discharge to the muscle spindle.

Skoglund (47) has shown that in healthy human subjects, two types of proprioceptive reflex responses to tapping can be demonstrated using needle electrodes in erector spinae muscles. In contrast, a pathophysiological reflex is described in which deep palpation of the muscle produces an initial burst of impulses followed by afterdischarges in patients with mechanical pelvic dysfunction. Occasionally this pathological erector spinae reflex (PESR) is seen weakly in the contralateral muscle as well. Manipulation restores the erector muscles to their normal responses. He proposes that mechanoreceptors in both skin and muscle (and possibly over vertebral column ligaments) may trigger this electromyographically demonstrable reflex, via increased motoneuron excitability causing long-lasting alterations in spinal reflex thresholds (segmental facilitation).

Simons and Hong (48) suggest that Skoglund's observations may reflect the previously reported local twitch response (LTR) seen in the "taut" band of a myofascial trigger point. They suggest that since a number of signs are similar to both PESR and LTR, they are part of the same general lesion (48):

1. Point tenderness;
2. Weak or pronounced contractions extending to adjacent muscles;
3. Reflex elicited by tapping the muscle in PESR (in LTR a sudden change in pressure on a trigger point is seen);
4. Trigger points associated with decreased stretch range of motion; PESR associated similarly with the Patrick test;
5. PESRs needle EMG findings identical to findings at LTRs in the quadriceps, deltoid, and peroneus longus muscles.

Simons and Hong (48) cited demonstration of LTRs after nearly complete interruption of both afferent and efferent neural pathways via both ischemic nerve compression and traumatic nerve injury. Hence, the myofascial trigger point, LTR, and PESR would be mediated locally as well as by the CNS reflex. They hypothesize that the "trigger point" itself may be the major source of

"continuous afferent bombardment" seen in LTR and PESR.

INFLAMMATORY/NEUROLOGICAL MODELS

While some models predict effects of SDF even in the absence of inflammatory changes, others combine both concepts to predict the potential outcome of the lesion. Some of these inflammatory/neurological models predict that SDF, like other physical or mental stressors, might evoke inflammatory changes and a local adaptation syndrome (LAS; see also Chapter 14).

Dvorak Model

Dvorak (49) summarized his work and others in proposing that SDF creates both the mechanical and the chemical stimulation necessary for activation of nociceptors and spinothalamic tract activity (Fig. 8.6). Key components of his model include:

1. SDF creates both articular pain and reflex muscular changes. The changes in muscle depend upon the type of muscle involved. Postural muscles such as the intertransverse muscles of the cervical spine contain a higher proportion of slow-twitch fibers (200–500 muscle spindles per gram of tissue) than are found in larger, phasic muscles such as rectus femoris (50 muscle spindles per gram of tissue). The smaller postural muscles tend to continue to shorten in response to SDF or when overly used; the fast-twitch phasic muscles respond to overuse with fatigue.
2. Increased muscle spindle activity after SDF results in a postcontraction sensory discharge via increased firing of Ia fibers (alpha motoneurons), which triggers further contraction of the same muscle and may ultimately change the spindle distribution.
3. Shortening of the postural muscles is also associated with histochemical changes that may help maintain the

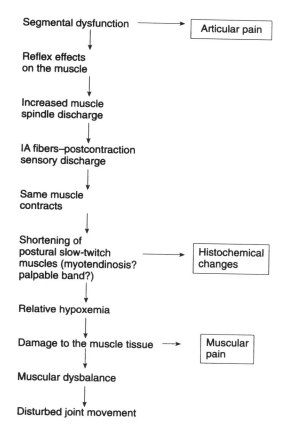

Segmental dysfunction → Articular pain

Reflex effects
on the muscle

Increased muscle
spindle discharge

IA fibers–postcontraction
sensory discharge

Same muscle
contracts

Shortening of
postural slow-twitch → Histochemical
muscles (myotendinosis?   changes
palpable band?)

Relative hypoxemia

Damage to the muscle tissue → Muscular pain

Muscular dysbalance

Disturbed joint movement

Figure 8.6. Dvorak's model for facilitation induced by segmental dysfunction (SDF). (Adapted from Dvorak J. Neurological and biomechanical aspects of pain. In: Buerger AA, Greenman PE, eds. Approaches to the validation of spinal manipulation. Springfield, Ill.: Charles C Thomas, 1985:241–266.)

postcontraction sensory discharge. These inflammatory changes might include changes in potassium concentrations within the muscles.

4. Relative hypoxemia and muscular dysfunction causing disturbed joint movement are consequences of these changes.

Gatterman/Goe Model

Gatterman and Goe (50) proposed a mechanism whereby traumatic or postural strain of skeletal muscle could generate a myofascial trigger point. Others (47, 48)

equate the paraspinal trigger point, taut band, and restricted spinal joint motion with SDF. If genesis of a myofascial trigger point at a spinal level is representative of SDF, then the Gatterman/Goe model is an interesting inflammatory/neurological model for SDF that initiates segmental facilitation (Fig. 8.7).

The Gatterman/Goe model includes tissue damage resulting in disruption of small blood vessels, with release of platelets and hence substances such as serotonin, which sensitizes nerve endings. Damage to connective tissues results in breakage of mast cells containing histamine, which also sensitizes and stimulates nerve endings. Additionally, a sustained local contraction creates a region of uncontrolled metabolism, additional mast cell liberation of histamine, and subsequent depletion of local adenosine triphosphate (ATP). Because energy from splitting ATP is required to reset the muscle spindle, as ATP is depleted, there is a progressive failure of relaxation, and eventually contracture, of the muscle (50).

By reducing local blood flow, the sustained contractions may stimulate autonomic nerves and a somatosomatic response; the result is local accumulation of metabolites such as prostaglandins, which further sensitize nerve endings (50). Gatterman and Goe (50) predict that this self-perpetuating cycle is painful, resists stretching, and decreases range of motion of adjacent joints.

Mense Model

Mense (51) holds that localized tenderness in muscle most likely results from sensitization of muscle nociceptors and other mechanosensitive receptive endings. His model predicts not so much the cause of the mechanical spinal lesion as it does the neurobiologic sequelae that might lead to facilitation and referral of muscle pain. He feels that sensitization probably results from the release of endogenous substances from damaged tissues, which reduces the stimulus threshold of nociceptors. Hence, even weak stimuli can excite nociceptive receptors and elicit muscle pain.

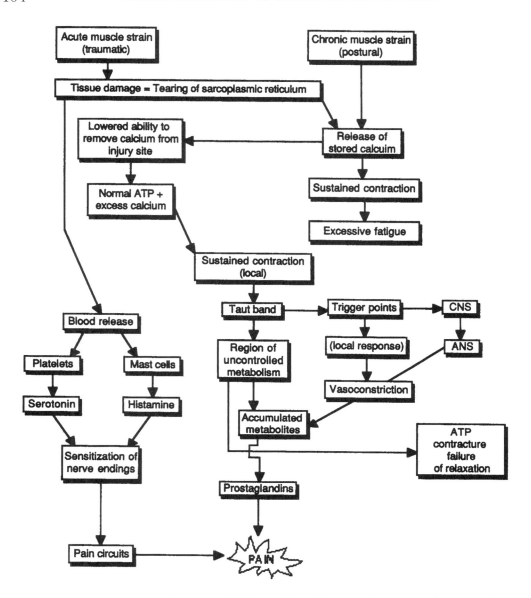

Figure 8.7. Gatterman and Goe's model for myofascial pain combines several concepts hypothesized by others to create facilitation. Chemical release sensitizing nerve endings, disturbed connective tissues, and a sustained local contraction are features of this model. (Adapted from Gatterman MI, Goe DR. Muscle and myofascial pain syndromes. In: Gatterman MI, ed. Chiropractic management of spine related disorders. Baltimore: Williams & Wilkins, 1990:285–329.)

Due to muscle overexertion or a mechanical spinal lesion, vasoneuroactive substances (e.g., bradykinin and PGE_2) are released, stimulating production of edema, with resultant ischemia that creates a vicious cycle (Fig. 8.8). Local ischemia further re-

sults from depletion of ATP, according to Mense (51), which triggers failure of the calcium pump, further contracture, and additional ischemia. Increases in muscle tone occur via descending pathways as well, adding to the muscle "spasm" and promoting facili-

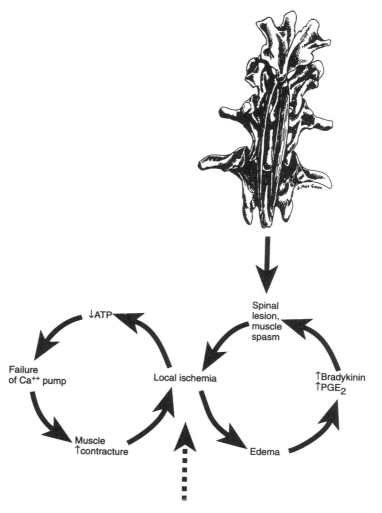

Figure 8.8. Mense's model predicts that a mechanical spinal lesion may cause release of vasoneuroactive substances that stimulate edema, ischemia, depletion of ATP, failure of calcium pump, further muscle contracture, and further ischemia. (Adapted from Mense S. Considerations concerning the neurobiological basis of muscle pain. Can J Physiol Pharmacol 1991;69:610–616.)

tation. His ideas regarding referral of pain and sensitization warrant exploration in some detail and are discussed in the next portion of this chapter.

Having reviewed both noninflammatory and inflammatory types of neurobiologic models of SDF, we now consider mechanisms that may modify the afferent bombardment of the dorsal horn expected as a result of such lesions.

Modulation of Spinal Reflexes

Neurophysiologists have identified a variety of mechanisms that would predictably modify, sensitize, or habituate spinal reflexes and the afferent bombardment expected from SDF. These mechanisms and anatomical considerations may well determine whether the host accommodates or succumbs to spinal trauma and lesions such as SDF.

CENTRAL MODULATION

Both the lateral fibers of the spinothalamic system and the medial fibers of the dorsal column system can be affected by facilitation, inhibition, convergence, divergence, synaptic afterdischarge, and synaptic fatigue (15). Both of these fiber tracts may be considered as individual neuronal pools. Some of these are centrally ordered mechanisms, which we shall refer to as *central modulation* of spinal reflexes.

As with other neuronal pools, these tracts may contain an unknown number of reverberating circuits that add to the effect of *synaptic afterdischarge.* (A postsynaptic potential develops in the neuron after discharge, and for many milliseconds, a sustained signal output ensues. This discharge lasts up to 15 msec in anterior neurons) (15). Generally, either temporal or spatial summation (or both) must occur before excitation threshold is reached. Subthreshold activity creates a state of facilitation in which the neuron is "ready" to begin discharging. More than one excitatory postsynaptic potential may reach the same neuron within 15 msec, either from the same presynaptic terminal (*temporal summation*) or from several presynaptic terminals (*spatial summation*). A maximally summated neuron discharges up to 1000 or more times/sec, while one that is barely summated may discharge 15–20 impulses/sec. These and other basic concepts in neurophysiology are important to understand the process of facilitation of an entire spinal segment and its implications for alteration of neural transmission.

All somatic sensations of a mechanoreceptive or a proprioceptive nature must enter the dorsal horn of the spinal column before proceeding to other higher neural centers. Holloway et al. (52) found that the phenomenon of descending inhibition can affect neural transmission in the dorsal horn cells. These cells may be inhibited by primary afferent depolarization (PAD), which gives rise to presynaptic inhibition of transmission at the interneuron level. The caudal reticular formation, lateral reticular forma-

tion, midbrain periaqueductal gray, and medial vestibular nucleus are involved in powerful suppression of dorsal horn responses to nociceptive and nonnoxious stimuli (52–54). Functionally different midbrain controls of descending inhibition have also been demonstrated (53, 54). Thus, whether or not pain impulses are permitted to pass from primary to second-order neurons is determined by a complex interaction of neural pathways and neurotransmitters.

Initially, for example, it was thought that 5-hydroxytryptamine was a direct neuronal inhibitor and that SP caused the release of endorphins thought to participate in inhibition. More recently, Bossut, Frenk, and Mayer (55, 56) have demonstrated in a series of experiments that while SP may act as a neuromodulator, it is neither necessary nor perhaps involved at all in the transmission of nociceptive information at the primary afferent synapse. Indeed, scratching and biting were the only behaviors produced by SP (57), and it was unlikely that these behaviors were produced by SP at the primary afferent synapse (56).

However, others have demonstrated recently that SP has an excitatory effect upon cat dorsal horn neurons and that certain structural analogues of SP can suppress this response (58). Further understanding of the role of neuropeptides comes from Tiseo and co-workers, who demonstrated a differential effect of noxious cold and heat on somatostatin and SP; noxious cold applied to the tail of male Sprague-Dawley rats caused a significant elevation in SP release into the cerebrospinal fluid, while exposure to noxious heat produced a significant increase in cerebrospinal fluid levels of somatostatin (59). Others have confirmed the excitatory effect of SP, recently, but have demonstrated that the excitatory effects of both SP and serotonin can be reversed in the nucleus tractus solitarius after prolonged conditioning by subsequent application of the other neurotransmitter (60).

Another type of central modulation involves the role of the the substantia gelatinosa in suppression of cranial spread of dorsal root potentials. Lupa and co-workers (61) found that ipsilateral dorsal root potentials that are produced by stimulation of the L5 dorsal root and spread caudally attain only 47% of the amplitude observed at the L6 dorsal root by the time that they have passed six segments. Conversely, cranially spreading dorsal root potentials decreased to zero by the time they had passed six segments.

Antidromic activity may also help to dampen afferent noxious bombardment of the dorsal horn. Curtis et al. (62) have shown that *antidromic discharge* (i.e., nerve conduction that is opposite the normal direction, as from axon toward dendrites) in the dorsal horn results from the extracellular flow of current that is generated by the propagation of action potentials. These transient depolarizations of types A alpha and beta afferent terminals synapsing on motoneurons lower the motoneuron threshold for conduction.

Further evidence that several phenomena dampen or depress the afferent bombardment associated with SDF was found by Calvin et al. (63). These researchers demonstrated alteration in sensitivity to synaptic currents when repetitive firing occurs within a neuron. Currents may be increased or decreased at the synapse by depression, facilitation, or posttetanic potentiation (63). Roby-Brami and co-workers (64) demonstrated that the nociceptive spinal flexion reflex (RIII reflex) could be inhibited with repeated electrical stimulation to the digital branches of the ulnar nerve in normal subjects, long past the normal conditioning period of 2 minutes. However, in tetraplegic patients, not only was the RIII reflex never decreased by the subsequent nociceptive stimulation, it was enhanced slightly. They concluded that heterotopic nociceptive stimulation in normal man is possibly centrally modulated by a complex loop within supraspinal structures (64).

Finally, with regard to central modulation we must remember that the concept of neuronal pools is important. Coote (12, 19) and others (24) have described the effect of seg-mental influences on incoming data. Kajander and Giesler (21) demonstrated sensitization of lateral cervical nucleus neurons to repeated noxious thermal stimulation in decerebrated and partially spinalized cats, indicating central modulation involving the spinocervicothalamic pathway. Then, a variety of central influences, both anatomical and physiological, appear to affect the course of dorsal horn bombardment after a spinal lesion, determining whether spinal reflexes will habituate or sensitize, and thereby influencing whether segmental facilitation will occur. Coote (12) envisions numerous pools of vasomotor preganglionic spinal cord neurons involved in the moment-by-moment regulation of various end organs, which are influenced by both supraspinal influences and by spinal afferents to effect behavioral goals.

PERIPHERAL MODULATION

Segmental facilitation may result from failure of damaged skeletal tissues to heal promptly, permitting prolonged bombardment of the dorsal horn to cause habituation of certain spinal reflex arcs. We refer to this concept of alterations in peripheral receptor fields affecting spinal reflexes as *peripheral modulation.*

One primary mechanism of peripheral modulation, briefly reviewed above, involves Mense's (13) concept of receptor field sensitization after trauma or muscular overexertion. His proposal explains focal deep tenderness and poor localization of muscle pain (see also "Pressure Pain Threshold" in Chapter 6); in an area of chronic segmental facilitation, where receptor fields are chronically activated, a new stimulus produces increased responsiveness in the dorsal horn because of long-lasting alterations in the central processing of pain. His model depends upon release of bradykinin, PGE_2, 5-hydrotryptamine, adrenaline, and possibly other peptides in edematous and damaged tissues. These chemically sensitize the peripheral receptor fields and promote segmental facilitation.

Peripheral modulation may be a consequence of anatomical considerations as well. Certain types of neurons exhibit properties that modulate excitatory postsynaptic potentials (EPSPs)(65). Hence, amplitude depression is seen at connections on small motoneurons that develop large EPSPs after high frequency bursts are delivered to single group Ia fibers. In contrast, positive modulation was seen at connections on large motoneurons that exhibit small EPSPs.

In addition to these mechanisms, both central and peripheral modulation may occur when certain stressors elicit the "alarm reaction" seen in the general adaptation syndrome (see Chapter 14). Such a reaction might further sensitize receptor fields and elicit a greater response in a spinal segment already facilitated.

Early in this chapter we asked how nature can fail to protect the spine from the effects of falls, accidents, and postures said to cause chronic spinal lesions? We have reviewed a number of neural mechanisms that nature does indeed appear to use to protect the spine from the effects of insults that create spinal lesions. Indeed, anatomical factors (including organization of the CNS into a system of neuronal pools), descending inhibition, and other mechanisms help the CNS discard unimportant information. It appears that only the more serious or more prolonged insults to this system can overcome nature's defense.

We can now address a second question we posed: How can mechanical spinal lesions (such as SDF and RDF) effect the diverse conditions purported to respond to CMT?

Somatoautonomic Dysfunction

If a variety of factors set the stage for SDF or RDF becoming chronic segmental facilitation, what next? What are the effects of this facilitative spinal lesion (clinical aspects of SDF and RDF are discussed in Chapter 9)? There is so much scientific literature on the role of the sympathetic nervous system in

disease that we can only briefly review it in this text (see also Section IV). Yet in introducing the subject of sympathicotonia as a factor in disease processes, Korr (66) pointed out that medical specialists often view sympathetic-mediated disease processes from a somewhat isolated perspective:

> Each discoverer of a sympathetic component seems, therefore, to regard it as peculiar to this or that disease within his or her area of specialization, rather than as part of a general theme (66).

Yet if some medical specialties still have difficulty believing that a chronic area of SDF, RDF, or segmental facilitation could detrimentally affect the sympathetic system, or if they have difficulty accepting the role of chiropractic in correcting that disorder, they appear to be aware of the effects of somatoautonomic dysfunction in general. Roizen (67), chair of the Department of Anesthesia and Critical Care at the University of Chicago, writes:

> Should we all undergo sympathectomy before operation, or perhaps, even sympathectomy at birth? Support for such a proposal might derive from the observations that, following sympathectomy, one might experience less myocardial ischemia, less hemodynamic alteration, and less arthritis; there are even implications of less inflammatory bowel disease, lower anesthetic requirements, a more stable perioperative course, and improved small vessel flow allowing less arteriolar and arterial thrombosis in the extremities. What's wrong with being sympathectomized at birth?

We characterize somatoautonomic dysfunction as aberrant sympathetic or parasympathetic activity associated with SDF, RDF, or VSC, discussed under the headings "Somatoautonomic Imbalance" and "Sympathicotonia."

SOMATOAUTONOMIC IMBALANCE

A number of investigators have discussed imbalance between the parasympathetic and sympathetic nervous systems as a factor in various disease processes. Some have further implicated activity from the somatic structures as initiating the aberrant neural response. This section focuses on syndromes in which parasympathetic tone predominates; somatoautonomic syndromes are referred to as somatoautonomic imbalance.

Early Evidence

Advocates of adjustment or spinal manipulation were not alone in the early decades of this century when they proposed that the chiropractic "bone out of place" or the osteopathic "vertebral lesion" could "pinch a nerve" and cause "altered tone" in the nervous system, or "dis-ease." For example, medical doctors Ussher (68, 69) and Wills and Atsatt (70) performed initial investigations of the "viscerospinal syndrome" in the 1930s, reporting 400 cases in the course of several years. The phenomenon involved severe pain in various viscera without signs of physical disease, severe asthmatic attacks, bronchial asthma, symptoms of angina, esophageal spasm (documented by barium fluoroscopic examination), pylorospasm and other gastrointestinal complaints, marked constipation, painful and frequent micturation, and a host of other conditions. Definite orthopaedic and roentgenographic findings of scoliosis, kyphosis, lordosis, and short-leg phenomena were reported, which when corrected—using heel lifts, physiotherapy, supports and muscle training—resulted in relief or cure of the symptomatology. Ussher (68) hypothesized:

> It may be that physiopathologic changes in these spinal structures actually produce an inhibition of sympathetic impulses. In turn this inhibition may allow parasympathetic tone to predominate, resulting in what appears to be an actual parasympathetic rather than sympathetic action on the viscera.

Other medical investigators reached similar conclusions. Murphy and Wilson (71) used osteopathic manipulation at T4 and T5 on 20 patients with severe asthmatic bronchitis that had failed to respond to injections of adrenalin and vaccine. Six were very much improved (90–100%), four had noticeable improvement (50–75%), and only five failed to report any improvement. Pottenger (72) advocated both somatovisceral and viscerosomatic reflexes as an explanation for a variety of clinical syndromes and diseases. For example, he studied the reflex effects of tuberculosis in a number of patients and found that it caused various aberrant reflexes resulting in secondary conditions: atrophy of the facial muscles, mucous membrane of the nose, and pharynx (mediated through the vagus and hypoglossal cranial nerves); atrophy of the tongue (also mediated through the vagus and hypoglossal nerves); and atrophy of the larynx (mediated through the laryngeal nerves). He found reflex relationships between the lung and other viscera mediated by the vagus nerve, and he recognized the segmental relationship of sympathetically mediated viscerosomatic and somatovisceral reflexes. In other studies, this recognized medical pathologist and author of *Symptoms of Visceral Disease* noted vagally mediated somatovisceral reflexes that resulted in asthma and bronchitis, and he suggested the possibility of this reflex in pulmonary collapse (acute pulmonary atelectasis) (72–74).

Acidity (Gastric)

From a review of osteopathic experimental studies performed through the early decades of this century, it almost seems that these researchers were trying to conclude that vertebral lesions in animal models can cause practically any one of a number of pathologies of a functional nature.

For example, gastric acidity was the focus of several osteopathic studies (75–77). There is now ample evidence to suggest that somatoautonomic pathways (cutaneovisceral) may certainly affect gastrointestinal tract function (78–82).

Angina Pectoris

Early osteopathic evidence that lesions can affect certain parameters of heart function and circulation is substantiated by more recent findings that somatoautonomic pathways (cutaneovisceral) may affect heart rate by altering vagal activity (66, 79–81, 83–85). In fact, more current evidence indicates that autonomic imbalance plays a strong role in the pathogenesis of spontaneous angina (excluding Prinzmetal's angina) (86). Matoba et al. (86) demonstrated complete relief of chest pain in 13 of 13 patients with angina who had augmented levels of autonomic activity and positive stress testing, by giving calcium antagonists orally. This finding supports the work of Rogers and Rogers (87), who demonstrated improvement in angiographic and electrocardiographic evidence of transient spasm of the coronary arteries—associated with angina pectoris—after osteopathic manipulation. These findings suggested an autonomic role in the pathogenesis of angina, according to these authors (86, 87).

Asthma

Early investigations into the role of vertebral lesions and various pulmonary disorders have been similarly substantiated in part by modern research (19, 66, 68–70, 79–81, 88, 89). For example, research on the mechanisms of allergic asthma and allergic rhinitis indicates a role for autonomic imbalance in the pathogenesis (90). There is a basic defect in patients with asthma that causes increased secretion of pulmonary mast cell mediators (e.g., histamine). This increased secretion leads to an alteration in autonomic activity, in autonomic receptors, or in effector mechanisms. Kaliner et al. (91) demonstrated autoantibodies to β-receptors in 24 patients with seasonal or perennial allergic rhinitis. These patients were found to have β-adrenergic hyporeactivity and cholinergic hypersensitivity. Since β-adrenergic agonists modulate the allergen-induced release of mast cell mediators that produce the inflammatory response, autoantibodies to these receptors would be expected to promote an allergic response. Autonomic activity is not the primary defect, since administration of β-blockers to normal subjects does not make them asthmatic (90). A role for stress and autonomic imbalance (includ-

ing spinal stress from a vertebral lesion), however, could be expected to enhance the allergic response (see Section 4). Either increased cholinergic or α-adrenergic activity or decreased β-adrenergic activity in the smooth muscles of the bronchial airways would be expected to enhance an asthmatic episode (89).

Emotions

The role of somatic sensations in alterating autonomic function has been dramatically demonstrated by Ekman and co-workers (92). They demonstrated that autonomic activity distinguishes between positive and negative emotions and even among different types of negative emotion. Such a powerful role for the autonomic nervous system had not been expected. They found that constructing facial prototypes of emotion, muscle by muscle, resulted in a more powerful autonomic response than the process of reliving past emotions. According to the authors, even biofeedback cannot produce such changes.

Epileptogenic Activity

An animal model of sudden infant death syndrome showed that epileptogenic activity correlated with changes in cardiovascular function and autonomic cardiac neural discharge; before death, an imbalance was found between sympathetic and parasympathetic cardiac neural discharges (see also Chapter 12)(93). Liu et al. demonstrated that whiplash can result in a somatoautonomic effect that causes epileptogenic activity (94). In their study of 16 monkeys subjected to whiplash, nearly all scalp, cortical, and subcortical EEG readings taken 6–8 weeks after trauma were normal. Shortly thereafter, a hippocampal spiking developed, which the authors categorized as a subclinical form of posttraumatic epilepsy (94).

Some syndromes have been briefly reviewed here in which autonomic imbalance has been hypothesized or parasympathetic tone has been said to predominate. However, the largest category of somatoautonomic reflexes said to effect disease (reviewed in the next discussion) involves specifically the somatosympathetic nerves.

SYMPATHICOTONIA

Why would a continuous, excessive discharge of sympathetic activity be such a cornerstone of nearly all somatoautonomic dysfunction? Early in his career, medical physiologist Dr. Arthur C. Guyton became completely convinced that all or almost all essential hypertension resulted from excessive sympathetic activity (95). Only recently has he recognized a genetic renal weakness as an important aspect of essential hypertension. However, he still holds that even a normal kidney, given stress of a sufficient magnitude and applied over a long enough time, might develop permanent changes that could sustain hypertension, even after sympathectomy (95).

Roizen (67) asks why evolution hasn't caused us to discard our sympathetic nervous systems, given our supposedly less survival-oriented lifestyles today and the potential for disease posed by overactive sympathetics.

Obviously the sympathetics play a critical role in the maintenance of a number of bodily functions necessary for survival, not the least of which is regulation of smooth muscle surrounding blood vessels, and including a role in immunocompetence (see Section 4).

One of the most deleterious effects of segmental facilitation occurs when SDF, RDF, or VSC is associated with hyperactive sympathetic function. Korr (66) referred to this as sympathicotonia, stating that this long-term hyperactivity may have general clinical significance as well as specific manifestations, depending upon which organs or tissues receive innervation from the involved sympathetic pathways.

Earlier in this chapter we reviewed the literature regarding a number of models for the development of spinal lesions, as well as neural receptors and spinal pathways which play a role in segmental facilitation. We now turn our attention to some selected areas of

clinical research on the effects of hyperactive sympathetics, specifically to evidence suggesting neural linkage of soma with viscus.

Arteriopathy

Sympathectomy and injuries to the peripheral and autonomic innervating nerves as well as neuroexcitation can enhance the development of arteriosclerosis. Gutstein et al. (96, 97) created experimental arteriosclerosis by stimulating the lesser splanchnic nerve in albino rats and found changes in the lower third of the abdominal aorta. Changes were observed in endothelial morphology, elastica, subendothelial cell proliferation, calcinosis, and in coagulation phenomena in the experimental animals receiving 2500 stimulations over 4 weeks but not in two control groups (96). A tendancy toward thrombosis seems to have been a factor. They noted that neuroexcitation always appears to be accompanied by local vasoconstriction and that it was not possible from their research to determine whether neuropharmacological substances, the physical effects of constriction, or both were responsible for the pathological changes observed.

Cardiovascular-Renal Disorders

Guyton (95) holds that in most persons with essential hypertension, a hereditary defect makes the kidneys susceptible to permanent functional changes. Hence, in some individuals with what he calls fragile kidney syndrome, various types of stresses—such as excessive sympathetic stimulation to the kidney, hormonal imbalance, or excess salt—acting alone or in combination, might alter the "set-point" of the kidney (the kidney–body fluid mechanism for pressure control) to a hypertensive level.

Support for his viewpoint regarding a hereditary defect in sympathetic activity in hypertensives comes from recent research by Ferrara et al. (98); they found that diastolic pressure increased significantly during mental arithmetic in children of hypertensive parents, compared with age- and sex-matched controls. This group also had significantly higher urinary excretion of cat-echolamine. They concluded that initial im-pairment of sympathetic activity is already detectable in young offspring of hyperten-sive patients.

Osteopathic researchers found evidence that spinal lesions were associated with my-ocardial infarction, in a randomized blinded trial (99). Twenty-five patients with con-firmed acute myocardial infarction and 22 without known cardiovascular disease were examined with osteopathic spinal palpation from T1 to T8 for increased firmness, warmth, ropiness, edematous changes, or heavy musculature paraspinally. Significant-ly more palpatory findings were noted, al-most entirely at the T1-T4 levels, in the pa-tients with known cardiovascular disease.

Finally, a sympathetic role for myocardial infarction is evidenced by the current de-bate in anesthesiology regarding the use of β-adrenergic blocking agents to induce chemical sympathectomy as part of overall anesthetic technique (67).

Immunocompetence

Changes in blood chemistry were associ-ated with spinal lesions affecting sympathet-ic tone to blood vessels that supply bone marrow, in early osteopathic research (100, 101). These effects included alteration of lymphocyte count as well as production of immature plasma cells by marrow. DePace and Webber (102) demonstrated that lumbar sympathetic stimulation results in stimula-tion of bone marrow to release reticulocytes and neutrophils. Others (103) had previous-ly shown that autonomic tone can have a neurovascular effect on bone marrow func-tion. Thus, it is not surprising that re-searchers have defined a role for sympathet-ic activity in immunocompetence, including direct innervation of the thymus by the sym-pathetics (see Section 4).

Neurogenic Pulmonary Edema

Severe pulmonary edema, accompanied by vascular congestion, atelectasis, intraalve-olar hemorrhage, and protein-rich fluid ap-pears rapidly after severe injuries to the head or CNS (66). This phenomenon is in-dependent of other pulmonary or cardiac disease and can be produced experimental-ly after head trauma or stimulation of the stellate ganglia (66).

Peptic Ulcer—Pancreatitis

Sympathetic stimulation alters mild, non-lethal, bile-induced pancreatitis to the hem-orrhagic, necrotizing, lethal form associated with vasoconstriction (66). A sympathetic component to peptic ulcers has been simi-larly identified (66).

Reflex Sympathetic Dystrophy

Reflex sympathetic dystrophy (RSD) in-volves a wide variety of similar clinical syn-dromes characterized by varying degrees of pain, autonomic dysfunction, sensory changes, loss of voluntary function, and pri-marily by causalgia (104). First named "causalgia" after the Greek word for burning pain, it was associated with the persistent burning pain and progressive trophic changes seen after gunshot wounds in the limbs of Civil War soldiers (104). More re-cently, it has been termed minor causalgia, Sudeck's atrophy, algodystrophy, acute bone atrophy, reflex neurovascular dystro-phy, shoulder-hand syndrome, posttraumat-ic pain syndrome, posttraumatic dystrophy, traumatic angiospasm, and minor causalgia (66, 104).

While most cases appear first after trau-ma, the initial precipitating event does not have to be severe, it can be a minor strain, sprain, or small cut (104). Pain scores in pa-tients with RSD correlate well with limb vol-ume in the affected extremity (measurement of edema), with joint pain by palpation, and with active range of motion assessment in the affected limb (105).

After surgery for a prolapsed lumbosacral disc, patients with postoperative sciatica have significantly more thermographic ab-normalities in the legs than patients without postoperative sciatica, indicating RSD (106). While there is no direct sympathetic outflow below L2 (so no direct irritation of sympa-thetic fibers by a prolapsing lumbosacral disc would be expected), anastomoses between the rami communicantes of the sympathetic chain and the posterior rami of the lumbar nerves, as well as nerve fiber connections between the IVD and the sympathetic chain, might provide the necessary linkage (106). Aside from physiotherapy and increasing joint range of motion, serial paravertebral sympathetic ganglion blockade is the medically recommended treatment for RSD (104)(see Chapter 9 for chiropractic treatment and RSDs).

Shock

Sympathetic discharge during traumatic shock appears to be a protective mechanism, yet it initiates processes that can be detrimental to survival. Pretreatment of experimental animals with β-adrenergic blocking agents or with sympathectomy protects them from the lethal effects of shock (66).

Type II Diabetes

There is mounting evidence of altered sympathetic activity in type II diabetes (107). Hyperresponsivity to epinephrine seems to be associated with an exaggerated insulin response to phentolamine in certain animals and in diabetic humans, suggesting enhanced sensitivity of α_2-receptors in the pancreas and possibly other sites (107).

Patients with type II diabetes appear to have higher levels of circulating catecholamines than do normal individuals, and elevated levels of endogenous opioid peptides have been found as well (107). According to Surwit and Feinglos (107), interventions to reduce sympathetic nervous system activity should, in theory, be useful in modulating hyperglycemia excursions. Patients with type II diabetes may be extremely sensitive to the effects of psychologic stress, and stress has been shown to precipitate hyperglycemia in several animal models of this disorder. Therefore α_2-blockade and relaxation training may benefit patients with this disorder, according to these researchers (107). This suggests a role for chiropractic intervention may be established as well.

Uterine Disorders

Unexplained obstetrical and gynecological conditions involving disturbances in uterine contractility may be related to abnormal sympathetic hyperactivity (66). Stimulation of the hypogastric nerve inhibited spontaneous uterine contractions in rabbits treated with estrogen and progesterone. This effect was reversed by adrenergic blocking agents; atropine and hexamethonium had no such effect (66).

Visual Disturbances

The protective effect of sympathectomy in experimentally induced trigeminal nerve interruption and in prevention of edema, hemorrhage, and thrombi formation after injection of systemic bacterial endotoxin in rabbits is profound (66). Sympathectomy prevents or suppresses other reactions to endotoxins in other areas of the body as well. Korr (66) feels that further research on the role of sympathetic innervation in glaucoma, uveitis, and iritis is well justified.

Increased sympathetic discharge has received significant attention in the scientific literature and has been only briefly reviewed here. Korr (66) states that one of the most significant aspects of sympathicotonia is that synaptic connections are made which are not normally used. Hence, somatic and visceral structures that are not functionally coupled in any normal bodily activity become linked, only because of the segmental proximity of their innervating neurons. According to Korr (66), this reflex "entanglement" is nonadaptive and harmful to each of the structures involved. Further anecdotal evidence for the linkage of soma with viscus comes from more recent osteopathic observations by Beal (109) and Johnston (110), who reported viscerosomatic reflex activity.

Discussion

While nature does indeed protect us from the effects of falls, accidents, and postures that cause spinal lesions—by organizing the CNS into neuronal pools that weigh groups of patterns, supraspinal pathways, descending inhibition, antidromic discharge, and by other protective mechanisms discussed in this chapter—if an aberrant stimulus is strong enough or is long lasting, adaptive mechanisms fail (39–43). Apparently, when these mechanisms fail, segmental facilitation triggers aberrant somatoautonomic reflexes that may be associated with a number of diverse conditions anecdotally said to respond to CMT (see Chapter 9 for current clinical research on CMT for somatoautonomic and organic syndromes).

Because the CNS involvement is complex, it is very difficult to predict the effect of any particular SDF, RDF, or VSC on autonomic or other function (15–27, 111). Guyton (3, 15) estimated that more than 99% of all the information that the brain receives is discarded as unimportant. The various phenomena described in this chapter function in processing unessential information, but the sympathetic reflexes and other somatic reflexes must certainly be affected to some degree by the somatic afferent bombardment seen in an area of SDF, RDF, or VSC (15–27, 39–43).

Certainly some combination of ischemic events—with subsequent receptor field sensitization such as is predicted by Mense (51)—might lead to the "spinal learning" that osteopathic researchers Patterson et al. observed (39–44). Indeed, many theoreticians suspect a role for endogenous substances released in damaged tissues, including histamine, bradykinin, prostaglandin, as well as for catecholamine. If the essence of SDF is a localized ischemic event, however, the buildup of these noxious substances enhances the development of segmental facilitation. This in turn is the lesion that may be most difficult for the body to overcome; central and peripheral modulation represent the next line of defense, but with repeat postural and/or traumatic strain, these too fail to totally protect the host.

Supraspinal excitation or inhibition is important in determining the response of the various sympathetic preganglionic neurons to the stimulus (12). Stimulus and the involved neuron are factors; hence, the segmental pathway is dominant in stimulating the smooth muscle of the gastrointestinal tract, and the suprasegmental pathway is more powerful in stimulating cardiac vascular and sudomotor neurons (12). Localized stimuli evoke somatosympathetic reflexes that are mediated by spinal reflex pathways, but the supraspinal pathway is favored in reflexes that involve a more generalized stimulus (12). These stimuli influence activity in the various levels of the neuroaxis, which in turn influences the sympathetic preganglionic neuron. Coote (12) has stated that such changes could well lead to altered autonomic motor responses.

Such observations are not entirely new. MacKenzie (112) reported that physicians have frequently used counterirritation in the pit of the stomach to allay vomiting and that retention of urine follows operations involving the skin of the perineum. He identified these "effects of the stimulation of the skin on the viscera" in 1893, before the first chiropractic adjustment was given.

The research reviewed in Chapters 5–7 and 9 as well as in this chapter shows that SDF and RDF are a logical premise from which to build the segmental facilitation hypothesis. Our knowledge of somatoautonomic dysfunction and sympathicotonia is based on a broad body of scientific study and observation.

Sympathicotonia appears to be the most prevalent type of somatoautonomic dysfunction. The role of SDF- or RDF-related facilitation in triggering aberrant somatoautonomic reflexes then appears to offer the most logical explanation for the use of adjustment or CMT for other than pain syndromes (16, 36–39, 66).

Amazingly, Palmer's (2) concept of altered "tone" of the nervous system being the cause of disease then has some support in the current neurophysiologic literature regarding facilitation and sympathicotonia.

Current clinical research on the effect of chiropractic and osteopathic manipulation for certain syndromes said to arise from these reflexes, moreover, appears to confirm these observations, as we shall see in the next chapter.

Summary

A brief review of joint, tendon, muscle, pressure, pain, and other receptors provides an understanding of potential sources of afferent activity that might generate "bombardment" of the dorsal horn necessary to facilitate a spinal segment.

Despite the arrangement of the CNS into a system of neuronal pools that sort and filter unessential information, and other neurophysiologic mechanisms such as descending inhibition, which modulate the incoming data (11, 15), there are a number of reasons why nature may fail to protect us from the effects of spinal lesions when exposed to sufficient postural or traumatic insults (12, 19). Both inflammatory/neurological and noninflammatory/neurological models have been proposed to explain chronic muscle spasm, a subliminal threshold or a state of segmental facilitation which results from SDF/RDF or VSC. Improper setting of muscle spindle gamma motorneuron "gain," endocoid release subsequent to tissue ischemia, and others have been proposed to explain facilitation or the "spinal learning" that occurs as a result of various stressors applied to the spine (36–44).

Once the facilitated segment is established, somatoautonomic imbalance or vagally dominated reflexes might predominate; or sympathicotonia with excessive discharge of sympathetic activity may occur instead, depending upon a number of factors (17–19, 36–38).

At least one anesthesiologist has suggested sympathectomy at birth might resolve a number of often serious disorders, including myocardial ischemia, inflammatory bowel disease, and arthritis (67). What role spinal lesions play in precipitating such deleterious reflexes—and likewise what role chiropractic adjustments play in ameliorating such disorders—remains to be fully established (see Chapter 9).

However, it appears that SDF is capable of initiating segmental facilitation and that certainly this is the most logical explanation for the use of adjustment or CMT for other than pain syndromes (16, 36–44, 66); certainly the segmental facilitation hypothesis is gaining greater acceptance and is based upon a large body of acceptable scientific research.

REFERENCES

1. Korr IM. The spinal cord as organizer of disease processes: some preliminary perspectives. J Am Osteopath Assoc 1976;76:89–99.

2. Palmer DD. Text-book of the science, art and philosophy of chiropractic. Portland, Ore.: Portland Printing House, 1910:18,19.

3. Guyton A. Basic human physiology. Philadelphia: WB Saunders, 1971.

4. Gardner E. Pathways to the cerebral cortex for nerve impulses from joints. Acta Anat [suppl] 1969;56:203–216.

5. Warwick R, Williams P, eds. Gray's anatomy. 35th ed. Philadelphia: WB Saunders, 1973: 784–786.

6. Wyke BD. The neurology of joints: a review of general principles. Clin Rheum Dis 1981; 7:223–239.

7. Giles LGF. Anatomical basis of low back pain. Baltimore: Williams & Wilkins, 1989: 58–64.

8. Novikoff AB, Holtzman E. Cells and organelles. New York: Holt, Rinehart & Winston, 1976.

9. Villee CA, Walker WF, Barnes RD. General zoology. 5th ed. Philadelphia: WB Saunders, 1978:372–374.

10. Burke D, Hagbarth K-E, Lofsedt L. Muscle spindle activity in man during shortening and lengthening contraction. J Physiol 1978; 277:131–142.

11. Singarajah KV. Neurophysiological evidence for manipulative therapeutic principles: involvement of synaptic interactions. Ann Swiss Chiro Assoc 1976;6:143–159.

12. Coote JH. The organization of cardiovascular neurons in the spinal cord. Rev Physiol Biochem Pharmacol 1988;110:147–265.

13. Mense S. Physiology of nociception in muscles. Adv Pain Res Ther 1990;17:67–85.

14. Kumazawa T, Mizumura K. Effects of synthetic substance P on unit discharges of testicular nociceptors of dogs. Brain Res 1979; 170:553–557.

15 Guyton AC. Textbook of medical physiology. 8th ed. Philadelphia: WB Saunders, 1991: 501–505.

16. Haldeman S. Neurophysiology of spinal pain syndromes. In: Haldeman S, ed. Modern developments in the principles and practice of chiropractic. New York: Appleton-Century-Crofts, 1980:119–141.

17. Chung JM, Kenshalo DR, Gerhart KD, Willis WD. Excitation of primate spinothalamic neurons by cutaneous C fiber volleys. J Neurophysiol 1979;42:1354–1369.

18. Schouenborg J, Dickenson A. Long-lasting neuronal activity in rat dorsal horn evoked by impulses in cutaneous C fibres during noxious mechanical stimulation. Brain Res 1988;439:56–63.

19. Coote JH. Somatic sources of afferent input as factors in aberrant autonomic, sensory and motor function. In: Korr IM, ed. The neurobiologic mechanisms in manipulative therapy. New York: Plenum, 1978:91–127.

20. Gardner E. Pathways to the cerebral cortex for nerve impulses from joints. Acta Anat [suppl] 1969;56:203–216.

21. Kajander KC, Giesler GJ Jr. Effects of repeated noxious thermal stimuli on the responses of neurons in the lateral cervical nucleus of cats: evidence for an input from A-nociceptors to the spinocervicothalamic pathway. Brain Res 1987;436:390–395.

22. Sato A, Schmidt RF. Somatosympathetic reflexes: afferent fibers, central pathways, discharge characteristics. Physiol Rev 1973;53: 916–947.

23. Sato A. The somatosympathetic reflexes: their physiological and clinical significance. In: Goldstein M, ed. The research status of spinal manipulative therapy. Washington, D.C.: Government Printing Office, 1975: 163–172.

24. King DW, Green JB. Short latency somatosensory potentials in humans. Electroenceph Clin Neurophysiol 1979;46: 702–708.

25. Goldberg LJ, Yoshio N. Production of primary afferent depolarization in group Ia fibers from the masseter muscle by stimulation of trigeminal cutaneous afferents. Brain Res 1977;134:561–567.

26. Haldeman S. Interactions between the somatic and visceral nervous systems. ACA J Chiropr 1971;5:57–64.

27. Whitwam JG, Kidd C, Fussey IV. Responses in sympathetic nerves of the dog evoked by stimulation of somatic nerves. Brain Res 1979;165:219–233.

28. Corbett JL, et al. Cardiovascular changes associated with skeletal muscle spasm in tetraplegic man. J Physiol 1971;215:381–393.

29. Collins G, Cohen MJ, Naliboff BD, Schandler SL. Comparative analysis of paraspinal and frontalis EMG, heart rate and skin conductance in chronic low back pain patients and normals to various postures and stress. Scand J Rehabil Med 1982;14:39–46.

30. Leach RA, Owens EF Jr, Giesen JM. Correlates of myoelectric activity detected in low back pain patients using hand held post-style surface electromyography. J Manipulative Physiol Ther 1993;16:40–49.

31. Ellestad SM, Nagle RV, Boesler DR, Kilmore MA. Electromyographic and skin resistance responses to osteopathic manipulative treatment for low-back pain. J Am Osteopath Assoc 1988;88:991–997.

32. Burgess PR, Perl ER. Myelinated afferent fibers responding specifically to noxious stimulation of the skin. J Physiol 1967;190: 541–562.

33. Bessou P, Perl ER. Response of cutaneous sensory units with unmyelinated fibers to noxious stimuli. J Neurophysiol 1969;32: 1025–1043.

34. Beacham WS, Perl ER. Background and reflex discharge of sympathetic preganglionic neurones in the spinal cat. J Physiol 1964; 172:400–416.

35. Denslow JS, Korr IM, Krems AD. Quantitative studies of chronic facilitation in human motoneuron pools. Am J Physiol 1947;150: 229–238.

36. Korr IM. Proprioceptors and the behavior of lesioned segments. In: Stark EH, ed. Osteopathic medicine. Acton, Mass.: Publication

Sciences Group, 1975:183–199.

37. Korr IM. Somatic dysfunction, osteopathic manipulative treatment, and the nervous system: a few facts, some theories, many questions. J Am Osteopath Assoc 1986;86: 109–114.

38. Korr IM. Osteopathic research: the needed paradigm shift. J Am Osteopath Assoc 1991; 91:156–171.

39. Patterson MM, Steinmetz JE. Long-lasting alterations of spinal reflexes: a potential basis for somatic dysfunction. Manual Med 1986; 2:38–42.

40. Patterson MM, Bartelt MJ, Johnson ES. Inhibition of persisting rat hindlimb flexion (spinal fixation) by contralateral hindlimb stimulation. Soc Neurosci Abstr 1991;17: 1047.

41. Johnson ES, Bartelt MJ, Johnson DA, Patterson MM. Dose-response effects of δ-amphetamine on persisting hindlimb flexion (spinal fixation) in rats. Soc Neurosci Abstr 1991;17:1047.

42. Bartelt MJ, Johnson ES, Patterson MM. Effects of repeated measures and stimulus interruptions on inducing persisting hindlimb flexion (spinal fixation) in rats. Soc Neurosci Abstr 1991;17:1046.

43. Patterson MM, Bartelt MJ, Johnson EJ, Howe A. Restraint stress increases induced persisting hindlimb flexion (spinal fixation) in rats. J Am Osteopath Assoc 1991;91:905.

44. Steinmetz JE, Beggs AL, Molea D, Patterson MM. Long-term retention of a peripherally induced flexor reflex alteration in rats. Brain Res 1985;327:312–315.

45. Fassbender HG. Der rheumatische schmerz. Med Welt 1980;31:1263–1267.

46. Schmidt RF, Kniffki KD, Schomburg ED. Der einfluss kleinkalibriger muskelafferenzen auf den muskeltonus. In: Bauer HJ, Koella WP, Struppler A, eds. Therapie der spastik. Munchen: Verlag fuer angewandte Wissenschaften, 1981:71–84.

47. Skoglund CR. Neurophysiological aspects on the pathological erector spinae reflex in cases of mechanical pelvic dysfunction. J Manual Med 1989;4:29–30.

48. Simons DG, Hong C-Z. Letter to the editor: the pathological erector spinae reflex, a local twitch response? J Manual Med 1989;4:69.

49. Dvorak J. Neurological and biomechanical aspects of pain. In: Buerger AA, Greenman PE, eds. Approaches to the validation of spinal manipulation. Springfield, Ill.: Charles C Thomas, 1985:241–266.

50. Gatterman MI, Goe DR. Muscle and myofascial pain syndromes. In: Gatterman MI, ed. Chiropractic management of spine related disorders. Baltimore: Williams & Wilkins, 1990:285–329.

51. Mense S. Considerations concerning the neurobiological basis of muscle pain. Can J Physiol Pharmacol 1991;69:610–616.

52. Holloway JA, Keyser GF, Wright LE, Trouth CO. Supraspinal inhibition of dorsal horn cell activity and location of descending pathways in the chicken (Gallus domesticus). Brain Res 1978;145:380–384.

53. Carstens E, Klumpp D, Zimmermann M. Differential inhibition from medial and lateral midbrain of spinal dorsal horn neuronal responses to noxious and nonnoxious cutaneous stimuli in the cat. J Neurophysiol 1980;43:332–342.

54. Carstens E, Bihl H, Irvine DRF, Zimmerman M. Descending inhibition from medial and lateral midbrain of spinal dorsal horn neuronal responses to noxious and nonnoxious cutaneous stimuli in the cat. J Neurophysiol 1981;45:1029–1042.

55. Bossut D, Frenk H, Mayer DJ. Is substance P a primary afferent neurotransmitter for nociceptive input? II. Spinalization does not reduce and intrathecal morphine potentiates behavioral responses to substance P. Brain Res 1988;455:232–239.

56. Frenk H, Bossut D, Mayer DJ. Is substance P a primary afferent neurotransmitter for nociceptive input? III. Valproic acid and chlordiazepoxide decrease behaviors elicited by intrathecal injection of substance P and excitatory compounds. Brain Res 1988;455: 240–246.

57. Bossut D, Frenk H, Mayer DJ. Is substance P a primary afferent neurotransmitter for nociceptive input? IV. 2-amino-5-phosphonovalerate (APV) and [D-Pro^2, D-Trp^{7,9}-substance P exert different effects on behaviors induced by intrathecal substance P, strychnine and kainic acid. Brain Res 1988;455: 247–253.

58. Randic M, Jeftinija S, Urban L, Raspantini C, Folkers K. Effects of substance P analogues on spinal dorsal horn neurons. Peptides 1988;9:651–660.

59. Tiseo PJ, Adler MW, Liu-Chen LY. Differential release of substance P and somatostatin in the rat spinal cord in response to noxious cold and heat; effect of dynorphin A(1–17). J Pharmacol Exp Ther 1990;252:539–545.

60. Jacquin T, Denavit-Saubié M, Champagnat J. Substance P and serotonin mutually reverse their excitatory effects in the rat nucleus tractus solitarius. Brain Res 1989;502: 214–222.

61. Lupa K, Wojcik G, Ozog M, Niechaj A. Spread of the dorsal root potentials in lower lumbar, sacral and upper caudal spinal cord. Eur J Physiol 1979;381:201–207.

62. Curtis DR, Lodge D, Headley PM. Electrical interaction between motoneurons and afferent terminals in cat spinal cord. J Neurophysiol 1979;42:635–641.

63. Calvin WH. Setting the pace and pattern of discharge: Do CNS neurons vary their sensitivity to external inputs via their repetitive firing processes? Fed Proc 1978;37: 2165–2170.

64. Roby-Brami A, Bussel B, Willer JC, LeBars D. An electrophysiological investigation into the pain-relieving effects of heterotopic nociceptive stimuli. Brain 1987;110:1497–1508.

65. Collins WF, Davis BM, Mendell LM. Modulation of EPSP amplitude during high frequency stimulation depends on the correlation between potentiation, depression and facilitation. Brain Res 1988;442:161–165.

66. Korr IM. Sustained sympathicotonia as a factor in disease. In: Korr IM, ed. The neurobiologic mechanisms in manipulative therapy. New York: Plenum, 1978:229–268.

67. Roizen MF. Should we all have a sympathectomy at birth? Or at least preoperatively? Anesthesiology 1988;68:482–484.

68. Ussher NT. Spinal curvatures—visceral disturbances in relation thereto. Calif West Med 1933;38:423–428.

69. Ussher NT. The viscerospinal syndrome—a new concept of visceromotor and sensory changes in relation to deranged spinal structures. Ann Intern Med 1940;54:2057–2090.

70. Wills I, Atsatt RE. The viscerospinal syndrome: a confusing factor in surgical diagnosis. Arch Surg 1934;29:661–668.

71. Murphy W, Wilson PT. A study of the value of osteopathic adjustment of the fourth and fifth thoracic vertebrae in a series of twenty cases of asthmatic bronchitis. Boston Med Surg J 1925;192:440–442.

72. Pottenger FM. Important reflex relationships between the lungs and other viscera. J Thorac Surg 1931;1:75–90.

73. Pottenger FM. The viscerospinal reflex. Calif West Med 1933;38(June).

74. Pottenger FM. Symptoms of visceral disease. St Louis: Mosby, 1953.

75. Burns L. Changes in the gastric juice and the mucosa of guinea pigs with upper thoracic lesions. Still Res Inst Bull 1931;7:27–36.

76. Burns L. Changes in the gastric juice and the stomach wall of guinea pigs with seventh and other lower thoracic lesions. Still Res Inst Bull 1931;7:37–41.

77. Burns L. Immediate effects of certain manipulations upon the secretion of hydrochloric acid. Still Res Inst Bull 1931;7:70–73.

78. Sato A. The somatosympathetic reflexes: their physiological and clinical significance. In: Goldstein M, ed. The research status of spinal manipulative therapy. Washington, D.C.: Government Printing Office, 1975: 163–172.

79. Sato A, Schmidt RF. Somatosympathetic reflexes: afferent fibers, central pathways, discharge characteristics. Phys Rev 1973;53: 916–947.

80. Appenzeller O. Somatoautonomic reflexology—normal and abnormal. In: Korr IM, ed. The neurobiologic mechanisms in manipulative therapy. New York: Plenum, 1978: 179–217.

81. Kiyomi K. Autonomic system reactions caused by excitation of somatic afferents: study of cutaneo-intestinal reflex. In: Korr IM, ed. The neurobiologic mechanisms in manipulative therapy. New York: Plenum, 1978:219–227.

82. Kuntz A, Haselwood LA. Circulatory reactions in the gastrointestinal tract elicited by localized cutaneous stimulation. Am Heart J 1940;20:743–749.

83. Deason J, Doron CL. Some immediate effects of bony lesions on vascular reflexes. Still Res Inst Bull 1916;1:128–132.

84 Wagnon RJ, Sandefur RM, Ratliff CR. Serum aldosterone changes after specific chiroprac-

tic manipulation. Am J Chiro Med 1988;1: 66–70.

85. Norman J, Whitwam JG. The vagal contribution to changes in heart rate evoked by stimulation of cutaneous nerves in the dog. J Physiol 1973;234:89P-90P.

86. Matoba T, Ohkita Y, Chiba M, Toshima H. Noninvasive assessment of the autonomic nervous tone in angina pectoris: an application of digital plethysmography with auditory stimuli. Angiology 1983;34:127–136.

87. Rogers JT, Rogers JC. The role of osteopathic manipulative therapy in the treatment of coronary heart disease. J Am Osteopath Assoc 1976;76:71–81.

88. Miller WD. Treatment of visceral disorders by manipulative therapy. In: Goldstein M, ed. The research status of spinal manipulative therapy. Washington D.C.: Government Printing Office, 1975:295–301.

89. Droste PL, Beckman DL. Pulmonary effects of prolonged sympathetic stimulation. Proc Soc Exp Biol Med 1974;146:352–353.

90. Editors. Autonomic abnormalities in asthma. Lancet 1982;1:1224–1225.

91. Kaliner M, Shelhamer JH, Davis PB, Smith LJ, Venter JC. Autonomic nervous system abnormalities and allergy. Ann Intern Med 1982;96:349–357.

92. Ekman P, Levenson RW, Friesen WV. Autonomic nervous system activity distinguishes among emotions. Science 1983;221: 1208–1210.

93. Schraeder PL, Lathers CM. Cardiac neural discharge and epileptogenic activity in the cat: an animal model for unexplained death. Life Sci 1983;32:1371–1382.

94. Liu YK, Chandran KB, Heath RG, Unterharnscheidt F. Subcortical EEG changes in rhesus monkeys following experimental hyperextension-hyperflexion (whiplash). Spine 1984;9:329–338.

95. Guyton AC. Hypertension a neural disease? Arch Neurol 1988;45:178–179.

96. Gutstein WH, LaTaillade JN, Lewis L. Role of vasoconstriction in experimental arteriosclerosis. Circ Res 1962;10:925–932.

97. Gutstein WH, Harrison J, Parl F, Kiu G, Avitable M. Neural factors contribute to atherogenesis. Science 1978;199:449–451.

98. Ferrara LA, Moscato TS, Pisanti N, Marotta T, Krogh V, et al. Is the sympathetic nervous system altered in children with familial history of arterial hypertension? Cardiology 1988;75:200–205.

99. Nicholas AS, DeBias DA, Ehrenfeuchter W, England KM, England RW, et al. A somatic component to myocardial infarction. J Am Osteopath Assoc 1987;87:123–129.

100. Cherrill K, Whiting LD, Tweed L, Still CE. Costogenic anemia. Still Res Inst Bull 1931;7: 156–166.

101. Cherrill K, Whiting LD, Tweed L, Still CE. Pigments of the blood plasma. Still Res Inst Bull 1931;7:174–179.

102. DePace DM, Webber RH. Electrostimulation and morphologic study of the nerves to the bone marrow of the albino rat. Acta Anat 1975;93:1–18.

103. Kuntz A, Richins C. Innervation of bone marrow. J Comp Neurol 1945;83:213–222.

104. Mandel S, Rothrock RW. Sympathetic dystrophies: recognizing and managing a puzzling group of syndromes. Postgrad Med 1990;87:213–218.

105. Davidoff G, Morey K, Amann M, Stamps J. Pain measurement in reflex sympathetic dystrophy syndrome. Pain 1988;32:27–34.

106. deWeerdt CJ, Journee HL, Hogenesch RI, Beks JWF. Sympathetic dysfunction in patients with persistent pain after prolapsed disc surgery. A thermographic study. Acta Neurochir 1987;89:34–36.

107. Surwit RS, Feinglos MN. Stress and autonomic nervous system in type II diabetes: a hypothesis. Diabetes Care 1988;11:83–85.

108. Varma JS, Smith AN. Neurophysiological dysfunction in young women with intractable constipation. Gut 1988;29:963–968.

109. Beal MC. Viscerosomatic reflexes: a review. J Am Osteopath Assoc 1985;85:786–801.

110. Johnston WL. Segmental definition: III. Definitive basis for distinguishing somatic findings of visceral reflex origin. J Am Osteopath Assoc 1988;88:347–353.

111. Bawa P, McKenzie DC. Contribution of joint and cutaneous afferents to longer-latency reflexes in man. Brain Res 1981;185–189.

112. MacKenzie J. Some points bearing on the association of sensory disorders and visceral disease. Brain 1893;16:321–354.

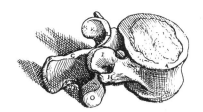

Chapter 9

Clinical Aspects of Spinal Dysfunction

*E*arly evidence suggests that joint dysfunction may involve a locked, entrapped, or pathological meniscus; abnormal paraspinal muscle function; and/or abnormal biochemical processes within the synovial joint, as we saw in Chapters 5 and 8. Moreover, as we shall see in the next section (see Chapter 10, Section 3), progression of spinal dysfunction leads to degenerative processes that predispose joints to subluxation. It is understandable then that chiropractic researchers—faced with mixed findings regarding reliability of chiropractic tests of dysfunction or subluxation—have studied the effectiveness of chiropractic manipulative therapy (CMT), using various outcome measures to assess improvement and using blinded tests of CMT effectiveness for various disorders or diseases, even in the absence of a radiographically demonstrable lesion. The present chapter reviews these studies. Later chapters explore spinal dysfunction associated with radiographically demonstrable malalignment or subluxation (see Section 3).

The chapter begins with a synthesis and plan for diagnosis of spinal dysfunction, both regional dysfunction (RDF) and segmental dysfunction (SDF), based upon studies cited in Chapters 6 and 7. While ongoing chiropractic research efforts may yield uni-

form diagnostic guidelines and outcome measurements for CMT in the future, the studies cited here conform to medical diagnostic criteria and generally reflect *medical philosophy* (as opposed to chiropractic or *holistic philosophy*).

The type M (musculoskeletal) disorders discussed are classified according to medical models: entrapment syndromes, mechanical syndromes, and muscular syndromes. Rather than identifying specific spinal dysfunction associated with these disorders, many chiropractic research investigations describe simply the medical disorder or diagnosis and the CMT used to treat it (unfortunately, some chiropractic investigators do not even specify the type of chiropractic technique used in the research). When specific RDF- or SDF-related outcome measures are used in these studies, they are cited. CMT and acute disc syndrome are presented in this chapter; however, progressive degenerative joint disease (with its chronic discal effects) is covered in Section 3.

Type N (neurological) disorders that have been subject to chiropractic investigation are presented next. As with all subject matter in this text, only literature published in peer-reviewed medical or chiropractic science journals or abstracted and presented at a scientific symposium is included (with the ex-

121

ception of research cited for historical interest; in such cases references will be acknowledged accordingly). Some additional type N disorders are discussed as they relate to subluxation in Chapters 11 and 12.

Type O (organic) disorders are covered in this section although they may be more applicable to chronic lesions discussed in the section on vertebral subluxation complex (VSC). However, because many of these conditions appear to respond to CMT whether or not actual subluxation is demonstrated, they are presented here. Remember, improvement in various medically diagnosed disorders after CMT does not prove the existence of VSC, SDF, RDF, nor necessarily of any manipulable lesion. Even when blinded controlled trials demonstrate effectiveness beyond the effects of placebo, these effects may be simply physiological sequelae of CMT (e.g., restoration of circulation or other phenomena that improve homeostasis). When researchers do associate improvement in specific outcome measures of SDF or RDF with improvement in these disorders after CMT, however, those measures are cited.

Finally, a discussion addresses the question, How does chiropractic work?

Diagnosing Spinal Dysfunction

Chiropractic researchers have started investigating reliability, specificity, and sensitivity of a variety of outcome measures clinically associated with the manipulable lesion, VSC, or SDF/RDF (see Chapters 6 and 7). We offer a model for assessment of spinal dysfunction, patterned loosely after the osteopathic model of Johnston (1), yet incorporating recent chiropractic research findings. Such a model could be used to explore the association between improvement in various disorders and improvement in spinal dysfunction. Of course the model must be tested to determine which test or tests best predict manipulative success.

The plan is to first perform a physical assessment, then to clinically scan regions of the spine first, hence the term *regional assessments* (Fig. 9.1). These assessments are tests that identify neuromusculoskeletal dysfunction in an isolated region of the spine (RDF; e.g., cervical, lower cervical, thoracolumbar).

After clinical tests have confirmed dysfunction in a spinal region, *segmental assessments* isolate the specific vertebral level (SDF; e.g., C2/3) that should receive intervention with CMT.

REGIONAL ASSESSMENTS

Chiropractic analysis generally begins with a routine physical examination of the patient. After physical disease and neurological disease are ruled out, mechanical and muscular disorders may be suspected, and regional chiropractic assessments may be made to quantify and qualify the suspected spinal dysfunction (Fig. 9.2). Positive findings based upon regional tests of spinal function would then indicate RDF.

Tests that are not specific to a single spinal segment but which confirm spinal dysfunction in a region include algometry (when applied in a regional scanning fashion: e.g., suboccipital, C5, T1, T6, T10, L3, L5/S1), passive range of motion (PROM: when applied as a regional assessment and not contacting a specific segment while testing), surface electromyography (sampling at one spinal level is considered an assessment of afferent input from several segments both above and below the placement of the electrodes), functional strength assessment (even isolated muscles generally have multiple segmental levels of innervation), thermography (considered to measure thermatomes with overlapping innervation), and other tests (e.g., straight leg raising, foraminal compression, which challenge the function of the spine by region)(see Chapters 6 and 7). Outcome assessments that are regional and/or segmental include back and neck pain questionnaires and pain scales and questionnaires. According to this assessment model, if all regional assessments are negative, the examiner rechecks physical

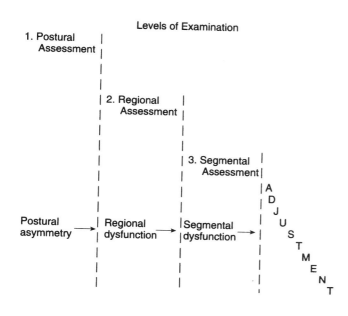

Levels of Examination

Figure 9.1. The plan for chiropractic assessment of spinal dysfunction. An initial postural assessment determines subtle or gross deformities and focuses examination procedures toward regions requiring further study. The second level of assessment is by region (e.g., cervical, dorsolumbar, sacroiliac) and uses specific tests (see text) known to reliably identify regional dysfunction. The third level of assessment includes tests (see text) that isolate specific segments of the spine; when positive, these identify segmental dysfunction amenable to chiropractic adjustment. (Adapted from: Johnston WL. Inter-rater reliability in the selection of manipulable patients. In: Buerger AA, Greenman PE, eds. Empirical approaches to the validation of spinal manipulation. Springfield, Ill.: Charles C Thomas, 1985:106–118.)

findings, orders additional laboratory tests or imaging, or makes a referral for additional examination (Fig. 9.1).

Algometry

As we saw in Chapters 6 and 7, a number of researchers have tried to establish normative values for the regional tests (Table 9.1). For example, normative data for pressure-pain threshold (PPT) has been established for a number of paraspinal and extraspinal sites that indicate myofascial pain (2, 3). PPTs significantly improve after trigger point injections and after manipulation (4, 5). Moreover, since diminished PPT at a muscle site probably reflects altered afferent responses from any one of several spinal levels corresponding to its innervation, used this way, this test should be considered to be a regional assessment for spinal dysfunction (Table 9.2).

Functional Strength Assessment

Another regional assessment, testing of isometric strength, has been receiving widespread attention recently, and tests of erector strength in the cervical and lumbar spine

represent promising approaches toward identification of RDF.

Vernon and co-workers (6) determined that the normal cervical extensor/flexor (E/F) ratio was 0.57, based on testing 40 asymptomatic young adults; Triano and Schultz (7) found an E/F ratio in the lumbar spine of 1.35. Lower cutoffs (1 standard deviation) were established at 2.5 mm Hg/sec for flexion and 4.5 mm Hg/sec for extension in Vernon's study using a modified sphygmomanometer dynamometer. All symptomatic subjects combined yielded an E/F ratio in the cervical spine of 2.01; whiplash patients showed an E/F ratio of 3.01 (6). In symptomatic patients with raw Oswestry scores below 8.5, Triano and Schultz (7) found trunk E/F ratios of 1.08, while E/F ratios were only 0.84 in LBP patients with raw Oswestry scores above 10.5. In addition, poor E/F trunk ratios correlated with loss of flexion/relaxation (F/R) in the lumbar spine at L3 ($p < .05$) (7).

Unfortunately, while a number of studies in the literature refer to improving E/F trunk ratios and "work hardening" to improve functional capacity for work, there are few

Figure 9.2. Proposed algorithm for the assessment of regional and segmental dysfunction (i.e., RDF, SDF). (Adapted from Leach RA. An algorithm for chiropractic management of spinal dysfunction. (In preparation).)

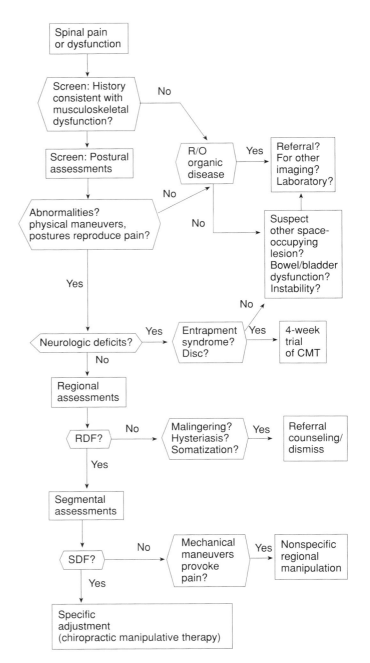

studies of the effect of CMT alone on E/F ratios in symptomatic patients.

Passive Range of Motion

Range of motion is generally assessed using goniometers or such recent technologies as digitized and/or computerized inclinome-

ters. Nansel and co-workers (8, 9) assessed passive range of motion (PROM), using goniometers, in several classic studies that established an association between level and side of cervical chiropractic adjustment and improvement in lateral and rotational cervical asymmetries. Adjustments to the lower

Table 9.1.
Outcome Assessments for Spinal Dysfunction[a]

Regional Assessments	Normative Values
Algometry	<2 kg asymmetry[b]
Electromyography	<3 mV during trunk flex[b]
Functional strength tests	E/F ratio 1.35 lumbar, 0.57 cervical
Range of motion (passive)	<10° asymmetry
Range of motion (active)	(See AMA Guidelines)
Straight leg raise	≥75° without pain
Thermography	≤1°C asymmetry

Segmental Assessments	Normative Values
Algometry	<2 kg asymmetry[b]
Motion palpation	No restricted end feel, w/o pt. perception of stiffness/restriction
Motion radiography	<3 mm translation during flexion/extension

Functional Assessments	Measures
Oswestry LBP Questionnaire	Activities of daily living disability due to lumbar pain/dysfunction
Neck Disability Index	Activities of daily living disability due to cervical and headache pain/dysfunction
Visual Analog Scale	Patient marks intensity of pain on a 10-cm line
McGill Pain Questionnaire	Patient answers questions regarding character and intensity of pain

[a]See text for references.
[b]Absolute minimum normative values also apply.

Table 9.2.
Pressure Pain Threshold (PPT)[a] Normative Values over 4 Sites Associated with the Spine[b]

Muscle	Average Value		84.1% Cutoff[c]	
	Male	Female	Male	Female
Upper trapezius[d]	4.8	4.0	2.9	2.0
Levator scapulae[e]	5.2	4.2	3.6	2.7
Gluteus medius[f]	6.4	5.9	4.3	3.7
Lumbar paraspinals[g]	8.0	5.7	5.6	3.8

[a]Measurements obtained by using a force gauge with 1 cm² plunger head, and rate of 1 kg/sec.
[b]Fischer AA. Pressure threshold meter: its use for quantification of tender spots. Arch Phys Med Rehabil 1986;67:836–838.
[c]The lowest PPT in 84.1% of normal subjects. One standard deviation, below which abnormal PPT is suggested.
[d]Measured approximately 6 cm lateral to C7.
[e]Measured approximately 4 cm lateral to T2.
[f]Measured approximately 2 cm under the posterior superior iliac crest at the level of L5.
[g]Measured 2 cm lateral to L4.

cervical spine on the side of restriction were significantly more effective when lateral flexion restrictions were identified in blinded studies; upper cervical adjustments on the side of restriction were significantly more effective for the correction of rotational asymmetries of more than 10° (see Chap-

ter 6). Their findings were confirmed recently by Tepe and co-workers (10) at the Logan College of Chiropractic.

Although PROM is generally thought to assess a region, general biomechanical principles and this chiropractic research suggest that certain segments thought to play the largest role in a given movement are more likely to be the dysfunctional units involved in motion asymmetry (e.g., cervical lateral flexion restriction is more likely due to lower cervical spinal dysfunction; thus, while we classify PROM as a regional assessment here, it may be more appropriate to think of it as a segmental assessment in some cases).

PROM has been found to be a reliable indicator of spinal dysfunction in osteopathic research as well (11). In contrast with *PROM tests*, in which the examiner physically moves the spinal region through a range of motion, the two-inclinometer method is advised in the *Guides to the Evaluation of Permanent Impairment* for assessing *active range of motion* (i.e., unassisted movement by the patient) (12).

Surface Electromyography

Surface electromyography (SEMG) may be considered to be a regional assessment because multiple segmental inputs are seen for any group of spinal muscles (13). Not only do individual spinal muscles have multiple levels of segmental innervation (it is generally understood that up to three or four segments above and below the site of SEMG paraspinal examination are being sampled), but assessment of the belly of the paraspinal muscles, for example, reveals myoelectric input from several surface muscles, using most standard SEMG equipment (14).

Leach, Owens, and Giesen (15) confirmed earlier research by Triano and Schultz (7) showing that SEMG tests of the lumbar erector spinae muscles in the standing, trunk-flexed position are significantly higher (a phenomenon termed "loss of F/R"; see Chapter 7) in patients with low back pain and correlate significantly with higher patient self-reports of disability (e.g., Oswestry Low Back Pain Questionnaire). Leach, Owens, and Giesen (15) also demonstrated that with hand-held post-style electrodes, loss of F/R in LBP patients correlated with the presence of myofascial trigger points (tender points assessed with algometry) and with tight straight leg raising (Table 9.3). In assessing the discriminability of the procedure, 9 of 10 LBP patients had much more than 3 microvolts of paraspinal activity during full flexion, while 5 of 6 controls had less than 3 microvolts in that same position. It was felt that the test would be a good regional indicator of lumbar spinal dysfunction, since it correlated well with other tests known to respond to manipulative therapy (15). Leach and co-workers assessed a number of predictors of low back pain in 30 consecutive cases of lumbar trauma as well (16). Of five clinical and myoelectric predictors (viz., straight leg raising,

Table 9.3.
Clinical Correlates of Myoelectric Dysfunction (Loss of Relaxation during Trunk Flexion) in the Lumbar Spine Paraspinal Muscles at L3[a]

Correlations[b]	Flex. (Av.) Right[c]	Flex. (Av.) Left
Pressure pain threshold, right	.5940***	.5148**
Pressure pain threshold, left	.3615*	.4821**
Pressure pain threshold, both	.5182**	.4575**
Oswestry disability	.4157*	.3443*
Straight leg raise, right	−.5042**	−.6465****
Straight leg raise, left	−.6204****	−.7427*****

[c] Significance:

*	p ≤.10
**	p ≤.05
***	p ≤.01
****	p ≤.005
*****	p ≤.0001.

[a] Adapted from Leach RA, Owens EF, Giesen M. Clinical correlates of myoelectric asymmetry in patients with acute LBP. J Manipulative Physiol Ther 1993 April (accepted for publication).
[b] Pearson's r.

pressure pain thresholds at L3 paraspinally, T10 minus L3 myoelectric activity (thoracolumbar asymmetry; $T - L/A$), trunk flexion as assessed with the two inclinometer method, and F/R assessed at L3), the two myoelectric indicators were most important in explaining variance in the patient's self-report of pain. Indeed, when the myoelectric measures were combined with data from the Oswestry LBP Questionnaire, 65% of the variance in patient's pain scores was explained (16). Unpublished observations following CMT in these 30 cases revealed highly significant (P <.0005) improvement in patients' self-report of pain, Oswestry disability scores, and lumbar flexion, and significant (P <.001) improvement in pressure pain thresholds at L3. However, data revealed no significant change in $T - L/A$ or in F/R after CMT, although F/R did improve from a pretreatment value of 5.12 microvolts to a posttreatment mean of 3.07 microvolts, which may have been a meaningful clinical change perhaps suppressed by a floor effect (see Chapter 7 for further discussion of postchiropractic SEMG changes). It should be noted that controversy over clinical applications of SEMG in chiropractic has yet to be resolved.

Thermography

In contrast with other outcome measures of SDF, RDF, or VSC, which have been in use for a relatively short time, thermography was first used as an assessment for subluxation by B. J. Palmer in 1924 (see Chapter 4). While Palmer supposed that a "break" in a Neurocalometer reading indicated upper cervical subluxation, more recent evidence supports the use of liquid crystal thermography or computerized infrared thermography as a regional indicator of spinal dysfunction (see Chapter 7). Some researchers argue that thermograms do not correlate well with dermatomal distribution of nerve root signs but instead reveal sympathetic-mediated dermatomal distribution (viz., autonome or thermatome)(18).

While other researchers have argued marginal reliability and poor specificity for thermographic evaluations, Uematsu and co-workers (19)—in a tightly controlled 5-year reliability study of computerized infrared thermography on 90 asymptomatic subjects—found excellent reliability and published normative values (Table 9.4). Feldman and Nickoloff (20) similarly reported excellent symmetry in most of 100 factory workers who were relatively asymptomatic. Paraspinal symmetry was within 0.3°C in 82% of these subjects, and side-to-side variation was less than 1.0°C in 94% of the subjects. The remaining six subjects had persistent asymmetries ranging from 1.0 to 1.6°C.

Post-CMT thermographic changes have been demonstrated in cases of lumbar disc herniation (21). Moreover, thermographic abnormalities have been documented in association with myofascial trigger points thought to be associated with SDF; thermograms made after CMT and after osteopathic manipulative treatment were improved in these cases (see Chapter 7).

Table 9.4.
Paraspinal Temperature Asymmetry in Normal Control Subjects[a]

Region	No. of Cases	Nerve (Dermatome)	δT ($\mp$C)[b]
Cervical	45	Cervical (C3–5)	0.23±0.16
Thoracic	46	Post. cutaneous (T2–12)	0.20±0.17
Lumbar	90	Dorsal div. spinal (T11–L3)	0.22±0.19
Sacral	90	Dorsal div. spinal (S1–S3)	0.28±0.19

[a]Adapted from Uematsu S, Edwin DH, Jankel WR, Kozikowski J, Trattner M. Quantification of thermal asymmetry. Part 1: normal values and reproducibility. J Neurosurg 1988;69:552–555.
[b]Mean ± one standard deviation of temperature difference between left and right sides of the spine tested with computerized infrared thermographic scanners.

Other Tests of Regional Dysfunction

Of course there are other tests that are used in chiropractic practice that may be considered to be indicators of RDF. The list is long and beyond the scope of the present discussion; however, two are used often enough in practice settings that they should be reviewed here. Moreover, there is some scientific research on the use of tests of leg length inequality and straight leg raising that we can draw upon.

The straight leg raising (SLR) test, used in chiropractic and orthopaedic settings, helps distinguish root-level lesions in the lumbar spine (viz., pain worse in the leg) from mechanical lesions of the lower back (viz., pain worse in the back) (22). Breen (22) stated that its reliability and validity have been established beyond question, and certainly no one would question that it has wide-spread acceptance in both medical specialties and chiropractic. Indeed, McCombe and colleagues (23) demonstrated that surgeons and a physiotherapist agree consistently when using the straight leg raising test to determine the onset of pain associated with SLR and when assessing the degree of maximum SLR. In addition, there was moderate to good agreement on the reproduction of back or leg pain using the SLR test ($K = 0.44–0.81$). Examiners also had fairly good agreement on pain during bending and during flexion, on tenderness over bone, flexion range, and lordosis measured in the lumbar spine (23).

A test pioneered by chiropractors, the Derefield pelvic leg check (DPLC), the Derefield-Thompson leg check, and other tests for leg length inequality are widely used in the profession. Some studies have shown marginal interexaminer and marginal to good intraexaminer reliability for these tests (24–26); however, the significance of short leg findings with the patient prone are in question because of a lack of correlation with any consistent post-CMT findings (see also Chapter 6) (27, 28). Moreover, leg length inequality does not correlate well with radiographically demonstrable scoliosis

(29). Thus the status of this test as an indicator of RDF remains in question. It is a phenomenon that remains poorly understood, and its continued clinical use must be discouraged. Indeed, Lawrence (42) concludes that chiropractic leg checks are not at all supported by research.

SEGMENTAL ASSESSMENTS

After a regional survey of the spine has identified RDF, the examiner then further characterizes and isolates the offending lesion. Tests that isolate and/or qualify the suspected spinal lesion include algometry, motion studies, motion palpation, and static palpation. Other tests, such as those for leg length inequality, often include a "challenge" to purportedly identify a specific SDF. In private practice, these tests are used to identify the specific site for the application of CMT. There are apparently no studies indicating which of these tests is used most in practice. However, this author speculates that some or most of these tests are used by nearly all chiropractors.

Algometry

While algometry can be used as part of a regional scan of muscle areas, algometry has also been successfully used to identify specific segmental sites of altered PPT (Table 9.2) (30). PPT improves significantly after CMT in cases of chronic neck pain (5), myofascitis (31), and sacroiliac joint syndrome (32). Moreover, research indicates that diminished PPT correlates with palpable sacroiliac fixations (6).

Both osteopathic and chiropractic studies of the reliability of soft tissue palpation of tender points have yielded encouraging data (33, 34). For example, Keating and co-workers (33) demonstrated marginal to good agreement beyond chance for palpatory pain over osseous structures and in paraspinal soft tissues. Moreover, weak but significant correlations were found between palpatory pain and detection of skin temperature differences (>1.5°F) between adjacent segments and between these findings and visual inspection for segmental abnormality as assessed by a composite joint abnormality index (33).

Hence algometric assessment of PPT and palpatory findings of tenderness and pain in general appear to be promising indicators of SDF. Normative values at some paraspinal sites have been established by Fischer (30) (see Chapter 7; see also Table 9.2).

Motion Palpation

Intraexaminer reliability for assessment of lumbar motion with passive palpatory tests was confirmed by Jull and Bullock (35) in a study of 20 subjects. Over two days this examiner made 580 decisions regarding mobility in the lumbar spine, and complete agreement was seen in 87.5% of the tests, which included flexion, extension, rotation, lateral flexion, and posteroanterior glide. Reliability of motion palpation using their method was confirmed in an interexaminer study of 10 subjects, where correlation coefficients for the different tests varied from 0.86 to 0.94 (35).

Support for these findings is found in the work of chiropractic investigators Nansel and co-workers (8–10) and Vernon and co-workers (6) (see Chapter 6), and while active and passive range of motion assessments have proved disappointing in some interexaminer studies of lumbar mobility (33, 36), other researchers have demonstrated that variation in lumbar mobility (estimated from flexicurve assessments) is best explained by the cumulative effects of age and sex. (Using multiple regression analysis, based on examination of 958 individuals, these variables accounted for one-third of the variation in mobility, while low back pain accounted for only an additional 1% (37).) Based upon their study of 200 asymptomatic subjects, Jull and Bullock (35) agreed that intersegmental lumbar mobility decreases with age, but unlike Burton and co-workers (37), they could not find a gender factor.

Based upon these and similar studies motion palpation, while clearly requiring additional investigation to assess outcome differences between researchers, seems to be a promising indicator of SDF. Jull and Bullock's criterion (35) (positive result is a restricted end feel of a joint corresponding with the patient's perception of stiffness or restriction) or that of Nansel and co-workers (38) (cervical rotational asymmetry or lateral bending asymmetry >10° indicates C2-3 or C5-7 SDF, respectively) may need to be used in clinical studies and practice until other techniques are more completely investigated.

Motion Studies

Radiographic studies of the spine during motion have been accomplished using videofluoroscopy and cineroentgenography, and roentgenography at the end-ranges of spinal motion (i.e., stress views) have used a plain-film x-ray technique available at most chiropractic offices. The primary purpose of these techniques in chiropractic settings is to find "motion disorders" or SDF; a secondary purpose is to rule out serious subluxation or unstable segments that might contraindicate CMT (see Chapters 7 and 10).

Promising techniques for isolating SDF include videofluoroscopic cervical studies for the detection of "fixation." Antos and co-workers (39) demonstrated strong (K = 0.80) and highly significant (P <.0001) agreement between two blinded chiropractors reviewing 48 videotapes of cervical flexion at the C4/5 interspace. During cervical forward flexion, "fixation" was deemed to be present when the spinolaminar junctions did not increase by more than 50% of the distance noted in the neutral position (39).

Stress or motion x-rays are generally deemed more reliable indicators of SDF in the cervical spine than in the lumbar spine, and the Penning (40) and Henderson (41) methods have been found reliable for differentiating hypomobile from normal segments in the cervical spine. Dvorak and co-workers (17) demonstrated a correlation between hypomobile segments in various groups of LBP subjects, as opposed to normal controls. However, other methods of assessing SDF in the lumbar spine have had poor interexaminer reliability (43), and some question using the techniques because of risks of "unnecessary" radiation exposure (44). Generally, medical radiologists agree that more than 3 mm of movement between adjacent segments of the spine during flexion/extension indicates aberrant spinal motion or hypermobility (see also Chapter 10).

Static Palpation

Throughout the chiropractic school clinical curriculum, the student is taught to palpate the patient's spine in prone, seated, and standing positions. Generally, students are taught to look for asymmetry in tissue texture, paraspinal muscle tension, or elasticity and to judge tenderness by the patient's verbal and nonverbal responses. Perhaps surprising to some, good to strong inter- and intraexaminer reliability has been demonstrated for soft tissue palpation of SDF in both osteopathic and chiropractic blinded studies of static palpation.

Keating and co-workers (45) demonstrated marginal to good agreement between chiropractic clinicians in palpatory pain over osseous structures and in paraspinal soft tissues. Johnston and co-workers (46) found absolute agreement between five osteopathic clinicians ranged from 79 to 86% for detecting segmental differences in deep muscular tension in 30 subjects at four marked and 10 unmarked spinal sites (positive finding was bilateral increased dullness/decreased rebound when paraspinal muscles were tapped deeply with the examiner's fingertips while the patient was standing).

Beal and Kleiber (47) demonstrated SDF using tissue texture assessments and motion assessments in patients with coronary artery disease and in controls. These SDF signs were present in the T1-T5 region on the left in most patients with coronary artery disease but not in the controls. Sensitivity of the test was 92%, specificity was 30%; predictive value of a positive test was 82%, and predictive value for a negative test was 57%.

Similar techniques of static palpation were combined with thermographic findings in a study of the T9–T12 region in pa-

tients with renal disease (48). Control groups included hypertensive and normotensive subjects without a history of renal disease. A significantly higher incidence of SDF was found in blinded assessments in the patients with renal disease only. These studies suggest that static palpation of abnormal muscle tension and palpable pain over muscle and bone are reliable indicators of SDF when used by trained clinicians.

Other Tests of SDF

Some specific tests of SDF associated with different chiropractic methods have received scrutiny recently. Initial investigations of inter- and intraexaminer reliability for diagnostic tests associated with chiropractic methods have been conducted for Sacro-Occipital technique (S.O.T.), Activator technique, and Toftness technique.

Gemmell and co-workers (49) showed poor interexaminer reliability for use of the Toftness radiation detector purported to detect SDF or spinal lesions. Similarly, Leboeuf (50) found generally poor interexaminer and poor to excellent intraexaminer reliability for specific S.O.T. diagnostic tests of spinal dysfunction.

In contrast, Youngquist and co-workers (25) demonstrated that an isolation test, used in conjunction with a prone leg length inequality test, for the identification of upper cervical subluxation (i.e., SDF) was repeatable and reliable. Interexaminer reliability for two groups of patients and two examiners was good and significant ($K = 0.52$, $p < .01$ and $K = 0.55$, $p < .001$). This test, however, remains to be correlated with other clinical indicators of upper cervical SDF.

Other tests used in chiropractic practice and by practitioners of manual manipulation include Mennell's sign, diminished hip flexion force, and Patrick's sign used to diagnose sacroiliac joint dysfunction. Poor agreement between these tests was found by a blinded examiner in patients with radiologically verified ankylosing spondylitis and verified sacroiliac inflammatory pathology (51).

A number of other tests probably remain in limited use, despite the lack of any research on their reliability. Until these diagnostic tests receive the attention of chiropractic researchers, clinicians should use them guardedly.

Summary: Diagnosing Spinal Dysfunction

The model for diagnosis of spinal dysfunction presented in this section is based loosely upon the work of Johnston (1) and studies by chiropractic and osteopathic investigators (Fig. 9.1). After pathological and nonmechanical lesions of the spine have been ruled out, examination begins with regional assessments, or tests that identify dysfunction in one or more segments within a region of the spine (Table 9.1). Once RDF has been identified, segmental assessments, or tests of SDF, are used to isolate the level of dysfunction (Fig. 9.2). It is not yet fully known which tests will best correlate with manipulative efficacy, although algometry, certain aspects of static palpation, certain types of motion palpation, and goniometric assessment of passive end range of motion asymmetries appear to hold promise for the chiropractic clinician.

CMT and Type M Disorders

Many researchers concede that the basic causes of back pain remain an enigma despite years of research at a cost in the millions. However, there is some consensus that certain indicators and signs are helpful and that broad categories are useful in the diagnostic process (52). For purposes of discussion, we will categorize research on efficacy of CMT by etiology. Type M (musculoskeletal) disorders are categorized as related to nerve (or root) entrapment, mechanical (related to joint dysfunction), related to muscular derangement, or undifferentiated. The effectiveness of CMT in treating degenerative disc disease is discussed in Chapter 10.

Any categorization of musculoskeletal syndromes is difficult because there is interplay of all spinal structures, and probably multiple components are at work in any given disorder. Nevertheless, this system remains useful, and the chiropractor should be aware that SDF most likely fits into this medical model under the subheading of "myofascitis" if one favors the muscular component, or under the subheading of "facet syndrome" if one favors the mechanical component. Similarly, RDF might be described medically as a region of myofascitis.

Setting these limitations and *medical orientation* aside, we will probe the research on effectiveness of CMT for these medically differentiated and undifferentiated disorders. In the final analysis, we are really evaluating CMT for groups of patients with certain types of symptoms and signs, because true causes remain obscure in many cases.

ENTRAPMENT SYNDROMES

Any cause of nerve root or nerve compression might be considered in this category. Space-occupying lesions of the spinal canal and intervertebral foramen are generally considered to be the most likely causes of true nerve entrapment, although entrapment occurs at many extraspinal sites as well. This discussion focuses primarily on disc syndrome as a lesion often amenable to CMT, although some evidence on other entrapment syndromes and CMT is presented as well.

Central Spinal Stenosis

Spinal stenosis can result from space-occupying lesions within the canal or intervertebral foramen. These disorders are thought to more commonly include central disc herniations and ossification of the posterior longitudinal ligament (OPLL). Seichi and coworkers (53) showed that development of cervical OPLL is associated with decreased intestinal calcium absorption, in a prospective study of 39 patients followed for 6 years. However, laminoplasty successfully controls progression of this disorder (53, 54), and surgical decompression is generally the medical treatment of choice.

In contrast Kirkaldy-Willis and Cassidy (55) reported on 11 patients with diagnosed central spinal stenosis who were unfit for surgery, had radiculopathy, and who reported to the orthopaedic hospital with leg pain. All of the patients were totally disabled with chronic pain and received two or three weeks of daily CMT (viz., side-posture lumbar high-velocity, low-amplitude thrust adjustments). While 46% experienced no significant improvement in clinical signs or symptoms, 54% had some significant improvement, including 18% who were pain free and back to work at 7 months follow-up. These patients had been on government disability, and their average duration of pain prior to chiropractic was 16.9 years. These researchers reject the idea that improvement after CMT is due to realignment of the spine; they hypothesize that results are due to either pain modulation based upon afferent stimulation or the breakup of fibrous adhesions about the chronically injured segments. That even a small number of patients with central stenosis could avoid surgery by receiving CMT is a significant finding that warrants further research (56).

Potter (57) reports a case of CT-confirmed central stenosis with lateral recess stenosis at L5/S1 responding to CMT; indeed the patient had failed back surgery and had back and left leg pain, with hypesthesia of S1 dermatome; nevertheless, a single adjustment brought "bizarre" sustained relief. In some cases CMT offers manual decompression of central stenosis, apparently via reduction in local ischemia and mechanical compression to chronically irritated nerve roots.

Intervertebral Disc Syndrome

A wealth of data accumulating on the role of CMT in the management of disc syndrome is well beyond the scope of this present work. However, a brief survey is certainly in order. The topic is important because of the high incidence of the disorder in the population, primarily in those 25–45 years of age (58). Major risk factors include frequent lifting more than 25 pounds (especially while twisting), cigarette smoking, exposure to whole body vibration (including operating motor vehicles), and narrow spinal canals (58).

Several important medical studies documented improvement in disc syndrome after various forms of spinal manipulation, generally of the side-posture rotational type. Matthews and Yates (59) demonstrated improvement after manipulation in epidurographic defects as well as symptomatic and clinical improvement in cases of lumbar disc prolapse. Nwuga (60) investigated 51 female patients with prolapsed lumbar intervertebral disc, confirmed by myelograms and electrodiagnosis, and clinical signs of low back pain coupled with radicular pain or numbness unilaterally. Only patients with a pain onset of less than 2 weeks prior to entrance and who had received no prior treatment were allowed in the study. Conventional treatment included shortwave diathermy and gentle pelvic tilt exercises combined with home care recommendations for 25 subjects. Lumbar oscillatory rotation was applied to the remaining 26 subjects. This form of manipulation involves contact on "the upper half of the buttocks in a push-relax sequence to the point of pain" (60). The manipulator's other hand contacts the patient's uppermost shoulder for stabilization. This is consistent with standard side-posture chiropractic low back adjusting procedure except instead of a high-velocity thrust, the manipulator rotates the pelvis to the point of pain only. This procedure (probably more analogous to *mobilization*) resulted in significant improvement in lumbar flexion and extension, lateral flexion, rotation of the trunk, and straight leg raising in the group receiving rotational manipulation over the group receiving conventional medical treatment, in blinded assessments.

In one of the larger observational studies to date, Yefu and co-workers (61) reported on reduction in lumbar disc prolapse in 1455 cases after traction and manipulation. Ellenberg et al. (62) and others (63) have presented case studies of lumbar disc herniation, indicating improvement in neurological and clinical/symptomatic signs after conservative treatments *whether or not* follow-up CT scans or MRI reveal significant discal reductions.

These medical findings are consistent with those of chiropractic investigators and joint chiropractic/medical teams. Quon et al. (64) report on an enormous centrally herniated L4/L5 disc treated with daily side-posture rotational chiropractic adjustments directed toward L4/L5 and L5/S1. Significant improvement in leg pain was seen within 2 weeks, and a follow-up 3 months after treatment ended revealed only mild calf pain reproducible at 60° of straight leg raising. Follow-up CT scan at that time revealed no change in the appearance of the central herniation, despite almost complete symptomatic and clinical recovery.

Similarly, Richards et al. (65) reported two cases of sciatic neuropathy associated with CT-confirmed disc herniations that responded symptomatically and clinically to low-force specific chiropractic adjustments (Activator technique) and high-voltage galvanic current, exercise, and pelvic blocking. In one case, CT examination after 39 treatments, 5 months from presentation, revealed complete reduction of a centrally herniated (4 mm diffuse, to right of midline) L4/L5 disc that had been observed initially with *multiplanar data imaging* (MPDI) CT. In another case, multiple disc herniations at L3/4 (4 mm central annular bulge) and at L4/5 (10 mm midcentral herniation without fragmentation) were documented initially with MPDI CT examination, which corroborated clinical signs of neurological loss. After 49 treatments and 10 months (she had been back to work for 6 months), all signs and symptoms were resolved, which of course may have been due to natural remission. One year after initial presentation, MPDI showed that a 4 mm diffuse central bulging at L3/4 was still present, while the herniation at L4/5 was reduced to 7 mm and had shifted away from the involved nerve root, according to the radiologist's report.

Perhaps the most dramatic chiropractic evidence to date is an observational report by Fonti and Lynch (66) on 3136 patients with apparently mildly herniated lumbosacral discs and lumbosciatalgia. Subjects with serious herniation were not deemed candidates for chiropractic, but these 2260 men and 876 women had all failed to gain appreciable improvement with pharmacotherapy and/or physiotherapy, and after examination revealed milder clinical signs, they received 15 consecutive sessions of CMT (undescribed technique) followed by mechanical traction. Fifteen additional sessions were performed at 15- or 30-day intervals, and orthopaedic examination was performed at the end of initial treatment, after 6 months, after 1 year, and after 2 years, at the Traumatologic and Orthopedic Hospital in Palermo, Italy. Examinations revealed that 1580 (50.4%) had complete resolution of painful relapses and complete resolution of Lasègue's sign after 3 years. An additional 1080 patients were defined as having a "good" response to treatment (i.e., only occasional relapses, which receded after subsequent treatment with no lasting neurological signs). Only 476 (15.2%) patients failed to see significant improvement in symptomatology, and these patients generally failed to comply with treatment prescriptions.

Fewer studies are available regarding CMT as an intervention for cervical disc herniation. One recent study, however, suggests that CMT is effective for "vertebrogenic" type cervical disc herniations (viz., neck and arm pain reflected in autonomic referred patterns as opposed to dermatomal distribution)(67). Twelve patients with MRI-confirmed cervical disc herniations (posterocentral or paracentral without nerve root compression) and infrared thermography (IRT)–documented nerve fiber dysfunction received an average of 5 to 6 months of cervical traction, cryotherapy, electrogalvanic stimulation, and CMT. They had all displayed typical signs and symptoms of cervical disc syndrome, with documented neurological deficits but without cord or extramedullary signs. Significant clinical and symptomatic improvement was seen after 30 days to 10 months. Most patients had totally symmetrical posttreatment thermograms; prior to CMT, an average of four areas of thermal asymmetry was seen in each case (e.g., lateral arm, anterior forearm,). The rest of the patients had only one area of post-CMT thermal asymmetry. The author concluded that IRT is useful in documenting thermatomal autonomic dysfunction associated with cervical disc herniation and as an aid to monitoring clinical improvement after CMT (67).

The chiropractic technique of choice for disc syndrome is under debate. Cox (68) has extensively researched correction of disc herniation using flexion-distraction, has advocated use of specialized tables for this purpose, and has developed a new method of calculating discal reduction. Others have demonstrated success combining flexion-distraction with rotational manipulation and extension mobilization (69). Still others advocate rotational or side-posture high-velocity, low-amplitude adjusting (55, 64, 70). Despite the interesting chiropractic debate (70, 71), recent medical research suggests that 80–90% of patients with lumbar disc herniations recover with conservative treatment (72, 73) and that there is no difference in outcome or costs in treating patients conservatively or with surgical intervention (74). Moreover, the only randomized controlled trial (RCT) demonstrated that rotational manipulation was superior to a regimen of heat, exercise, and postural education (60). There are no comparative RCTs of chiropractic flexion-distraction.

Nerve Root Syndromes

Kirkaldy-Willis and Cassidy (55) reported on 60 patients with nerve root entrapment syndrome. In their prospective trial, after CMT (side-posture adjustments), 50% of patients—with a 7-year history of low back and leg pain with total work disability—had returned to work by 14 months of follow-up. Similarly, five additional patients with both nerve root entrapment and lumbar instability saw significant improvement after CMT and were able to return to work (aver-age follow-up, 12.6 months; average duration of pain before CMT, 11.5 years).

Rossi, Martini, and Hornbeck (75) demonstrated improvement in *somatosensory evoked potentials* (SEPs) in peroneal and median nerves of patients with *lumbosciatalgias* and *cervicobrachialgias*, respectively, after an average of 20 sessions of CMT. That at least two-point discrimination is influenced by chiropractic adjustments was similarly demonstrated by Cleveland (76). These data suggest sensory and motor functions are affected by CMT.

Adams (77) presented a case report of a patient with numbness in both hands, neck pain, and loss of grip strength. Cervical hypolordosis was visualized, along with C5/6 congenital blocked vertebrae, retrolisthesis of C3 on C4, and atlantodental arthrosis on cervical x-rays. Positive findings of *Adson's test* (diminished right radial pulse with rotation and extension of the neck), diminished sensation in the C6 dermatome, and diminished biceps and brachioradialis reflexes led to the diagnosis of cervicobrachialgias probably associated with *thoracic outlet syndrome*. After the first adjustment, improved deep tendon reflexes were confirmed by an intern and a clinician. After a second session of CMT, changes were noted in the perception of sharp and dull sensation in the C6 dermatome. Improvements were maintained, and after 4 weeks of adjustments, improvement in subjective pain was recorded using the McGill Pain Questionnaire. While this case report is typical of many clinical experiences this author has seen in 14 years of practice, few chiropractic studies are available on this subject, although numerous studies using physiotherapeutic mobilization and other conservative therapies have been cited in the literature (78).

Double crush syndrome has been reported to respond to chiropractic intervention as well (79). Thus, rather than searching for a single cause to explain a patient's symptom complex, the clinician is encouraged to search for more than one source of nerve entrapment. Mariano et al. (79) present a case of concomitant cervical radiculopathy and carpal tunnel syndrome that responded satisfactorily to CMT, ultrasound, electrical nerve stimulation, traction, and a wrist splint.

RAND researchers, reviewing scientific literature on manipulation for low back and leg pain syndromes, concluded that generally there is more consensus for manipulative intervention in cases with few or no neurological deficits (80). (See also type N disorders later this chapter.)

MECHANICAL SYNDROMES

A number of etiologic classifications of low back and other joint pains are accorded to mechanical disorders. Most of these have received attention in both chiropractic and medical literature and are considered treatable with conservative or nonsurgical interventions. The following is a sample of some that have received attention in the recent literature.

Adhesive Capsulitis

Frozen shoulder syndrome has been generally considered to be self-limiting, with the natural history suggesting remission in most cases within 2 years, even without treatment (81). Hill and Bogumill (81) followed 15 patients who were nonresponsive to physical therapy for this condition and were work disabled. Within 2.6 months of manipulative intervention, 70% had returned to work, and 100% had significant improvement in shoulder flexion and abduction. The authors felt that manipulation caused a significant change in the natural history for these patients. Even before their observations, chiropractors treated this condition with CMT and have anecdotally reported successes (82).

Facet Syndrome

Facet syndrome (i.e., posterior joint syndrome) has been generally accepted as a primary indicator for CMT for a number of years in both medical and chiropractic literature (83, 84). Helbig and Lee (85) proposed a scoring system to better predict which patients would obtain significant long-term improvement in low back pain after facet joint

injection. Of 100 points possible, scoring is as follows: back pain associated with groin or thigh pain, +30 points; paraspinal tenderness that is localized, +20 points; pain reproduced by extension and rotation, +30 points; radiographic changes including facet imbrication usually associated with degenerative changes, +20 points; and pain below the knee, −10 points. A score greater than 60 points indicates a high probability that pain will be relieved by facet joint injection (or CMT?).

Early attempts at identifying referred pain from facet joint pain include the efforts of Mooney and Robertson (86), who in 1976 used arthrography during facet joint injections in conjunction with pain pattern drawings. While injection of 6% hypertonic saline into the joints caused typical patterns of pain and abnormal myoelectric activity in the hamstring muscle, complete obliteration of the pain and myoelectric abnormalities was achieved in every case with subsequent injection of 2–5 ml of 1% Xylocaine.

More recent studies suggest that relief of facet joint pain after manipulation is not due to an opioid response, since subsequent intravenous injection of 0.4 mg naloxone does not afford equivalent relief (although control subjects subsequently given placebo intravenously had an even poorer response) (87).

While few chiropractic studies using strict diagnostic criteria are available on the effectiveness of CMT for facet syndrome, Cox (68) and others have concluded that a significant portion of patients who respond successfully to CMT in chiropractic practice have this disorder (55, 83, 84) (see also Chapter 5).

Meralgia Paresthetica

Meralgia paresthetica, compression of the lateral femoral cutaneous nerve as it passes under the inguinal ligament, has responded well to CMT in several case reports (88–90). Ferezy (90) reported a case medically diagnosed after electromyography, thermography, and CT scanning were negative and antiinflammatory medications were ineffective.

After four sessions of CMT to correct SDF at the L2–L3 and right sacroiliac joints, the patient reported significant relief of LBP and almost complete alleviation of paresthesias for the first time in 2 years. Sixteen adjustments were administered over a 6-week period before the patient was dismissed without LBP and with only mild residual hypesthesia (90).

Rib Fixation

Bronston and Larson (91) reported a new approach to upper rib fixation mobilization, which they have used when a rotational manipulation is indicated for the upper five ribs at the costosternal articulation. They find that an audible and palpable release accompanies the CMT in cases of dysfunction in these joints, and immediate improvement in pain is appreciated.

Sacroiliac Joint Syndrome

Sacroiliac joint syndrome has received the attention of a number of chiropractic researchers. Gemmell and Jacobson (92) studied the incidence of sacroiliac joint (SIJ) dysfunction in 83 physically fit college students who had been or were currently engaged in varsity sports or activity classes, ages 18 to 26. Blinded examiners assessed history of LBP, SIJ pain, and SIJ function using the modified *Gillet-Liekens method* of motion palpation. The examiner places one thumb over the second sacral tubercle and the other thumb on the posterior superior iliac spine (PSIS) on the side of the joint to be tested, with the subject standing. The subject flexes the knee and hip, bringing the thigh to the abdomen. Normally the ilium rotates posteriorly and inferiorly on the sacrum, with respect to the second sacral tubercle; reduced or absent SI mobility is demonstrated when the thumb on the PSIS moves cephalad or does not move at all. Using this test and blinded historical information, 26.5% of the subjects had a history of LBP, and 19.3% demonstrated either unilateral or bilateral SIJ dysfunction. Males reported a history of LBP less often (23.1%) than females (38.9%), and of individuals in-

dicating LBP, 27.3% were diagnosed as having SIJ dysfunction. No association was found between the incidence of LBP and SIJ syndrome.

Fifty subjects were assessed by two independent chiropractors using both the Gillett motion palpation test and the modified Gillet-Liekens method, and SIJ dysfunction was graded as mild, moderate, or severe in a study by Herzog et al. (93). Thirty-seven met the study criteria and were included: chronic SIJ dysfunction confirmed by both examiners, between the ages of 18 and 50, ambulatory, and not extremely obese. Blinded assessments included Oswestry LBP Questionnaires, visual analog pain scales (VAS), and weekly SIJ assessments. Patients were randomly assigned to back school classes or CMT using side-posture diversified technique. Sixteen patients followed through with up to 10 sessions of CMT, and 13 followed through with up to 10 sessions of back school (viz., exercise and posture training). Gait analysis was tested before and after each session, using a force platform (Kistler, Inc., Winterthur, Switzerland) and six repeat trials. Pain and Oswestry disability ratings were significantly improved in the back school–treated group over those receiving CMT. Oswestry scores dropped from 22 to 14% in the CMT group after treatment, and from 17 to 8% in the group receiving back school sessions. Gillet scores improved equally in both groups, but gait symmetry improved significantly to normal in the group receiving CMT, while back school patients had no significant improvement in gait symmetry after the sessions. The researchers concluded that the greater improvement in pain scores in the back school group may have resulted from the interaction with the physiotherapist during the 30-minute sessions, as opposed to 5-minute sessions in the chiropractor-treated group. They concluded that CMT was more effective than back school in restoring normal gait symmetry in chronic sacroiliac joint patients.

Osterbauer and co-workers (94) treated nine subjects with SIJ syndrome, using an

Activator instrument three times per week for 5 weeks. The patients were between the ages of 25 and 50, of both sexes, and had had predominantly unilateral SIJ pain for more than 6 months. A 1-week pretreatment baseline was used and VAS, PPTs assessed using an algometer, postural sway assessed using a plumb line, and SIJ mobility tests (Gillet) and Oswestry disability scores were recorded. Statistically significant improvement was seen in the number of positive orthopaedic tests in 70% of the subjects, in VAS pain scores (mean score improved from 27 to 14), in PPT over bone (pretreatment, 2.6 kg/cm^2/sec; posttreatment, 3.5 kg/cm^2/sec), and in Oswestry scores (pretreatment, 28% ADL disability; posttreatment, 13% ADL disability). The authors concluded that the suggested improvement in this chronic population warranted further research of CMT for this condition.

Two other studies merit attention. Vernon and colleagues (6) demonstrated correlations between SIJ dysfunction and reduced PPTs in a blinded evaluation (see Chapter 6), and Grimston and co-workers (95) demonstrated in 18 female long-distance runners with SIJ dysfunction, that while CMT (side-posture diversified SIJ adjustment) significantly improved lumbopelvic asymmetry seen on x-ray and while 83% maintained or increased training mileage during care, there was no change or a slight increase in SIJ symptomatology assessed in blinded examinations. In contrast, when individualized exercise regimens were subsequently instituted in these athletes, all reported significant reductions in pain, five reported personal records for 10 km, and two patients reported personal records for marathon runs. Hence, the clinical utility of an initial course of CMT, followed by exercise to aid in neuromuscular reeducation and rehabilitation was emphasized.

Temporomandibular Joint Syndrome

Temporomandibular joint syndrome has received considerable attention in the non-peer-reviewed chiropractic literature, but with rare exception, has not received atten-

tion in the chiropractic scientific literature to date (96–98). This is unfortunate, since chiropractors often treat TMJ disorders with manipulation and/or soft tissue therapies.

Weinberg (96) reviewed the pathoanatomy, history, diagnosis, and treatment of TMJ injuries and the importance of a team approach, including chiropractic and dentistry, in managing the disorder.

Curl (97) describes the Visual Range of Motion Scale, which involves gait analysis and is used to identify aberrant motion of the TMJ. TMJ gait analysis can be used as a screening procedure for head pain patients or whenever TMJ syndrome is suspected. The scale, especially when used in conjunction with compressive, distractive, and other tests, is useful in documenting gait status before and after CMT, in communicating with other health care providers, and in differentiating between different types of TMJ disorders (e.g., helping to rule out an ankylosed articular disc).

Curl (98) also describes manipulation with thrust, traction, and patient assistance for the reduction of closed lock of the TMJ. He states that anecdotal reports of improvement of TMJ syndromes after CMT or other manipulation have been generally described poorly in the literature but that there is good evidence for the effectiveness of manipulative intervention for the disorder, including success rates as high as 72% in one study of TMJ closed lock.

MUSCULAR SYNDROMES

Certainly there is a consensus in the literature that muscular disorders comprise the majority of conditions amenable to CMT, despite the protestations of mechanists and other theorists (99). The reader should refer back to "spinal learning" as a likely cause of segmental facilitation after SDF to gain appreciation for this viewpoint (see Chapter 8). Here we will review some conditions typically associated with "muscle tension" or other muscle-related dysfunction, as they have been reported to respond to CMT. Having stated this, a disclaimer is necessary because of the complicated interactions involved in spinal disorders. Hence, our very first subject, cervicogenic headache, while thought to be related to muscle tension due to stressful postures and trauma to the cervical joints, responds well to percutaneous nerve block of the cervical facets, suggesting a facet (or mechanical) lesion as the primary cause of the muscular disturbance (100). The fact that cervicogenic headache responds well to other nonmanipulative and biofeedback measures demonstrates the difficulty with categorizing spinal disorders causally (101). Nevertheless, our effort to do so will continue unabated.

Cervicogenic Headache

Most researchers appear to favor dysfunction of the upper cervical muscles, tendons, ligaments, joints, and other structures as the primary cause of pain referred to the head in the most common of all headache types, *cervicogenic headache* (CEH) (102). Bogduk (102) holds that only structures innervated by the cervical sympathetics from C1 to C3 can initiate this type of headache. Furthermore, SDF was documented in 11 patients with CEH in a study by Jaeger (103). Significantly more myofascial tender points were documented on the symptomatic side in these patients as well, and trigger point palpation clearly reproduced the headache in 8 of the 11 patients. Five of the 11 subsequently received a course of conservative therapy for SDF and myofascial pain, and 2 years later this subgroup reported significantly less frequent and intense headaches. Typically, the patient suffers from one-sided headaches, precipitated and intensified by mechanical maneuvers (104). A number of patients experience ipsilateral lacrimation, conjunctival injection, lip edema, and visual blurring, and less often phono- and photophobia, nausea, and vomiting. These symptoms respond favorably to biofeedback and blockade of the upper cervical sympathetics, particularly at C2 (100, 104).

Within the past decade, a number of chiropractic investigations have focused on the response of CEH to CMT. Vernon (105) reviewed the literature and found five clinical studies of manipulative intervention for CEH. When manipulation was compared with mobilization, no treatment, and other therapies, it was consistently found to be the most effective treatment. Indeed, successful outcomes were reported in from 75 to 90% of the cases in these investigations, better than with any other treatments.

A type of CEH, *occipital headache*, was the subject of a retrospective evaluation by Droz and Crot (106). Of 10,321 case histories reviewed by an independent evaluator, 332 patients were found to have an entrance complaint of occipital headache. Most of these cases responded well after 5 to 10 chiropractic adjustments on the side of restricted cervical movement. Indeed, 93% reported a reduction in headache intensity and frequency, with 79.5% reporting very good results (viz., only slight pain once per month after chiropractic). Only 5% of these patients reported a worsening of the headache after chiropractic care, and no cases of neurological or spinal accidents such as Wallenburg syndrome were reported.

Currently, a randomized comparative clinical trial of CMT and amitriptyline for CEH is ongoing at the Northwestern College of Chiropractic. Initial findings presented at a recent conference suggest that patients receiving CMT maintain their improvement in reduction of headache pain after CMT is discontinued, while patients receiving amitriptyline revert back to their pretreatment pain scores (107). Moreover, chiropractic-treated patients no longer require over-the-counter (OTC) medications after a trial of CMT, while patients receiving amitriptyline continue to rely on OTC drugs.

Hence, while the profession awaits more studies using careful quantification and qualification of patients suffering from CEH, with more descriptive accounts of the type of CMT used, sufficient data exist to suggest that CMT for patients with this often disabling disorder appears promising and may be a treatment of choice. Of course, chiropractors often consider managing their patients with dietary and stress-management advice as well (108). Such a wholistic approach combined with CMT may afford our patients even greater long-term improvements.

Fibrositis Syndrome (Myofascitis, Fibromyalgia)

Fibrositis is the term used in rheumatology to describe a noninflammatory disorder of the soft tissues that results in tender points in the body (109). Early research associated the presence of numerous tender points at specific sites in the body with a sleep disorder (109). Dolorimetry (algometry, see also pressure pain threshold in Chapter 7 and earlier in this chapter) was used in early research to quantify these points.

Masi and Yunus (110) held that multiple host and environmental factors contribute to fibrositis and that it is seen commonly in patients with concomitant irritable bowel syndrome and tension headache syndrome, as well as with other disorders suggestive of a psychoneurophysiologic etiologic mechanism. Hence, they suggest stressors, noise, injuries and allergens as agents affecting host adaptive mechanisms. Further, nutritional, socioeconomic, and occupational factors might affect the sleep disturbance associated with the syndrome, accounting for remissions and exacerbations apart from the influences of medical intervention. As fatigue and a sleep disturbance are central to the disorder, they suggest that anxiety as a precursor to muscle tension and spasm might begin a cycle causing even more anxiety. Behavioral factors and personality influences are deemed important in this regard as well.

In 1990, the results of a multicenter criteria committee were released, after a prospective blinded investigation involving more than 550 fibrositis patients at multiple clinic and hospital out-patient settings across the U.S. (111). Tender points confined to a specific region and associated with specific muscles were referred to as *myofascitis*, while patients with generalized tender points associated with a sleep disturbance, in the presence of wide-spread pain for at least 3 months, are now classified as having *fibromyalgia*. The study committee adopted specific definitions (Table 9.5) for use in making the diagnosis, and qualified the tender point sites to be used in the examination process. Patients are asked how often they awaken unrested in the morning and how often they feel fatigue throughout

Table 9.5.
American College of Rheumatology 1990 Criteria for the Classification of Fibromyalgia[a]

---

1. History of widespread pain; must have all of the following:
   a. Pain in both sides of the body
   b. Pain above and below the waist
   c. Axial skeletal (cervical, thoracic, lumbar, or anterior chest) pain
2. Pain at 11 of 18 sites (bilateral) using an approximate force of 4 kg. (see Fig. 9.3):
   a. Occiput—at suboccipital muscle insertions
   b. Lower cervical—at anterior aspects of intertransverse spaces at C5–C7
   c. Trapezius—at midpoint of the upper border
   d. Supraspinatous—at origins above scapula spine near medial border
   e. 2nd rib—at second costochondral junctions lateral to junctions on upper surfaces
   f. Lateral epicondyle—2 cm distal to epicondyles
   g. Gluteal—in upper outer quadrants, in anterior fold of muscle
   h. Greater trochanter—posterior to trochanteric prominence
   i. Knees—at medial fat pad proximal to joint line
3. History of widespread pain for at least 3 months. The presence of another disorder does not exclude the diagnosis of fibromyalgia.

---

[a]Adapted from: Wolfe F, Smythe HA, Yunus MB, et al. The American College of Rheumatology 1990 criteria for the classification of fibromyalgia: report of the Multicenter Criteria Committee. Arthritis Rheum 1990;33:160–172.

the day. Before the diagnosis is made, the patient must acknowledge pain in at least 11 of 18 proscribed tender point sites (Fig. 9.3).

Freundlich and Leventhal (112) criticized the use of the study committee's question about refreshing sleep on fibromyalgia patients, suggesting that probably 25% of their patients with fibromyalgia deny having a sleep disorder and say they awaken refreshed. Yet upon further questioning, these

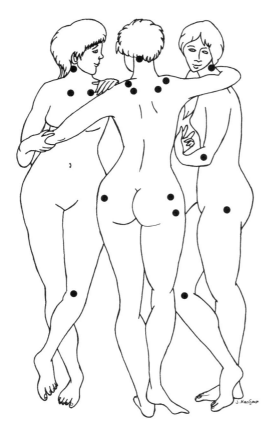

Figure 9.3. Sites for tender point examination, as established by the American College of Rheumatology in 1990, for the classification of fibromyalgia. Early evidence suggests that chiropractic may be more effective than traditional medical treatments for fibromyalgia, a sleep disorder related to widespread joint pains and often associated with posttrauma onset. If 11 or more of these sites are painful with 4 kg of pressure, then the tender point portion of the examination is considered positive. (Adapted from Renault's *The Three Graces.*)

patients admit they are light sleepers who have multiple awakenings at night or otherwise acknowledge that their sleep could be better. Moreover, others have no sleep complaints but have been shown to have alpha wave intrusion on sleep studies. Hence, these authors feel that light sleepers; women with young, nocturnally active children; patients with inflamed joints who can't find a comfortable position in bed; patients taking diuretics who have nocturia; and patients with a spouse who snores loudly are all prone to developing fibromyalgia.

In an unusual twist, the role of chiropractic for treatment of this disorder apparently caught the attention of medical researchers before it received the attention of chiropractic clinicians who have probably been inadvertently treating the syndrome with CMT since the inception of the profession. Hence, when Wolfe (113) studied 81 patients with fibrositis having chronic, generalized musculoskeletal aching or pain, seven or more tender points (of 14 possible), without concomitant disease (other than age-related degenerative joint disease) and 81 age- and sex-matched controls, he might have been surprised to learn that chiropractic care was deemed more successful than physical therapy and seven different pharmacologic therapies in affording patients relief. Dr. Wolfe is the rheumatologist who later chaired the multicenter criteria study committee on fibromyalgia.

In his blinded study, questionnaires indicated that patients with fibrositis received moderate to great improvement 45.9% of the time with chiropractic and some improvement 37.9% of the time; only 16.2% of the time did patients indicate chiropractic care was ineffective. Patients indicated that nonsteroidal antiinflammatory drugs (NSAIDs), narcotics, steroid injections, tranquilizers, antidepressants, cyclobenzaprine, and amitriptyline (low-dose bedtime therapy) were less effective than chiropractic. Moreover, 48.7% of the patients had tried chiropractic, while more than 50% had tried each of the other medications, except tranquilizers. Hence, patients who used chiropractic more than likely had compared it fa-vorably to more than one medication. In his study, only "rest" fared better than chiro-practic care in gaining relief for these pa-tients (113).

Chiropractors have begun discussing fi-bromyalgia, but no case studies or trials have been published to date (114–115). However, based upon Wolfe's initial obser-vations, further research on chiropractic care for patients with fibromyalgia is cer-tainly indicated, and his data suggest that chiropractic may be the treatment of choice for this disorder.

Snapping Hip Syndrome

Myofascial trigger points (TPs) in the ten-sor fascia lata and gluteus medius/minimus muscles were associated with snapping hip and knee pain in a marathon runner in a case presented by Schneider (116). By con-tacting the TPs, Dr. Schneider was able to reproduce lateral thigh to left lateral knee pain in the 32-year-old athlete. The patient had previously reported pain in the hip and lateral knee, especially when running, and a "snapping" noise in his hip joint, especially when running hills. He had been unrespon-sive to antiinflammatory medications, and arthroscopic surgery had been suggested. Double-thumb pressure, gliding across the bellies of the involved muscles, and firm, consistent pressure with the thumb over hard, nodular areas applied for 5–10 sec-onds (viz., Nimmo and Vannerson tech-niques) was applied to the patient, followed by abductor stretching in the side-lying po-sition. Dramatic relief of pain and the "snap-ping" sensation was appreciated after the first treatment. After four treatments, he could do a 20-mile run without pain or snapping, and he was discharged after six sessions.

This case is an example of extraspinal muscle dysfunction treated by nonmanipula-tive technique. Comparison of nonmanipula-tive TP techniques with standard high-veloc-ity low-amplitude controlled thrust CMT should prove interesting for SDF, based upon this report and similar case studies.

Strain/Sprain Injuries

Elsewhere in this chapter, neck and low-er back pain of undifferentiated etiology as it responds to chiropractic care is discussed. Here, our focus is on studies of CMT for acute injury, primarily to the lumbar spine. Indeed, some of the first objective informa-tion regarding the effectiveness of CMT for LBP came from reviewing workers' compen-sation files in various states and comparing worker time loss as a function of disability, and costs of chiropractic care as opposed to medical care for the treatment of lumbar strain/sprain injuries on the job (117). Re-cent estimates are that LBP costs industries in the U.S. $11.1 billion annually in com-pensation costs and time loss from work; therefore, it is a significant socioeconomic as well as medicolegal issue (117).

Recent examples of comparisons be-tween medical, osteopathic, and chiroprac-tic treatment of work-related neck and/or back strain/sprain injuries are found in the current literature and consistently indicate that chiropractic care results in less worker time loss (118–120). In addition, most stud-ies report workers treated by chiropractors incur less total expense than workers treat-ed by medical or osteopathic physicians (118–120).

For example, Johnson, Schultz, and Fer-guson (118) evaluated cost of care and num-ber of days lost due to work-related injury in a postal card survey sent to all Iowa back or neck injury claimants (sprain/strain) on record for 1984. The analysis focused on those workers who lost enough time to qualify for compensation (at least 4 days in Iowa), whose cases were closed, and who received all their care from one health care professional. Of 266 cases treated by D.C.'s, the mean number of compensated work-loss days was at least 2.3 less than for those who were treated by M.D.'s (n = 494; p <.025) and at least 3.8 days less than for those who were treated by osteopaths (n = 102; p <.025). Provider care cost data were incomplete, so an accurate cost comparison was unavailable; however, for the data available, median provider cost was highest for D.C.-treated patients, while mean costs were highest for those who saw M.D.'s. When a change in providers occurred, time loss and cost of care varied widely, but generally when chiropractic was included in the flow of care, worker time loss was reduced, and lower disability compensation and provider costs were incurred.

A study funded by the Foundation for Chiropractic Education and Research and conducted by Wolk (119) reviewed a much larger sample of work-related low back strain/sprain injuries incurred during Florida's fiscal year 1985–1986. Only cases that were closed by April 30, 1987 were included in the results, producing data on 17,198 claimants. In addition, only claimants receiving care from one provider (D.C., D.O., M.D.) and who had a compensable injury (viz., 7 or more work days lost) were included. *All claimants in this study had freedom of choice to select their physicians.* Worker time loss (average days of temporary total disability) was 48.7% longer for nonsurgery M.D.-treated patients than for nonsurgery D.C.-treated patients, and was 51.3% longer for surgery/M.D.-treated patients than for surgery/D.C.-treated patients. Similarly, compensation costs and physician costs were significantly higher in the M.D.-treated groups. For example, nonsurgery M.D.-treated patients incurred $1558 average physician costs, and surgery/M.D.-treated (all M.D.-treated patients combined) patients incurred $1593 average physician costs. In comparison, nonsurgery and surgery/D.C.-treated patients incurred average physician costs of $1003. Another factor strongly influencing total care costs was hospitalization. Since 1 in 2 M.D.-treated patients underwent some hospitalization (regardless of whether surgery was later performed) and since only 1 in 5 chiropractic patients underwent hospitalization (same percentage for patients later receiving surgery as for patients not requiring subsequent surgery), significantly lower insurance expenditures were incurred by chiropractor-treated claimants. In addition, M.D.-treated

patients incurred higher drug and medical supply costs, transportation costs, and miscellaneous costs than D.C.-treated patients, in both surgery and nonsurgery groups. Both groups of claimants, when treated by chiropractors, had just under half the total care cost of both groups of M.D.-treated patients.

Jarvis, Phillips, and Morris (120) reviewed 3063 neck and back injury claims in Utah for 1986. Claimants later requiring surgery were eliminated, as were claimants requiring the services of more than one provider. Costs in the database included physician fees, emergency care, hospital care, drugs, radiographic and laboratory costs, appliances, and physical therapy. Worker time loss was 2.4 days in the D.C.-treated group (1210) and 20.7 days in the M.D.-treated group (1643). Hence total compensation costs were higher in the M.D.-treated group ($668.39) than for D.C.-treated patients ($68.38). While chiropractors gave significantly more treatments (12.9 as opposed to 4.9) and cared for their patients over a longer period of time (54.5 days as opposed to 34.3), physician costs also were significantly lower for D.C.-treated patients (D.C., $527; M.D., 684; p = .009).

Nyiendo (117) used a novel approach to studying M.D.- versus D.C.-treated work-related back injury claimants in Oregon during 1985. Rather than using ICDA diagnosis codes to group patients, as some other studies have done, an independent investigator made a random sampling of 94 D.C.-treated cases and 94 M.D.-treated cases, and evaluated the physician's case notes and copies of daily notes to classify the patients, based on the presence or absence of neurological signs, orthopaedic findings, and referral of pain. Median worker time loss was 9 days for D.C.-treated and 11.5 days for M.D.-treated patients, primarily because a higher proportion of D.C.-treated cases are returned to work with 1 week or less of time loss, regardless of the disorder classification. However, Nyiendo (121) found that in contrast with prior studies, mean total chiropractic care costs were $1712, while mean M.D. total care costs were $1112. Nyiendo explained that differences in care costs were primarily caused by significantly more patients with a history of prior episodes of disabling back pain seeking chiropractic care as opposed to medical care. Indeed, these chronic cases incurred most of the chiropractic care costs. When only patients with no prior history of LBP were compared, D.C. care costs were lower than M.D. care costs.

In summary, chiropractor-treated workers' compensation patients in various studies incur lower total and physician costs, have significantly less time loss, and accumulate lower compensation costs than M.D.-treated claimants (118–120). Chiropractors apparently treat their patients longer and more often to attain these results. They hospitalize their patients less often and may only incur greater physician expense when treating patients with a history of prior disabling back pain (117, 119, 121).

Torticollis

Bolton (122) reviewed medical and chiropractic literature regarding torticollis and concluded that despite efforts to classify this lesion according to etiology, in most cases it results from a cervical spine muscle dystonia. This postural deformity may be caused by congenital, benign paroxysmal, spasmodic, acute discal prolapse, hysterical, and other specific causes such as tumors and infections (122, 123).

Wood (124) outlined chiropractic therapy and management of acute torticollis, emphasizing use of cryotherapy prior to chiropractic adjustment involving either seated diversified technique (the treatment of choice for the author, as it conforms readily to the patient's antalgic posture), prone cervical technique (advantage to this is that the patient is in a non-weight-bearing position), or supine cervical break (if patient can tolerate this position and rest the head comfortably in the doctor's stabilizing hand). Wood (124), Sandoz (125), and others (36, 38) have emphasized that initially the adjustment should be given in the direction offering least resistance and that is least

painful. Most authors feel that manipulative attempts to reduce lateral flexion or extension malpositions are contraindicated in acute torticollis because of the painfulness of the procedure (124, 125). Instead, after adjusting the side of least resistance, the patient is given a soft collar to stabilize the lesion for up to 72 hours, home use of cryotherapy up to 20 minutes per hour is prescribed, and the patient returns for daily adjustments, usually for 3 or 4 days, until the pretorticollis range of motion and posture return (124). Follow-up adjustments every other day are indicated for up to 2 weeks, when tenderness, increased muscle tone, lack of proper passive or active range of motion, and other findings persist (124). Acute torticollis responds well to chiropractic adjusting, according to these anecdotal reports (123–125).

UNCOMPLICATED/COMPLICATED SCIATICA

Studies indicate that the most common form of sciatica (viz., *uncomplicated sciatica*, unrelated to pathology and without accompanying neurological deficit) responds well to manipulative intervention in the form of side-posture, high-velocity low-amplitude thrust technique (55, 80, 126, 127). This disorder favors workers involved with concrete reinforcement (over house painters), workers reporting prior history of low back injury, and workers with a prior history of low back pain (128). A prior history of low back pain was the most powerful prospective predictor of sciatic pain in one study of over 300 workers followed for 5 years. Another predictor was history of stress episodes. Degenerative changes in the lumbar spine seen by radiography were related to sciatic pain in retrospect, as was back muscle strength (128).

Arkuszewski (126) demonstrated significant reductions in time of treatment, improvement in six signs and symptoms (posture, mobility, pain severity, gait, manual examination of the whole spine, and neurological examination), greater ability to continue professional employment, and significantly less worker disability in 50 patients receiving manual treatment (Lewit manipulative technique, muscle energy or postisometric relaxation techniques) than in 50 patients for whom bed rest, 1500 mg aspirin, 6 mg diazepam, massage, and electrical muscle stimulation were prescribed. Fully 84% of these patients had nerve root signs and/or neurological deficits associated with their sciatica.

While RAND researchers favor using CMT primarily for uncomplicated sciaticas, Sandoz (127) reported that even the paretic sciaticas (radicular and pseudoradicular)— probably 10% of all sciaticas demonstrate partial L5 or S1 motor deficits of the foot and leg muscles—involving the S1 neurological level generally respond to conservative measures (fully 90% of cases recover completely within 2 years). The distinction between paresis and paralysis is apparently unclear to some neurosurgeons, and L5 neurological deficits (viz., foot drop, weak toe extensors) require immediate neurosurgical referral if they do not begin to show reduction of deficits and lessening of hypothermia within 10 days of the onset of chiropractic adjustments. Sandoz (127) states that in cases of continuing L5 paresis, the patient should be admitted without additional delay for neurosurgical intervention, usually to repair a herniated L4–5 disc.

Fonti and Lynch (66) demonstrated improvement in fully 85% of 3136 cases of lumbosciatalgia treated with adjustments (see also "Intervertebral Disc Syndrome" above). Moreover, Rossi, Martino, and Hornbeck (75) demonstrated improvement in somatosensory evoked potentials after chiropractic adjustments, and Caruso, LoMonaco, and Pizzetti (129) demonstrated improvement in the EMG H-reflex (ratio Hmax: Mmax) after chiropractic adjustments in cases of lumbosciatalgia as well. Generally, these medical doctors and chiropractors use a preliminary EMG to determine the extent of neurological involvement, refer cases of frank herniation to neurosurgery, and have demonstrated significant differences in H-reflex activity between the limb with sciatica and the healthy limb. Further, good improvement in the H-reflex is seen after chiropractic adjustments in these sciatica cases (129). These findings appear to have been confirmed by more recent research at the National College of Chiropractic and elsewhere (see Chapter 7).

UNDIFFERENTIATED CERVICAL END-RANGE MOTION ASYMMETRIES

Significant improvement is seen in lateral flexion and rotational asymmetries in the cervical spine after side-specific and level-specific chiropractic adjustments in blinded studies (see Chapter 6 and "Regional Assessments," above).

UNDIFFERENTIATED GAIT DISTURBANCES

There is good initial evidence that CMT is effective in correcting gait asymmetries associated with spinal dysfunction and LBP. Dr. Fred Illi explored the effects of chiropractic adjustment on locomotion (130). He used a combination of full-spine upright radiography, static balance (i.e., patient stands on weight scales that register distribution of body weight in four quadrants), and an orthodyn (i.e., patient stands or walks on a platform that is either inclined or level) to assess postchiropractic gait changes. Torsional disturbances, scoliotic deformities, and antalgic postures due to LBP were investigated, and improvements after chiropractic were documented in an overview of his work by Illi and Sandoz (130).

Lorez (131) used the computerized gait-analysis laboratory at the Solbad Rehabilitation Clinic in Rheinfelden, Switzerland, to assess a patient with left sacroiliac joint fixation and pain of 9-weeks duration after trauma. The patient was videographed from both right and left sides while walking on a treadmill at constant speeds of 1.3, 1.5, 2, 4, and 4.5 km/hr before and after a side-posture high-velocity low-amplitude thrust adjustment (viz., anteroinferior direction with slight torque for a left sacral base anterior list), followed by 2 minutes of heavy thumb pressure applied to the left sacrotuberous ligament. The patient was pain-free immediately, and computed data revealed longer steps; diminished foot- and knee-lift in the swing-phase was documented after the single session of CMT. Speed and acceleration maxima of the malleolus marker increased, while those of the knee point decreased. These improvements were confirmed in follow-up computer-assisted tests 1 year later, and the patient continued to be pain free. Gait improvements were especially notable on the right side, suggesting apparently paradoxical improved body stability after correction of the lesioned left side (131).

Recent investigations have shown that LBP patients exhibit significantly more postural sway and keep their center of force more posteriorly than do subjects with healthy backs (132). In addition, LBP patients are significantly less likely to be able to balance on one foot with both eyes closed, according to Byl and Sinnott (132). More subjectively, the 20 LBP subjects were more likely to fulcrum about the hip and back to maintain an erect stance when challenged by imbalance. In contrast, 25 healthy controls maintained their fulcrum for center of force about the ankle.

In another study, eight patients with mild sacroiliac joint pain and dysfunction were monitored for changes in gait while wearing an intertrochanteric support belt during the support phase of gait using a force-platform (133). The gait patterns did not differ significantly with the intertrochanteric support belt in a normal or an abnormal position (placebo, nonsupport position) from their gait patterns without the belt.

Finally, Herzog, Conway, and Willcox (134) compared CMT and physiotherapy as treatments for chronic sacroiliac joint dysfunction and pain. Patients (n = 37) were randomly assigned to receive sacroiliac side-posture thrust technique adjustments or physiotherapy in the form of back school education with stretching and postural exercise sessions. Patients were released from

the study when they had achieved complete recovery (viz. visual analog pain score = 0; Oswestry score <6%; and complete range of motion, as assessed by Gillet motion palpation tests) or after 10 sessions of CMT or physiotherapy. Both groups had significant improvement in pain, Oswestry disability, and mean Gillet motion palpation scores (tests by blinded chiropractors). Physiotherapy-treated patients had significantly less pain and Oswestry disability than did patients receiving CMT; however, CMT-treated patients had significantly greater improvement in Gillet motion palpation scores. Patients were monitored with six gait trials before and after each treatment session. They were required to walk at an average horizontal speed of 1.5 m/sec, and ground reaction force was measured during the stance phase of one step. There was significant improvement in the vertical, mediolateral, and anteroposterior components of ground reaction force measurements in the patients receiving CMT; back school/exercise patients actually fared slightly worse after their last treatment session than after their first. The authors concluded that the objective measures (computerized gait analysis) clearly revealed that CMT-treated patients' gait patterns returned to normal values after care, while back school and exercise administered by a physiotherapist was ineffective. They also concluded that the additional time spent by the physiotherapist (30-min physiotherapy sessions vs. 5-min CMT sessions) might have influenced the responses of the patients to the Oswestry Questionnaire and Visual Analog Pain Scale.

UNDIFFERENTIATED LOW BACK PAIN

A number of studies have favorably compared CMT with physiotherapy, placebo, and medications for the treatment of LBP. RAND researchers reviewing the literature and participating in a controlled panel discussion rated CMT for appropriateness for over 1500 indications relating to LBP (80). In addition, a recent meta-analysis revealed 23 RCTs of the effectiveness of spinal manipulative therapy and 34 mutually exclusive, discrete samples (135). Spinal manipulative therapy was consistently more effective than any of the comparison treatments, including mobilization, for the treatment of low back pain.

It is beyond the scope of this work to detail the individual results of these trials and other investigations of manipulative efficacy in cases of LBP; good references analyze them in some detail (80, 135–137). There is probably more research and justification of chiropractic for the treatment of LBP than for most procedures used in medical practice today (99). However, several studies stand out and will be reviewed here briefly.

Randomized Controlled Trials

Matthews and co-workers (138) studied the effect of rotational side-posture manipulation in 33 acute LBP patients without restriction in straight leg raising (SLR), 132 acute LBP patients with restriction in SLR, and 126 control subjects, in an RCT. Up to 2 weeks of daily manipulations were compared with the effect of infrared heat treatments applied three times per week for 2 weeks in control subjects.

Recovery was about 10% better for manipulated patients without restricted SLR (marginally significant). However, after 2 weeks, 98 of 123 (80%) manipulated patients with restricted SLR had recovered, compared with 56 of 84 (67%) control subjects (P <.05). Using survival statistics, the difference in recovery rates was nearly 30% after 6 days and was highly significant (P <.01). Both sexes responded equally, except that women under age 45 benefitted more from manipulation than did older women and men of all ages (138).

One of the earlier randomized trials and the first offered by chiropractic investigators Waagen and co-workers (139) demonstrated significant improvement in acute LBP for patients receiving CMT (side-posture technique).

In one of the few randomized studies comparing physiotherapeutic mobilization to side-posture manipulative procedures, Had-

ler et al. (140) demonstrated that patients with LBP of less than 2 weeks' duration fared similarly (mobilized patients, n = 13; manipulated patients, n = 13). However, significantly more improvement was seen in manipulated patients with pain of 2–4 weeks' duration. In the first week of treatment, based on the Rowland-Morris Questionnaire, functional impairment improved more (P = .009) and more rapidly (p <.025). Manipulated patients (n = 13) achieved 50% reduction in Rowland-Morris scores 3 days after their first treatment session more often than did patients receiving mobilization (n = 15).

One of the important studies to be released recently apparently inadvertently compared CMT with physiotherapeutic manipulative procedures. When Meade et al. (141) studied the effect of CMT or physiotherapy on 741 patients aged 18 to 65 years with low back pain of mechanical origin in an RCT in Britain, they discovered that most physical therapists and the chiropractors used a form of manipulation. Apparently, physical therapists widely used Cyriax (12%) and Maitland (72%) forms of manipulation or mobilization, while chiropractors administered side-posture high-velocity, low-amplitude thrust adjustments in 99% of their cases. After 2 years, Oswestry disability scores were 7.2% lower in patients treated at one of the 11 chiropractic facilities. Patients received an average of 6.3 physiotherapy treatments or 9.1 chiropractic adjustments. Physiotherapy departments used more exercise and modalities than the chiropractors, who saw their patients for a longer period of time. Surprisingly, patients with chronic or more severe forms of LBP had greater success with CMT (as opposed to physical therapy) than patients with less chronic and more acute pain, where differences between treatment approaches were not as great. Moreover, this reduction in activities of daily living disability remained 3 years after initial care had ended (Oswestry disability at 3 years was 9.6% less in the group receiving CMT) (141).

Assendelft, Bouter, and Kessels (142) took issue with this landmark study on several grounds. For example, subsidiary outcome measures (straight leg raising, lumbar flexion) were made at 6 weeks by a coordinating nurse who was not blinded. These authors reported that not all patients in the Meade et al. (141) study had completed 2 years of care at the time the study was released (a point refuted by Meade (143)), and provided potential statistical weaknesses associated with publishing interim data. Other inaccuracies and problems with interpretation and generalizability were reported as well; however, some may have actually caused an underestimation of the beneficial effect of CMT (142). On balance, Assendelft, Bouter, and Kessels (144) provide information suggesting that despite these limitations, the Meade et al. (141) research was one of the better conducted of 35 RCTs of manipulation for LBP studied in a recent meta-analysis.

Results of the Meade et al. (141) study received publicity and had the public relations value chiropractic associations have so often sought. (This one study was reported by newspapers across the U.S., by magazines, and by network television newsmagazines in the U.S.). However, Koes and co-workers (145) presented a much more efficient comparison of manual manipulation and general practitioner, physiotherapy, and placebo care, in an RCT.

In the Koes et al. (145) trial, 256 patients with chronic (at least 6-weeks' duration) back and neck pain and limitations in range of back or neck motion were randomly assigned to receive either physiotherapy (heat, electrotherapy, ultrasound, or shortwave diathermy at the discretion of the therapist; mean number of sessions = 14.7), manual therapy (mobilization or manipulation carried out by members of the Dutch Society for Manual Therapy and not by physiotherapists; mean number of sessions = 5.4), continued treatment by the general practitioner (GP: analgesics, NSAIDs, advice about posture, home exercises, and other recommendations; mean number of office visits = 1), or placebo treatment (physical examination followed by 10-minute sessions of detuned

shortwave diathermy and detuned ultrasound, twice per week for 6 weeks). Follow-up blinded examinations were performed 3, 6, and 12 weeks after randomization and consisted of a set of spinal motions measured by an inclinometer (Cybex EDI 320) to assess overall physical function. In addition, pain was rated. Of the patients entering the study, 56% reported LBP, 25% complained of neck pain, and 19% complained of both. Mean age was 43, and 52% of the subjects were female. Two separate statistical approaches (one that accounted for a high drop-out rate among patients treated by general practitioner and placebo interventions) both revealed that manual therapy was significantly more effective at 3 weeks than all other treatment approaches. Moreover, at 6 and 12 weeks, the group receiving manual therapy still had significantly higher scores for improvement in physical functioning than GP and placebo groups, but not significantly higher than physiotherapy-treated patients.

Finally, recent RCTs by chiropractic investigators are providing fundamental information about chiropractic adjustment for LBP. For example, Hsieh, Phillips, Adams, and Pope (146) demonstrated that the Roland-Morris Activity Scale was more sensitive to postchiropractic improvement than was the Oswestry questionnaire. Eighty-five patients with LBP of 3 weeks to 6 months' duration received either CMT (hot packs and diversified adjustments to the lumbar and/or sacroiliac joint areas), stroking massage, corset, or transcutaneous muscular stimulation (8 hours/day with weekly follow-ups for 3 weeks). Both CMT and massage groups received 3 weeks of thrice-weekly sessions. Both disability questionnaires revealed significant improvement in patients receiving CMT (compared with massage) after 3 weeks (P = .05). However, the Rowland-Morris instrument also showed significant differences between CMT and TMS groups and between the corset and massage groups.

Endocrine changes after chiropractic care were first proposed by Vernon and co-workers (147) after seeing small but significant rises in beta endorphins after cervical adjusting in 27 asymptomatic males. In an RCT, Sanders and co-workers (148) studied 18 subjects (9 males, ages 22–56, and 9 females, ages 24–48) with acute LBP of less than 2 weeks' duration for changes in pain scores and in plasma beta endorphins before and 5 minutes after a single high-velocity, low-amplitude adjustment at L5/S1, a sham (viz., only light physical touch at L5/S1), or no intervention (control subjects). No significant group differences in plasma beta endorphin levels were seen after the procedures. In contrast, subjects receiving CMT reported statistically significant pain reduction more so than subjects in the control and placebo groups. The authors did speculate that changes in cerebrospinal fluid levels of beta endorphins might occur after CMT, despite the lack of significant changes peripherally.

Other Studies

Valentini (149) profiled 2 years' cases of "lumbar disc syndrome" he had seen in a private chiropractic practice in a retrospective review. Unfortunately, patients with neurological signs were not distinguished from patients with antalgia, limited movement, and positive Lasègue test only. He cited 194 subjects, (118 male, 76 female, av. age 42), who were adjusted using side-posture rotary technique, generally toward the opposite side of the antalgic position, and were given home care instructions and cryotherapy. After an average of 7 adjustments, 90 males and 62 females were asymptomatic for more than 6 months follow-up. An additional 15 males and 4 females had initial success but relapsed within the 6-month follow-up. Of 23 failures, six males and four females required surgery subsequent to the chiropractic intervention. While it is difficult to distinguish from the report whether these patients had undifferentiated low back pain or true disc syndrome, it was, nevertheless, an important retrospective review.

Kirkaldy-Willis and Cassidy (50) observed 54 patients with chronic (av. duration of pain, 5.6 years; av. follow-up, 9.2 months) disabling LBP attributed to the posterior joints; 79% had good to excellent recovery after CMT and could return to work. CMT included high-velocity, low-amplitude thrust technique in the side-posture position.

More improvement in erector spinae muscle strength in low back pain and disc syndromes is seen in patients receiving manual therapy than in patients receiving standard physiotherapy, according to Kinalski, Kuwik, and Pietrzak (150). Since increasing lumbar and hip mobility is more important to relieving chronic low back pain than is an exercise strengthening regimen, it may be that adjustments to the spine allow erector strength to improve faster (151). Indeed, LBP patients receiving flexor exercises do not improve significantly faster than when receiving extensor exercises (152), suggesting that some other factor (e.g., joint locking) must be addressed first.

Muscular imbalances and spinal dysfunction mimicking organ disorders and disease have been the subject of numerous investigators, and undifferentiated LBP can certainly be a source of noxious stimuli triggering somatosomatic and somatoautonomic reflexes (see also Chapters 5 and 8). For example, Lewit (153) discusses the role of the iliopsoas muscle in causing *pseudovisceral* symptoms (gall bladder, pancreas, appendix, etc.) and the quadratus lumborum in simulating kidney pain (viz., *somatovisceral reflexes*). Szlazak and Nansel (154) reviewed 350 studies over 75 years of literature and proposed that noxious stimuli from spinal lesions might mimic a host of visceral diseases; they proposed that CMT might reduce these aberrant reflexes, which were not actually associated with disease.

A number of studies better quantify the characteristics of patients' responses to chiropractic intervention. For example, Triano, Hondras, and McGregor (155) studied 241 patients with acute, subacute, or chronic LBP and found that 1–22 sessions of CMT were needed to achieve maximum results. Chronic complaints took longest to achieve resolution (mean, 8.2 sessions), and thoracic disorders required half the treatment that cervical and lumbar lesions needed before dismissal. In contrast, by grouping patients according to entrapment, mechanical, or muscular pain syndromes, no significant differences in number of sessions was found. All but 25 cases were resolved within 6 weeks. These cases required a mean of 3.8 (range, 1–11) additional treatment sessions.

Other issues in undifferentiated back pain include psychosocial factors and the inability of researchers to identify tests that discriminate a specific lesion. For example, Lee et al. (156) demonstrated that patients who recover from LBP uneventfully have better incomes, report more satisfaction with medical personnel, and had prolonged pain-free periods. In contrast, those with poor work role adjustment and severe pain complaints were identified as immigrants, engaged in heavy manual labor, involved in compensation claims for work-related injuries, manifesting high anxiety and depressive symptoms, with lower incomes, and hostile toward medical personnel. Two of the most important indicators of poor outcome were the patient's conviction that his

or her problem was serious and the feeling that people were not taking the illness seriously. These psychosocial factors have been suggested to explain at least some of the successes doctors of chiropractic have over other medical interventions in cases of undifferentiated LBP, as chiropractors are said to interact with their patients more than their medical counterparts do, offering plausible explanations for their patients' illnesses more often than medical practitioners do, generally (see Appendix A: "Social Theory of Chiropractic").

Finally, some researchers continue to lament the inability of known clinical tests to reliably identify a single spinal lesion responsible for LBP. Hence, despite Haldeman's (157) argument that there does not have to be simply one cause of undifferentiated LBP, Waddell and co-workers (158) investigated physical and behavioral indicators of chronic undifferentiated LBP and found no single underlying dimension to the physical tests entering into the regression model (Table 9.6), leading them to doubt a structural or anatomical basis for physical impairment associated with chronic LBP. They suggest that clinical findings are not related to disease but are due to functional limitation that might relate better to a biopsychosocial model of disability (158).

Table 9.6.
Regression Analysis of LBP Disability[a] (correlations of Rowland-Morris Disability Questionnaire with physical tests conducted on 120 CLBP patients and 70 control subjects) and cutoffs for normal for seven best outcome assessments entering the regression model)

Outcome Measure	Rowland-Morris % Variance Explained	Cutoff (1 SD)
Total flexion	20.9	<87°
Lumbar flexion	18.3	NA
Lateral flexion	11.3	<24°
Sit-up	10.9	<5 sec
Total extension	10.2	<18°
Straight leg raise	9.7	F <71, M <66
Pelvic flexion	9.5	NA
Spinal tenderness	9.0	Positive
Bilateral active SLR	NS	5 sec

[a]Adapted from Waddell G, Somerville D, Henderson L, Newton M. Objective clinical evaluation of physical impairment in chronic low back pain. Spine 1992;17:617–628.

UNDIFFERENTIATED NECK PAIN

Dozens of randomized trials of manipulation for the treatment of undifferentiated lower back pain exist but relatively few for the cervical corollary to this disorder. The paucity of data on manipulation—chiropractic or medical—for cervical syndromes and undifferentiated neck pain seems even more inexplicable given the disability and cost associated with motor vehicle trauma and given the high cost to industry of worker time loss because of "muscle tension headache" in the U.S., especially given early data that suggest chiropractic may be an optimal intervention for such disorders.

Randomized Controlled Trials

Koes and colleagues (145) randomly assigned patients with chronic neck complaints and limited neck motion to receive either manual manipulation (n = 23), physiotherapy (n = 22), placebo therapy (n = 18), or general practitioner care (n = 21). Patients receiving physiotherapy received significantly more treatment sessions during the 12-week study (mean, 14.7) than did patients receiving manual manipulation sessions (mean, 5.4). Most patients in the general practitioner group paid one visit to their doctor (for analgesics and NSAIDs), while placebo-treated patients received physical examination and detuned shortwave diathermy (10 minutes) and detuned ultrasound (10 minutes) two times per week for 6 weeks. Follow-up assessments at 3, 6, and 12 weeks revealed more improved physical functioning and range of motion in the group treated with manual manipulation than in the other groups. Only patients treated with manual manipulation had improved lateral cervical-flexion range of motion during all three follow-up assessments, and physical functioning was most improved in the manual manipulation patients at all three follow-up examinations, based on the intention-to-treat analysis. After 6 weeks, patients had the opportunity to discuss the results of the treatment with their general practitioners and to decide whether to continue, change, or stop the treatment. Contamination at this point occurred mainly in the placebo and GP-treated patients, a considerable number of whom switched at that time from their assigned therapy. Proof of adequate blinding was found by asking the patients after 6 weeks of care whether they thought they received "the treatment which professionals would expect to provide no effect." Half the patients in the GP-treated group, 29% of the placebo-treated patients, 23% of the patients receiving manual therapy, and 7% of the physiotherapy patients answered affirmatively. At all follow-up examinations, the drop-out rate was lowest for those receiving manual therapy, followed by physiotherapy, GP, and placebo-treated patients, respectively. These medical authors concluded that the main difference between treatments occurred at the 3-week assessment, where manually manipulated patients fared significantly better than physiotherapy, placebo, and GP-treated groups.

In a pilot randomized trial of nine neck pain sufferers, (onset, 2 weeks to 8 years; av. <3 months), Vernon and co-workers (5) used assessment of PPT as a clinical outcome measure to distinguish improvement after CMT or oscillatory mobilization. Four tender points were evaluated above, below, contralateral to, and ipsilateral to the site of perceived hypomobility, by a blinded assessor using the Fischer (2–4, 30) method, before and after CMT or the mobilization. Improvement in PPT was 40–55% higher at all four points around the fixation level in the group receiving CMT. In contrast, there was virtually no change in PPT before and after mobilization (F = 26.052, p <.0001). These investigators felt that this robust clinical change after a single cervical adjustment, despite the small number of subjects studied, was clear evidence that manipulation produced immediate and higher increases in PPT surrounding fixation in the cervical spine than sham adjusting (oscillatory mobilization) and argues against small fiber coactivation as the mechanism whereby adjustments bring relief from spinal pain.

Others have found spinal manipulation to be effective for neck pain (159) and for neck pain concomitant with LBP (160). In an open randomized trial, Arkuszewski (160) found that when cervical joint dysfunction (especially atlantooccipital) associated with neck pain was treated with spinal manipulation, improvement in neurological signs associated with LBP was greater in patients also receiving manipulative therapy for their LBP. In contrast, patients with LBP and concomitant neck pain who received spinal manipulation only to their lumbosacral region had less significant long-term improvement.

Other Studies

Leboeuf et al. (161) examined 38 subjects who responded to a newspaper advertisement and fulfilled criteria for *repetitive strain injury* (RSI) of the upper limb. These were randomly assigned to receive either CMT or CMT and soft tissue therapy (i.e., manual massage to tender and tight areas of the neck, shoulder girdle, and upper limbs). Patients were scheduled for twice-weekly sessions for 5 weeks. Patients in both groups had good clinical improvement in pain severity and the frequency of symptoms after care.

Other researchers have investigated epidemiology of cervical spine injuries and conclude that motor vehicle trauma can have serious long-term effects; 1% of soft tissue injuries without fracture/dislocation in Switzerland result in permanent disability, and 4 to 7 years postinjury, nearly one third of patients who did not receive pensions continue to report pain and other complaints (162).

Chiropractic researchers are beginning to focus on the intrinsic parameters of cervical spine adjusting as well. For example, the toggle method of chiropractic adjusting with a magnetic drop headpiece was used to quantitatively assess forces imparted to the cervical spine during CMT, in a study by Kawchuk, Herzog, and Hasler (163). With this technique, they found that two experienced chiropractors used a *mean peak force* of 117.7 newtons (N) with a mean duration

of 101.7 msec (based on three assessments over a 2-week period on one of their patients). The authors state that typical of CMT, much is known or hypothesized about the clinical and physiological effects of adjustments, while little is understood of the intrinsic parameters of CMT. To assess forces generated during CMT, a force-measuring "pad" was inserted between the doctor's contact hand and the previously marked spinal level of the subject. Follow-up study by these investigators on 71 patients, using five different chiropractic techniques (viz., toggle recoil, cervical break, rotary break, Gonstead P-A thrust, and Activator (Reg.TM) thrust) and four separate chiropractors, revealed a peak force range of 62.8 N (Activator (TM) thrust) to 141.7 N (lateral to medial thrust) (164). Normalizing all preload forces to zero, forces ranged from 40.5 N (rotational thrust) to 117.6 N (lateral to medial thrust). No single adjustment force exceeded 210 N. The mean time to peak force ranged from 31.8 msec (Activator (TM) thrust) to 91.9 msec (Gonstead P-A thrust). Their early conclusion was that there is little relationship between force delivered, practitioner mass, and/or patient mass. There are similar force/time characteristics to all chiropractic short-lever, high-velocity thrust techniques checked thus far, having similar *slope profiles* (i.e., the rise in force over time; Fig. 9.4) and stopping at a low force (e.g., Activator (TM) instrument adjusting, rotary break) or at a higher force (e.g., lateral to medial thrust, Gonstead).

Similarly, Triano and Schultz (165) investigated myoelectric responses to chiropractic adjusting technique (cervical break) and compared light and heavy thrust procedures. In general, myoelectric activity in longissimus colli, sternocleidomastoideus, semispinalis capitus, and trapezius muscles increased significantly during manipulation and mildly immediately after CMT. These and ongoing studies to quantify the adjusting procedures are needed to determine which techniques are useful and for which applications. Moreover, these studies will complement outcomes research that further

Figure 9.4. In an effort to quantify the forces generated on the cervical spine during CMT, Kawchuk, Herzog, and Hasler (163) used a force measuring "pad" (EMED Inc., Munich, Germany) placed between the doctor's contact hand and the patient's neck prior to administration of adjustments. The force-time profile shown above was typical of those observed between two doctors adjusting two patients on three occasions. (From Kawchuk GN, Herzog W, Hasler EM. Forces generated during spinal manipulative therapy of the cervical spine: a pilot study. J Manipulative Physiol Ther 1992;15: 275–278. Reprinted by permission.)

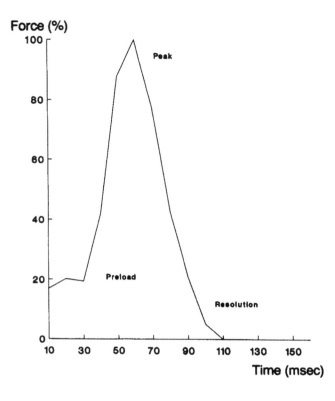

evaluates the effectiveness of CMT for cervical pain trauma and pain syndromes.

CMT and Type N Disorders

While there is no clear consensus regarding the role of CMT for type N (neurological) disorders in general, nor even for lower back and leg pain complicated by minor neurological deficits (166), some of the strongest statements in the classic chiropractic literature are reserved for the effectiveness of chiropractic in these often serious cases. Hence, while RAND researchers were in total agreement that CMT is extremely inappropriate in cases of LBP with any major neurological deficit (e.g., progressive unilateral muscle weakness and/or motor loss documented by repeat examinations prior to CMT)(166), D. D. Palmer (167) claimed that a janitor deaf for 17 years regained his hearing immediately after a single spinal adjustment. Because of a lack of research on the role of CMT in type N disorders, this

subject can be expected to remain controversial.

BARRÉ'S SYNDROME

Eleven patients with Barré's syndrome and concomitant cervical arthrosis were examined before and after cervical CMT for changes in levels of *beta-endorphin* and *calcitonin*, dosed by antiserum A, in an Italian study by medical doctors and chiropractors (168). Luisetto et al. (168) hoped to demonstrate nonclinical changes that might reflect upon hormonal mechanisms associated with CMT. These patients reported, to varying degrees, paresthesias, cervicalgias, cephalgias, vertigo, and tinnitus, along with radiographically confirmed osteoarthritis, and had no prior CMT. After 10 sessions of CMT, paresthesias were partially reduced in 4 patients and totally resolved in the remaining 4. Cervicalgias were unreduced in 1 of 11 patients, partially reduced in 4, and totally resolved in the remaining 6 after CMT. Cephalgia was unresolved in 1 of 10 patients, partially resolved in 5 others, and totally resolved after CMT in the remaining 4. *Vertigo*, initially present in 7 patients, was unchanged after CMT in 1, partially resolved in 3, and totally resolved in the final 3 patients. *Tinnitus* was partially resolved in 1 patient and totally resolved after CMT in the only other patient (168). The researchers found no significant change in plasma beta endorphin levels after 10 sessions of cervical CMT—in agreement with Sanders and colleagues (148)—but there were marked reductions in plasma levels of calcitonin dosed with antiserum A (pretreatment: 290±384 pg/pl SD; posttreatment: 242±396 SD) in 8 of the 11 subjects (p <.02), compared with a reference group. No changes in calcitonin dosed with antiserum B were found before and after CMT compared with a reference group. The authors speculate that since only the immunoreactive form of calcitonin, found in the pituitary and thought to be influenced by pain, was modified by CMT, pain modulation was via an endocrine mechanism (see also Chapter 14).

BELL'S PALSY

While there is no clinically proven treatment for facial nerve paralysis at this time, Palmieri (169) reviewed the literature and offered an algorithm and rationale for chiropractic intervention. Chiropractors have reported significant improvement in the natural course of Bell's palsy after CMT, in anecdotal reports published in trade journals. These reports parallel this author's experiences in private practice. Unfortunately, it is difficult to document success with disorders known to have high rates of spontaneous remission, such as Bell's palsy. Indeed, 86% of patients will recover completely within weeks to 2 to 4 months from the date of onset. This recovery usually occurs within 10 to 21 days of onset of paralysis. Immediate referral for electrodiagnostic testing is advocated within 2 weeks of onset, as patients with 90% or greater loss in amplitude within 10 days have a 50% chance of poor recovery, and referral for surgical consultation may be indicated (169). Otherwise, cranial and cervical adjusting procedures to relieve trigger points in the spine and facial muscles may help the disorder, and stress management procedures may be beneficial (most cases are thought to be viral).

DOWN'S SYNDROME

Some chiropractors claim that CMT is helpful in the management of Down's syndrome according to anecdotal reports, but there is clear evidence that CMT could be potentially fatal if administered to a patient with associated atlantoaxial instability (see Chapter 12) (170, 171). LaFrancis (171) reviewed the available literature and noted that atlantoaxial instability occurs in 15–50% of Down's syndrome cases. (An atlantodental interval (ADI), based on neutral lateral, flexion, and extension cervical x-rays under 3 mm suggests low risk and above 4.5 mm indicates great risk. In addition, any neurological signs attributable to the cervical spine add to the risk of cervical instability.) Despite the lack of any published report of an accident in Down's patients after CMT, LaFrancis recommends light force adjustments such as Nimmo and Activator, when CMT is being contemplated. The role of CMT in Down's cases has yet to be established, but clearly the chiropractor should assume that all Down's syndrome patients have atlantoaxial instability until proven otherwise.

DYSPHAGIA

Although dysphagia is associated with myelopathy and vertebrobasilar insufficiency (see Chapters 12 and 13), there are no studies or reports in the peer-reviewed indexed literature of its remission in conjunction with CMT.

HEADACHE: MIGRAINE TYPE

Headache is often classified by etiology into broad categories such as organic, vascular, and somatic. Barbuto (172) classifies headache as cervicogenic, ligamentous, greater occipital neuralgia, posttraumatic (including muscle contraction, vasodilation, scar formation, intracranial hemorrhage and hematoma, and concussion), vascular, cluster (sphenoplatine neuralgia), intracranial disorders (including neoplasms and other space-occupying lesions), intracranial hemorrhage, and ocular. Of these types, the most common cervicogenic (CEH) or "muscle tension" and migraine types have been reported to respond well to intervention with CMT. Vernon (173) prefers to characterize "muscle tension" headache sufferers according to the degree of vertebrogenic involvement. Hence, when the vertebrogenic component is etiological, great relief can be expected from CMT. In contrast, less relief would be expected in sufferers whose vertebrogenic component is synergistic or negligible. (Efficacy of CMT for CEH is discussed above.)

In a review of articles published from 1964 to 1982 on migrainous headache, Vernon (173) describes chiropractic work by Wight (174) and by Parker, Tupling, and Pryor (175) in detail. Consensus from the nonrandomized trials of CMT and spinal manipulation for migrainous headache was that manipulation provides relief of both so-called classic migraine and common migraine in 75–90% of cases after 9 to 10 adjustments (173). In the only medical randomized trial of CMT for migraine, Parker and co-workers (176) documented a 47% success rate 20 months after chiropractic intervention. Patients receiving CMT reported significantly less severe pain than did patients assigned to physiotherapeutic mobilization or to medical manipulation (176). In an uncontrolled study, medical researchers have more recently demonstrated that in 31 patients with cervicogenic migraine (functional "blockade" or motion restriction at the occipitoatlantal junction, migraine headache, neck pain, dizziness, and positive Hautant's or past-pointing test), after Lewit-type mobilization and manipulation, significant improvement in cervical rotation was seen immediately ($p < .02$) and 1 week later

($p < .05$), along with improvement in headache intensity, neck pain intensity, frequency of dizziness, and the Hautant test (177). Another test of dizziness, the two-weight test (difference in weighting of the right and left lower extremities), was abnormal significantly less often immediately after manipulation and 1 week later ($p < .001$).

Cervical joints can play a direct role in headache; 25–38% of patients with significant neck pain receive relief from zygapophyseal joint blocks at specific levels, and their pain is aggravated by injection of saline into the joint(178). A *vertebrogenic migraine* has been cited in the medical literature, documented by plethysmographic analysis of the superficial temporal artery during resting and stressful conditions in 9 subjects having migrainous headaches and in 9 age- and sex-matched controls (179). Abnormal vasoconstriction as a response to stressors, and other asymmetric reactions were seen only in the migraine sufferers (179). That the superior cervical ganglia influence cerebral arterial flow is well documented. Vasospasm may occur because of the release of vasoactive substances such as 5-HT, adenine nucleotides, oxyhemoglobin, and arachidonate metabolites, and both vasoconstriction and vasodilation of cerebral arteries are mediated by α_2-adrenoceptors in the dog and cat (180). Clinical evidence that headache sufferers gaining relief after CMT also gain increased pressure-pain thresholds suggests that simple physical tests (e.g., algometry) may be able to quantify improvement in pain sensitivity in these subjects, which might be directly related to improvement in zygapophyseal function (181). Further research will hopefully identify clinical protocols to better identify the migrainous patients who are the best candidates for CMT and elucidate the neurobiologic mechanisms whereby CMT brings relief to them.

MYOCLONUS

A single case report in the chiropractic literature describes a 24-year-old female suffering from posttraumatic spinal myoclonus who appeared to recover after CMT (182). She had apparently suffered continuous rhythmic focal involuntary jerking movements in her abdomen and inner thighs for 17 years after she dove into a pool with her spine in a hyperextended position at age 7. She had immediate lower back pain. Initial EEG examination had been normal. Her mother reported that the jerking persisted during sleep and was intensified by sitting, volitional movement, and emotional stress. She did not respond to pharmacotherapy. Immediately before chiropractic intervention, the patient reported that the persistent muscular jerks of her abdomen were more intense, she was beginning to vomit occasionally after eating, and she could not sit comfortably. Chiropractic examination revealed a moderately overweight subject with exaggerated spinal curvatures. After a single session of dorsal and lumbar CMT, there was a gradual reduction of abdominal myoclonus over the next few hours. These rhythmic jerks were replaced by intermittent asynchronous contractions. On follow-up 6 days later, abdominal myoclonus had ceased, and one to three irregular involuntary contractions in her left thigh could be elicited by active or passive muscle stretching. Weekly adjustments were administered for persistent backache for the next month, and at 3-month follow-up, back pain and myoclonus were abolished; however, irregular, low-amplitude, short-duration, involuntary contractions of her left adductor could still be elicited by muscle stretching. Woo (182) suggests spinal cord ischemia as the pathophysiological mechanism in this case (see also Chapter 12). While spinal myoclonus from a diving accident is rare, spinal hyperextension strains in diving are common. The author recommended trials of early spinal manipulation for selected patients with spinal myoclonus before invasive decompressive laminectomy.

NYSTAGMUS

Some researchers have identified nystagmus as a sequela of vertebrobasilar syn-

drome (see Chapter 13). While associated with subluxation posttrauma, according to these researchers, it may also result from a host of other causes. Nevertheless, perhaps the only investigators to use electronystagmography to evaluate the effects of CMT in patients with confirmed cervical arthrosis and vertigo determined that nystagmus decreased in 28 patients, disappeared in 28, and was unchanged in the 8 remaining patients (183). These patients received unspecified CMT to the cervical spine over the course of 15 days to 2.5 months.

REFLEX SYMPATHETIC DYSTROPHY

Sympathetic dystrophies are a poorly understood phenomenon first observed in Civil War soldiers after gunshot wounds (184). Generally, trauma involving an extremity results in C-fiber hyperactivity, dorsal horn facilitation, subsequent sympathetically mediated activation of peripheral A-mechanoreceptors, and resultant spontaneous pain, hyperesthesia, and allodynia (184). The disorder progresses in stages, which can last from weeks to years; stages are classified as acute, dystrophic, and atrophic. Thermography has been accepted as a primary method for diagnosis of this disorder, termed reflex sympathetic dystrophy (RSD) (185).

Some cases are now appearing in the chiropractic literature regarding effectiveness of CMT for the disorder. For example, Ellis and Ebrall (186) found significant improvement after CMT in a 13-year-old female with chronic inversion and plantarflexion of the foot, left foot pain preventing weight bearing, and a feeling of "cold" in the foot, who presented after medical treatment, including crutches and a molded plastic orthotic supporting her foot. Treating her 14 weeks postinjury, passive stretch (dorsiflexion) held 10 seconds and repeated twice, Gonstead technique CMT to the pelvis and lumbar spine, and ankle adjustments achieved complete remission that physiotherapy and passive stretch alone could not achieve in this case (186). (After 6 weeks of chiropractic, strength in the extensor hallucis longus was back to 4/5; after 3.5 months, she could walk without aid of a support; and at 1 year, function and performance were assessed by an independent evaluator at 95% of normal.) Prior to chiropractic, she had been getting progressively worse. Certainly more research is needed to elucidate the role of chiropractic in the management of RSD.

SEIZURE DISORDERS

While there have been anecdotal case reports in chiropractic trade journals about improvement in various forms of epilepsy after CMT, little has been reported in our science journals (187–189). Goodman and Mosby (188) reported that after correction of occipitoatlantoaxial complex, a 5-year-old female with Lennox-Gastaut seizure disorder had a significant reduction of seizures from 30–70 per day to 6 per day. Chiropractic findings included cervical paravertebral palpable spasms with restricted right lateral cervical flexion and atlas subluxation. Also noted was a 3/4 to 1-inch leg length deficiency. Multiple side-posture upper cervical adjustments were administered over a 3-day period, after atlas misalignment was determined from line-marking analysis of upper cervical radiographs. Initially, the seizures abated and postadjustment x-rays revealed improved postural alignment. However, 17 days posttreatment, she experienced more than 100 seizures, and some seizure activity remained through the 27th day, when they again abated for 4 weeks. At the time the case report was written, seizures had diminished to 6 per day, and her carbamazepine dose was reduced by one half. As the patient's medical prognosis was grave and a significant remission in this case was preceded by chiropractic intervention, the authors concluded that CMT was responsible for altering the natural course of this disorder.

Evidence that whiplash can result in a somatoautonomic effect that causes subcortical EEG changes has been presented by Liu et al. (189). In their study of 16 monkeys subjected to whiplash (including control animals in which electrodes were implanted after whiplash), nearly all scalp, cortical, and subcortical EEG readings taken 6 to 8 weeks after the trauma were normal. Shortly thereafter, hippocampal spiking developed, which the authors categorized as a subclinical form of posttraumatic epilepsy. Certainly, whiplash-type injuries are commonly treated in chiropractic practice, and this may be a causal mechanism for some epilepsy successfully treated by chiropractors. However, more research on CMT for this and other seizure disorders is needed to show what role, if any, chiropractic may play in management of these disorders.

SPASMODIC DYSPHONIA

Spasmodic dysphonia (focal laryngeal dystonia) is thought to be associated with neurological or psychogenic illness, although its precise etiology is unknown (190). Apparently, an adductor-type spasmodic dystonia (ASD) involves strain-strangle phonation. The patient attempting conscious speech shows hyperadduction of the vocal folds, which closes the glottis and creates a "choked, pressed, or over-pressured" effort (190). Wood (190) reports a case of ASD involving a 46-year-old male with a 6-month history of total inability to produce speech. He was unable to pass air through the glottis because of vocal cord hyperadduction when he attempted to speak. His symptoms started as hoarseness after a common cold and progressed as various specialists diagnosed ASD and prescribed medications. Finally, specialists concluded that his condition was due to hysteria and recommended psychiatric therapy. Chiropractic evaluation revealed atlas/axis motor unit dysfunction (after motion and static palpation, C-spine x-rays, and other chiropractic tests), and after two treatments of atlas/axis CMT, the patient could phonate; within 2 weeks and five adjustments, there was complete resolution of ASD symptoms. Complete resolution of upper cervical pain, stiffness, and headache was noted as well. A partial recurrence resulting in hoarseness 5 months later required four sessions of CMT, with no other recurrence in the subsequent 4 years, prior to writing the case history (190). Given the reluctance of this disorder to respond favorably to surgical and medical interventions reported in the medical literature, this singular case history should prompt further investigation. Moreover, CMT should be considered an optional conservative therapy prior to use of relatively ineffective surgical interventions (190).

TOURETTE'S SYNDROME

A chronic familial neuropsychiatric disorder, Tourette's syndrome is associated with chemical imbalances in the brain. While the etiology is unknown, the patient with this disorder develops motor tics and uncontrolled vocalizations that vary in intensity. Medical treatment often consists of haloperidol, and of 80% of patients who are responsive to this medication, long-term compliance drops to 33% (191). Moreover, side effects include extrapyramidal symptoms; tardive dyskinesia may develop with long-term use of the drug and is irreversible (191). While anecdotal reports of improvement after chiropractic have appeared in chiropractic trade journals, no case reports have appeared in the chiropractic scientific journals until recently.

Trotta (191) reported a case of Tourette's syndrome that was treated with Life Upper Cervical adjustive technique and followed for 3 months. Outcome assessments included the Tourette's Syndrome Association (TSA) symptom survey, Stress Audit Profiles, infrared paraspinal thermographic readings, and upper cervical spine x-rays. Review of assessments for this 31-year-old male with a 27-year history of Tourette's suggested little change in the TSA symptom survey and continuing atlas misalignment on follow-up x-ray. In contrast, the 12 weekly adjustments produced clinically significant improvement in the Psychological Stress Audit Test. Pretreatment testing revealed significant stress in 9 of the 16 component factors, while posttreatment profiles suggested significant stress in only one component. The author suggested that more frequent chiropractic adjustment sessions and/or variation in the application of chiropractic technique might have produced more desirable results in the posttreatment TSA symptom survey and greater reduction in atlantoaxial misalignment (191). Until more is known about management of Tourette's with CMT in case-controlled studies such as this, patients should be advised that there is no conclusive evidence that CMT is effective for this disorder.

VERTIGO (CERVICOGENIC)

For some time, medical and chiropractic sources have recognized cervical trauma (notably whiplash), cervical arthritis, and other joint-related disorders as potential causes of imbalance, vertigo, and other inner ear disturbances. Chester (192) postulated that damage to the inner ear labyrinthine structures after trauma caused a central disorder of postural control, thereby causing abnormal muscular tension in the cervical spine. However, his demonstration of equilibrium disorders in 42 of 48 posttrauma (rear-end collision) patients, using six-step sensory-interaction trials, and of abnormal motor response strategies in 20 of those patients, using moving platform posturography, did not examine whether subsequent loss of postural control was causally related to cervical muscle spasms. Indeed, his hypothesis goes against the traditional medical theory that irritation of the cervical sympathetics, abnormal neck reflexes, or deflection or irritation of the vertebral arteries causes posttraumatic vertigo (193).

The latter hypotheses are supported by Fitz-Ritson (193), who demonstrated a test for cervicogenic vertigo and demonstrated ablation of vertigo after CMT in 90.2% of 112 patients who tested positive. The first part of the test involves having the patient sit on a stool that rotates, with thighs parallel to the floor. With eyes closed, the patient is asked to rotate ("shake") the head from side to side, as far and as quickly as possible. Some patients, due to pain, will have very little side-to-side movement. With this procedure, vertigo could originate either from vestibular nuclei or from muscles and joints in the cervical spine.

In the second part of the test, the patient sits upright on the same rotating stool or chair, with feet 15–18 inches apart. The feet are used to rotate the entire body on the stool from side to side. After practicing several times, the doctor stands behind the patient and holds the head steady while the patient repeats the procedure with eyes closed (Fig. 9.5). The doctor places a little cephalad traction to prestretch the cervical spine. If the patient experiences vertigo, it is from the tissues of the cervical spine. (With the head held stationary, there is no movement to affect the semicircular canals. Instead, this movement would affect the vestibular nuclei.) The examiner should be prepared for severe reactions to the test such as vomiting or a quick veer to one side with the patient falling.

Some 123 females and 112 males were assessed posttrauma for vertigo with this test. Of 112 patients testing positive for cervicogenic vertigo, 101 were symptom free after 18 sessions of CMT, and 6 had decreased vertigo. Only 5 reported no change in vertigo after CMT. In addition, of the 112 testing positive, 73 tested positive for cervical fixations as well (193).

These dramatic findings mirror those of Zerillo and Lynch (183), who reported that of 80 patients presenting with vertigo (verified by nystagmography) and headache secondary to cervical arthrosis, 64 had complete resolution and the remaining 16 had decreased vertigo after CMT. Moreover, spontaneous nystagmus and cervical nystagmus were dramatically decreased or resolved after CMT, according to otoneurologic tests, with only 3 of 46 cases of spontaneous nystagmus unchanged and only 8 of 64 cases of cervical nystagmus unchanged after adjustments. Tinnitus improved dramatically after CMT as well, in their series. Certainly these findings should fuel longer-term and broader investigations in this area.

In general, a number of disorders considered typically in the domain of neurology may respond to CMT. For some of these, CMT may prove to be a superior form of care; however, research is just beginning to scratch the surface of questions of efficacy. Meanwhile, chiropractors treating patients with type N disorders should use careful documentation, follow good rules of doctor-patient communication, and work with other physicians or specialists whenever indicated.

CMT and Type O Disorders

As with use of CMT for the treatment of type N disorders, many type O (organic) disorders, including primarily stress syndrome disorders, have long been treated by chiropractic methods, with numerous references of effectiveness reported anecdotally in the chiropractic trade journals. In the United States, annual surveys by the American Chiropractic Association reveal that chiropractors are increasingly focusing their practices on treatment of LBP and musculoskeletal syndromes; however, in Australia, more than half of respondents to a scientific survey favored chiropractic for migraine, asthma, hypertension, or dysmenorrhea (194). It is common knowledge that outside the chiropractic profession, use of CMT for these disorders remains controversial, and third party payors generally do not reimburse for such care. Despite these objections, good evidence is beginning to accumulate in peer-reviewed journals that CMT may be effective for a number of these conditions.

In another chapter of this text, one of the coauthors (RBP) states that research may eventually establish chiropractic as an effective treatment for two broad areas of illness: spinal and extraspinal joint and muscle syndromes and stress syndrome disorders (see Appendix A). While research is now beginning to shed light on the clinical effectiveness of CMT for some type O disorders, studies are also helping us to understand the experimental basis for these results.

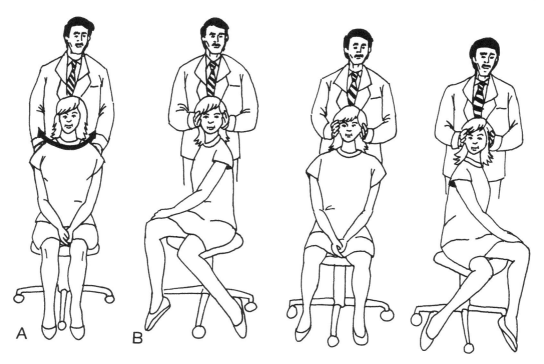

Figure 9.5. In the first part of the test for cervicogenic vertigo, the patient, seated on a stool, closes her eyes and shakes her head from side to side as far and as quickly as possible, while the doctor stands behind her and stabilizes her shoulders with his hands. (*A*). Vertigo could arise from muscles and joints of the cervical spine or from the vestibular nuclei. In the second part of the test, the doctor grasps the patient's head to stabilize it while she uses her feet to rotate her entire body on the stool from side to side. (*B*). If after practicing the procedure, the patient closes her eyes and experiences vertigo during this maneuver, it is thought to originate from the spinal tissues, since there is no head movement to affect the semicircular canals. Instead, this movement would affect the vestibular nuclei. Of 235 patients with cervical trauma, 112 were positive for this test. Of these, 90.2% were free of vertigo after 18 adjustments, in one retrospective study. (Adapted from Fitz-Ritson D. Assessment of cervicogenic vertigo. J Manipulative Physiol Ther 1991;14:193–198.)

For example, the work of Sato (195) has, for more than two decades, helped lay a framework for our understanding of somatovisceral reflexes. Under experimental conditions, after eliminating emotional factors following somatic sensory stimulations, his studies and others have clearly demonstrated effects on the cardiovascular and gastrointestinal systems, the urinary bladder, and the adrenal medulla (see also Chapter 8). Sympathetics are dominant during some responses; for others, parasympathetics are dominant. Some responses are characterized by propriospinal and segmental reflexes,

while others are supraspinal or are generalized. Nevertheless, Sato (195) contends that these somatovisceral responses may explain some of the purported effects of CMT in conscious humans.

CARDIOVASCULAR DISEASE

While modern research on chiropractic care for dysrhythmias, essential hypertension, and angina pectoris has been reported in peer-reviewed journals and at a symposium and is summarized below, probably the most fascinating evidence for a role for

CMT in cardiovascular disorders came from the Correlative Research Department of the Palmer Chiropractic College in 1949 (196). Under the direction of B. J. Palmer, 1500 cases seen in the outpatient clinic were examined ex post facto to determine what electrocardiographic changes occurred after specific upper cervical chiropractic technique. Arguably, these might be considered controlled or at least semicontrolled observations because of the procedures they used in collecting data (others argue that these were uncontrolled observations at best). Moreover, their results should be reviewed here because of the sheer size of the sample, and the historic value of Palmer's efforts should be acknowledged as well. These findings are reported below in light of our current understanding of coronary physiology, along with the aforementioned studies on CMT for dysrhythmias, essential hypertension, and angina pectoris.

Coronary Pathophysiology

In the 1980s, researchers began to accept a powerful role for the sympathetics in generating life-threatening arrhythmias in patients with myocardial infarction (197). Surgical removal of the left-sided cardiac sympathetic nerves was found to have anti-ischemic and antifibrillatory effects (197). A central nervous system mineralocorticoid receptor is known to play a crucial role in certain forms of hypertension, but its role in clinical disease remains obscure (198).

While afferents from arterial and cardiopulmonary baroreceptors and chemoreceptors play the greatest role in regulation of moment-to-moment cardiovascular function, afferents from other viscera contribute significantly to both cardiovascular regulation and abnormalities such as hypertension (199). For example, sensory fibers from renal parenchyma project through dorsal root ganglia to the dorsal horn of the spinal cord, and activation of renal afferents through central relays increases sympathetic activity and arterial blood pressure. In addition, much attention has been given to the role of somatosensory afferents in making cardio-

vascular adjustments during exercise (see also Chapter 8) (199). A role for the sympathetics is so well documented that β-blockers are routinely used to prepare patients for coronary bypass surgery (see also Chapter 8) (197).

Angina Pectoris

Acute ischemic coronary episodes resulting in chest pain are termed angina pectoris. Traditional medical therapy for this disorder includes prompt patient rest, administration of nitroglycerin or amyl nitrate, and observation until the ischemic episode passes (200). In contrast, several investigators have suggested a role for CMT or OMT in management of this disorder.

Palmer and co-workers (196) observed improvement in 4 of 5 cases of persistent angina pectoris after upper cervical (viz., atlas/axis using HIO technique) adjustment, the first chiropractic investigation of CMT for this disorder to be verified by electrocardiography.

Rogers and Rogers (201) showed that in ischemic heart disease with angina pectoris, transient spasm of the coronary arteries ceased immediately after OMT. These findings were confirmed by angiography and electrocardiography. They hypothesized that manipulation is of value in correcting the function of the autonomic nervous system, thereby influencing cellular metabolism and vasomotor dynamics of the coronary arteries. They challenged the idea that atherosclerotic phenomena are responsible for both angina pectoris and myocardial infarction, and suggested that autoregulatory control of coronary artery flow is of principal importance in meeting the increased metabolic needs of the myocardium. The work of Matoba et al. (202), demonstrating complete relief of chest pain in 13 of 13 patients with angina who had augmented levels of autonomic activity and positive stress testing, after administration of calcium antagonists orally, supports Rogers and Rogers (201) findings in suggesting an autonomic role in the pathogenesis of angina. Moreover, experimental research has shown that sympathectomy, injuries to the peripheral and autonomic innervating nerves, and neuroexcitation can enhance the development of arteriosclerosis (see Chapter 8).

Johnson (203) reported in the osteopathic literature on using a left second rib technique that quickly relieved acute coronary symptoms. In the acupuncture literature, Sherwood (204) discussed seven cases in which improvement in coronary artery spasm was associated with three treatments (ultrasound, faradism, massage and spinal remobilization) per week for 3 weeks, after a 3-month follow-up examination. In contrast, Tilley (205) reported unsatisfactory responses of patients with angina to OMT. Based on these preliminary reports, further research on the use of CMT in the management of angina is indicated, and outcome assessments including stress profiles might be beneficial in further discriminating which patients with this disorder might respond best to CMT.

Dysrhythmias

According to Balduc (200), common *dysrhythmias* (i.e., sinus dysrhythmia, sinus bradycardia, sinus tachycardia, paroxysmal atrial and nodal tachycardias, atrial premature beats, ventricular premature beats, and ventricular tachycardia) are generally associated with coronary symptoms such as precordial pain, palpitations, dyspnea, syncopy, racing or fluttering of the heart, and breathlessness. However, noncardiac symptoms may be missed without thorough examination, including dizziness, numbness, paralysis, urinary frequency, oliguria, abdominal pain and distention, and weakness. These symptoms are due to ischemia related to the myocardium, brain, kidney, and gastrointestinal tract (200). They are important because they can reduce cardiac output, lower blood pressure, and interfere with oxygen perfusion of tissues, and they may herald heart failure, myocardial infarction, angina pectoris, pulmonary edema, cerebral thrombosis, and poor cerebral perfusion (200).

Unblinded observations at the B. J. Palmer Chiropractic Clinic (196) included assessment of 1500 patients by electrocardiography. Altogether, 816 male and 684 females, primarily in the 41–50 and 51–60 age groups were tested before and weekly after the onset of Palmer HIO technique (viz., side-posture adjustment of atlas/axis on a drop-piece table after assessing upper cervical misalignments on x-rays). Final assessment in the average case was made 3.6 weeks after the start of treatment. Sinus tachycardia was found in 78 cases, and 52 of these demonstrated improvement after upper cervical adjustments. Sinus bradycardia was observed in 36 cases, and significant improvement after HIO adjustments were seen in half ($n = 18$) of these patients. Sinus arrhythmia was seen in 256 cases, and 141 were demonstrably improved after HIO. Auricular flutter was found in 32 cases, and 17 were improved after HIO. Auricular flutter fibrillation was seen in 5 cases; 3 were improved after HIO. Ventricular extrasystole was found in 155 cases; 100 were improved after HIO.

Most of these patients had no reported manifestations of coronary disease. Patients were only selected if a heart irregularity had occurred for 5 years or longer and if they had been receiving medication for a coronary condition. Of all dysrhythmias cited by these researchers, a worsening of the ECG was observed in only 7 cases. However, most patients with auricular extrasystole, auricular tachycardia, auricular fibrillation, A-V nodal rhythm, A-V nodal tachycardia, and ventricular tachycardias did not improve (196). This is the largest chiropractic investigation to date of the effectiveness of a chiropractic technique for specific dysrhythmias as assessed by ECG examination. While these controlled observations are not conclusive (no blinding of ECG assessments, no control population was used to observe normal variation over time, and no placebo group was used to observe the effect of doctor-patient interaction), they nevertheless provide some evidence (given the 5-year histories and prior medical intervention) that this technique may be effective in ameliorating these disorders.

Spano and Darling (206) demonstrated a relationship between cervical arthrosis and cervicobrachialgias and first-degree A-V block, nodal rhythm, tachycardia, and extrasystole seen on ECG. Cardiac dysrhythmias improved after chiropractic adjustments to the cervical spine, which they reasoned caused sympathetic stimulation and a peripheral arterial response. However, in their controlled case series of 97 cases, patients were prepared for chiropractic with pharmacological prophylaxis, including an antidystonic drug two or three days prior to the adjustment, when cervical maneuvers (i.e., forced movement of the head in flexion, extension, or rotation; compression of the eyeballs or the carotid sinus) were positive for paroxysmal tachycardia or extrasystole and a slight increase in humeral pressure followed by a hypotensive phase. These researchers felt that when repeated cervical maneuvers produced these cardiac alterations, sympathetic lability was demonstrated, and antidystonic prophylaxis prior to chiropractic was indicated. Vertebropathy related to substenosis associated with osteophytic encroachments was cited as the mechanism whereby changes in heart activity occur after cervical arthrosis, in some cases causing brainstem hypoxia (demonstrated also by EEG when insufficient carotid compensation occurred).

In addition to these studies, a number of osteopathic case presentations and uncontrolled observations appear in the literature (200, 203). Balduc (200) reviewed 14 papers, including at least one controlled trial revealing that significantly more right upper thoracic lesions occur in patients with dysrhythmias, in blinded tests. Many other investigators favor increased frequency of lesions in the upper cervicals as well, and at least one researcher cites T9–T12 lesions in patients with these disorders. However, largely left unanswered by this body of research is whether these lesions result in somatoautonomic reflexes that adversely affect coronary function, from viscerosomatic

reflexes (in which case CMT might not be expected to have much long-term effect), or both. Nevertheless, further research using control groups is certainly warranted, given the potential benefit of having a nondrug intervention for dysrhythmias.

Myocardial Infarction

While a role for prevention of *sudden cardiac death* by correction of spinal joint dysfunction using CMT has been proposed (207) and is supported indirectly by experimental research demonstrating a deleterious influence on cardiovascular regulation by aberrant somatosympathetic reflexes (195), no clinical evidence supports this hypothesis. Indeed, research from B. J. Palmer's laboratory appears to contradict this hypothesis (196).

Evidence from 1500 cases seen from 1935 to 1949 at the B. J. Palmer Chiropractic Clinic suggests that the more stress-related coronary conditions such as sinus tachycardia, bradycardia, and sinus arrythmias improved after specific upper cervical technique (viz. HIO adjustments) according to pre- and posttreatment electrocardiograms (ECGs) (196). In contrast, the vast majority of ECGs demonstrating bundle brand blocks, myocardial infarction, auricular or ventricular dilation, mitral and aortic stenosis and/or regurgitation, low-voltage QRS complex, inverted T and T waves 1 and 2, abnormal notching and slurring of QRS in all leads, and other signs of structural damage to the heart or of clotting demonstrated no improvement on post-CMT ECGs (196).

One would not expect an already structurally damaged heart to respond to CMT, and this research by Palmer et al. (196) appears to confirm that expectation. Improvement in post-CMT ECGs occurred in only 16.8% of 1500 patients presenting to his clinic with ECG abnormalities, and most of the improvement occurred in patients having dysrhythmias (see above).

This research is important historically since B. J. Palmer was willing to publish research that really did not support his hypotheses at the time (see Chapter 4), which lends some credibility to his other published work. It is also the largest-scale investigation ever made using ECG observations before and after manipulation or CMT (196).

Balduc (200) reported on 19 studies, primarily case presentations and at least two controlled blinded osteopathic investigations, demonstrating upper thoracic spinal lesions significantly more often in coronary patients than in noncoronary patients (see also Chapter 8). Moreover, several of these investigators reported improved ECG tracings and reduced pain, oppression, fatigue, and dyspnea after manipulation of upper thoracic and other spinal lesions in unselected patients with coronary disease. It is not known whether these lesions precede coronary pathology or to what extent manipulation effects such changes. From the observations of Palmer and co-workers (196), however, if one in nine patients with ECG and other manifestations of chronic coronary disease receives benefit from short-term use of chiropractic, one might expect even better results using chiropractic as a preventive measure and over a longer term.

Essential Hypertension

Studies of CMT or osteopathic manipulative therapy (OMT) for the management of essential hypertension have shown mixed results. Since Palmer and co-workers (196) showed in 1949 that after an average of 3.6 weeks of CMT, only 6 of 57 patients with hypertensive heart disease improved, a number of osteopathic and chiropractic investigations of essential hypertension have appeared in the literature.

After Tran and Kirby (208, 209) demonstrated a marginal reduction in blood pressure after adjustments to asymptomatic students, Dulgar and co-workers (210) used Logan basic technique in a pilot investigation and demonstrated a significant hypotensive effect over placebo treatment in patients with hypertension. Their study was the first chiropractic investigation in the modern era to use hypertensive subjects.

Morgan and colleagues (211) were the first to use a controlled randomized crossover trial to investigate the effectiveness of OMT in reducing blood pressure in patients with hypertension. Twenty-nine subjects were randomly assigned to receive either weekly spinal manipulation of the occipitoatlantal joint, T1 through T5, and T11 through L1 or sham manipulation in the form of soft tissue massage of T6 through T10 and from L4 to sacrum. Procedures were crossed over after 6 weeks and stopped after 12. Neither procedure reduced or controlled elevated systemic blood pressure in hypertensive adults already receiving medication. This research has been criticized since subjects were manipulated in both upper cervical and upper dorsal regions, which might be expected to both stimulate and inhibit cardiac activity simultaneously (personal communication, Dana Lawrence).

Yates, Lamping, Abram, and Wright (212), at the Canadian Memorial Chiropractic College, studied the effectiveness of Activator instrument adjusting on 21 hypertensive patients, the first randomized chiropractic investigation of manipulative effectiveness for this disorder. Patients were randomly assigned to receive active treatment (viz., Activator mechanical adjusting device delivering a 28-pound thrust within 1/300th second to the T1–T5 segments as needed), placebo treatment (viz., Activator instrument in the off position), or no treatment.

Blinded blood pressure (BP) and state anxiety (State-Trait Anxiety Inventory) assessments were made twice before and once after the interventions. There were no treatment group differences on baseline and pretreatment-dependent measures, but active treatment significantly reduced systolic BP ($p < .0001$), diastolic BP ($p < .0001$), and State anxiety ($p < .005$). Moreover, post hoc Newman-Keuls multiple comparisons indicated that systolic BP decreased significantly (14.71 mm Hg; $p < .05$) following active treatment, compared with the other two groups (both placebo and control groups experienced slight increases in systolic BP).

Similarly, diastolic BP decreased significantly (13 mm Hg) in the active treatment group, but decreased only 1.43 mm Hg in the placebo group and rose 0.71 mm Hg in the control group. The investigators concluded that the results supported the hypothesis that blood pressure is reduced following chiropractic treatment. They suggested that the long-term effects of chiropractic for this disorder should be studied (212).

Maloney and co-workers (213) at Logan College of Chiropractic investigated the effectiveness of sacro-occipital technique (SOT) in reducing hypertension, in a randomized trial. Thirty hypertensive patients not taking medication were recruited (15 male and 15 female subjects; ages 23 to 57; mean age = 36.7, SD = 10.43) and were randomly assigned to receive occipitomastoid suture adjustment (the medial mastoid suture line is grasped with the thumbs free and held for 20 seconds, followed by 20 seconds of rest—procedure repeated six times) by a certified craniopath who is also an SOT instructor, a sham treatment (light pressure on the upper trapezius held for an equal amount of time, approximately 4 minutes), or a control procedure (doctor physically present in room with patient for 4 minutes but with no patient contact). Two pretreatment and two posttreatment or postsham/postcontrol blinded BP assessments were made. ANOVAs revealed no significant pretreatment differences between groups in any of the dependent variables. Posttreatment comparisons revealed no significant treatment effect and no significant group differences for diastolic, systolic, and pulse rate assessments. Almost all variables decreased slightly after treatment/placebo/control interventions. These researchers argued that the clinical effectiveness that Major Bertrand DeJarnette claimed for SOT (i.e., reductions in posttreatment BP on the order of 20 mm Hg) was not replicated in this empirical investigation.

Finally, the investigation of Nansel and co-workers (214) that showed no hypotensive effect of adjustments in asymptomatic normotensive students, while not in agreement with the findings of Tran and Kirby (208, 209), is not comparable with the randomized trials on hypertensive subjects just cited (211–213). In addition, Corbett et al. (215) demonstrated that muscle spasms in the upper dorsal spine caused increased blood pressure in tetraplegic patients. Perhaps the effectiveness of CMT in hypertensive subjects with upper dorsal muscle spasms or RDF should be examined, to determine if there is a more robust and/or longer-lasting treatment effect in such individuals.

While chiropractic care for cardiovascular disorders may be expected to remain controversial so long as research findings are inconclusive, ample evidence exists to warrant serious research in this area. Moreover, for patients who are offered this option in full knowledge of the limitations of chiropractic research of these disorders, CMT may remain a viable nondrug intervention for some.

GASTROINTESTINAL DISORDERS

There is now ample evidence of somatoautonomic influences upon gastrointestinal function (see Chapter 8). Of course, such observations are not entirely new. MacKenzie (216) reported that physicians frequently used counterirritation in the pit of the stomach to allay vomiting and that retention of urine followed operations involving the skin of the perineum. He identified these "effects of the stimulation of the skin on the viscera" in 1893, before the first chiropractic adjustment was given.

While a great deal of modern neurophysiological research has elucidated some mechanisms whereby chiropractic adjustments could influence gastrointestinal function, exact descriptions of the neurological and neurohumoral mechanisms remain unknown (195). For example, we know that both innervated and denervated fundic mucosa release acid and pepsin after pentagastrin stimulation, and this is inhibited by doses of epinephrine and isoproterenol that produce unequivocal cardiac stimulation (217). However, gastric secretions stimulated by food, histamine, bethanechol, or methacholine are not inhibited by epinephrine and isopro-terenol (217). Moreover, sympathectomy seems to increase the responsiveness of the fundus to acid stimuli. However, it is too early to know the specific actions in this regard of either sympathetic stimulation or ablation:

> This subject, at present unfashionable for research, represents a black hole in our knowledge. Confusion has resulted from failure to interpret results from conscious and acute preparations separately, in the former also from failure to recognize that the basal state is a regularly fluctuating control, and finally from the rush to study modern complicated synthetic catecholamines, before we know anything about the nerves and the naturally occurring neurohormones in physiologic concentrations (217).

DeBoer, Schultz, and McKnight (218), at the Palmer College of Chiropractic, followed up on earlier osteopathic attempts to create an animal model for subluxation, to determine its effect upon gastrointestinal myoelectric activity. EMG activity was recorded from the serosa of the gastric antrum and duodenal bulb in 22 normal California rabbits before and during application of spinal manipulation for 2.5 minutes. When the manipulation-induced acute vertebral lesion was applied at T6, dramatic inhibition of slow-wave and spike-burst EMG activity from the upper GI tract occurred. Similar interventions at T1, T12, and L3 had progressively weaker effects. Moreover, control and pain-producing skin stimuli applied over these same areas had no effect on GI EMG. This study supported findings by Sato (195) and others (219), who have demonstrated a lesion-specific gastrointestinal response in the middorsal region.

Taken collectively, experimental research strongly supports the notion that gastrointestinal viscerosomatic and somatovisceral reflex relationships may be influenced by CMT or OMT. A brief review of clinical studies of this hypothesis follows.

Bowel and Bladder Dysfunction

Falk (220) presented three cases describing bowel and bladder dysfunction secondary to *lumbar dysfunctional syndrome.*

Two of the three patients had sciatalgias with antalgia. A third patient had sacroiliac joint pain. All three had a tight and painful straight leg raise; in addition, one presented with left testicular pain and bladder pain and difficulty voiding, a second had dysuria, while a third had constipation. In each case, bowel and bladder complaints appeared within hours of the back and/or leg pain. Side-posture adjustments were administered to the involved lumbosacral areas, in addition to cryotherapy and other therapies, on a daily basis; bowel and bladder dysfunction was totally resolved within 5 days in the two patients with dysuria, and within 6 weeks in the patient with constipation, although more regular bowel movements started within 3 days. Falk (220) reviewed the literature and suggested that these cases might be explained by nerve root irritation secondary to discal lesions. He hypothesized that chiropractic might change the vascularity of the visceral organs with sympathetic or parasympathetic stimulation, improving their function or that constipation might be due to voluntary suppression of the urge, associated with aggravation of the LBP. In such cases a positive Valsalva maneuver and thorough history could confirm the diagnosis (220).

In a good review of the literature including his own studies, Browning (221) describes the syndrome of *pelvic pain and organic dysfunction* (PPOD) secondary to *lower sacral nerve root compression* (LSNRC). Typically, according to medical and chiropractic literature, women are much more commonly affected than men and often with a broad range of involved pelvic symptomatology. Falls, accidents, pregnancy, and delivery are associated with the onset of the syndrome, and patients frequently deny the existence of an association between PPOD and the back or leg pain.

Medical and chiropractic literature cite LSNRC symptomatology as including urinary frequency, urgency, incontinence, retention, nocturia, sluggishness, dysuria, difficulty or inability in emptying the bladder, and chronic bladder infection. In addition, vaginal discharge, painful and irregular menstruation, prostatovesiculitis, impotence, decreased sexual sensitivity, miscarriage, loss of ability to achieve orgasm, dyspareunia, chronic pelvic pain, and constipation have been associated with LSNRC in the empirical literature. More recently, proctalgia, excessive flatus, anal sphincter spasm, pelvic pain during orgasm, deficient precoital lubrication, menstrual migraine, vaginal spotting, spontaneous bowel discharge, and loss of ability to perceive rectal filling were associated with LSNRC in chiropractic case studies (221).

Improvement in the symptomatology generally parallels improvement in pain associated with LSNRC after CMT (generally side-posture manipulation or lumbar flexion-distraction techniques). Sensory, reflex, motor, and pain provocation examination procedures are suggested to identify PPOD secondary to LSNRC. In addition, production or aggravation of inguinal or suprapubic cramping or mild to sharp pain on straight leg raise suggests PPOD secondary to LSNRC. Browning (221) carefully considers examination procedures to rule out nonmechanical causes of PPOD, such as organic pathology, as well. For example, pelvic pain with digital pressure not reproducible in adjacent areas indicates the absence of intraabdominal disease. Conversely, pain on deep rebound pressure over the abdomen indicates intraabdominal sources of pain. Finally, pelvic or abdominal rebound pain with digital pressure during active bilateral straight leg raise suggests involvement of the abdominal wall (221). In such cases, further testing or referral is indicated.

Gastritis

Anecdotal reports of improvement in gastritis, dyspepsia, hiatal hernia, and even gastric ulcers after CMT have appeared in chiropractic trade journals through the years but have not appeared in the recent chiropractic science journals. Indeed, while the trend is toward chiropractors treating primarily neuromusculoskeletal disorders, ACA member surveys consistently reveal that approximately 8% of chiropractic cases consist of "viscerosomatic" disorders (222). Most of these are so-called stress syndrome disorders such as gastritis (see Chapter 14). The hypothesis is that adjustments "normalize" the balance between sympathetic and parasympathetic activity, thereby relieving these disorders.

As an initial test of this theory, Wiles (223) made electrogastrograms (viz., surface electrodes 2 inches to the left and 1 inch above the navel, with a ground wire attached to the right leg) before, during, and after motion palpation ($n = 7$), palpation with C1 adustment ($n = 4$), or palpation with C2 adjustment ($n = 2$). Recording sessions lasted from 15 to 30 minutes, and adjustments were given at C1 or C2 in the middle-aged subjects only if motion palpation revealed restricted movement.

Frequency and peak amplitude did not vary between groups as a result of the intervention or the mobilization that occurred with movement palpation. In contrast, a significant (χ_2 test: $P = .01$) elevation in "displacement" (viz., averaged for all baseline changes in a recording) occurred in the normal subjects receiving C1 adjustments only. According to Wiles (223), this suggested an increase in gastric tone following upper cervical manipulation, possibly due to increased efferent vagal activity, probably via indirect neural connections. In addition, significant improvement in wave shape, or clarity, occurred only in two of four subjects receiving C1 adjustment. Certainly, these preliminary results favor a role for CMT in normalizing autonomic tone to the stomach and suggest that other viscera might be similarly influenced. Further research is warranted by these findings.

GENITOURINARY DISORDERS

Anecdotal reports of improvement in renal and bladder infections, in female infections, and in a wide variety of other genitourinary disorders have historically appeared in the chiropractic trade literature but not in the more recent chiropractic science journals (i.e., since 1978).

Palmer, Sherman, and Coulter (224) published a fascinating study of 2006 cases seen at the B. J. Palmer clinic from 1935 to 1949 in which urinalysis was conducted before and at weekly intervals after upper cervical specific adjustments were administered. Without regard for diagnosis, and acknowledging that this represented a small sample of the total patients seen at the clinic during that time period, the data offer historical value if limited clinical application. For example, there is no control for natural history nor for placebo effect; furthermore, there is no mention of menstruation and at what point in the cycle recordings were made.

Despite these significant limitations, the findings should be explored further, if only because this is the largest pre- and postadjustment urinalysis sample—using somewhat controlled methodology—ever conducted in chiropractic. To their credit, they published data that suggests relative ineffectiveness of adjustments for many measures associated with urinalysis. With regard to physical changes, for example, the data clearly show that for all ages, male and female, most urinalyses were unchanged, and some worse, after the adjustments (224). Indeed, only 5% of all females and 9% of all males had normal physical appearance to their urine after CMT when preadjustment urinalysis had revealed abnormality. In males, exactly 50% of acetone and albumin tests were better or normal after adjustments; 50% were unchanged or worse. Similarly, microscopic four-field investigation for bacteria revealed 57% better or negative after adjustments, but 43% unchanged or worse, potentially explainable by natural remission alone. The finding of leukocytes in the urine initially with a negative postassessment examination occurred in 8% of cases; an additional 41% were somewhat better, 11% were unchanged, and 40% were worse after adjustments. Given the limitations previously cited, these observations are not encouraging.

In contrast, specific gravity improved in 73% of all cases abnormally elevated, 19% worsened, and only 8% were unchanged, as assessed by the Fischer urinometer. Perhaps most surprisingly, in males with blood in the urine on entrance to the clinic, 11% had less blood after adjustments, and 67% had no blood in final urinalysis. Similarly, pH returned to normal in 71–86% of cases.

Sugar was positive in the urinalysis initially and negative after adjustments in 63% of the cases (27% unchanged or worse, 10% some better) (224). One would certainly not expect a natural remission in sugar to occur that often in a sample of this size. While there is no controlled research suggesting CMT can result in remission of diabetes mellitus, sympathoneuronal activity in diabetics is diminished in comparison with patients with peripheral arterial obstructive disease (PAOD) stage II (225). Further, lumbar sympathectomy has only temporary value in improving hemodynamics in both diabetic and nondiabetic patients with PAOD (225). Nevertheless, experimental evidence that chemical sympathectomy affects renal counterbalance supports the notion that adjustments could, at least hypothetically, improve physiological mechanisms associated with some measures assessed with urinalysis (226).

Finally, research on CMT applied to the dorsolumbar transition in cases of genitourinary disorders remains to be completed (with the exception of cases of PPOD associated with LSNRC cited previously in "Bowel and Bladder Dysfunction"). Whether or not dorsolumbar adjustments will be more effective in influencing renal health than the Palmer and co-workers (224) upper cervical adjustment remains to be seen.

Chiropractors typically use a variety of "wholistic" remedies in conjunction with adjustments, which remain to be tested as well. For example, more than one practitioner has observed that many acute mild kidney and/or bladder infections have spontaneous remissions and others clear up quickly with dietary advice such as avoiding caffeinated beverages and increasing the intake of cranapple juice and water. In addition, some chiropractors employ counseling, biofeedback, and modern psychological techniques to gain improvement in genitourinary disorders such as adult diurnal enuresis (227). It remains for chiropractors using such approaches to demonstrate their effectiveness or abandon their use in favor of more traditional medical approaches to these disorders.

GYNECOLOGICAL DISORDERS

In addition to a wide range of pelvic disorders that may mimic gynecological pain, a variety of female disorders that occur secondary to mechanical lumbopelvic syndromes have been described in the literature. Sandoz (228) observes that a number of causes of intrapelvic distortion, aside from the pelvic instabilities of pregnancy and puerperium, involve the sacroiliac joints. However, Szlazak and Nansel (229) state that since nociceptive afferents arising from somatic structures converge on the same neuronal pools that receive input from visceral structures, claims of cures of visceral symptoms after CMT may be unwarranted. To establish CMT as being effective for gynecological symptoms, improvement must be demonstrated in clinical signs that correlate with female pain syndromes. Below is a synopsis of studies of CMT for several female syndromes. Emphasis is given to the pain of female disorders and to other more objective measures as well.

Dysfunctional Uterine Bleeding

Stude (230) reports on the use of CMT for *dysfunctional uterine bleeding* (DUB), which is characterized by a variety of anovulatory cycles and bleeding manifestations. The 40-year-old female reported LBP radiating into her posteromedial thighs. Her chronic lumbosacral pain had been treated symptomatically 2 years earlier by chiropractic; however, she had no prior history of leg pain. Other than a D & C performed after a miscarriage 17 years earlier, she had no significant gynecological history. Her LBP had progressively worsened since the onset of spotting 3 months prior to her first adjustment. Immediately before her chiropractic

visit, her gynecologist advised her that her uterus was the size associated with a 10-week pregnancy and that there was evidence of a cervical polyp. She was instructed to schedule for a D&C and possible hysterectomy the following week. The chiropractic diagnosis was L5 intervertebral disc syndrome (contained), S1 and S2 nerve root compression syndrome, and dysfunctional uterine bleeding. After two side-posture adjustments administered to both T12/L1 and L4/S1 segments, she experienced no further pain or bleeding for a 6-month follow-up period. About 1 year later, she returned with reported recurrence of a 2-week bout of DUB without back or leg pain, which resolved within 2 weeks, after seven adjustments. Follow-up gynecological examination was normal, and she continued to be free of DUB 6 weeks later. The author concluded that while a causal relationship between cessation of DUB and CMT cannot be inferred from this case study, obviously the relationship of the two appears to be more than coincidental. Further research is warranted.

Dysmenorrhea

Primary dysmenorrhea is characterized by painful menstruation from a local dysfunctional cause, without organic pelvic pathology (231). Arnold-Frochot (232–233) reports on five female patients, aged 18 to 23, with primary dysmenorrhea. They were adjusted for 2 or 3 months, and Menstrual Syndrome Questionnaire (234) was used as an outcome measure. Two patients were almost completely relieved of menstrual pain, one responded to other chiropractic pelvic therapy, and two had no benefit. The author could not explain why three seemed to benefit while two others did not.

Hains, Batt, Bellis, and Martel (235), at the Canadian Memorial Chiropractic College, attempted to identify a somatic lesion that would correlate with primary dysmenorrhea, in a double blinded study. Fifty women, aged 21 to 42, were evaluated by written questionnaires to determine the type and intensity of dysmenorrhea and LBP.

Twenty subjects were considered to be nondysmenorrheic; 26 subjects were considered dysmenorrheic. A second blinded investigator measured PPT of each subject at 14 different sites located bilaterally over the posterior spinal joints, at a control area (T8–9), and at the thoracolumbar junction (T10–L2), thought to be somatically related to dysmenorrhea.

Tender points were defined operationally as sensitive at less than 4.5 kg or with a pain threshold 2 kg less than the contralateral spinal pressure point. Four subjects were excluded because of uniformly low PPTs over the entire experimental area (considered to be due to a confounding disorder such as fibromyalgia). There was no significant association between dysmenorrhea and low back pain at the time of the study (p = .629). Yet, the average number of tender points at the thoracolumbar junction was 0.75 (SD = .851) in the nondysmenorrheic group and 1.58 (SD = 1.528) in the dysmenorrheic group. Unpaired t tests revealed this to be a significant difference between the groups (p = .025). Moreover, PPTs in the control area were not significantly different between groups (p = .521). They concluded that the results suggest a significant increase in the number of tender points at the thoracolumbar junction in subjects with dysmenorrhea (as opposed to controls). The absence of a correlation with LBP suggests that the tender points were related to some other somatic component (e.g., a somatoautonomic or viscerosomatic reflex). The authors advocated further research using a questionnaire with known validity and reliability and suggested measuring prostaglandin levels as an improved outcome assessment (235).

Kokjohn, Schmid, Triano, and Brennan (231) did measure prostaglandin levels (viz., plasma prostaglandin F_2 metabolite, 15-keto-13, 14-dihydroprostaglandin (2a)) 15 minutes before and 60 minutes after the experimental procedures, and used the *Menstrual Distress Questionnaire* (MDQ) (236) and the Visual Analog Scale. Forty-five women with a history of primary dysmenor-rhea, aged 20 to 49, were randomly assigned to receive either side-posture adjustments at clinically relevant levels between T10 and L5/S1 (n = 24) or a sham procedure (n = 20; patients side-lying receive thrust over sacrum with both knees bent and adjacent to each other).

Results indicated no significant group differences before treatment in terms of three outcome measures. The group receiving CMT had significantly less LBP (F = 4.44; p = .04), significantly less abdominal pain (F = 5.92; p = .02), and lower MDQ scores (F = 9.97; p = 0.003) than those receiving the sham procedure. There was a significant reduction in plasma levels of $KDPGF_{2a}$ in the subjects receiving CMT (t = 3.276; p = .002), but an equally impressive reduction in prostaglandin levels occurred in the control group as well.

The authors suggested that improvement in prostaglandin levels in the sham-treated group might have occurred because thrust forces were not monitored and some manipulation might have taken place. Further, higher (although not significant statistically) pretreatment $KDPGF_{2a}$ levels were observed in the sham-treated group, which might have influenced the outcome. Also, decreased prostaglandin levels have been observed after administration of placebo drugs in other trials. Finally, physiological measures of organic pain, such as 2a may not be directly related to the perception of pain. They advocated studies with more subjects followed over a longer time frame, with rigorous control of the threshold force in the sham manipulation (231). Nevertheless, the finding of significantly less back and abdominal pain—as well as less menstrual distress—only in the group receiving adjustments adds to the growing evidence favoring a role for CMT in the management of dysmenorrhea.

Pelvic Pain and Organic Dysfunction (Female)

This chapter has reviewed PPOD associated with LSNRC in terms of bowel and bladder dysfunction, but some female-specific aspects deserve further consideration here.

Browning (237) reports on treating a 39-year-old female with chronic pelvic pain and dyspareunia but without LBP. At about age 18, she fell down a flight of stairs and shortly thereafter developed pelvic pain in the inguinal region. As a result of her pain, an appendectomy was performed without relief. Following the appendectomy, she developed severely painful menstruation and continuous diarrhea. She was rehospitalized, the diagnosis of irritable bowel secondary to stress was made, and she was discharged without relief. Within 2 to 3 years, she developed vaginal discharge and recurrent genitourinary disorders that were treated as yeast and bladder infections, with temporary benefit each episode. Genital pain radiating into the labia and clitoris made it painful and sensitive to touch or any contact. Her menstruation became increasingly painful and more irregular, with excessive bleeding. Estrogen afforded no appreciable relief, and at age 26 she married, although unable to attain orgasm because of her pain.

With difficulty, LBP, and paresthesias, she became pregnant three times: she carried the first to full-term delivery, had a spontaneous miscarriage after 5 1/2 months, and delivered a child 2 months prematurely. Because of her problems, exploratory surgery was performed but was negative; however, partial hysterectomy was performed at about age 29. Unfortunately, she developed bladder dysfunction while still hospitalized after the hysterectomy, with total urinary retention and complete loss of vesical sensory perception. She was self-catheterized to aid in emptying the bladder and was subsequently discharged, whereupon her diarrhea, bleeding, and mucous discharge worsened. Diagnosed as having proctalgia fugax and bleeding rectal fissures, she began to have nocturnal encopresis several times per week, and her left inguinal pains worsened. Eight weeks later her left ovary was removed, and cysts were documented. The right ovary was found to be normal. However, her inguinal pains persisted on both

sides, prompting removal of her right ovary 1 year later (237).

Four years later, urinary incontinence developed, accompanied by return of recurrent bladder infections. Bladder suspensory surgery helped this difficulty for about 1 year, but self-catheterization was still required. A second suspensory surgery provided initial relief of incontinence and infections, but without change in her loss of vesical sensory perception or urinary retentive state. Six months later she fell twice, and within 24 hours urinary incontinence returned. After several surgeries she was able to accept a supportive mesh implant for her bladder, which resolved her incontinence. At no time did her vesical sensory perception return.

Upon entrance she denied any LBP since her pregnancy, yet lumbosacral pain was provoked by numerous orthopaedic maneuvers (viz., extremes of lumbar ROM, Kemp test, straight leg raising, etc.). Moreover, inguinal and suprapubic pelvic pain was provoked by these same maneuvers. On neurological examination, a mild paresis of right hip abduction, slightly diminished right ankle jerk, and hypesthesia of the left L5, S1, S2, and S3 dermatomes was demonstrated. Pain provocation examination revealed palpatory hyperpathia over the left and right inguinal, ischial, medial popliteal, posteromedial leg, symphysis and para-anal regions. Radiographs were normal, with no degenerative processes. A working diagnosis of an "asymptomatic," well-defined, central L5 annular protrusion with bilateral LSNRC and secondary PPOD was made; daily distractive decompressive manipulation (flexion-distraction) to the lumbosacral spine, cryotherapy, a lumbosacral appliance, lumbar spine curve-reducing exercises, and strict bed rest brought rapid relief. Within 4–6 weeks, all her pelvic and genital pains were completely relieved. Vesical sensory loss, diarrhea, enuresis, and decreased rectal sensory perception all returned within 4 weeks as well. Rectal and mucous discharges stopped within 10 weeks, and genital sensory perception returned. By 12 weeks, precoital lubrication returned along with libido; by 19 weeks, she no longer felt pain with coitus; and by 30 weeks, she had her first orgasm (237).

The case was deemed important not only for the misdirected surgeries and treatments, which were performed for incorrect diagnoses, but because the patient presented with PPOD subsequent to LSNRC but without LBP (237). Dobrik (238) suggested that malfunction of the iliopsoas muscle was another source of dysfunction of the internal genitalia and gynecological disease. He states that spasm of the iliopsoas can directly influence blood flow through adjacent vessels, affecting blood and lymph flow to the pelvis and presenting symptoms mimicking inflammation. Moreover, he holds that inflammation of the adnexa, parametritis, and adhesive processes in the environment of the internal genitalia are often accompanied by iliopsoas m. spasm. Despite the somewhat dismissive observations of Szlazak and Nansel (229) that somatic lesions may mimic pain of visceral disease and that therefore most "cures" are not of actual visceral disorders, the cases offered by Browning (221, 237) and others (230) suggest a possible causal relationship between gynecological disease and LSNRC in some cases, which may be effectively managed by chiropractic care. Further research is certainly warranted in this area.

Pregnancy-related Low Back Pain

A number of good investigations and controlled trials offer increasing evidence that gravid patients with LBP benefit significantly with pre- and postpartal chiropractic care. Good trials are helping us to identify those at risk. For example, Östgaard and Andersson (239) followed 429 pregnant patients with a prior history of LBP and 375 patients with no history of LBP to delivery. Back pain occurred twice as often in the group with a prior history, and prevalence was three times greater; pain lasted longer as well. Women were more at risk for LBP during pregnancy if they had been pregnant previously (and multiparity predicted longer

periods of LBP as well) and if they were young. Pain intensity was worse in early pregnancy. Moreover, patients with sacroiliac joint pain had increased pain as pregnancy progressed, while other pain presentations remained stable or decreased throughout the pregnancy (240). True sciatica occurred in only 10 of 855 women. Numerous chiropractic techniques for the gravid female are available, documented, and apparently safe to apply throughout pregnancy (241).

One of the first chiropractic-medical investigations of the effectiveness of CMT for postpartal LBP was reported by Mantero and Crispini (242). After an average of 15 adjustments applied to 120 patients, 25% were cured, 50% were feeling very well, 15% were somewhat improved, and only 10% claimed no improvement. Of those who did not respond to CMT, uterine inflammation, fibromas, and cysts were subsequently suggested as the source of their postpartal complaints and reflex pain in the lumbar spine. Further uses of chiropractic for postpartal care, according to these authors, include restoring tone to the abdominal musculature, improving tone of the pelvic floor to prevent prolapse and urinary incontinence, avoiding alterations in venous circulation to the lower limbs, and correction of altered lumbopelvic posture.

In a more recent retrospective study of 400 consecutive pregnancies and deliveries presenting to five chiropractic offices, back pain was reported during 170 (42.5%) of the pregnancies and 179 (44.7%) of the deliveries (243). There was a statistically significant association between back pain during these events (P <.001). Of 170 pregnancies with reported back pain, 122 (72%) reported back labor. A subsample of those who reported back pain received CMT and experienced less pain during labor (P <.001).

A similar retrospective review of 100 consecutive pregnancies at a rural medical practice revealed back pain spontaneously reported to the physician in 23 cases (244). Eleven of the 23 met diagnostic criteria for sacroiliac subluxation (viz., absence of lumbopelvic pathology, pain in the sacral region, positive Piedallu's sign (asymmetrical movement of the posterior superior iliac spines during trunk flexion), positive pelvic compression test, and asymmetry of the anterior superior iliac spines) and were treated with rotational manipulation of the sacroiliac joints (side-posture maneuver). Ten of the 11 had relief after manipulation: 7 after the first session (3 of those had recurrences at 3, 4, and 13 weeks, respectively) and 4 after two sessions (a second was required at 1, 2, 5, and 7 weeks). One woman had a third manipulation but continued to have recurring pain. These medical authors conclude:

> The diagnosis and treatment of sacroiliac subluxation can be learned in a few hours. The manipulative technique requires only simple equipment and can be practiced without harm on persons without sacroiliac subluxation.
> The results of this preliminary study are encouraging and should be confirmed by a larger prospective study of the diagnosis and treatment of low-back pain in pregnancy (244).

Certainly we can expect that as more benefits of chiropractic become known in the medical and physiotherapy professions, advice such as that given by Daly and coworkers (244)—however simplistic it may appear to the doctor of chiropractic—will be increasingly observed. Chiropractic research of pre- and postpartal pain is necessary to further elucidate the diagnostic and adjustment procedures that will be most effective.

Premenstrual Syndrome

Following up on anecdotal reports of improvement in premenstrual syndrome after chiropractic, Stude (245) provided a case report with objective methodology to provide a framework for future research. *Premenstrual syndrome* (PMS) comprises the symptomatology (including insomnia, mastalgia, nausea, vomiting, diarrhea, or constipation), fluid retention, and mood alterations associated with the female menstrual cycle (246).

Diagnosis was based on finding (*a*) symptoms occurring during the luteal/postovulatory phase of the menstrual cycle that are re-

lieved sometime during the menstrual period (viz. days 1–5), (*b*) symptoms worsening progressively during the symptom cycle, (*c*) a symptomless interval during the follicular/preovulatory phase of the cycle (minimal occurrence during a 7–10 day duration), (*d*) symptoms recurring at least minimally for no less than three consecutive menstrual cycle intervals, (*e*) at least one somatic and one psychological complaint, generally reported during the luteal phase, (*f*) a PMT-Cator (a measure of menstrual distress used to objectively quantify symptomatology associated with PMS) score suggestive of PMS, and (*g*) absence of confounding factors such as psychiatric, hormonal, and/or treatment with medications that could directly and/or indirectly affect the hypothalamic/pituitary/ovarian axis or thyroid function (245).

A pretreatment baseline of recorded symptoms during three consecutive menstrual cycles prior to CMT was compared with symptoms during three consecutive cycles after CMT, using the PMT-Cator instrument. The PMT-Cator measures such symptoms as crying spells, forgetfulness, heart pounding, breast tenderness, backache, headache, abdominal cramping, low back pain, abdominal bloating, and dizziness/lightheadedness. In the case presented, the 3-month pretreatment baseline average PMT-Cator score was 62 (any score above 10 suggests PMS), while the scores during treatment were 0, 9, and 8 (av. 5.67). While single case studies must of course always be interpreted with caution, the findings were suggestive. Moreover, side-posture lumbar adjustments were the principal treatment, as the patient had previously tried dietary and medical treatments without success. Certainly this study provides a protocol for further randomized trials or single subject designs that more accurately control for threats to internal and external validity (such as the multiple baseline across subjects design—see Section 5) (245).

OPHTHALMOLOGIC DISORDERS

Anecdotal reports of improved vision after chiropractic have not appeared in the indexed scientific literature, although some have observed improvement in vertical phorias and tropias accompanying neck pain, after adjustments to the cervical spine (247). Nonetheless, Gilman and Bergstrand (247) report a case of loss of vision following head trauma. A 75-year-old patient with lung cancer and a coronary condition presented to an optometrist on 4/4/88 seeking treatment for blindness. His ophthalmological record included cataract removal and intraocular lens implantation for the left eye; postsurgical corrected acuities were OD 20/50, OS 20/50, and OU 20/40. Satisfactory results of the surgery 2 years earlier were observed, and other than bilateral macular degeneration and the aforementioned medical conditions, he had no other confounding medical problems, and medications had not changed in the 6 months prior to presentation. A month prior to presentation, the patient reported falling between two logs and striking both sides of his head; he felt immediate head pain and dizziness and awoke the next morning without vision. A CT scan was negative and helped rule out a hematoma or stroke as the cause.

Optometric findings were pupils 1–2 mm and unreactive to light, although he walked with a cane and gave some indication of light perception. Fundus revealed bilateral slight optic atrophy and mild macular degeneration. The intraocular lens in the left eye was in position, with no signs of inflammation or other problems; intraocular pressure was 15 OD and 15 OS (mm Hg). It was not possible to measure visual acuities, and distance and nearpoint retinoscopy showed a dull, distorted reflex in each eye. Attempts to induce retinoscopic reflex changes with small and large dioptric lens changes were unsuccessful. Retinoscopy reflexes were a dull reddish-orange. Tentative diagnosis was blindness due to head trauma (247).

Ophthalmologic confirmation of the diagnosis was obtained on 7/13/88. At that time bilateral light perception was the only visual response, and refractive evaluation did not show any improvement. Clinical impression from the ophthalmologist was that vision loss was permanent.

As the patient sought any treatment that might improve his condition, and as both authors had observed patients reporting vision changes after receiving adjustments, referral for chiropractic intervention was made. Chiropractic evaluation included observation of restricted atlantoaxial motion, and palpable taut and tender suboccipital muscles. X-ray findings were consistent with the patient's age. Diagnosis was cervical subluxation complex with autonomic nervous system involvement. Eleven adjustments of the atlas vertebra were made over the next 3 months, with the patient noting vision changes after the third treatment session (247). First he observed shades of gray instead of just black, and by the sixth session, he noted seeing blue swirling circles. Later, he saw yellow areas, and finally, light coming through a window.

Optometric examination on 11/28/88 revealed distance visual acuities of OD 20/50, OS 20/100, and OU 20/50. Pupils were 1–2 mm and slightly reactive to light and near-far stimulus. Retinoscopic reflexes improved significantly. Distance retinoscopy was OD +3.00–4.50 × 97 and OS + 1.75–2.75 × 74. Subjective refraction was OD + 2.50–4.75 × 99 with 20/40 and OS + 1.00–3.00 × 72 with 20/100. Complete optometric findings were cited, including distance phoria, nearpoint findings, and nearpoint acuities. Additional progress evaluation on 1/9/89 revealed acuities of 20/50++, 20/100, and 20/50++. The patient reported he could again read comfortably, and he was continuing his chiropractic care.

While caution should be used in reaching conclusions about single cases, the authors did not feel that spontaneous remission was an appropriate explanation for the somewhat immediate and dramatic improvement seen after the onset of CMT in this case. Two hypotheses offered were that CMT induced changes in vascularity of the optic nerve via the cervical sympathetic influence on cerebral blood flow or that CMT induced direct somatoautonomic changes influencing optic nerve function. Further, they suggested that this case is probably not as uncommon as the paucity of literature would indicate and that further research of visual changes after chiropractic is warranted (247).

PEDIATRIC DISORDERS

Nothing seemingly angers detractors of chiropractic more than talk of giving adjustments to children, who are too young to say "no" and whose "misguided" parents are unaware of the "dangers" of chiropractic. Hence, when *Consumer Reports* advised parents not to subject their children to an unproven remedy, it seemed as though the fourth estate was offering advice that truly protected the public (248).

However, in the nearly two decades since that article appeared, a number of investigations are offering initial evidence that CMT may offer children effective help with a variety of disorders related to the spinal and extraspinal joints and nerves; some are presented below. And, while there is no strong evidence that adjustments alone can stop the progression of idiopathic scoliosis, for example, chiropractors have had apparent success with cases of infantile colic, attention-deficit hyperactivity, some undifferentiated learning and behavioral disorders, pediatric trauma, and perhaps with enuresis and even certain chronic respiratory infections and disorders (see next section, this chapter). While the jury is still out regarding chiropractic pediatrics, there is growing evidence that some role for CMT for children will one day be scientifically validated.

Attention Deficit Hyperactivity Disorder

Attention deficit hyperactivity disorder (ADHD), according to the DSM-III-R (249), is evidenced by developmentally inappropriate inattention, hyperactivity, and impulsiveness. The disorder appears in most situations and is typically worse when prolonged attention is required, such as listening to a teacher. Improvement is seen when the person is receiving frequent reinforcement or very strict control or is in a new environment or playing a video game. Features associated with this disorder include low self-esteem, mood lability, low frustration tolerance, and temper outbursts. Academic underachievement is common. Complete diagnostic criteria have been operationally defined (249).

There is growing knowledge of the clinical course of ADHD, and good evidence that its effects last into adulthood. For example, Fischer and co-workers (250) prospectively followed 100 hyperactive children meeting diagnostic criteria and 60 control children over an 8-year period, and found that hyperactive children tended to remain chronically impaired in academic achievement, in inattention, and in behavioral disinhibition well into their late adolescent years. Moreover, Mannuzza et al. (251) followed up on their earlier work on late adolescent hyperactives with a blinded investigation that confirmed the earlier findings. Hence, in 94 18-year-old boys who had been previously diagnosed (mean age at initial diagnosis, 7.3 years) as hyperactive (ADHD), blinded interviews by clinicians revealed significantly more ADHD (43 vs. 4%), antisocial disorders (32 vs. 8%), and drug use disorders (10 vs. 1%) in the probands than in 78 normal controls.

Evidence for etiology of ADHD was reported recently in the *New England Journal of Medicine* by Zametkin et al. (252). Knowing that the premotor cortex and superior prefrontal cortex had been earlier shown to be involved in the control of attention and motor activity, these researchers measured glucose metabolism in 25 adults with histories of hyperactivity who continued to have symptoms (and who were also the biologic parent of a hyperactive child), and in 50 normal controls. Whole-brain and regional rates of glucose metabolism were measured by tomography (Scanditronix positron-emission tomograph after administration of fluoro-2-deoxy-D-glucose intravenously) and revealed lower global metabolism in adult hyperactives and significantly reduced glucose metabolism in 30 of 60 specific regions of the brain (p <.05). The premotor cortex and superior prefrontal cortex experienced some of the greatest reductions in glucose metabolism. While not offering a hypothesis about this finding, the authors suggested that it was consistent with others that suggest a role for the frontal lobe in the pathophysiology of ADHD, while not ruling out a more general role for abnormal "arousal" in this disorder.

Certainly the prevailing paradigm for the treatment of children with hyperactivity is that the child has abnormally low arousal levels (as evidenced by electrodermal tests, for example) and that stimulant medications (primarily, methylphenidate (Ritalin)) cause a "paradoxical" increase in arousal and thereby improved performance in school (253). However, Whalen and Henker (253), in a recent review of their own research and other literature, suggested that what has been called a paradoxical "calming" effect of Ritalin in ADHD children may be neither paradoxical nor specific to individuals with biological dysfunctions. They cite studies showing that ADHD children, normal children, and adults are all capable of stimulant-induced behavioral and task improvements. Due to the multiproblem nature of ADHD, they call for multipronged treatments, including psychosocial treatment (254). They contend that stimulant medication may undermine or facilitate other treatments and that the relative advantages and disadvantages of the pharmacologic approach need further investigation (253).

Early chiropractic investigators observed significant improvement in children with hyperkinetic behaviors, as well as in children with other learning and behavioral impairments, after adjustments, in a clinical case study at College Station, Texas (255, 256). The study was directed by E. V. Walton, Ph.D., Sc.D., M.D., director of Psychoeducational and Guidance Services, and included a clinical psychologist and a superintendent of schools (see further discussion below). In this investigation, 12 ADHD students (grade school through high school) receiving stim-

ulant medication were compared with a group of 12 ADHD students receiving CMT. Initially, medication seemed to be effective in 9 of the 12 in controlling hyperactivity and improving attention span, while not improving fine and gross motor coordination. However, increasing dosages of stimulant medication were required to maintain this effect. Moreover, 50% of subjects receiving stimulant medication had personality alterations, loss of appetite, and insomnia related to their treatment (256).

In contrast, not only did CMT improve hyperactive behaviors, ADHD students receiving chiropractic had concomitant improvement in a wider range of 13 symptom or problem areas assessed by the investigators than did students receiving stimulant medication alone. While reduction in hyperactivity and improvement in attention span were approximately equal initially, the effectiveness of medication alone in these two symptom areas was not as sustained as chiropractic treatment effects. Statistically, CMT was 20–40% more effective than medications. These researchers concluded that the improvement in impairment rating (especially in relieving nervous tension), effort, and motivation was associated with chiropractic care (256).

Following up on this work and anecdotal observations, Giesen, Center, and Leach (257) used the multiple-baseline-across-subjects design to evaluate seven consecutive previously diagnosed ADHD school-aged children before and after CMT. (In this design, first the subject's pretreatment baseline is established, then that subject receives treatment; after the first subject's treatment baseline is established, a second subject is introduced. For further discussion see Section 5.) Using an Activator instrument set in the "off" position as a placebo treatment in these subjects who had no prior chiropractic experience, the pretreatment baseline was actually a "placebo" condition. Consecutively, the patients were introduced to diversified full-spine technique at all applicable segments. Data were analyzed visually and with nonparametric statistical methods.

Five of 7 children showed improvement in mean behavioral scores from placebo care to treatment (P <.03). Four of seven showed significant decreases in arousal levels (p = 0.009) (Fig. 9.6), which were initially elevated—a finding not inconsistent with some other studies and in contradiction to those suggesting Ritalin use for supposed "paradoxical effects." Despite interexaminer blinding and problems with two confounding patients who had less than 2 weeks of active treatment before the study ended (school was starting and they were scheduled to restart their stimulant medications), three of the four principal tests used to detect improvement (parent ratings of activity, motion recorder scores, electrodermal measures, and x-rays of spinal distortions) agreed, either positively or negatively, for all seven children. Parent ratings of hyperkinesity were dramatically reduced in four of the seven children as well (Fig. 9.7).

The authors concluded that considering the short duration of chiropractic intervention (viz., 5, 4, 3, or 2 weeks of thrice-weekly sessions) and considering the short domains tapped by the four primary outcome measures, the results suggest a clinically significant effect of CMT on hyperactivity and its autonomic substrate in these hyperactive patients. The results point to CMT as a possible nondrug intervention for children with hyperactivity (257).

Colic (Infantile)

There are reports that chiropractic has been used for the treatment of *infantile colic*, a disorder seen in approximately 20% of all infants, characterized by uncontrollable crying generally starting at age 1–4 weeks and resolving spontaneously at age 3–4 months (258). Apparently, CMT has been used in Denmark for years, with anecdotal reports of success (258). In a questionnaire study, Nilsson (259) retrospectively found that 90% of infants with colic treated with CMT had satisfactory results.

To more accurately assess the possible effect of CMT on the course of infantile colic, Klougart, Nilsson, and Jacobsen (258) pro-

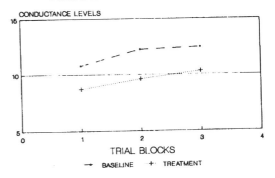

Figure 9.6. Electrodermal activity was reduced in children with hyperactivity, in a trial by Giesen, Center, and Leach (257). Using a single-subject research design, subjects had significantly lower (P = .009) arousal levels when receiving CMT than during intervention with a placebo treatment in the baseline phase. In addition, movement of the children as assessed by motion recorders was reduced significantly (Walsh test: P <.03) (not shown) while under chiropractic care. (From Giesen JM, Center DB, Leach RA. An evaluation of chiropractic manipulation as a treatment of hyperactivity in children. J Manipulative Physiol Ther 1989;12:353–363. Reprinted by permission.)

spectively followed 316 cases seen at 50 chiropractic clinics. Of 569 patients with symptoms of colic, 316 met strict inclusion criteria (viz., age 2–52 weeks; no symptoms or signs other than colic; at least one violent crying spell per day lasting at least 1.5 hr for 5 of the last 7 days; weight gain at least 150 g/week; motoric unrest during colic with frequent flexing of knees toward abdomen and/or backward bending of head and trunk; and inability to be comforted during colic by being picked up, diaper change, or food or other aid) and did not meet any of the exclusion criteria (i.e., they had no spinal functional disturbance on chiropractic examination), and their parents accepted participation. The median age at debut of colic in the study sample was 2 weeks. The median age at the onset of CMT was 5.7 weeks. Before CMT, 51% of the infants in

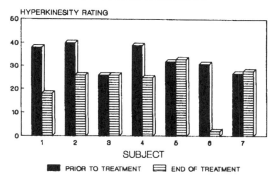

PARENTAL RATINGS
OF HYPERKINESITY

Figure 9.7. Parental ratings of hyperkinetic activity were assessed with the Werry-Weiss-Peters scale, in a study of children with hyperactivity receiving CMT. Robust clinical improvement after CMT was indicated by four of the seven sets of parents; 1 year after the treatment, follow-up tests revealed that two of the four children had sustained permanent reduction in hyperkinetic behaviors, despite no follow-up care. (From Giesen JM, Center DB, Leach RA. An evaluation of chiropractic manipulation as a treatment of hyperactivity in children. J Manipulative Physiol Ther 1989;12:353–363. Reprinted by permission.)

the study sample had other forms of treatment, primarily dimethicone.

Mothers were given a diary and recorded symptoms daily; structured assessment by the chiropractor was used 1, 2, and 4 weeks after the start of CMT. Chiropractic technique generally consisted of nonaudible light or no-thrust adjustment forces, usually applied with one finger, to restore intersegmental mobility. According to assessment forms completed by the chiropractors, 94% of infants received CMT to the upper cervical articulations, and 53% received only upper cervical adjustments. Midthoracic adjustments (T4/5 to T8/9) were administered 41% of the time in addition to occipitoatlantoaxial adjustments. Only 6% of infants received adjustments to other spinal areas without upper cervical CMT.

There was clinically significant improvement after 1 week (35% colic stopped, 56% colic improved, 8% no change, 1% worse);

after 2 weeks and an average of three adjustments, very impressive clinical results were achieved (60% colic stopped, 34% colic improved, 4% no change, 2% worse). As colic is considered to be potentially life threatening—the authors point out that uncontrollable crying may provoke acts of violence toward the infant—the resolution of colic after 2 weeks of care and very early in the normal 2- to 3-month course of this disorder, suggests that CMT altered its natural history and is an effective treatment (258). Further research on CMT in the management of this potentially serious disorder is certainly warranted, given these findings.

Dyslexia

Brzozowske and Walton (255) cited the case of an obese 13-year-old white male with a psychiatric diagnostic workup of dyslexia, impaired visual memory imprint, response formulation lag (reading), impaired mental coordination and finger pursuit, marked equilibrium impairment, and mixed dominance (residual), with severe emotional overlay (the patient had not been in school for 2 years because of separation anxiety). Apparently, a severe hysteria attack at school 2 years earlier (after a major family trauma) was construed as an epileptic seizure, and his doctor had prescribed a mild tranquilizer. He also had psychosomatic problems, hypoventilated, and had infantile regression (he had been allowed to sleep with his mother for 2 years). CMT was instituted. All learning disabilities except the dyslexia disappeared. He reenrolled in school and has continued chiropractic and started family counseling. However, when therapy was discontinued, infantile regression recurred (255).

Lefkowitz and Lefkowitz (unpublished observations) followed 21 subjects (16 school-aged) with histories of dyslexia and learning disability. Seven additional subjects did not complete treatment (four dropped out, two moved, and one completed care but was unavailable for retest). Consecutive patients seen in the chiropractic clinic from April 1987 to August 1988 with reports of perceptual disorder, known dyslexia or learning disabilities, and generally poor school performance were examined with the Woodcock Reading Mastery Test (260), which tests for five functions of reading (word attack, word comprehension, passage comprehension, word identification, and letter identification). A variety of chiropractic applied kinesiology and diversified adjusting techniques were used on the subjects, from short-lever high-speed adjusting to light touch (nutritional advice, treatment of extraspinal sites, exercises such as cross-crawl for in-home use, and continuation of daily practicing of reading and writing were among many other treatments used). Improvement in reading scores in at least one area was noted in 18 of 21 subjects; indeed, in these the grade-level function jumped 1 year or more during the 3-month study period, between pre- and post- chiropractic care assessments. The remaining three subjects had no improvement or lower scores on retest. Thirteen returned for at least a 1-year assessment, and all these retained their improvement in school work and grades. Two subjects in their fifth decade were functioning at the third and fourth grade levels despite remedial help throughout school; after 3 months of chiropractic, both were functioning at the 12.9 grade level. Despite these encouraging results, further controlled trials are still necessary to determine whether benefits were derived more from CMT, from daily reading and writing practice, or from placebo. Nevertheless, the findings warrant research, given the large cost to society of dyslexia.

Enuresis

Enuresis is characterized by involuntary voiding at least twice per month in 5- or 6-year-old children and at least once per month in older children (261). Following up on anecdotal observations reported in the chiropractic literature, Gemmell and Jacobson (261) used a time series descriptive design to evaluate improvement in enuresis after CMT, in a 14-year-old white male who had never experienced a dry night despite

medical intervention, including an alarm system (bell and pad or dry bed training). Examination revealed palpable tenderness and movement dysfunction of the L5/S1 joints. Otherwise, findings were normal.

For 2 weeks, a pretreatment baseline was established in which placebo adjusting (i.e., touching and gentle massage of the low back) was used. Then one or two adjustments per week for 4 weeks followed by two biweekly treatments were given using toggle recoil technique applied only to L5/S1. A daily diary of wet/damp/dry bed conditions was kept by the patient throughout the trial. A dramatic partial remission was seen immediately after the onset of CMT but not during the placebo intervention. Indeed, after the onset of chiropractic 5 consecutive nights were dry for the first time ever, and 1 month later, there had been 12 additional dry nights, 8 damp nights, and only 6 wet nights, according to preset criteria. While not permitting definitive conclusions, the large and abrupt change in a previously stable pretreatment condition suggested that CMT was responsible for the observed improvement (261).

In a thorough follow-up to such case studies Leboeuf et al., (262) at the School of Chiropractic, Phillip Institute of Technology, prospectively evaluated 171 children (aged 4 to 15) to investigate the effectiveness of CMT for enuresis. These children met inclusion criteria and did not meet exclusion criteria that eliminated 21 additional subjects, all of whom responded to advertisements in the local press and letters to local primary schools.

Subjects were divided into two groups, both of which received a 2-week preintervention baseline assessment. Then one group received unspecified chiropractic adjustments while the other was further observed for an additional 2-week baseline prior to CMT. Specific chiropractic adjustments to areas of abnormal spinal motion detected on each visit were accomplished by fifth year chiropractic students. Treatment continued until the parent recorded fewer than two wet nights over a 2-week period while the child was on unrestricted fluid intake. Success was operationally defined as a reduction of 50% or more in wet nights per week during intervention. Due to a skewing in the distribution of wet nights between subject groups, nonparametric statistical tests were used (viz., Mann-Whitney U test) for analysis. Of the 120 boys and 51 girls included in the study, mean age 8.3 years, more than 80% were classified as primary enuretics (i.e., they had never had a dry night) (262).

Results revealed a reduction in wet nights from 6 to 5 during intervention in the first group; the group receiving an additional 2-week pretreatment baseline dropped during intervention from 5 to an average of 3 wet nights per week. While improvement in both groups was considered statistically significant (p <.0001), without a control group, the placebo effect cannot be ruled out as an explanation for the results. Moreover, only 25% of these cases met the preset operational definition for successful outcome, and only 15.5% were "dry" after CMT. Other interventions have achieved similar or much better outcomes in terms of dry nights: psychotherapy (10%), periodic waking (11%), spontaneous improvement while placed on a waiting list (14%), psychotherapy plus placebo (40%), bell and pad (80%), and dry bed training (100%). The authors concluded that since "dry" nights after CMT were not much more frequent than spontaneous improvement while on a waiting list, the changes observed were likely a placebo effect.

Several drawbacks to this research were the lack of descriptive data regarding the chiropractic technique involved (and what spinal levels were most often adjusted), length of time receiving CMT, and number of adjustments administered. Without these data, it is difficult to compare these results with cases observed in private practice and hard to know if adequate (dosage) care comparable with our practice experiences was even administered. The question of CMT for enuresis remains unresolved. Use of CMT for this disorder remains experimen-

tal for the time being, and patients should be advised accordingly.

Learning and Behavioral Disabilities

In a pilot investigation, Brzozowske and Walton (255) studied the effects of CMT on 13 children with learning and behavioral impairments resulting from neurological dysfunction. Of 20 patients initially recruited, 7 did not pass exclusion criteria including concomitant medical care. The remaining 13 all met inclusion criteria including indicators of associative learning disabilities and emotional overlay.

Five of the 13 had previously received extensive medical care and treatment without apparent benefit; these were also seriously emotionally disturbed (suicidal, schizophrenia, etc.). Symptoms of emotional disturbance disappeared and have not recurred in four of these five, after up to several months of chiropractic care. The remaining subject could not remain under chiropractic care long enough for more than temporary amelioration of symptomatology (255).

Eight of the remaining nine subjects had some prior medical and other remedial assistance for their conditions. Generally, symptoms of neurological and/or brain dysfunction affecting behaviors and academic progress were effectively reduced or eliminated in these cases. In all cases where neurological impairments remained after CMT, coping abilities improved. This investigation spurred follow-up investigations on the effect of adjustments on children with ADHD by Brzozowske and Walton (256) and by Giesen, Center, and Leach (257) (see above), with favorable results. However, further research on CMT for pediatric patients with severe emotional and learning disabilities has not been forthcoming, despite two nonprofit chiropractic institutions that treat children with multiple handicaps and disabilities, often with great but only testimonial-type reports of success (i.e., the Kentuckiana Children's Center, Dr. Lorraine M. Golden, Exec. Administrator, 3700 Georgetown Place, Louisville, KY

40256–0039; and Oklahaven Children's Chiropractic Center, Dr. Bobby Doscher, President, 2245 N.W. 12th Street, Oklahoma City, OK 73107).

Scoliosis

A number of anecdotal and uncontrolled case history presentations suggesting correction of scoliosis after adjustments have appeared in the chiropractic nonindexed literature through the years. Generally these studies and observations do not define the type/location/severity of the scoliosis or the risk of progression and the prognosis (263).

In an initial case report in the indexed literature, Aspergren and Cox (264) used CMT (flexion-distraction with lateral flexion to reduce the apical curvature and stretch-shortened tissues on the concave aspect of the curve) with neuromuscular stimulation in a 14-year-old female with idiopathic scoliosis. Her rate of progression was 1° per month for the 9 months prior to onset of CMT. After 3 months of distraction/stimulation her curvature was reduced from 27° (Cobb) to 17°; after 9 months of follow-up nighttime stimulation, the curvature was 23°. The authors hypothesize that distractive manipulation may increase the flexibility of spinal curvatures and further potentiate the effects of transneural stimulation (TNS). Comparing prior results from investigators using neuromuscular stimulation only with findings in this case, the authors concluded that excellent and improved clinical results were obtained by combining distractive manipulation with neuromuscular stimulation. Further research on this innovation is warranted.

Significant leg length inequalities (LLI; anatomical short leg syndrome) can promote scoliosis, and Specht and DeBoer (265) confirmed findings of a number of medical investigators regarding this effect. With LLI greater than 6 mm, 53% had either scoliosis, hyperlordosis, or hypolordosis of the lumbar spine. Finding significantly greater incidence (p = .01) of these spinal abnormalities in cases of LLI >6 mm matched results of prior investigators and suggested the need for correction with heel lift therapy.

While there is good evidence that LLI-induced scoliosis should be corrected with heel lift therapy, chiropractic researchers question the use of adjustments to correct idiopathic scoliosis, since there is no good evidence that adjusting the apices of curvatures reduces scoliosis (266, 267). Use of adjustments to increase joint mobility in conjunction with heel lift therapy, neuromuscular stimulation, or bracing may have validity but needs full evaluation (263). As these other approaches are fully described in medical journals, they are not reviewed here, although they do generally fall within the domain of chiropractic practice.

Trauma (Pediatric)

Hinwood and Hinwood (268) reviewed the myriad of potential traumatic causes of spinal lesions in children cited in the chiropractic literature, including falls, accidents, sports, exertion, and birth. Throughout this chapter (and in later sections of this book; see also Chapter 12) the response of traumatically induced spinal lesions to CMT has been reviewed in some detail. Many of these cases and studies involve pediatric trauma, and very often the outcome of chiropractic management has been entirely successful. For example, although the sufferer of traumatic spinal myoclonus cited earlier in this chapter was 24 on entrance to the chiropractor, she suffered the diving injury that started her ordeal at age 7 (182). The interested reader should search for pediatric trauma under specific etiologic classifications.

RESPIRATORY DISORDERS

If chiropractic management of pediatric disorders is considered controversial, especially outside chiropractic circles, then management of respiratory disorders with CMT is probably an outrage! While asthma, for example, is not generally a life-threatening disorder, in certain cases nontreatment can be disastrous. Hence, when ABC's "20/20" program featured a program on chiropractic, it reported that asthma was not a condition that could be treated by chiropractic, implying that any chiropractor who claimed to treat asthma was a quack (269). Nevertheless, from early anecdotal reports in the chiropractic and osteopathic literature to case reports now appearing in peer-reviewed journals, there is growing evidence that certain respiratory disorders—many of them pediatric—appear to show sustained improvement after CMT.

Allergies

There are no case studies in the chiropractic peer-reviewed literature regarding CMT for the management of patients with allergies or sinusitis. However, several articles have appeared in a chiropractic trade journal. Management of *Candida albicans* allergy, *allergic rhinitis (sinusitis)* associated with C1-C3 segmental dysfunction, and differentiating neurogenic triggers for the allergic reaction versus atopic IgE-mediated allergy, were reported in the *Digest of Chiropractic Economics*, according to a search in the *Index to Chiropractic Literature* (270).

It is discouraging for those of us in chiropractic who feel we have personally benefited from chiropractic management of allergies and sinus disorders to find that as of this writing, there still are no case reports on CMT and these conditions in the chiropractic scientific literature. However, growing evidence that chiropractic adjustments (but not placebo treatments) influence natural killer cell production and influence immunity (see Chapter 14) offers hope that confirmation of an allergy-suppressing influence or homeostatic benefit of CMT in allergic individuals can be established as well.

Asthma/Asthmatic Bronchitis

Childhood asthma is indeed a devastating disease. Requiring 200,000 hospitalizations and 10.1 million missed days of school annually, researchers claim it is the leading cause of days lost from school and costs society about $6.2 billion per year (271). Even worse, the disease is potentially fatal, and mortality has risen about 46% in the 1980s to about 4700 deaths in 1989. Scientists are unsure why asthma is on the rise despite advances in treatment and in our understanding of the disorder (271).

Kaliner and co-workers (272) demonstrated autoantibodies to β-receptors in 24 patients with seasonal or perennial allergic rhinitis. These patients were found to have β-adrenergic hyporeactivity and cholinergic hypersensitivity. Since β-adrenergists modulate the allergen-induced release of mast cell mediators that produce the inflammatory response, autoantibodies to these receptors would be expected to promote an allergic response. The autonomic activity is not the primary defect, since administration of β-blockers to normal subjects does not make them asthmatic (273). Stress and autonomic imbalance (including spinal stress from a vertebral lesion), however, could be expected to enhance an allergic response (see Chapter 14). Either increased cholinergic or α-adrenergic activity or decreased β-adrenergic activity in the smooth muscles of the bronchial airways would be expected to enhance an episode of allergic asthma (274). Therefore, some combination of spinal stress with facilitation and aberrant somatoautonomic reflexes, with superimposed genetic predisposition to allergic asthma, may be responsible for especially marked episodes of the disease and may account for the mechanism whereby chiropractic manipulation may be of benefit in its treatment.

While a number of observations of impressive improvement after chiropractic treatment of asthma have been reported anecdotally in the nonrefereed literature, few have appeared in the indexed scientific literature (269).

A study in the *Boston Medical Journal* (now the *New England Journal of Medicine*) by Murphy and Wilson (275) in 1925 was published as part of an ongoing investigation of osteopathy and chiropractic. Twenty patients were chosen who had suffered nearly continuous attacks of asthma, had failed to respond to vaccine therapy, and had only minimally responded to adrenalin injections. Instead of determining whether each patient had an osteopathic lesion, the investigators assumed that one existed at the fourth and fifth dorsal level (the segments presumed to be responsible for sympathetic nerve supply to the bronchial tubes and, hence, circulation). These patients were treated with 10–70 sessions of OMT. No control patients were used to assess the psychosomatic involvement. Fifteen of 20 patients experienced at least some temporary relief, and five reported no change. Six of the 15 who reported relief of symptoms were very much improved (90–100%), and another four reported noticeable improvement (50–75%). No conclusions were drawn by the authors, but it is noteworthy that even without locating the exact osteopathic lesion, these investigators could treat the area of the spine segmentally associated with the visceral disturbance and achieve significant results in 75% of these patients in whom medical treatments had previously failed.

Modern chiropractic investigations were conducted by Jamison et al. (276) Nilsson and Christiansen (277), and Lines, McMilan, and Spehr (278) in Australia. In a pilot investigation of asthma at the Phillip Institute of Chiropractic, researchers determined that lung volume and peak flow did not improve significantly after CMT. However, all patients (n = 15) reported satisfaction with chiropractic care and indicated that they believed chiropractic had benefitted their condition. In addition, while under CMT, six patients voluntarily elected to reduce their medications and another stopped medication altogether (276).

These findings mirrored results published by Miller (279) on 44 patients with chronic obstructive pulmonary disease. While 92% of 22 patients receiving OMT in addition to medication reported definite subjective improvement in their physical work capacity, there were no significant collateral improvements seen in pulmonary function studies, compared with a group receiving medication only. Only vital capacity (nearly identical in both groups prior to interventions) improved, 0.5 liters in the manipulated group,

as opposed to 0.1 liters improvement in the control group, but even this effect was not statistically significant because of the small number of patients investigated.

Nilsson and Christiansen (277) reviewed consecutive records (n = 79) of asthma cases and found that the age of onset of asthma was a significant factor in predicting improvement after CMT. Younger patients had a greater response to CMT than did older patients, and improvement was seen after five treatments over the course of at least one month. The authors concluded that younger patients with milder forms of asthma appeared to respond best to CMT.

More recently, Lines, McMilan, and Spehr (278) examined a technique first reported in the osteopathic literature, but widely used in chiropractic practice as well, to determine its benefit in enhancing forced vital capacity (FVC), forced expiratory volume in one second (FEV 1), and FEV1/FVC% in 30 asymptomatic subjects. While there was no significant improvement in the group as a whole after four sessions using soft tissue and Chapman's neurolymphatic reflex stimulation of the diaphragm, a subgroup of eight subjects with lower than expected initial FVC and FEV 1 values improved significantly from the first pretreatment FVC to the last posttreatment FVC (paired t test P = .02). Five of these eight subjects reported a past history of asthma or bronchitis. The authors suggested that traditional CMT and reflex techniques may have therapeutic value in the treatment of patients who have below average respiratory function. Certainly, these findings should spur additional chiropractic research to elucidate what role CMT may have in the management of these potentially serious respiratory diseases.

Somatic Dyspnea

Masarsky and Weber (280) presented six cases of dyspnea that improved following CMT, along with objective spirometric assessment of expiratory volume. These cases primarily were associated with orthopaedic complaints. For example, patients presented with any combination of the following: low back pain, headaches, TMJ syndrome, stiffness of the rib cage, interscapular pain, and/or a history of chronic obstructive lung disease. They were given high-velocity low-amplitude diversified chiropractic technique; neurovascular treatment according to Bennett/Goodheart, including "light touch" to specific muscles based upon muscle testing; Meridian treatment including accupressure; and treatment of the pterogoid muscle after palpable hypertonicity was found there in every case, as well as Chapman's reflex technique. Results of treatment were reported based on spirometric evaluation of forced vital capacity (FVC) and forced expiratory volume in one second (FEV-1). From their prior research and these data, the authors suggest mild clinical improvement in the functional capacity of the lungs after CMT. Calculations based on available data indicate that in addition to good to excellent symptomatic results in these cases (n = 6), there was modest improvement in FVC (average increase of 0.4 liters in FVC after a course of CMT) and in FEV-1 (average increase of 0.5 liters in FEV-1 after a course of CMT). While strong conclusions cannot be drawn from case histories, the response to manipulative intervention was sometimes so dramatic and rapid, even in long-standing somatic dyspnea, that the authors felt compelled to suggest that a strong linkage between the dyspnea and the primary presenting complaint was likely.

Discussion

Prior editions of this text extensively reviewed osteopathic experimental studies performed since the turn of the century that outlined a role for experimentally induced spinal lesions causing a wide variety of somatovisceral responses in animals (281). Due to space limitations, that material was eliminated from this revision. However, current experimental research cited in this chapter (see also Chapter 8) along with human clinical studies provide a strong basis for arguing that many human disorders are affected by somatic lesions, even if causation cannot yet be inferred. Indeed, in the years since the first edition of this text appeared, the arguments grow stronger that SDF with concomitant facilitation remains the most likely justification for the use of CMT for other than pain syndromes.

Studies cited in this chapter are beginning to zero in on operational definitions of SDF-related autonomic imbalance as well. For example, evidence continues to mount from blinded studies that certain physical measures of SDF (restricted range of motion and paraspinal tenderness as assessed by algometry) correlate well with each other and are present at spinal sites reflexly related to certain visceral disorders (coronary artery disease, renal disease, primary dysmenorrhea) (6, 35, 47, 48, 235). These studies used preset criteria for documentation of a spinal lesion or SDF. Future studies can begin to prospectively follow patients meeting these criteria to determine if ablation of these signs following chiropractic care results in improvement in the related visceral disturbances.

How does CMT work? As we saw earlier, not all early chiropractors held to bone-out-of-place as the primary mechanism to explain spinal lesions and their effects. D. D. Palmer himself—while obviously a proponent of bone-out-of-place—also held that too much or not enough "tone" in the nervous system caused disease (see Chapter 4).

Certainly current models of SDF and RDF presented in the past few chapters do not point exclusively to mechanical hypotheses such as entrapped meniscus but suggest a role for biological and physiological mechanisms as well (see section in Chapter 8, "Neurobiologic Models of SDF"). Even neurophysiologists argue that the nervous system plays a considerable role in inflammation and inflammatory disease (282). Hence, Basbaum and Levine (282) indicate that norepinephrine release is associated with a decreased plasma extravasation, which is associated with increased severity of disease. Acute inflammation, in their view, is an attempt by the body to repair damaged tissues, especially in diseases like arthritis. Moreover, sympathetic postganglionic nerve terminals contain substances that are proinflammatory (i.e., enhance plasma extravasation) and others that participate in the development, severity, and longevity of tissue injury (Fig. 9.8). With our current level of understanding we can only speculate, but certainly evidence suggests that mechanists and biologists should join hands: the chiropractic lesion is probably both a mechanical and a biological problem! Moreover, D. D. Palmer's concept of "tone" may not be far off the mark.

In a randomized trial of passive joint movement versus placebo therapy, Zusman, Edwards, and Donaghy (87) found no support for the hypothesis that relief of joint pain is due to the release of opioid peptides, although they could not rule out involvement of centrally activated "nonopioid" pain control. The authors speculated that inhibition of reflex muscle contraction and/or some temporary decrease in somatic afferent bombardment of the dorsal horn might accompany passive joint mobilization (and similarly, CMT). Chiropractic researchers have had mixed findings about a proposed CMT-initiated release in other endogenous opioids such as beta endorphins; however, researchers have not yet looked for a central release of this substance following CMT (see Chapter 8).

Thoren and co-workers (283) propose that prolonged rhythmic exercise and acupuncture activate central opioid systems by triggering increased discharge from mechanosensitive afferent group III or A-delta nerve fibers arising from skeletal muscle. They held that this would explain many of the cardiovascular, analgesic, and behavioral effects of exercise. Indeed, such diverse conditions as anorexia, essential hypertension, and depression have improved in subjects receiving regular exercise, and there are known benefits for immunity and pain control as well. A central mechanism for beta endorphin release after CMT has never been investigated and remains an interesting possibility. Such a mechanism

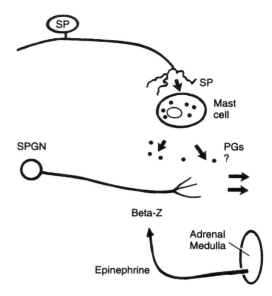

Figure 9.8. Major peripheral nervous system elements thought to mediate the neural contribution to plasma extravasation. Plasma extravasation is a major feature of acute inflammation. Peptides (e.g., substance P; *SP*) are released from primary afferent fibers and act upon mast cells that influence sympathetic postganglionic neuron (*SPGN*). This initiates the release of a number of substances, such as prostaglandin (*PG*), which causes plasma extravasation. A role for stress is proposed whereby epinephrine released by the adrenal medulla acts as a β_2-receptor on the terminals of the SPGN. Several recent trials have shown that adjustments affect plasma levels of SP. (Adapted from Basbaum AI, Levine JD. The contribution of the nervous system to inflammation and inflammatory disease. Can J Physiol Pharmacol 1991;69:647–651.)

would go far in explaining many of the purported somatovisceral benefits of CMT. While the beta endorphin question remains, chiropractic researchers have made great strides recently in documenting other biological mechanisms related to CMT.

Brennan and colleagues (284) at the National College of Chiropractic found, in a randomized trial, that the zymosan-stimulated chemoluminescence response of both polymorphonuclear neutrophils and monocytes was stimulated by CMT but not by sham or soft-tissue interventions. Further, radioimmunoassay of substance P from plasma demonstrated significant elevations after CMT but not after sham intervention. They determined that this is a short-term (greatest increase 15 minutes after manipulation) response and that mononuclear cells were also primed for enhanced endotoxin-stimulated tumor necrosis factor production by CMT (see also Chapter 14) (285). Such provocative findings suggest complex biological events surround the act of chiropractic manipulation, which we are only now beginning to explore. Does this activity relate to the intraarticular gaseous and fluid exchange associated with the manipulative event (see Chapter 5)? The work of Brennan and co-workers (284, 285) does suggest that a minimum of force during manipulation is necessary to effect the biological events they noted. Certainly joint coaptation (the audible release or "crack") associated with manipulation is the supreme clinical sign of effectiveness used throughout the profession, and it may be the primary instigator of these biological phenomena.

The role of somatic sensations in causing alterations of autonomic function was dramatically demonstrated by Ekman et al. (286). They demonstrated that autonomic activity distinguishes between positive and negative emotions and even distinguishes among different types of negative emotion. Such a powerful role for the autonomic nervous system had not been previously expected. Their study found—using trained actors—that constructing facial prototypes of emotion, muscle by muscle, resulted in a more powerful autonomic response than did the process of reliving past emotions. According to the authors, even biofeedback cannot produce such changes.

Generally, CMT as a valid treatment for disorders other than pain syndromes remains to be fully validated. Yet evidence is clearly emerging that a wide variety of stress-related disorders appear to benefit from CMT. No one would dispute that the vast majority of named medical conditions in this chapter might be considered related to stress syndrome (see also Appendix I).

Researchers in chiropractic should continue to explore the role of CMT in the management of these and similar disorders, and the reader is urged to stay abreast of developments in the chiropractic scientific peer-reviewed journals.

Given a role for SDF and RDF in creating facilitation, sympathicotonia, and autonomic dysfunction, what role do these lesions play in self-progression or degeneration? Are these precursors to spondylosis and so-called subluxation degeneration? Is SDF maintained by facilitation a precursor to medical subluxations? These and other questions are addressed in the next section of this text.

Summary

This chapter began by presenting a plan for diagnosing spinal dysfunction based upon available chiropractic and osteopathic scientific literature. Regional assessments (i.e., algometry, functional strength assessment, passive range of motion, surface electromyography, thermography, etc.) identify neuromusculoskeletal dysfunction in an isolated region of the spine, while segmental assessments (i.e., algometry, motion palpation, motion studies, static palpation, etc.) isolate dysfunction at a specific vertebral level.

The role of CMT in the management of type M (musculoskeletal) disorders was discussed under the subheadings entrapment syndromes (primarily disc syndrome), mechanical syndromes (such as adhesive capsulitis, facet syndrome, and sacroiliac joint syndrome), and muscular syndromes (i.e., cervicogenic headache, fibrositis, and strain/sprain injuries). Sciaticas and undifferentiated neck and back pain disorders were reviewed in light of research using manipulation or CMT as well.

Improvement in type N (neurological) disorders after CMT was similarly reviewed. Barre's syndrome, Bell's palsy, migraine headache, seizure disorder, reflex sympathetic dystrophy, and similar disorders were reviewed in this section.

CMT and type O disorders (organic) were surveyed as well. Subheadings included cardiovascular, gastrointestinal, genitourinary, gynecological, ophthalmologic, pediatric, and respiratory.

The chapter ends with a discussion that suggests that reduction of SDF and RDF by adjustment probably involves both mechanical and biological mechanisms. While evidence for a centrally acting opioid mechanism after CMT remains to be explored, researchers have demonstrated significant increases in substance P, and in natural killer cells after CMT but not after sham or soft-tissue interventions in control subjects. Such mechanisms could account for the diverse visceral effects of CMT reported throughout this chapter. Generally, CMT remains to be fully validated as a treatment for disorders other than pain syndromes.

REFERENCES

1. Johnston WL. Inter-rater reliability in the selection of manipulable patients. In: Buerger AA, Greenman PE, eds. Validation of spinal manipulation. Springfield: Charles C Thomas, 1985:106–118.

2. Fischer AA. Pressure threshold meter: its use for quantification of tender spots. Arch Phys Med Rehabil 1986;67:836–838.

3. Fischer AA. Pressure algometry over normal muscles. Standard values, validity and reproducibility of pressure threshold. Pain 1987; 30:115–126.

4. Fischer AA. Pressure threshold measurement for diagnosis of myofascial pain and evaluation of treatment results. Clin J Pain 1987; 2:207–214.

5. Vernon HT, Aker P, Burns S, Viljakaanen S, Short L. Pressure pain threshold evaluation of the effect of spinal manipulation in the treatment of chronic neck pain: a pilot study. J Manipulative Physiol Ther 1990; 13:13–16.

6. Vernon H, Cote D, Beauchemin D, Bonnoyer B. A correlative study of myofascial tender points and joint fixations in the lumbopelvic spine in low back pain. Proceedings 1990 International Conference Spinal Manipulation, Washington, D.C., May 11–12, 1990: 236–240.

7. Triano JJ, Schultz AB. Correlation of objective measure of trunk motion and muscle function with low-back disability ratings. Spine 1987;12:561–565.

8. Nansel D, Peneff A, Quitoriano J. Effectiveness of upper vs. lower cervical adjustments with respect to the amelioration of passive rotational vs. lateral-flexion end range asymmetries in otherwise asymptomatic subjects. Proceedings 1991 International Conference Spinal Manipulation, Washington, D.C., April 12–13, 1991:21–25.

9. Nansel D, Peneff A, Jansen R, Cremata E, Carlson J, et al. Time course considerations for the effect of lower cervical adjustments with respect to the amelioration of cervical lateralflexion passive end-range asymmetries, and on blood pressure, heart rate, and plasma catecholamine levels. Proceedings 1990 International Conference Spinal Manipulation, Washington, D.C., May 11–12, 1990; 345–351.

10. Tepe R, Cook P, Cook L, Koontz T, Steets C. Rangiometer readings of lateral flexion asymmetry in the cervical spine before and after a diversified cervical adjustment. Proceedings 1992 International Conference Spinal Manipulation, Chicago, Ill., May 15–17, 1992:148.

11. Johnston WL, Elkiss ML, Marino RV, Blum GA. Passive gross motion testing: part II. A study of interexaminer agreement. J Am Osteopath Assoc 1982;81:304–308.

12. Editors. Guides to the evaluation of permanent impairment. 3rd ed. Chicago: American Medical Association, 1988:75–95.

13. Cram JR. Clinical EMG for surface recordings: vol 2. Seattle: Clinical Resources, 1990.

14. Denslow JS, Korr IM, Krems AD. Quantitative studies of chronic facilitation in human motoneuron pools. Am J Physiol 1947;105: 229–238.

15. Leach RA, Owens EF, Giesen JM. Correlates of myoelectric asymmetry detected in low back pain patients using hand held poststyle surface electromyography. J Manipulative Physiol Ther 1993;16:140–149.

16. Leach R, Trusty J, Lay M, Owens E, Beck R. Myoelectric and clinical predictors of low back pain in consecutive cases of lumbar trauma. Proceedings 1992 International Conference Spinal Manipulation, Washington, D.C., May 15–17, 1992:92–94.

17. Dvorak J, Panjabe MM, Chang DG, Theiler R, Grob D. Functional radiographic diagnosis of the lumbar spine: flexion/extension and lateral bending. Spine 1991;16:562–571.

18. Ben Eliyahu DJ. Infrared thermography in the diagnosis and management of sports injuries: a clinical study and literature review. Chiro Sports Med 1990;4:46–53.

19. Uematsu S, Edwin DH, Jankel WR, Kozikowski J, Trattner M. Quantification of thermal asymmetry. Part I. Normal values and reproducibility. J Neurosurg 1988;69:552–555.

20. Feldman F, Nickoloff E. Normal thermographic standards in the cervical spine and upper extremities. Skeletal Radiol 1984;12: 235–249.

21. Ben Eliyahu D. Infra-red thermographic assessment of chiropractic treatment in patients with lumbar disc herniations—a clinical study. Proceedings 1990 International Conference Spinal Manipulation, Washington, D.C., May 11–12, 1990:405–411.

22. Breen A. The reliability of palpation and other diagnostic methods. J Manipulative Physiol Ther 1992;15:54–56.

23. Troup JDG. Straight-leg-raising (SLR) and the qualifying tests for increased root tension. Spine 1981;6:26–27.

24. DeBoer KF, Harmon RO, Savoie S, Tuttle CD. Inter- and intra-examiner reliability of leg-length differential measurement: a preliminary study. J Manipulative Physiol Ther 1983;6:61–66.

25. Youngquist MW, Fuhr AW, Osterbauer PJ. Interexaminer reliability of an isolation test for the identification of upper cervical subluxation. J Manipulative Physiol Ther 1989;12: 93–97.

26. Rhudy TR, et al. Inter-examiner reliability of functional leg length assessment. Am J Chiro Med 1990;3:63–66.

27. Shambaugh JP, Sclafani L, Fanselow D. Reliability of the Derifield-Thompson test for leg length inequality, and use of the test to demonstrate cervical adjusting efficacy. J Manipulative Physiol Ther 1988;11:396–399.

28. Falltrick DR, Pierson SD. Precise measurement of functional leg length inequality and changes due to cervical spine rotation in pain-free students. J Manipulative Physiol Ther 1989;12:364–368.

29. Hoikka V, et al. Leg-length inequality has poor correlation with lumbar scoliosis: a radiological study of 100 patients [analysis by Donald D. Aspergren]. DC Tracts 1990;2: 28–29.

30. Fischer AA. Documentation of myofascial trigger points. Arch Phys Med Rehabil 1988; 69:286–291.

31. Hsieh J, Hong C. Effect of chiropractic manipulation on the pain threshold of myofascial trigger point: a pilot study. Proceedings 1990 International Conference Spinal Manipulation, Washington, D.C., May 11–12, 1990: 359–363.

32. Osterbauer P, Fuhr A, Widmaier R, Petermann E, DeBoer K. Preliminary clinical and biomechanical assessment of patients with chronic sacroiliac syndrome. Proceedings 1990 International Conference Spinal Manipulation, Washington, D.C., May 11–12, 1990: 403–404.

33. Keating JC Jr, Bergmann TF, Jacobs GE, Finer BA, Larson K. Interexaminer reliability of eight evaluative dimensions of lumbar segmental abnormality. J Manipulative Physiol Ther 1990;463–470.

34. Johnston WL. Interexaminer reliability studies: spanning a gap in medical research—Louisa Burns Memorial Lecture. J Am Osteopath Assoc 1982;81:819–829.

35. Jull G, Bullock M. A motion profile of the lumbar spine in an aging population assessed by manual examination. Physiother Pract 1987;3:70–81.

36. Nansel DD, Peneff AL, Jansen RD, Cooperstein R. Interexaminer concordance in detecting joint-play asymmetries in the cervical spines of otherwise asymptomatic subjects. J Manipulative Physiol Ther 1989;12:428–433.

37. Burton AK, Tillotson KM, Troup JDG. Variation in lumbar sagittal mobility with low-back trouble. Spine 1989;14:584–590.

38. Nansel DD, Peneff A, Quitoriano J. Effectiveness of upper versus lower cervical adjustments with respect to the amelioration of passive rotational versus lateral-flexion end-range asymmetries in otherwise asymp-

tomatic subjects. J Manipulative Physiol Ther 1992;15:99–105.

39. Antos JC, Robinson Gk, Keating JC Jr, Jacobs GE. Interrater reliability of fluoroscopic detection of fixation in the mid-cervical spine. Chiro Technique 1990;2:53–55.

40. Dvorak J, Panjabi MM, Chang DG, Theiler R, Grob D. Functional radiographic diagnosis of the cervical spine: flexion/extension and lateral bending. Spine 1991;16:562–571.

41. Yeomans SG. The assessment of cervical intersegmental mobility before and after spinal manipulative therapy. J Manipulative Physiol Ther 1992;15:106–114.

42. Lawrence DJ. Chiropractic concepts of the short leg: a critical review. J Manipulative Physiol Ther 1985;8:157–161.

43. Haas M, Nyiendo J, Peterson C, et al. Interrater reliability of roentgenological evaluation of the lumbar spine in lateral bending. J Manipulative Physiol Ther 1990;13:179–189.

44. Phillips RB, Howe JW, Bustin G, Mick TJ, Rosenfeld I, Mills T. Stress x-rays and the low back pain patient. J Manipulative Physiol Ther 1990;13:127–133.

45. Keating JC, Bergmann TF, Jacobs GE, Finer BA, Larson K. Interexaminer reliability of eight evaluative dimensions of lumbar segmental abnormality. J Manipulative Physiol Ther 1990;13:463–470.

46. Johnston WL, Allan BR, Hendra JL, et al. Interexaminer study of palpation in detecting location of spinal segmental dysfunction. J Am Osteopath Assoc 1983;83:839–845.

47. Beal MC, Kleiber GE. Somatic dysfunction as a predictor of coronary artery disease. J Am Osteopath Assoc 1985;85:302–307.

48. Johnston WL, Kelso AF, Hollandsworth DL, Karrat JJ. Somatic manifestations in renal disease: a clinical research study. J Am Osteopath Assoc 1987;87:22.

49. Gemmel HA, Heng BJ, Jacobson BH. Interexaminer reliability of the toftness radiation detector for determining the presence of upper cervical subluxation. Chiro Technique 1990;2:10–12.

50. Leboeuf C. The reliability of specific sacro-occipital technique diagnostic tests. J Manipulative Physiol Ther 1991;14:512–517.

51. Rantanen P, Airaksinen O. Poor agreement between so-called sacroiliacal joint tests in ankylosing spondylitis patients. J Manual Med 1989;4:62–64.

52. Triano JJ. The subluxation complex: outcome measure of chiropractic diagnosis and treatment. Chiro Technique 1990;2:114–120.

53. Seichi A, Hoshino Y, Ohnishi I, Kurokawa T. The role of calcium metabolism abnormalities in the development of ossification of the posterior longitudinal ligament of the cervical spine. Spine 1992;17:S30–32.

54. Kawaguchi H, Kurokawa T, Hoshino Y, Kawahara H, Ogata E, Matsumoto T. Immunohistochemical demonstration of bone morphogenetic protein-2 and transforming growth factor-β in the ossification of the posterior longitudinal ligament of the cervical spine. Spine 1992;17:S33–36.

55. Kirkaldy-Willis WH, Cassidy JD. Spinal manipulation in the treatment of low-back pain. Can Fam Physician 1985;31:535–540.

56. Kirkaldy-Willis WH. The relationship of structural pathology to the nerve root. Spine 1984;9:49–52.

57. Potter GE. The diagnostic clinical trial. J Manual Med 1989;4:31.

58. Kelsey JL, Golden AL, Mundt DJ. Low back pain/prolapsed lumbar intervertebral disc. Rheum Dis Clin North Am 1990;16:699–716.

59. Matthews JA, Yates DAH. Treatment of sciatica. Lancet 1974;1:352.

60. Nwuga VCB. Relative therapeutic efficacy of vertebral manipulation and conventional treatment in back pain management. Am J Phys Med 1982;61:273–278.

61. Yefu L, Jixiang F, Zuliang L, Zhengian L. Traction and manipulative reduction for the treatment of protrusion of lumbar intervertebral disc—an analysis of 1,455 cases. J Tradit Chin Med 1986;6:31–3.

62. Ellenberg M, Reina N, Ross M, et al. Regression of herniated nucleus palposus; two patients with lumbar radiculopathy. Arch Phys Med Rehabil 1989;70:842–4.

63. Dreyer P, Lantz C. Chiropractic management of a herniated disc: reduction of disc protrusion and maintenance of disc integrity as substantiated by MRI. Proceedings 1991 International Conference Spinal Manipulation, Foundation for Chiropractic Education and Research, Arlington, Va., 1991:57–59.

64. Quon JA, Cassidy JD, O'Connor SM, Kirkaldy-Willis WH. Lumbar intervertebral disc hernia-

tion: treatment by rotational manipulation. J Manipulative Physiol Ther 1989;12:220–227.

65. Richards GL, Thompson JS, Osterbauer PJ, Fuhr AW. Low force chiropractic care of two patients with sciatic neuropathy and lumbar disc herniation. Am J Chiro Med 1990;3:25–32.

66. Fonti S, Lynch M. Etiopathogenesis of lumbosciatalgia due to disk disease. Chiropractic treatment (statistics on 3,136 patients). In: Mazzarelli JP ed. Chiropractic interprofessional research. Torino, Italy: Edizioni Minerva Medica, 1985:53–58.

67. Ben Eliyahu DJ. The efficacy of chiropractic treatment for MRI documented cervical disc herniations: a case study. Proceedings 1991 International Conference Spinal Manipulation, Foundation for Chiropractic Education and Research, Arlington, Va., 1991:26–27.

68. Cox JM. Low back pain, mechanism, diagnosis and treatment. 4th ed. Baltimore: Williams & Wilkins, 1985.

69. Hubka MJ, Taylor JAM, Schultz GD, Traina AD. Lumbar intervertebral disc herniation: chiropractic management using flexion, extension, and rotational manipulative therapy. Chiro Technique 1991;3:5–12.

70. Cassidy JD, Quon JA, Kirkaldy-Willis WH. Letter to the editor: in reply. J Manipulative Physiol Ther 1990;13:40–41.

71. Cox JM. Letter to the editor. J Manipulative Physiol Ther 1990;13:36–40.

72. Saal JA, Saal JS. Nonoperative treatment of herniated lumbar intervertebral disc with radiculopathy: an outcome study. Spine 1989;14:431–437.

73. Weber H. Lumbar disc herniation: a controlled prospective study with ten years of observation. Spine 1983;8:131–140.

74. Shvartzman L, Weingarten E, Sherry H, Levin S, Persaud A. Cost-effectiveness analysis of extended conservative therapy versus surgical intervention in the management of herniated lumbar intervertebral disc. Spine 1992;17:176–182.

75. Rossi A, Martino G, Hornbeck R. Influence of chiropractic on lumbosciaticas and cervicobrachialgias studied through the somatosensorial evoked potentials (SEP). In: Mazzarelli JP, ed. Chiropractic interprofessional research. Torino, Italy: Edizioni Minerva Medica, 1985:1–6.

76. Cleveland CS. Spinal correction effects on motor and sensory functions. In: Mazarelli JP, ed. Chiropractic interprofessional research. Torino, Italy: Edizioni Minerva Medica 1985:21–32.

77. Adams E. Post adjustment motor and sensory changes in cervical brachial syndrome. Proceedings 1990 International Conference Spinal Manipulation, Foundation for Chiropractic Education and Research, Arlington, Va., 1990:391–392.

78. Liebenson CS. Thoracic outlet syndrome: diagnosis and conservative management. J Manipulative Physiol Ther 1988;11:493–499.

79. Mariano KA, McDouble MA, Tanksley GW. Double crush syndrome: chiropractic care of an entrapment neuropathy. J Manipulative Physiol Ther 1991;14:262–265.

80. Shelkelle PG, Adams AH, Chassin MR, Hurwitz EL, Phillips RB, Brook RH. The appropriateness of spinal manipulation for low-back pain: project overview and literature review. Santa Monica, Calif.: RAND, 1991:7–13.

81. Hill JJ Jr, Bogumill H. Manipulation in the treatment of frozen shoulder. Orthopedics 1988;11:1255.

82. Schafer RC. Clinical biomechanics: musculoskeletal actions and reactions. Baltimore: Williams & Wilkins, 1987:647–654.

83. Haldeman S. Spinal manipulative therapy in the management of low back pain. In: Finneson BE. Low back pain. 2nd ed. Philadelphia: JB Lippincott, 1980:245–275.

84. Keim HA, Kirkaldy-Willis WH. Low back pain. Ciba Clin Symp 1980;32:13.

85. Helbig T, Lee CK. The lumbar facet syndrome. Spine 1988;13:61–64.

86. Mooney V, Robertson J. The facet syndrome. Clin Orthop 1976;115:149–156.

87. Zusman M, Edwards BC, Donaghy A. Investigation of a proposed mechanism for the relief of spinal pain with passive joint movement. J Manual Med 1989;4:58–61.

88. Ebrall PS. Meralgia paraesthetica part 2: a clinical update. J Aust Chiro Assoc 1990;20:15–16.

89. Dudley WN, Merritt RW. Meralgia paresthetica and the superior popliteal space. J Chiro 1990;27:45–47.

90. Ferezy JS. Chiropractic management of meralgia paresthetica: a case report. Chiro Technique 1989;1:52–56.

91. Bronston LJ, Larson KM. A new approach to upper rib fixation mobilization. Chiro Technique 1990;2:39–44.

92. Gemmell HA, Jacobson BH. Incidence of sacroiliac joint dysfunction and low back pain in fit college students. J Manipulative Physiol Ther 1990;13:63–67.

93. Herzog W, Conway PJW, Willcox BJ. Effects of different treatment modalities on gait symmetry and clinical measures for sacroiliac joint patients. J Manipulative Physiol Ther 1991;14:104–109.

94. Osterbauer PJ, Fuhr AW, Widmaier RS, Petermann EA, DeBoer KF. Preliminary clinical and biomechanical assessment of patients with chronic sacroiliac syndrome. Proceedings 1990 International Conference Spinal Manipulation, Foundation for Chiropractic Education and Research, Arlington, Va., 1990:403–4.

95. Grimston SK, Engsberg JR, Shaw L, Vetanze NW. Muscular rehabilitation prescribed in coordination with prior chiropractic therapy as a treatment for sacroiliac subluxation in female distance runners.Chiro Sports Med 1990;4:2–8.

96. Weinberg LA. Temporomandibular joint injuries. In: Whiplash injuries: cervical acceleration/deceleration syndrome. Baltimore: Williams & Wilkins, 1988:347–383.

97. Curl DD. The visual range of motion scale: analysis of mandibular gait in a chiropractic setting. J Manipulative Physiol Ther 1992; 15:115–122.

98. Curl DD. Acute closed lock of the temporomandibular joint: manipulation paradigm and protocol. Chiro Technique 1991;3: 13–18.

99. Shekelle P. The appropriateness of spinal manipulation for low back pain. Chiro Technique 1992;4:5–7.

100. Hildebrandt J, Argyrakis A. Percutaneous nerve block of the cervical facets—a relatively new method in the treatment of chronic headache and neck pain. Manual Med 1986;2:48–52.

101. Vernon H. Vertebrogenic headache. In: Vernon H, ed. Upper cervical syndrome. Baltimore: Williams & Wilkins, 1988:152–188.

102. Bogduk N. The anatomical basis for cervicogenic headache. J Manipulative Physiol Ther 1992;15:67–70.

103. Jaeger B. Are cervicogenic headaches due to myofascial pain and cervical spine dysfunction? Cephalgia 1989;9:157–64.

104. Pfaffenrath V, Dandekar R, Pöllmann W. Cervicogenic headache—the clinical picture, radiologic findings and hypotheses on its pathophysiology. Headache 1987;27:49–499.

105. Vernon HT. Spinal manipulation and headaches of cervical origin. J Manipulative Physiol Ther 1989;12:455–468.

106. Droz JM, Crot F. Occipital headaches: statistical results in the treatment of vertebrogenous headache. Ann Swiss Chiro Assoc 1985;8:127–136.

107. Boline PD. Chiropractic treatment and pharmaceutical treatment for muscle contraction headaches: a randomized comparative clinical trial. Proceedings 1991 International Conference Spinal Manipulation, Foundation for Chiropractic Education and Research, Arlington, Va., 1991:303–304.

108. Lewith GT. Headache and its management; a personal review. Ann Swiss Chiro Assoc 1985;8:7–16.

109. Smythe H. Tender points: evolution of concepts of the fibrositis/fibromyalgia syndrome. Am J Med 1986;81:2–6.

110. Masi AT, Yunus MB. Concepts of illness in populations as applied to fibromyalgia syndromes. Am J Med 1986;81:1– 25.

111. Wolfe F, Smythe HA, Yunus MB, et al. The American College of Rheumatology 1990 criteria for the classification of fibromyalgia: report of the multicenter criteria committee. Arthritis Rheum 1990;133:160–172.

112. Freundlich B, Leventhal LJ. Letter to the editor. Arthritis Rheum 1990;33:1863.

113. Wolfe F. The clinical syndrome of fibrositis. Am J Med 1986;81:7–14.

114. Taylor MR. Fibromyalgia syndrome: literature review. Proceedings 1991 International Conference Spinal Manipulation, Foundation for Chiropractic Education and Research, Arlington, Va., 1991:207–209.

115. Boline PD, Anderson AV, Berk R. The various components and treatment of fibrositis: a review. Chiro Technique 1989;1:133–139.

116. Schneider MJ. Snapping hip syndrome in a marathon runner: treatment by manual trigger point therapy—a case study. Chiro Sports Med 1990;4:54–58.

117. Nyiendo J, Lamm L. Disabling low back Oregon Workers' Compensation claims. Part I: methodology and clinical categorization of chiropractic and medical cases. J Manipulative Physiol Ther 1991;14:177–184.

118. Johnson MR, Schultz MK, Ferguson AC. A comparison of chiropractic, medical and osteopathic care for work-related sprains and strains. J Manipulative Physiol Ther 1989;12: 335–344.

119. Wolk S. Chiropractic versus medical care: a cost analysis of disability and treatment for back-related workers' compensation cases. Arlington, Va.: Foundation for Chiropractic Education and Research, 1988.

120. Jarvis KB. Phillips RB, Morris JD. Cost per case comparison of back injury claims of chiropractic versus medical management for diagnostically similar conditions. Proceedings 1990 International Conference Spinal Manipulation, Arlington, Va.: Foundation for Chiropractic Education and Research, 1990: 131–139.

121. Nyiendo J. Disabling low back Oregon Workers' Compensation claims. Part II: time loss. J Manipulative Physiol Ther 1991;14: 231–239.

122. Bolton PS. Torticollis: a review of etiology, pathology, diagnosis and treatment. J Manipulative Physiol Ther 1985;8:29–32.

123. Mawhiney RB. Chiropractic treatment procedure in a case of spasmodic torticollis with associated scoliosis. Chiropractic 1990;3: 18–21.

124. Wood KW. Acute torticollis: chiropractic therapy and management. Chiro Technique 1991;3:105–108.

125. Sandoz R. A classification of luxations, subluxations, and fixations of the cervical spine. Ann Swiss Chiro Assoc 1976;6:219–276.

126. Arkuszewski Z. The efficacy of manual treatment in low back pain: a clinical trial. Manual Med 1986;2:68–71.

127. Sandoz RW. The paretic and paralysing sciaticas. Ann Swiss Chiro Assoc 1989;9: 133–148.

128. Riihimaki H, Wickstrom G, Hanninen K, Luopajarvi T. Predictors of sciatic pain among concrete reinforcement workers and house painters—a five-year follow-up. Scand J Work Environ Health 1989;15:415–423.

129. Caruso I, LoMonaco M, Pizzetti M. EMG and H-reflex in the diagnosis and evaluation of chiropractic treatment of lumbosciatalgia (preliminary study). In: Mazarelli JP, ed. Chiropractic interprofessional research. Torino, Italy: Edizioni Minerva Medica, 1985:37–40.

130. Illi C, Sandoz RW. Spinal equilibration; further developments of the concepts of Fred Illi. Ann Swiss Chiro Assoc 1985;8:81–126.

131. Lorez E. Computer assisted quantification of gait improvement after a chiropractic adjustment. Ann Swiss Chiro Assoc 1989;9: 209–232.

132. Byl NN, Sinnott PL. Variations in balance and body sway in middle-aged adults: subjects with healthy backs compared with subjects with low-back dysfunction. Spine 1991;16: 325–330.

133. Conway PJW, Herzog W. Changes in walking mechanics associated with wearing an intertrochanteric support belt. J Manipulative Physiol Ther 1991;14:185–88.

134. Herzog W, Conway PJW, Willcox BJ. Effects of different treatment modalities on gait symmetry and clinical measures for sacroiliac joint patients. J Manipulative Physiol Ther 1991;14:104–109.

135. Anderson R, Meeker WC, Wirick BE, Mootz RD, Kirk DH, Adams A. A meta-analysis of clinical trials of spinal manipulation. J Manipulative Physiol Ther 1992;15:181–194.

136. Gatterman MI. Chiropractic management of spine related disorders. Baltimore: Williams & Wilkins, 1990.

137. Shekelle PG, Adams AH, Chassin MR, et al. The appropriateness of spinal manipulation for low-back pain. Santa Monica: RAND, 1991.

138. Mathews JA, Mills SB, Jenkins VM, et al. Back pain and sciatica: controlled trials of manipulation traction, sclerosant and epidural injections. Br J Rheum 1987;26:416–423.

139. Waagen GN, Haldeman S, Cook G, et al. Short term trial of chiropractic adjustments for the relief of chronic low back pain. Manual Med 1986;2:63–67.

140. Hadler NM, Curtis P, Gillings DB, Stinnett S. A benefit of spinal manipulation as adjunctive therapy for acute low-back pain: a stratified controlled trial. Spine 1987;12:703–6.

141. Meade TW, Dyer S, Browne W, Townsend J, Frank AO. Low back pain of mechanical origin: randomised comparison of chiropractic and hospital outpatient treatment. Br Med J 1990;300:1431–1437.

142. Assendelft WJJ, Bouter LM, Kessels AGH. Effectiveness of chiropractic and physiotherapy in the treatment of low back pain: a critical discussion of the British randomized clinical trial. J Manipulative Physiol Ther 1991;14:281–286.

143. Meade TW. Letter to the editor. J Manipulative Physiol Ther 1991;14:444–445.

144. Assendelft WJJ, Bouter LM, Kessels AGH. In reply. J Manipulative Physiol Ther 1991;14: 445–446.

145. Koes BW, Bouter LM, Knipshild PG, et al. The effectiveness of manual therapy, physiotherapy and continued treatment by the general practitioner for chronic nonspecific back and neck complaints: design of a randomized clinical trial. J Manipulative Physiol Ther 1991;14:498–502.

146. Hsieh C-YJ, Phillips RB, Adams AH, Pope MH. Functional outcomes of low back pain: comparison of four treatment groups in a randomized controlled trial. J Manipulative Physiol Ther 1992;15:4–9.

147. Vernon HT, Dhami MSI, Howley TP, Annett R. Spinal manipulation and beta-endorphin: a controlled study of the effect of a spinal manipulation on plasma beta-endorphin levels in normal males. J Manipulative Physiol Ther 1986;9:115–124.

148. Sanders GE, Reinert O, Tepe R, Maloney P. Chiropractic adjustive manipulation on subjects with acute low back pain: visual analog pain scores and plasma β-endorphin levels. J Manipulative Physiol Ther 1990;13: 391–395.

149. Valentini E. Acute lumbar syndromes under chiropractic care. A two year statistical study. Ann Swiss Chiro Assoc 1981;7:67–84.

150. Kinalski R, Kuwik W, Pietrzak D. The comparison of the results of manual therapy versus physiotherapy methods used in treatment of patients with low back pain syndromes. Manual Med 1989;4:44–46.

151. Mellin B, Hurri H, Harkapaa K, Jarvikoski A. A controlled study on the outcome of inpatient and outpatient treatment of low back pain. Part II. Effects on physical measurements three months after treatment. Scan J Rehabil Med 1989;21:91–95.

152. Elnaggar IM, Nordin M, Ali Sheikhzadeh MA, Parnianpour M, Kahanovitz N. Effects of spinal flexion and extension exercises on low-back pain and spinal mobility in chronic mechanical low-back pain patients. Spine 1991;16:967–972.

153. Lewit K. Muscular pattern in thoraco-lumbar lesions. Manual Med 1986;2:105–107.

154. Szlazak M, Nansel D. Simulation of visceral disease brought about by somatic pain referral and common associated reflex patterns: a more plausible explanation for presumed chiropractic "cures" of true organic visceral disease. Proceedings 1992 International Conference Spinal Manipulation, Arlington, Va.: Foundation for Chiropractic Education and Research, 1992:45.

155. Triano JJ, Hondras MA, McGregor. Differences in treatment history with manipulation for acute, subacute, chronic and recurrent spine pain. J Manipulative Physiol Ther 1992;15:24–30.

156. Lee PWH, Chow SP, Lieh-mak F, Chan KC, Wong S. Psychosocial factors influencing outcome in patients with low-back pain. Spine 1989;14:838–842.

157. Haldeman S. Why one cause of back pain? In: Buerger A, Tobis J, eds. Approaches to the validation of manipulation therapy. Springfield, Ill.: Charles C Thomas, 1977: 187–197.

158. Waddell G, Somerville D, Henderson I, Newton M. Objective clinical evaluation of physical impairment in chronic low back pain. Spine 1992;17:617–628.

159. Sloop PR, Smith DS, Boldenberg SRN, Dore C. Manipulation for chronic neck pain: a double-blind controlled study. Spine 1982;7:532–535.

160. Arkuszewski Z. Involvement of the cervical spine in back pain. Manual Med 1986;2: 126–128.

161. Leboeuf C, Grant BR, Maginnes GS. Chiropractic treatment of repetitive strain injuries: a preliminary prospective outcome study of

SMT versus SMT combined with massage. J Aust Chiro Assoc 1987;17:11–14.

162. Dvorak J, Valach L, Schmid St. Cervical spine injuries in Switzerland. J Manual Med 1989;4: 7–16.

163. Kawchuk GN, Herzog W, Hasler EM. Forces generated during spinal manipulative therapy of the cervical spine: a pilot study. J Manipulative Physiol Ther 1992;15:275–278.

164. Kawchuk G, Herzog W, Hasler E. Various manipulative techniques and their transmission of force to the cervical spine. Proceedings 1992 International Conference Spinal Manipulation, Chicago, Foundation for Chiropractic Education and Research, 1992:51.

165. Triano J, Schultz A. Muscle response to manipulation of the neck. Proceedings 1990 International Conference Spinal Manipulation, Washington, D.C., Foundation for Chiropractic Education and Research, 1990:352–355.

166. Shekelle PG, Adams AH, Chassin MR, et al. The appropriateness of spinal manipulation for low-back pain: indications and ratings by a multidisciplinary expert panel. Santa Monica, Calif.: RAND, 1991:22–30.

167. Palmer DD. The science, art and philosophy of chiropractic. Portland, Ore.: Portland Printing House, 1910:18.

168. Luisetto G, Tagliaro D, Spanò D, Darling P, Steiner W, Campacci R. Plasma levels of beta-endorphin and calcitonin before and after manipulative treatment of patients with cervical arthrosis and Barré's syndrome. In Mazzarelli JP, ed. Chiropractic interprofessional research. Torino, Italy: Edizioni Minerva Medica, 1985:47–52.

169. Palmieri NF. Idiopathic facial paralysis: mechanism, diagnosis, and conservative chiropractic management. Chiro Technique 1990;4:182–187.

170. McMullen M. Handicapped infants and chiropractic care: Down syndrome. Int Chiro Assoc Rev 1990;46:32–35.

171. La Francis ME. A chiropractic perspective on atlantoaxial instability in Down's syndrome. J Manipulative Physiol Ther 1990;13: 157–160.

172. Barbuto LM. Differential diagnosis of headaches. In: Vernon H, ed. Upper cervical syndrome: chiropractic diagnosis and treatment. Baltimore: Williams & Wilkins, 1988: 141–151.

173. Vernon H. Vertebrogenic headache. In: Vernon H, ed. Upper cervical syndrome: chiropractic diagnosis and treatment. Baltimore: Williams & Wilkins, 1988:152–188.

174. Wight JS. Migraine: a statistical analysis of chiropractic treatment. J Am Chiro Assoc 1978;12:36– 67.

175. Parker GB, Tupling H, Pryor DS. A controlled trial of cervical manipulation for migraine. Aust NZ J Med 1978;8:589–593.

176. Parker GB, Pryor DS, Tupling H. Why does migraine improve during a clinical trial? Further results from a trial of cervical manipulation for migraine. Aust NZ J Med 1980;10: 192–198.

177. Stodolny J, Chmielewski H. Manual therapy in the treatment of patients with cervical migraine. J Manual Med 1989;4:49–51.

178. April C, Bogduk N. The prevalence of cervical zygapophyseal joint pain. Spine 1992; 17:744–747.

179. Figar J. Jansky M. Studies of vascular reflexes in cases of vertebrogenic migraine. Acta Univ Carol 1964;(suppl 21):76–79.

180. Motohatsu F, Tsukahara T, Taniguchi T. α-Adrenoceptors in human and animal cerebral arteries: alterations after sympathetic denervation and subarachnoid hemorrhage. Trends Pharmacol Sci 1989;10:329–332.

181. Vernon H, Gitelman R. Pressure algometry and tissue compliance measures in the treatment of chronic headache by spinal manipulation. J Can Chiro Assoc 1990;34:141–144.

182. Woo C-C. Traumatic spinal myoclonus. J Manipulative Physiol Ther 1989;12:478–481.

183. Zerillo G, Lynch M. Importance of chiropractic on oto- vestibular pathology. In: Mazzarelli JP, ed. Chiropractic interprofessional research. Torino, Italy: Edizioni Minerva Medica 1985:69–76.

184. Mandel S, Rothrock RW. Sympathetic dystrophies: recognizing and managing a puzzling group of syndromes. Postgrad Med 1990; 87:213–218.

185. Uematsu S, Hendler N, Hungerford D, Long D, Ono N. Thermography and electromyography in the differential diagnosis of chronic pain syndromes and reflex sympathetic dystrophy. Electromyogr Clin Neurophysiol 1981;21:165–182.

186. Ellis WB, Ebrall PS. The resolution of chronic inversion and plantarflexion of the foot: a pediatric case study. Chiro Technique 1991;3:55–59.

187. Hospers LA, Sweat RW, Hus L. Response of a three-year-old child to upper cervical adjustment. Today's Chiro 1987;15:6–70.

188. Goodman RJ, Mosby JS Jr. Cessation of a seizure disorder: correction of the atlas subluxation complex. Chiropractic: J Chiro Res Clin Invest 1990;6:43–46.

189. Liu YK, Chandran KB, Heath RG, Unterharnscheidt F. Subcortical EEG changes in rhesus monkeys following experimental hyperextension-hyperflexion (whiplash). Spine 1984;9:329–338.

190. Wood K. Case study: resolution of spasmodic dysphonia (focal laryngeal dystonia) via chiropractic manipulative management. Proceedings 1990 International Conference Spinal Manipulation, Arlington, Va.: Foundation for Chiropractic Education and Research, 1990:50–53.

191. Trotta N. The response of an adult Tourette patient to life upper cervical adjustments. Chiro Res J 1989;1:43–48.

192. Chester JB. Whiplash, postural control, and the inner ear. Spine 1991;16:716–720.

193. Fitz-Ritson D. Assessment of cervicogenic vertigo. J Manipulative Physiol Ther 1991; 14:193–198.

194. Jamison JR, McEwen AP, Thomas SJ. Chiropractic adjustment in the management of visceral conditions: a critical appraisal. J Manipulative Physiol Ther 1992;15:171–180.

195. Sato A. The reflex effects of spinal somatic nerve stimulation on visceral function. J Manipulative Physiol Ther 1992;15:57–61.

196. Palmer BJ, Macfarlane AJ, Sherman LW, Coulter WW. Electrocardiograph changes under specific chiropractic adjustment: research on 1500 cases in the B.J. Palmer Chiropractic Clinic. Davenport, Ia.: Palmer School of Chiropractic, 1949.

197. Schwartz PJ. Cardiac sympathetic innervation and the prevention of sudden death. Cardiologia 1990;35(suppl 1):51–54.

198. Sanchez G. What is the role of the central nervous system in mineralocorticoid hypertension? Am J Hypertens 1991;4:374–381.

199. Varagic VM, Prostran MS, Stepanovic S, Savic J, Vujnov S. Transmitter interactions in the central cholinergic control of blood pressure regulation. Drug Metab Drug Interactions 1991;9:50–69.

200. Balduc HA. Chiropractic cardiology. In: Sweere J, ed. Chiropractic family practice. Gaithersburg, Md.: Aspen, 1992:31–37.

201. Rogers JT, Rogers JC. The role of osteopathic manipulative therapy in the treatment of coronary heart disease. J Am Osteopath Assoc 1976;76:71–81.

202. Matoba T, Ohkita Y, Chiba M, Toshima H. Noninvasive assessment of the autonomic nervous tone in angina pectoris: an application of digital plethysmography with auditory stimuli. Angiology 1983;34:127–136.

203. Johnson FE. Some observations on the use of osteopathic therapy in the care of patients with cardiac disease. J Am Osteopath Assoc 1972;72:87–92.

204. Sherwood P. Effective prevention of coronary heart attacks. Am J Acupunct 1984;12: 321–326.

205. Tilley RM. The somatic component of heart disease. Osteopath Ann 1974:May:30–37.

206. Spano D, Darling P. Cardiovascular changes in degenerative cervicopathy. Chiropractic treatment. In: Mazzarelli JP, Chiropractic interprofessional research. Torino, Italy: Edizioni Minerva Medica, 1985:77–88.

207. Jarmel ME. Possible role of spinal joint dysfunction in the genesis of sudden cardiac death. J Manipulative Physiol Ther 1989;6: 469–477.

208. Tran TA, Kirby JD. The effects of upper thoracic adjustment upon the normal physiology of the heart. ACA J Chiro 1977;11:25–28.

209. Tran TA, Kirby JD. The effects of upper cervical adjustment upon the normal physiology of the heart. ACA J Chiro 1977;11:58–62.

210. Dulgar G, Hill D, Sirucek A, Davis B. Evidence for a possible anti-hypertensive effect of basic technique apex contact adjusting. ACA J Chiro 1980;14:S97-S102.

211. Morgan JP, Dickey JL, Hunt HH, Hudgins PM. A controlled trial of spinal manipulation in the management of hypertension. J Am Osteopath Assoc 1985;85:308–313.

212. Yates RG, Lamping DL, Abram NL, Wright C. Effects of chiropractic treatment on blood pressure and anxiety: a randomized, controlled trial. J Manipulative Physiol Ther 1988;11:484–488.

213. Maloney P, Rambacher L, Owens P, Johnston V, Jackson M. Assessing the effectiveness of chiropractic adjustment for lowering blood pressure. Proceedings 1990 International Conference Spinal Manipulation, Arlington, Va., Foundation for Chiropractic Education and Research, 1990:356–358.

214. Nansel D, Jansen R, Cremata E, Dhami MSI, Holley D. Effects of cervical adjustments on lateral-flexion passive end-range asymmetry and on blood pressure, heart rate and plasma catecholamine levels. J Manipulative Physiol Ther 1991;14:450–456.

215. Corbett JL, et al. Cardiovascular changes associated with skeletal muscle spasm in tetraplegic man. J Physiol 1971;215:381–393.

216. MacKenzie J. Some points bearing on the association of sensory disorders and visceral disease. Brain 1893;16:321–354.

217. Magee DF. The role of sympathetic innervation and sympathomimetics in gastric secretion in vivo. Mount Sinai J Med 1989; 56:272–277.

218. DeBoer KF, Schultz M, McKnight ME. Acute effects of spinal manipulation on gastrointestinal myoelectric activity in conscious rabbits. Manual Med 1988;3:85–94.

219. Burns L, Chandler L, Rice R. Pathogenesis of visceral disease following vertebral lesions. Chicago: Still Research Institute, 1948: 193–211.

220. Falk JW. Bowel and bladder dysfunction secondary to lumbar dysfunctional syndrome. Chiro Technique 1990;2:45–48.

221. Browning JE. The recognition of mechanically induced pelvic pain and organic dysfunction in the low back pain patient. J Manipulative Physiol Ther 1989;12:369–373.

222. Vear HJ. Chiropractic standards of practice and quality of care. Gaithersburg, Md.: Aspen, 1992:63.

223. Wiles MR. Observations of the effects of upper cervical manipulations on the electrogastrogram: a preliminary report. J Manipulative Physiol Ther 1980;3:226–229.

224. Palmer BJ, Sherman LW, Coulter WW. Urological changes under specific chiropractic adjustment: research on 2006 cases in the B.J. Palmer Chiropractic Clinic. Davenport, Ia.: Palmer School of Chiropractic, 1949.

225. Huber KH, Rexroth W, Werle E, Koeth T, Weicker H, Hild R. Sympathetic neuronal activity in diabetic and non-diabetic subjects with peripheral arterial occlusive disease. Klin Wochenschr 1991;69:233–238.

226. Chevalier RL. Counterbalance in functional adaptation to ureteral obstruction during development. Pediatr Nephrol 1990;4:442–444.

227. Keating JC, McCarron K, James J, Gruenberg J, Lonczak RS. Urobehavioral intervention in the rehabilitation of lower urinary tract dysfunction: a case report. J Manipulative Physiol Ther 1985;8:185–189.

228. Sandoz RW. Structural and functional pathologies of the pelvic ring. Ann Swiss Chiro Assoc 1981;7:101–160.

229. Szlazak M, Nansel D. Simulation of visceral disease brought about by somatic pain referral and common associated reflex patterns: a more plausible explanation for presumed chiropractic "cures" of true organic visceral disease. Proceedings 1992 International Conference Spinal Manipulation, Arlington, Va.: Foundation for Chiropractic Education and Research, 1992:45.

230. Stude DE. Dysfunctional uterine bleeding with concomitant low back and lower extremity pain. J Manipulative Physiol Ther 1991;14:472–477.

231. Kokjohn K, Schmid DM, Triano JJ, Brennan PC. The effect of spinal manipulation on pain and prostaglandin levels in women with primary dysmenorrhea. J Manipulative Physiol Ther 1992;15:279–285.

232. Arnold-Frochot S. Investigation of the effect of chiropractic adjustments on a specific gynaecological symptom: dysmenorrhea (part 1). J Aust Chiro Assoc 1980;11:6–10,17.

233. Arnold-Frochot S. Investigation of the effect of chiropractic adjustments on a specific gynaecological symptom: dysmenorrhea (part 2). J Aust Chiro Assoc 1981;12:14–16.

234. Chesney MA, Tasto DL. The development of the menstrual symptom questionnaire. Behav Res Ther 1975;13:237–244.

235. Hains F, Batt R, Bellis S, Martel J. Association between primary dysmenorrhea and pain threshold at the thoracolumbar junction. Proceedings 1991 International Conference Spinal Manipulation, Arlington, Va.: Foundation for Chiropractic Education and Research, 1991:106–109.

236. Moos RH. Perimenstrual symptoms: a manual and overview of research with the men-

strual distress questionnaire. Stanford University School of Medicine, 1985.

237. Browning JE. Mechanically induced pelvic pain and organic dysfunction in a patient without low back pain. J Manipulative Physiol Ther 1990;13:406–411.

238. Dobrik I. Disorders of the iliopsoas muscle and its role in gynecological diseases. J Manual Med 1989;4:130–133.

239. Östgaard HC, Andersson GBJ. Previous back pain and risk of developing back pain in a future pregnancy. Spine 1991;16:432–436.

240. Östgaard HC, Andersson GBJ, Karlsson K. Prevalence of back pain in pregnancy. Spine 1991;16:549–552.

241. Esch S, Zachman Z. Adjustive procedures for the pregnant chiropractic patient. Chiro Technique 1991;3:66–71.

242. Mantero E, Crispini L. Static alterations of the pelvic, sacral, lumbar area due to pregnancy. Chiropractic treatment. In: Mazarelli JP, ed. Chiropractic interprofessional research. Torino, Italy: Edizioni Minerva Medica, 1985: 59–68.

243. Diakow PRP, Gadsby TA, Gadsby JB, Gleddie JG, Leprich DJ, Scales AM. Back pain during pregnancy and labor. J Manipulative Physiol Ther 1991;14:116–118.

244. Daly JM, Frame PS, Rapoza PA. Sacroiliac subluxation: a common, treatable cause of low-back pain in pregnancy. Fam Pract Res J 1991;11:149–159.

245. Stude DE. The management of symptoms associated with premenstrual syndrome. J Manipulative Physiol Ther 1991;14:209–216.

246. Stude DE. Female organic reproductive dysfunction: conservative intervention. In: Sweere JJ, ed. Chiropractic family practice: a clinical manual. Gaithersburg, Md.: Aspen, 1992:1–20.

247. Gilman G, Bergstrand J. Visual recovery following chiropractic intervention. J Behav Optom 1990;3:73.

248. Botta JR, ed. Chiropractors healers or quacks? Part 2: How chiropractors can help—or harm. Consumer Reports 1975;40: 606–610.

249. Spitzer RL, Williams JB, eds. Diagnostic and statistical manual of mental disorders. 3rd ed. Washington, D.C.: American Psychiatric Association, 1987:50–53.

250. Fischer M, Barkley RA, Edelbrock CS, Smallish L. The adolescent outcome of hyperactive children diagnosed by research criteria: II. academic, attentional, and neuropsychological status. J Consult Clin Psychol 1990; 58:580–588.

251. Mannuzza S, Klein RG, Bonagura N, Malloy P, Giampino TL, Addalli KA. Hyperactive boys almost grown up. Arch Gen Psychiatry 1991;48:77–83.

252. Zametkin AJ, Nordahl TE, Gross M, et al. Cerebral glucose metabolism in adults with hyperactivity of childhood onset. N Engl J Med 1990;323:1361–1366.

253. Whalen CK, Henker B. Therapies for hyperactive children: comparisons, combinations, and compromises. J Consult Clin Psychol 1991;59:126–137.

254. Erhardt D, Baker BL. The effects of behavioral parent training on families with young hyperactive children. J Behav Ther Exp Psychiatry 1990;21:121–132.

255. Brzozowske WT, Walton EV. The effect of chiropractic treatment on students with learning and behavioural impairments resulting from neurological dysfunction (part 1). J Aust Chiro Assoc 1980;11(7):13–18.

256. Brzozowske WT, Walton EV. The effect of chiropractic treatment on students with learning and behavioural impairments resulting from neurological dysfunction (part 2). J Aust Chiro Assoc 1980;11(8):11–17.

257. Giesen JM, Center DB, Leach RA. An evaluation of chiropractic manipulation as a treatment of hyperactivity in children. J Manipulative Physiol Ther 1989;12:353–363.

258. Klougart N, Nilsson N, Jacobsen J. Infantile colic treated by chiropractors: a prospective study of 316 cases. J Manipulative Physiol Ther 1989;12:281–288.

259. Nilsson N. Infantile colic and chiropractic. Eur J Chiro 1985;33:264–265.

260. Woodcock RW. Woodcock reading mastery test. Circle Pines, Minn.: American Guidance Service, 1974.

261. Gemmell HA, Jacobson BH. Chiropractic management of enuresis: time-series descriptive design. J Manipulative Physiol Ther 1989;12:386–389.

262. Leboeuf C, Brown P, Herman A, Leembruggen K, Walton D, Crisp TC. Chiropractic

care of children with nocturnal enuresis: a prospective outcome study. J Manipulative Physiol Ther 1991;14:110–115.

263. Danbert RJ. In reply. J Manipulative Physiol Ther 1989;12:406.

264. Aspergren DD, Cox JM. Correction of progressive idiopathic scoliosis utilizing neuromuscular stimulation and manipulation: a case report. J Manipulative Physiol Ther 1987;10:147–156.

265. Specht DL, De Boer KF. Anatomical leg length inequality, scoliosis and lordotic curve in unselected clinic patients. J Manipulative Physiol Ther 1991;14:368–375.

266. Danbert RJ. Scoliosis: biomechanics and rationale for manipulative treatment. J Manipulative Physiol Ther 1989;12:38–45.

267. Plaugher G, Cremata EE, Phillips RB. A retrospective consecutive case analysis of pretreatment and comparative static radiologic parameters following chiropractic adjustments. J Manipulative Physiol Ther 1990;13:498–506.

268. Hinwood JA, Hinwood JA. Children and chiropractic: a summary of subluxation and its ramifications. J Aust Chiro Assoc 1981;11:18–21.

269. Fysh PN. Do chiropractors really treat asthma? MPI's Dynamic Chiropractic May 22, 1992, pp 12,86.

270. Irvine K, ed. Index to chiropractic literature 1985–1989. Portland, Ore.: Western States Chiropractic College Library (Chiropractic Library Consortium), 1990:6,245.

271. Taylor WR, Newacheck PW. Impact of childhood asthma on health. J Pediatr 1992;90:657–662.

272. Kaliner M, Shelhamer JH, Davis PB, Smith LJ, Venter JC. Autonomic nervous system abnormalities and allergy. Ann Intern Med 1982;96:349–357.

273. Editors: autonomic abnormalities in asthma. Lancet 1:1224–1225, 1982.

274. Droste PL, Beckman DL. Pulmonary effects of prolonged sympathetic stimulation. Proc Soc Exp Biol Med 1974;146:352–353.

275. Murphy W, Wilson PT. A study of the value of osteopathic adjustment of the fourth and fifth thoracic vertebrae in a series of twenty cases of asthmatic bronchitis. Boston Med Surg J 1925;192:440–442.

276. Jamison J, et al. Asthma in a chiropractic clinic: a pilot study. J Aust Chiro Assoc 1986;16:137–143.

277. Nilsson N, Christiansen B. Prognostic factors in bronchial asthma in chiropractic practice. J Aust Chiro Assoc 1988;18:85–87.

278. Lines DH, McMilan AJ, Spehr GJ. Effects of soft tissue technique and Chapman's neurolymphatic reflex stimulation on respiratory function. J Aust Chiro Assoc 1990;20:17–22.

279. Miller WD. Treatment of visceral disorders by manipulative therapy. In: Goldstein M, ed. The research status of spinal manipulative therapy. Washington, D.C.: Government Printing Office 1975:295–301.

280. Masarsky CS, Weber M. Somatic dyspnea and the orthopedics of respiration. Chiro Technique 1991;3:26–29.

281. Leach RA. The chiropractic theories. 2nd ed. Baltimore: Williams & Wilkins, 1986:132–146.

282. Basbaum AI, Levine JD. The contribution of the nervous system to inflammation and inflammatory disease. Can J Physiol Pharmacol 1991;69:647–651.

283. Thoren P, Floras JS, Hoffman P, Seals DR. Endorphins and exercise: physiological mechanisms and clinical implications. Med Sci Sports Exerc 1990;22:417–28.

284. Brennan PC, Kokjohn K, Kaltinger CJ, et al. Enhanced phagocytic cell respiratory burst induced by spinal manipulation: potential role of substance P. J Manipulative Physiol Ther 1991;14:399–408.

285. Brennan PC, Triano JJ, McGregor M, Kokjohn K, Hondras M, Brennan DC. Enhanced neutrophil respiratory burst as a biological marker for manipulation forces: duration of the effect and association with substance P and tumor necrosis factor. J Manipulative Physiol Ther 1992;15:8–89.

286. Ekman P, Levenson RW, Friesen WV. Autonomic nervous system activity distinguishes among emotions. Science 1983;221:1208–1210.

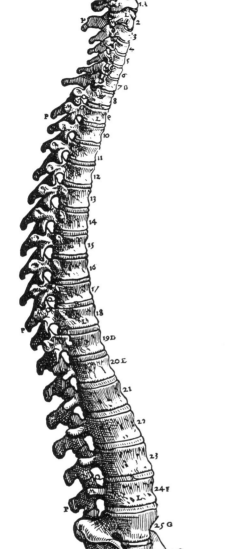

Section 3

Pathophysiology of Vertebral Subluxation Complex

There is but one sure road of access to truth—the road of patient, cooperative inquiry operating, by means of observation, experiment, record, and controlled reflection.

John Dewey

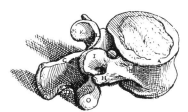

Chapter 10

Vertebral Subluxation Complex Hypothesis

"*B*one out of place," the primary hypothesis to explain the clinical effects of chiropractic since its inception was termed "subluxation" and was proposed by the founder, D. D. Palmer (1). Palmer and others in chiropractic held that subluxations may be caused by acute trauma (e.g., falls, strenuous posture), poisons, and other insults (1–5). The medical profession also recognizes that trauma (e.g., accidents, postural stresses) may result in subluxations and/or arthroses of the spinal column (6–9). If the medical profession does not recognize that poisons may result in subluxations of vertebrae, clearly infections of various kinds may cause reflex spinal subluxations by some viscerosomatic pathway(s) (10–16).

What is less clear is the clinical distinction between *intervertebral subluxation*—operationally defined in the medical literature as translations on motion radiography, and as significant alterations in bony alignment with other imaging techniques—and the chiropractic *vertebral subluxation complex* (VSC), which implies alteration in function and structure (see definitions Chapter 3).

Indeed a critical problem for the chiropractic profession at this time is the lack of a universally accepted operational definition of VSC that would distinguish it clinically

from the medical intervertebral subluxation. Hence, each chiropractic technique system (see also Chapters 1 and 3) offers different operational definitions of VSC, and to date, few of these have been subjected to studies of inter- and intraexaminer reliability (see also Chapters 6 and 7). Compounding this problem, government use of outdated and rigid definitions of chiropractic subluxation (e.g., the federal Medicare operational definition of chiropractic subluxation in the U.S., mandating x-ray validation of the lesion) perpetuates the simplistic model of "bone out of place" for the public and for the chiropractic profession.

However, despite differing definitions and lack of uniformity in descriptions of this lesion, much of our present understanding of both VSC and intervertebral subluxation comes from biomedical research.

The chiropractic profession accepts that VSC is a common occurrence; some within the medical profession would disagree (20), probably because of discrepancies between definitions. Medical definitions generally imply translations with more than 3 mm of bone misalignment, often associated with myelopathy or neurological deficits, occurring relatively infrequently, and often treated with surgery. In contrast, the chiropractic

VSC may or may not have radiologic mani-festations (i.e., x-ray findings of misalign-ment and degeneration may develop later in the pathogenesis of spinal lesions) and may include common forms of soft tissue dys-function for which chiropractic has been shown to be a superior intervention (see Chapter 9). The *vertebral subluxation com-plex hypothesis* is that segmental dysfunction commonly progresses to intervertebral sub-luxation and spinal degeneration.

Many nonpartisan medical authors have reported the causes, development, and progress of intervertebral subluxations using the medical radiologic criteria. This chapter attempts to clarify the concept of VSC by re-viewing the various reports and the various causes of subluxations: trauma, aging, pos-tural influences, arthrosis, and others. These may help to explain why correction of sub-luxation after surgery or chiropractic is not permanent in many cases (e.g., disc degen-eration, unilateral arch defects, ligamentous damage, and erosive arthritides) (10–12, 17–19).

The localized pathological sequelae of subluxation and the concept of immobiliza-tion degeneration are also reviewed. This is the concept that has led to widespread use of the phrase "phases of degeneration" in the profession.

Before this review, however, a discussion of the principal methods that chiropractors use to differentiate subluxations will be helpful.

Spinography and Imaging in Chiropractic

Spinography has been used extensively in the chiropractic profession; its use was pio-neered by B. J. Palmer (*spinography* is the term for radiographs taken while the patient is standing upright) (21). Spinographic ex-amination is necessary to assess the postural and biomechanical integrity of the spine for indicators of intervertebral subluxations (22–24). Various analytical techniques may be used for visual identification of spinal subluxations on radiographs (Table 3.1) (22). It has long been the chiropractic viewpoint that postural status is a major factor in the pathogenesis of subluxation, so spinography is the method of choice for its analysis (25).

However, the use of radiographs and imaging (e.g. magnetic resonance imaging; MRI) has been questioned in cases of acute low back pain, since neither can discrimi-nate patients with LBP from subjects without pain (26, 27). Phillips (26) feels that the lit-erature fails to justify the use of x-ray to identify biomechanical lesions as well, and instead he proposes other criteria (after the work of R. Deyo and A. K. Diehl) for the jus-tification of x-rays (Table 10.1). He cites studies that failed to support the use of stress x-rays to identify aberrant motion, since these films failed to correlate with sacral base angles, the presence of scoliosis, the presence of degenerative change, or ev-idence of foraminal encroachment. In addi-tion, abnormalities on films failed to corre-late with abnormal range of motion and orthopaedic and palpatory findings (26).

Phillips and co-workers (28) found good interobserver reliability for detection of many radiographic findings, including de-generative joint disease and spondylolisthe-sis (Table 10.2), which might arguably influ-ence the type of intervention used by the chiropractor.

Problems such as premature degenera-tion of the spine cannot be established with-out imaging, and MRI evaluations find this abnormality in 35% of subjects aged 20 to 39 (27). And, even when medical radiologists admit that MRI cannot distinguish LBP from nonpain subjects in blinded evaluations, they do not claim that such evaluations should be abandoned for patients in acute pain. Instead, they conclude that abnormal-ities on MRI should be correlated with age and clinical signs and symptoms before op-erative treatment is contemplated (27).

Moreover, according to the current chiro-practic definitions (see Chapters 3 and 9), while identification of intervertebral sublux-ation can be made from a radiograph, diag-nosis of VSC must include physical assess-

Table 10.1.
Recommended Indications for Use of Diagnostic X-rays in Chiropractic Practice[a]

1. Age >50 years
2. Significant trauma
3. Neuromotor deficits
4. Unexplained weight loss
5. Suspicion of ankylosing spondylitis
6. Drug or alcohol abuse
7. History of cancer
8. Use of corticosteroids
9. Temperature >100°F
10. Recent visit for same problem unimproved
11. Patient seeking compensation for pain

[a] Adapted from Phillips RB. Plain film radiology in chiropractic. Manipulative Physiol Ther 1992;15:47–50.

Table 10.2.
Chiropractic Radiology Dependent Variables Associated with Good, Fair, and Poorest Interobserver Reliability, from a Total of 56 Investigated in a Blinded Trial[a,b]

Variable	α
Good agreement between examiners	
Sacral base angle	0.980
Ferguson's weight-bearing line	0.896
Lumbarization	0.860
Short leg discrepancy	0.854
Spondylolysis	0.834
Spondylolisthesis	0.834
Fair agreement between examiners	
Short leg	0.763
L2–3 disc space narrowing	0.756
Intercrestal line	0.735
L4–5 disc space narrowing	0.708
Spondylosis L4	0.705
L5–S1 disc space narrowing	0.690
Spondylosis L3	0.681
Spina bifida	0.671
Inferior pelvic inclination	0.661
Lumbar deviation to side of unlevel pelvis	0.645
Lordosis	0.639
Lumbar deviation with compensatory rotation	0.626
Plane asymmetry of facets	0.613
L3–4 disc space narrowing	0.605
Poorest agreement between examiners	
Pelvic rotation	0.298
Wedged vertebrae	0.119
Shortened pedicles/narrow canal	0.119
Innominate subluxation	0.000

[a] Adapted from Phillips RB, Frymoyer JW, MacPherson BJ, Newberg AH. Low back pain: a radiographic enigma. J Manipulative Physiol Ther 1986;9:183–187.
[b] Variables demonstrating only poor agreement not included; statistical analysis used Cronbach's alpha.

ments that identify a correlation with abnormal segmental function.

Other types of imaging used in chiropractic have been described elsewhere in this text (see Chapter 7). Although used primarily through referral, chiropractors now avail themselves of MRI, videofluoroscopy, and computerized axial tomography (CT scan), as well as spinography (22–25, 29).

Etiologies of Intervertebral Subluxation

In the medical literature, a number of causes for intervertebral subluxation have been proposed. Postural, traumatic, and aging effects are cited most often as most important, but genetic, developmental, and infectious processes have been cited as well. Intervertebral subluxation as cited in the medical literature is considered to be the phase of instability of the VSC (discussed below).

POSTURE AND BIPED MAN

One reason for the high incidence of spinal subluxations is associated with the theory of evolutionary development of man from a quadruped to a biped (30). The quadruped animal's skeleton is built like a cantilever bridge. The vertebrae form an arch, which is supported by the four limbs; in this case, the trunk and abdomen are the load that is supported and suspended by the well-balanced arch (31).

According to the theory of evolution, man developed an upright stance, or became biped. To accommodate to this new mechanical imbalance, man developed several anteroposterior (AP) curves. This proposed evolutionary scene is replayed during infancy, when the first, or primary, single-arch curve is broken into the secondary lordotic curves as children learn to hold their heads up and as they begin to walk (32).

Because of the biped stance, man can perform tasks that no other animal is capable of, but this freedom has been gained at

a cost to the spine. For example, the lumbar vertebrae have been remodeled, with a thicker edge anteriorly and a thinner edge posteriorly. Although this provides a greater range of motion, it also weakens the low back, which causes more lumbar lesions (subluxation) (33).

Beyond the postural difficulty associated with this upright stance is the difficulty brought on when a person does not maintain this stance. Jackson (34) reported that occupations that require prolonged cervical hyperflexion or hyperextension or prolonged or repeated rotation or lateral bending of the neck may result in symptoms of foraminal encroachment. Further, unilateral subluxations may occur when a person turns over in bed during sleep, with the neck muscles relaxed. Her findings indicate that although an upright posture has its inherent weaknesses, an improper posture presents even more difficulties. Certainly, postural stresses are a major factor in the pathogenesis of subluxations (30–34).

TRAUMA

From the medical profession, there is ample acknowledgment that trauma can cause subluxations. Hadley (10) recognized the occurrence of unilateral forward and rotary subluxations in the cervical spine when the patient's head is turned in an unguarded moment during an auto accident. Jacobson and Adler (7) reported that injuries to the atlas-axis joint may result in subluxations there. Their patients included those in auto accidents and one who fell down a staircase. Schleehauf and co-workers (35) demonstrated that computed tomography had good sensitivity for detecting unstable cervical injuries in 104 consecutive high-risk cases; however, all false-negative studies involved atlantoaxial rotary subluxation.

Maigne (36), in a review of the literature, reported that the posterior branches of the spinal nerves are affected by any derangement of the posterior joints. He claimed that acute or chronic derangement may result in traction on the nerves; furthermore, other factors such as edema, periarticular hematoma, or ligamentocapsular tears may be involved.

Birney and Hanley (37) reviewed 84 consecutive cases of pediatric cervical spine injuries treated over a 10-year period at the Children's Hospital of Pittsburgh. Injuries were classified into four groups of relatively equal incidence: atlantoaxial rotary subluxation (n = 23), occiput to C2 ligamentous or bony lesions (n = 24), C3 to C7 fractures and fracture/dislocations (n = 19), and spinal cord injuries without radiographic abnormality but with neurological deficits (n = 18).

Upper cervical injuries occurred primarily in younger children (mean age, 6.2 years); lower cervical spine injuries were more likely to occur in older children (mean age, 13.6 years). These serious injuries occurred most often after falling from a height (n = 32), while motor vehicle accidents and pedestrian-auto accidents accounted for an additional 14 cases. Other common injuries included recreational, athletic, and diving accidents. Forceps delivery was associated with cervical injury in one case. Of the 84 patients, 37 had neurological deficits, including 9 immediate, complete, and permanent deficits.

Of the trauma cases theoretically most amenable to chiropractic, atlantoaxial rotary subluxation was associated with only mild to moderate trauma, and no neurological deficits were associated with this injury. Halter traction with soft collar follow-up or cervical bracing were the medical treatments used, and generally symptoms resolved within weeks. It remains to be demonstrated whether this type of subluxation will respond even more favorably to chiropractic intervention. This study provided a larger series than was previously available from which to better understand neck injuries in these age groups.

Hughes (8) reported that blows to the head may result in cervical subluxation. He stated that hyperflexion of the cervical spine may tear the interspinous and dorsal column ligaments; the annulus fibrosus of intervertebral discs may also be torn. Sunderland (17)

called attention to acute traumata affecting the spinal nerve roots when neighboring structures are displaced or deformed. Braakman and Penning (9) documented the case of a 12-year-old boy who developed an anterior C2-C3 subluxation after diving into shallow water. Kovacs (38) reported on cervical subluxations resulting from traumata or chondrosis. Seletz (6) reported that in whiplash injuries, a momentary posterior subluxation occurs and sometimes persists; he believed, however, that persistent symptoms result from nerve and blood vessel involvement.

Seletz also believed that the axis is especially vulnerable in whiplash injuries. Other medicolegal authorities now accept that subluxations may occur in whiplash injuries; excellent sources outline in great detail the pathophysiology of this injury, its diagnosis, and prognostic indicators for chiropractic clinicians (39). Jackson (34) reported that cervical hypolordosis is found in 76% of all cervical spine injuries after motor vehicle trauma. Epilepticogenic activity has been associated with the whiplash injury, as well as brainstem involvement, even without fracture/dislocation (see Chapter 9).

Trauma resulting in dorsal, lumbar and sacral subluxations has also been reported in the medical literature (10, 40, 41). According to Dussault and Lander (40), while the lumbar facet joints normally are responsible for only a small portion of weight bearing (during erect standing posture a lumbar facet loaded in axial compression is responsible for 16% of normal weight bearing), this increases during extension, and with disc narrowing these joints may carry as much as 70% of the compressive forces.

Studies of facet joint injection with saline to provoke pain and with anesthesia and corticosteroid to attain pain relief have offered insight into the facet syndrome; common after trauma, prospective studies can validate this diagnosis (see Chapters 6 and 10) in only 16% and 29% of cases, respectively (40). *Facet subluxation* in medical studies is often operationally observed by displacement of the superior articulating process of the inferior vertebra to above the inferior vertebral endplate of the superior vertebra. Pain generally extends only to the hip and thigh or is localized to the back. Some authors question the use of large amounts of anesthetic in these studies (>1.5 ml), because extravasation into the epidural space via the superior recess foramina might result in a combined facet joint and epidural block. These authors conclude that the facet joints are sites of microtrauma that lead to degenerative changes, as well as subluxation, dislocation, and fracture (40).

According to studies cited by Giles (41), trauma is directly related to the onset of LBP or sciatica in only 5.5% of cases; osteoarthritis is blamed in 25.6% of cases; and disc syndrome in 22.3% of cases (no cause listed in 27.2% of 2000 cases).

Finally, Warwick and Williams (42) suggest that pregnancy may induce pelvic rotational subluxations, and Lounavaara (43) cited traumatic birth as a cause of subluxation in the newborn infant (see also Chapter 12). Although chiropractors have generally believed that trauma is the most significant single cause of subluxations, medical researchers have implicated many other factors.

DISC DEGENERATION

The intervertebral disc is considered to be a key factor in the etiology of subluxations. The disc is composed of a semigelatinous nucleus pulposus center (a network of collagen fibrils supporting a protein polysaccharide gel complex) and a surrounding dense annulus fibrosus (interlacing fibers of collagen attached to the adjacent vertebral bodies) (10, 41). The discs are avascular (except for their periphery, which may be supplied by nearby blood vessels) and receive their nourishment by diffusion from the adjacent vertebrae (41).

Normally, through the second decade of life, the discs are strong enough that traumata displace the vertebrae rather than the disc (41). Yet, aging takes its toll on the structure; one of the first changes is deterio-

ration of the nucleus pulposus and replacement of it with coarse collagen fibrils (10, 41, 44). As this occurs, the disc loses some of its water content, which decreases the intradiscal pressure. This allows the cartilage plates to come closer together, with resultant discal bulging (10, 44). Normally, the nucleus pulposus acts as a hydrostatic ball bearing, supporting and cushioning the spine; these changes, however, promote instability and more thinning and bulging (10, 44). Instead of the nucleus pulposus carrying the superimposed weight, the annulus fibrosus must increasingly perform this function. Tension is placed on the longitudinal ligaments by the discal bulging, which may stimulate the production of bony spurs to stabilize the joint (10, 44).

From the third decade of life on, injury, postural stresses, and trauma enhance this process (10, 41, 44). Therefore, disc degeneration, thinning, and bulging result from trauma and the general aging process. Scoliosis will cause even more degenerative changes and spur formation (10) (Figs. 10.1 and 10.2).

The literature is replete with references to the effects of disc degeneration. Hadley (10) noted that if the disc becomes thinned in the lumbar region because of degeneration and the posterior articulations of the vertebrae remain intact, the superior vertebra will likely displace posteriorly (posterior subluxation or retrospondylolisthesis). Epstein et al. (45) reported on 15 patients who experienced sciatica. None showed disc herniation, but nerve root entrapment in the lateral recess beneath the superior articular facet of the inferior vertebra was documented operatively. They concluded that the patients' symptoms were caused by trauma, which resulted in disc thinning that allowed posterior subluxations to occur. Sunderland (17) recognized disc thinning as a predisposing factor to subluxation in both the lower cervical and the lower lumbar spine:

Narrowing of the intervertebral disc would lead to subluxation of the joint so that the superior articular process of the subjacent vertebra would move upward to-

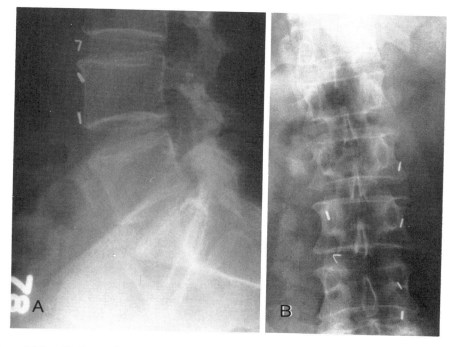

Figure 10.1. Radiographs of a middle-aged man who presented with objective signs of sciatica. The fifth lumbar vertebra is seen subluxating posteriorly on the sacrum, with a minor degree of L5-S1 disc narrowing (**A**). Minor osteoarthritic changes include only minor lipping spurs and sclerosis of the lumbosacral apophyseal joints. The AP view (**B**) shows development of a simple scoliosis, the postural factor. There is developing lumbosacral instability, and future chronic L5 subluxation and/or spondylosis and chronic lumbar osteoarthritis (see VSC phase 3, later this chapter) is to be expected. (The metal clips are from vascular surgery.)

ward the pedicle of the vertebra above, thereby encroaching on that part of the foramen containing the nerve. Kim et al. (46) used nonlinear three-dimensional finite element models of a two-segment ligamentous spine specimen to predict that disc degeneration at L4-5 causes increased intradiscal pressure at an intact L3-4 disc. This predictably triggers degeneration at L3-4 over time, in accordance with *Wolff's law* (viz., living tissue responds to chronic changes in stress and strain). Finite-element models also predict that loss of the fluids within the nucleus palposus (as occurs with aging) further predisposes the annular layers to lateral instability and degeneration; in addition, facets are subjected to significant additional load bearing, which predisposes them to subluxation (47).

Disc degeneration occurs more rapidly in men than in women, beginning as early as the second decade, perhaps because of more mechanical stress and longer nutritional pathways (48). As laminas degenerate, fraying, splitting, and loss of collagen fibers are observed; this may promote disc pathology (49). Perhaps the earliest signs of aging cannot be seen by radiography but occur on a molecular level. Proteoglycan in the annulus fibrosus shifts from larger to smaller moieties in older (but not in younger) dog motion segments subjected to cyclic stress (50).

Recent findings by researchers establishing the presence of nerve fibers as deeply as the outer third of the anulus fibrosus (51) have been supported by others demonstrating structures (resembling Pacinian

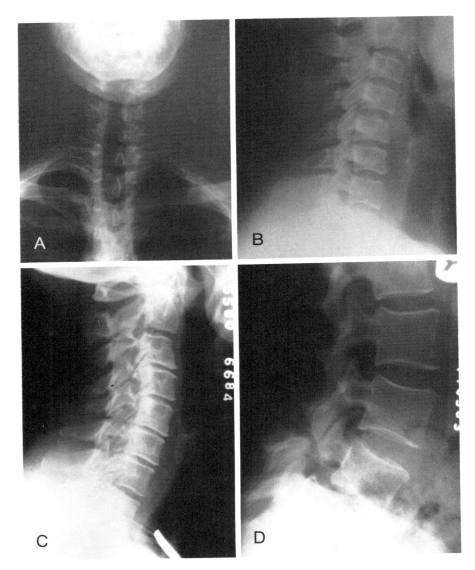

Figure 10.2.   A-D. Radiographs show subtle postural deviations (**A**) and (**B**) reversal associated with whiplash trauma (whiplash with resultant so-called reversed cervical curvature). The young man, who was left unconscious after he was struck by a collapsing roof, has developed significant degenerative joint disease at the level of reversal subluxation (the C3-C4 vertebral motor unit) less than 3 years after the accident (**C**). A defect in the pars interarticularis permits spondylolisthesis of the L5 vertebra in (**D**) a young woman who developed severe radiculitis after falling from a horse; this proved to be unstable and later required surgery. The final result of trauma, postural faults, chronic unreduced subluxation, etc. is often severe multiple spondylosis (degenerative joint disease).

corpuscles and Golgi tendon organs) that function as sensory and mechanoreceptors (52, 53) (see also Fig. 8.1).

Thus disc degeneration, especially when combined with trauma or postural stress, can result in posterior subluxation (displacement, retrolisthesis, retrospondylolisthesis) of the vertebral body above the discopathy when it occurs in the lower cervical or lower lumbar spines. A more detailed explanation of factors predisposing discs to degeneration follows below.

EROSIVE ARTHRITIDES

The erosive arthritides have also been implicated as causes of subluxation, especially in the cervical spine. The primary disease now clearly linked to upper cervical subluxation is *rheumatoid arthritis*. *Stedman's Medical Dictionary* (54) defines this disease as:

> a systemic disease, occurring more often in women, which affects connective tissue; arthritis is the dominant clinical manifestation, involving many joints, especially those of the hands and feet, accompanied by thickening of articular soft tissue, with extension of synovial tissue over articular cartilages, which become eroded; the course is variable but often is chronic and progressive, leading to deformities and disability.

Atlas-axis subluxation and upward translocation of the odontoid are found in one fourth of all patients with rheumatoid arthritis (19). Rana et al. (19) found that 41 of 49 such patients had subluxations, and 8 others had upward translocation of the odontoid. Davidson et al. (18) found atlas-axis subluxation in a case of brainstem compression. Rheumatoid arthritis may cause atlas-axis or other cervical subluxations, and other erosive arthritides have been implicated as causes of subluxations (including rheumatoid spondylitis, Reiter's syndrome, and spondylitis deformans) (10; see Chapter 12).

It is suggested that some unknown factor causes a destructive synovitis of the atlas-axis articulations. This allows the atlas to subluxate, and in some cases, the odontoid becomes translocated. Brainstem compression often accompanies subluxation or translocation of the odontoid, with subsequent bulbar dysfunction. (These findings are discussed in Chapter 12.)

INFECTIONS

Infections are commonly complicated by subluxations (10–16). Grogono (11) reported on a 4-year-old boy with forward subluxation of the atlas on the axis (which occurred 1 week after tonsillectomy) and a retropharyngeal abscess. He lay on his bed with his neck flexed and his head buried in a pillow, complaining of neck stiffness. Grogono reported on a 10-year-old girl with anterior subluxation of the atlas that developed 1 week after a sore throat. Sullivan (13) recognized the occurrence of subluxation with inflammatory lesions of the neck, rheumatic fever, cervical gland infection, pharyngitis, retropharyngeal abscess, influenza, rheumatoid arthritis, and tonsillectomy. Grogono (11) claimed that spontaneous rotary dislocation (subluxation) was the most common type of lesion to affect the atlas and axis. Hess et al. (12) reported on atlas-axis dislocations in which trauma had not occurred recently but inflammatory foci were hypothesized as the initial cause. Hadley (10) also has recognized the role of inflammation in the pathogenesis of subluxation.

Grisel's syndrome is the term used broadly to describe any atlantoaxial subluxation that is associated with inflammatory ligamentous laxity (as discussed above) (14). Rare and primarily a disease of children and young adults, it occasionally occurs in adults as well; patients generally seek treatment for progressive throat and neck pain. Clinically, it is associated with torticollis and subluxation; neurological complications (in as many as 15% of all cases) range from radiculopathy to myelopathy and death (14). From 1981 to 1988, eleven cases were reported.

Reports (15, 16) of atlantoaxial subluxation following oral, head, and neck surgery have been detailed. Atlantoaxial subluxation has been reported following pharyngoplasty and subsequent infection, following otitis media without surgery, and following surgical repair of choanal atresia and adenoidectomy. How inflammation causes displacement is not clearly explained. Ligaments, muscles, and associated structures of the vertebral motor unit may be significant or critical to the pathogenesis in these cases.

A case of brucellosis creating an unstable cervical spine with atlantoaxial subluxation (9 mm atlantodental space) was reported in the chiropractic literature (55). Human brucellosis is rare in the United States. The 62-year-old insurance adjuster entered with low back pain and stiffness, which improved within 2 weeks of CMT. He began to complain of neck stiffness and soreness, although he had not received any neck adjustments. After x-rays confirmed atlantoaxial subluxation, he admitted that until 3 years earlier, he had suffered bouts of brucellosis symptoms and tested serologically positive. He apparently was infected 40 years previously, when an open leg wound came into contact with infected cattle. His back exercise program was altered and trigger point therapy and pulsed ultrasound was used to restore the cervical spine to an almost asymptomatic state. Regular adjustments were contraindicated, and surgery was not necessary as there were no neurological findings and symptoms abated. Brucellosis more commonly occurs after consumption of raw milk or related products such as cheese.

CONGENITAL AND DEVELOPMENTAL FACTORS

Various congenital and developmental structural faults have been associated with subluxation.

Spondylolisthesis

A defect in the isthmus of the neural arch in the lumbar region, or separation of the pars interarticularis, may be complicated by a type of subluxation known as *spondylolis-*

thesis (anterior subluxation, anterolisthesis). This break was formerly thought to be a congenital deformity, but Hadley (10) has not found a single case of congenital defect in the isthmus among some 600 fetal, stillborn, and newborn subjects. Hadley concluded that the problem is developmental and results from a combination of pressure (as the normal lumbar lordosis develops) and trauma. These cause the vertebral body to "slip" forward at the level of the defect.

In reviewing 530 lumbar radiographs, chiropractic investigators Leboeuf, Kimber, and White (56) found spondylolisthesis in 5.1%. A number of orthopaedic investigators have concluded that further slippage occurs with or without fusion surgery to stabilize the vertebra; indeed, even after 40 years, conservative management of spondylolisthesis is just as effective as surgery, which has no significant effect on progression (57–59). In one investigation on 134 girls (mean age, 13.8) and 138 boys (mean age, 14.9) who were followed on average for 14.8 years, 90% of the slip seen on follow-up assessment, on average, had been observed during the first examination. In 62 patients, more than a 10% progression occurred within the first year after surgery or entrance, and no prognostic value for predicting progression was given to female gender, dysplasia (spina bifida), a wedge form of L5, or sacral rounding (57). The conclusion was reached that conservative therapy should be used for the management for this condition whenever progression has not been demonstrated (59). Ventura and Justice (60) propose that CMT is not contraindicated if used specifically at sites of joint hypomobility, usually above and/or below the slip, when the spondylolisthesis is stable. They hold that CMT may prove to be diagnostic as well as therapeutic.

Ligamentous Instability

Ligaments and muscles have also been mentioned as important factors in the pathogenesis of subluxation. Damage to the posterior interspinous ligament, according to cadaver studies by Hadley (10), may predispose the spine to forward or anterior subluxation.

A number of congenital and developmental disorders lead to ligamentous laxity that can cause even potentially fatal subluxation. For example, in *Down's syndrome*, an increase in the atlantodental interval is seen during extension as a potential serious form of subluxation (61–63). But Stein and colleagues (61) found atlantoaxial subluxation of this nature in only two of 14 cases, whereas atlantooccipital subluxation (AOS) occurred in all but one case (see Chapter 12).

Normally, the basion (the midsagittal point of the anterior portion of the foramen magnum) is immediately (approximately 5–10 mm in children) above the odontoid, and typical radiographic procedures fail to discriminate AOS satisfactorily (61). Instead, Stein et al. (61) assess the presence and degree of AOS by observing the position of the occipital condyles with regard to the lateral masses and anterior arch of C1 and by the position of the superior surface of the clivus to the odontoid. Others also report difficulty with normal radiographic analyses for AOS in Down's syndrome cases (62).

Unfortunately, while there appear to be no accurate clinical or radiographic predictors, as many as 1.5% of Down's syndrome patients may have AOS that may cause myelopathy (62). There are potentially fatal consequences to performing adjustments in such cases (63). While conservative chiropractic care may be appropriate in some Down's cases, all subjects should be assumed to have AOS until proven otherwise and be treated accordingly (61–63).

Congenital Anomalies

Other congenital structural problems may give rise to subluxation. For example, in many people the lumbar articulating facets face more anteroposteriorly than laterally, which predisposes that vertebra to posterior displacement (10).

Ritterbusch et al. (64) found subluxation of 5 mm or more in 5 of 20 cases of radiographically documented pediatric *Klippel-*

Feil syndrome. This syndrome is associated with a congenital fusion of two cervical vertebrae, resulting in a characteristically shortened neck. MRI documented stenosis of 9 mm or less below C1 in five and cord abnormalities in three of the patients. Ten patients had symptoms; four reported only occasional neck pain, two had intermittent quadriparesis (one of those also reported arm tingling and neck pain, and the other had documented stenosis), and another had severe headaches with tingling in arms and legs and neck pain (64).

Thus, there are congenital and developmental factors that should be considered when the pathogenesis of subluxations is differentiated.

Vertebral Subluxation Complex Model

There is a growing consensus in the profession, based upon the medical and scientific literature, that intervertebral subluxation occurs as a result of numerous postural and traumatic insults—initially creating segmental dysfunction with its motion disturbance and purported inflammatory and ischemic sequelae (see Chapters 5 and 9)—and subsequently results in joint instability, spinal degeneration, and stabilization, as the final attempt by the body to ameliorate the spinal lesion.

Attempts have been made to quantify the degenerative process, and terms such as "phase of subluxation degeneration" have been commonly used to identify the lesion by stage of development. Unfortunately, there is no commonly accepted operational definition for this process. Nevertheless, we will use the term *vertebral subluxation complex* (VSC) to describe this lesion, regardless of stage, and a model is proposed to describe three phases of VSC, which takes into account the work of several investigators. Since *VSC is associated with pathophysiological sequelae of the manipulable lesion* regardless of the "phase" or stage of degeneration with which it has been associated, a three-phase model will be described.

Much of what we know or suspect about progression through phases or stages of degeneration comes from analyzing mechanical and physiological components of the facets and discs. Other information comes from research on immobilization degeneration. These concepts are briefly reviewed below.

ZYGAPOPHYSES AND INTERVERTEBRAL DISCS: FACTORS PREDISPOSING TO DEGENERATION

Several properties of the zygapophyses and discs help explain their exposure to stresses and strains that might lead to subsequent derangement and degeneration. This section also reviews some factors known to interact with disc degeneration and low back pain (LBP).

Comparing the human literature with results of their canine research, Zimmerman et al. (65) concluded that the posterior elements (i.e., the facet joints) provided a significant amount of torsional rigidity and structural support in axial loading for the spine. During axial compression, canine spinal ligaments are structurally more significant at L2-3 than at L5-6. These researchers stated that discal loading studies of human spines fail to differentiate and provide normative data for individual disc levels, averaging data for all discs instead. They compared various discal levels and found that L5-6 had greater torsional stiffness than L2-3, with the posterior elements equalizing the difference. That the zygapophyseal joints have a special role in weight bearing has long been known, but further research is necessary to determine variances at different spinal levels. This role in weight bearing probably exposes the facets to the effects of repeated stresses and strains, as well as to postural insult over time.

Variants of normal anatomy can predispose disc and cartilage to derangement and degeneration. Noren and co-workers (66) found that 54 back pain patients with *tropism* (i.e., asymmetry in the geometric configuration of zygapophyseal joints) had

significantly more disc degeneration at all lumbar spine levels examined (L3-4, L4-5, L5-S1) by CT and MRI. Similarly, collaborative chiropractic and medical research by Singer, Giles, and Day (67) demonstrated that variations in hyaline articular cartilage from 102 thoracolumbar junction zygapophyseal joints were associated with tropism, with the presence of a mortise joint, or with degenerative changes with or without tropism.

Finite-element simulation of changes in the fluid content of human lumbar discs predicts that a loss in nucleus-confined fluid disrupts the normal mechanical function of the nucleus; anulus layers are then predisposed to lateral instability, disintegration, and further degeneration (68). Because loss of nuclear material created this instability, significant additional loads are subsequently borne by the zygapophyses, and stresses are distributed differently to the vertebral bodies. Hence, aging and trauma to the discs and subsequent fluid loss of the nucleus (and perhaps fluid loss associated with percutaneous nucleotomy) places further stress on the facets.

Fluid content of the disc is important in determining its mechanical response and is critical to transport and biological properties (69). In postmortem studies on 32 human lumbar discs, proteoglycan content fell with age and was lowest in the L5/S1 disc. Proteoglycan content influences fluid content and the relationship of external load to the disc's swelling pressure; hydration of the discs fell with age, with L1-L2 and L5-S1 discs showing the lowest hydration (69). However, the relationship between hydration change and swelling pressure depended more on disc composition than on age or degree of degeneration, and it could be predicted satisfactorily for a disc of known collagen and proteoglycan content. The two-dimensional Poisson equation predicts that maximum cell density in the disc is determined by nutrient supply, and exchange area and disc thickness are critical parameters (70).

Evidence that intraosseous elevated pressure, venous dilatation, and abnormalities of pH, pCO_2, and pO_2 are associated with pain in patients with osteoarthritis led to MRI investigations by Moore and co-workers (71). Vertebral bodies with abnormal MRI signals had intraosseous pressures 55% higher than vertebral bodies with homogeneous signals, along with significantly decreased pH and increased pCO_2. They felt that the findings further supported the concept that abnormalities of intraosseous pressure or blood gas concentrations may be related to pain production in some patients with back pain (71). It appears that such changes would, in addition, predispose the zygapophyses to further degenerative changes.

Swedish researchers investigated elite male gymnasts (n = 24) by MRI and compared degenerative changes in the thoracolumbar spine with findings in male nonathletes (n = 16)(72). Disc degeneration (i.e., reduced MRI signal intensity, associated with loss of water content) was found in 75% of the athletes and only 31% of the nonathletes, a significant difference. There were also significantly more MRI abnormalities in the athletes' spines, and significant correlation was found between the other abnormalities, including abnormal vertebral configurations and reduction in signal intensity of the disc. The authors concluded that male elite gymnasts run a high risk of developing severe abnormalities of the thoracolumbar spine, and they often have a history of back pain (72).

Another factor predisposing the spine to degenerative changes (and therefore to VSC?) is smoking, according to award-winning research by Battié and co-workers (73). Prior to their research, cigarette smoking had been implicated, but not clearly established, as a risk factor for back pain. Using pairs of identical twins highly discordant for the independent variable, MRI examinations revealed 18% greater disc degeneration in the smokers, and the degenerative changes appeared uniformly. The effect of cigarette smoking was clearest at L1-2, where spinal stresses are thought to be less. Finding few other lifestyle variances between the twins that could account for such changes, these researchers suggested that impaired discal circulation secondary to smoking was responsible for the advanced disc degeneration seen in the smokers. Further support for this hypothesis comes from their observation that 38 of the 40 twin pairs in their investigation had undergone duplex sonography of the carotid arteries one year previously for assessment of carotid arteriosclerosis; smokers had larger arteriosclerotic plaques, a finding that reflects the status of the circulatory system in general (73).

Andersson (74) concludes that seven occupational factors are associated with increased risk of low back pain and sciatica: heavy physical work, static work postures, frequent bending and twisting, lifting, pushing and pulling, repetitive work, and vibrations. Individual factors have been identified as well: the literature suggests that aging is most important, sex (women have higher prevalence of LBP with age, but men have twice the risk of disc hernia surgery in their early 40s), smoking, and others (posture, anthropometry, muscle strength, physical fitness, and spinal mobility) (74).

Clinical issues are raised by these studies, confirming the multifactorial etiology of back pain and suggesting a multiplicity of factors contributing to spinal degeneration. For instance, the finding that limitation of straight leg raising (SLR) does not correlate with the size or position of discal hernia further confirms that other factors such as inflammation about the nerve root (see Chapters 9 and 11) are more responsible for the pain and limited SLR associated with discal hernia than is the hernia itself (75). Predisposition to inflammation might be affected by circulatory and other factors discussed in this section, and similar mechanisms might be predicted to occur in the cervical and dorsal spine as well. Reduction in herniated discal material after chiropractic (flexion-distraction combined with physiotherapeutics and nutritional supplements or after side-posture adjustments) may be due to a reduction in inflammatory processes, improvement in discal position, stretching and reduction in multifidus muscle spasm and trigger points, or other unknown mechanisms (see Chapter 9) (76–78).

IMMOBILIZATION DEGENERATION AND PHASES OF SUBLUXATION COMPLEX

Sandoz (79) may have articulated the natural history of VSC more thoroughly than any other chiropractic theorist. In his paper "The Natural History of a Spinal Degenerative Lesion", he summarized the concept of articular overstress proceeding to instability, fixations, and stabilization, and correlated these concepts with the medical term intervertebral subluxation and with what chiropractors have termed subluxation or VSC (79). What follows is a modification of Sandoz's important work (Table 10.3), including concepts presented earlier in this text regarding segmental dysfunction (SDF) and regional dysfunction (RDF), presenting a unified model for phases of VSC. The role of immobilization degeneration in the genesis of spinal pathophysiology is reviewed as well.

Unified Model for Phases of Vertebral Subluxation Complex

In the most recent model proposed by Sandoz (his first work was published in 1960) (79), similar to what was forwarded by Kirkaldy-Willis (80), during the first phase, spinal degenerative lesions begin as articular overstress. We will term this *vertebral subluxation complex phase 1* (VSC phase 1), and it represents the *phase of segmental dysfunction* essentially described earlier in Section 2 of this text.

Mechanical overstress exists whenever excessive compression (static type) or overstretching (dynamic type) affects one or more elements of the three-joint complex (i.e., intervertebral disc and two zygapophyseal articulations). This *articular overstress* can result from congenital hypermobility such as seen in Ehlers-Danlos syndrome, may be acquired through training since childhood, or may be compensatory, adjacent to a congenital lesion such as Klippel-Feil syndrome. Strains can be *elastic* (i.e., immediately recoverable), *viscoelastic* (i.e., recoverable over time), or *plastic* (i.e., irreversible) and are measurable deformations resulting from stress (79). Symptoms and clinical signs of articular overstress include clinical signs suggested by Sandoz (79) as well as those relating to SDF.

VSC phase 2 refers to the *phase of instability* of spinal dysfunction and is associated with radiographic signs of instability. Typically it is heralded radiographically by traction spurs and other initial signs of degenerative joint disease—and seen with other imaging as simple protrusion or bulging of the nucleus pulposus—and in more serious forms seen radiographically by listhesis and angular deformities suggesting ligamentous

Table 10.3
Unified Model for Phases of Vertebral Subluxation Complex (VSC)[a]

VSC Phase	Description	Major Features
1	Phase of segmental dysfunction	Preradiologic[b]
2	Phase of instability	Cartilage destroyed, ligament damage, radiologic lesions (intervertebral subluxations may develop that meet radiologic criteria), some degeneration
3	Phase of stabilization	Predisposed to dynamic overstress in adjacent segments, significant osteoarthritis, (even ankylosis) seen on x-ray

[a] Modified from Sandoz RW. The natural history of a spinal degenerative lesion. Ann Swiss Chiro Assoc 1989;9:149–192.
[b] Plain film radiology will not detect this lesion, but films made during dynamic bending or videofluoroscopy may reveal hypo- or hypermobility.

disruption (79). Intervertebral subluxation by medical radiographic criteria may or may not develop.

According to the Sandoz model, phase 3 is associated with episodic fixations (79). A *vertebral fixation* occurs when a vertebra becomes temporarily immobilized in a position that it may occupy during any phase of physiological spinal movement (79). In Sandoz's model, this may occur at any time before the final stage of degeneration, when stabilization occurs; instead, we include this aspect of the spinal lesion as a type of SDF (see chapters 5–7, and 9) included in VSC phase 1.

The final stage of spinal dysfunction is termed *VSC phase 3*, the *phase of stabilization*, the final phase of repair (Fig. 10.3), again after Sandoz (79). This phase is characterized by signs of advanced degenerative joint disease such as ossification of the longitudinal ligaments, formation of uncovertebral arthrosis, and in the most advanced cases, vertebral ankylosis (80).

Sandoz (79) suggests that phases of VSC be kept for intraprofessional use only and that medical terminology (medical radiographic operational definitions) be used to identify intervertebral subluxation and for interprofessional communication and dialogue. Hence, use of the term *vertebral subluxation complex* should at least be further qualified by additional precise description in terms current in the scientific community. As the chiropractic research community continues to focus on this lesion, it is hoped that at least a "global" operational definition of VSC will evolve, which will permit greater inter- and intraprofessional use of the term.

Since hypomobility is such a central component of SDF, a brief review of scientific literature regarding the role of immobilization in promoting spinal dysfunction and degeneration will be helpful to our discussion of phases of VSC.

Immobilization Degeneration

Much is known of the role of immobilization in the promotion of spinal degeneration. Yoshida (81) experimentally induced facet joint cartilage osteoarthrosis in 49 Wistar rats using lumbar-pelvic distraction for 2–12 weeks. After 2 weeks of distraction, histological examinations revealed early regressive degeneration in superficial layers of the facet joint cartilage. Progressive degeneration ensued with subsequent distraction; between 4 and 8 weeks the effects of distraction became irreversible, and after release of the immobilization, facet joint cartilage developed osteoarthritic changes (81). Similarly, in six clinical cases of thoracolumbar spinal fracture treated by posterior instrumentation without arthrodesis, following removal of the instrumentation, spinal mobility returned temporarily then gradually decreased again. The human facet joints showed pathological changes similar to those in the experimental animals. Yoshida concluded that the spine without arthrodesis appears to develop symptomatic degenerative lesions by a process of internal fixation (81).

The role of immobilization on the intervertebral disc and cartilaginous tissues was similarly investigated. Experimental spondylosis in the mouse was created by surgically removing the posterior paravertebral muscles and by resectioning the spinous processes and the supraspinous and interspinous ligaments without the muscles (82). In several experiments covering 12 months, experimental animals experienced changes including proliferation of cartilaginous tissue and fissures in the anulus fibrosus, shrinkage of the nucleus pulposus, herniation of disc material, and osteophyte formation (82).

Muscular atrophy following immobilization has been investigated as well. In an excellent review of the literature, Appell (83) described strength, electromyographic, and contraction characteristics before and after immobilization in humans. In addition to functional, structural, and biochemical properties of immobilization, he discussed oxygen supply and use, connective tissue changes, and recovery from immobilization. He concluded that after immobilization, atrophy develops quickly during the first days of muscle disuse. Apparently, early loss of

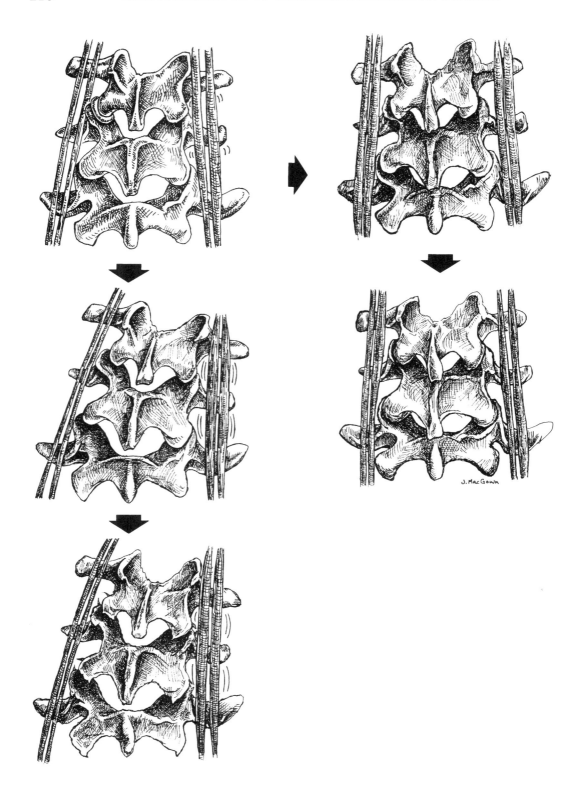

mitochondrial function causes protein breakdown, perhaps secondary to ischemia and perfusion. Postural muscles (slow muscle fibers) appear to be most susceptible to these effects, perhaps due to a higher rate of protein turnover and a greater need for regular oxygen. He concludes that although muscle structure, metabolism, and function are severely impaired after immobilization, the physiological responses and biochemical and contractile properties are largely recoverable through retraining. The time needed for this recovery, however, may depend on such factors as age and sex of subjects, duration of immobilization, length at which the muscle was immobilized, degree of disuse compared with normal use, preimmobilization treatment, preexisting muscle weakness or atrophy, muscle fiber types, and extensor versus flexor activity (83).

In human research, the role of immobilization in promoting osteoarthritis and impeding healing is well established, according to Videman (84). Immobilization promotes thickening of the joint capsule and results in increased capsular tension, compression of articular cartilage, subsequent disturbance of chondrocyte metabolism, fibrillation, depletion of glycosaminoglycans, and finally, arthrotic changes to the joint. Pain can trigger the immobilization and can result from the arthritic changes as well, thus completing a deleterious cycle (84).

There is strong clinical evidence—based upon an award-winning literature review by Waddell (85)—that the immobilization produced by bed rest deters the healing of mechanical back disorders. Conversely, there is strong evidence that increased activity promotes increased bone mineral density, and indeed that muscle strength is an independent predictor of bone mineral density in young women (86, 87). These studies, the postmortem examinations of Hadley (10), and others cited in this chapter show that the earliest phase of VSC (SDF with its primary characteristic of restricted joint mobility) can create both the second phase of VSC—the instability often associated with the radiographically demonstrable intervertebral subluxation—and the stabilizing and immobilizing final phase of VSC, the response referred to as osteoarthrosis or degenerative joint disease.

Figure 10.3. Schematic drawings (L3-L5 vertebra; erector spinae muscle fibers) depict various aspects of the unified model for phases of vertebral subluxation complex (VSC). VSC phase 1 (*upper left*) shows segmental dysfunction (SDF) with inflammation of the left zygapophyseal joint at L3, resulting in antalgic spasm of the contralateral erectores; alignment of the vertebrae is within normal limits. (The slight off-centering to the right does not indicate that adjustment should be applied on the right side; restricted movement will be to the left due to the blockage there.) VSC phase 1 generally is equated with manipulable lesions not discernible by plain film x-ray, but videofluoroscopy or motion studies may reveal fixation (see Chapter 7). It is generally thought that this progresses to VSC phase 2 (*middle left*—the phase of instability), as prolonged muscle contractures promote facilitation, and repeat episodes of trauma produce ligamentous instability. Initial radiographic findings are now present on plain films, including sclerotic endplates and margins, initial osteophytes (not shown), and abnormal curvatures or translations (not shown). The final stage of stabilization is VSC phase 3 (*lower left*), with contractures of the erector spinae muscles (perhaps much less intense) and significant osteoarthritis and in severe cases ankylosis. Alternatively, SDF can theoretically result in impaired joint and adjacent muscle circulation and ischemia, with chronic muscle contracture (*upper right*) but no misalignment discernible by x-ray (see Chapters 5 and 8). Later, although alignment remains normal and ischemia abates somewhat through adaptive mechanisms, a facilitative lesion remains (*middle right*). This might skip VSC phase 2 and proceed to phase 3 with advanced osteoarthritis at levels of involvement but without misalignment (not shown). This may be the most common type of manipulable lesion, according to this hypothesis (see text).

CHIROPRACTIC REDUCTION OF VSC

Chapter 9 focused on the role of chiropractic adjustive and therapeutic techniques in correcting differentiated and undifferentiated mechanical disorders of the spine and in treating lesions most likely meeting the clinical criteria of SDF and RDF (VSC phase 1). This current discussion will outline what is known of chiropractic correction of radiographically definable lesions (VSC phases 2 and 3). Several types of spinal lesions will be discussed: abnormal spinal curvatures (including short leg syndrome), cervical hypolordosis, idiopathic scoliosis, innominate tilt, kyphosis, retrolisthesis, spondylolisthesis, and upper cervical subluxation. Pediatric scoliosis (idiopathic) was reviewed in Chapter 9 and will be only briefly addressed here. Sacro-Occipital technique adjusting is discussed in Chapter 12.

Although purported chiropractic correction of subluxation is continually reported in chiropractic *trade journals*, as in all sections of this text, only peer-reviewed, scientific journals are cited here. Unfortunately, comparatively little *scientific literature* is available to validate the use of adjustive procedures to reduce radiographically demonstrable subluxations. Nevertheless, this section reviews what is known about adjustive reduction or nonsurgical correction of these lesions using chiropractic methods.

Abnormal Curvatures

It is universally accepted in the chiropractic and orthopaedic literature that faulty posture creates mechanical strain and weakness of the human spine; many medical and chiropractic authors have proposed criteria for the correction of a number of radiographically demonstrable abnormalities of curvature and imbalance in the spine (Table 10.4) (88).

Compensatory Scoliosis Secondary to Leg Length Inequality

Panzer, Fechtel, and Gatterman (88) point out that leg length inequality (LLI) contributing to compensatory scoliosis can

Table 10.4
Treatment of Leg Length Inequality: Common Distortions and Related Shoe Lift Applications[a]

Type	Lateral Distortions Ipsilateral Application	Contralateral Application
Lumbar scoliosis (convexity)	Heel lift	Sole lift/heel drop
Sacral anteroinferiority	Heel lift	Sole lift/heel drop
Sacral posterosuperiority	Sole lift/heel drop	Heel lift
Iliac anterosuperiority	Sole lift/heel drop	Heel lift
Iliac posteroinferiority	Heel lift	Sole lift/heel drop
Unilateral pelvic anteriority	Sole lift/heel drop	Heel lift
Unilateral pelvic posteriority	Heel lift	Sole lift/heel drop
Unilateral low femur head	Plantar lift	
Unilateral short ischium	Ischial lift	

Type	Anteroposterior Distortions Application
Sprung back (lumbar)	Bilateral heel lifts
Kissing spines (lumbar)	Bilateral sole lifts/heel drops
Lumbar hyperlordosis	Bilateral sole lifts or heel drops
Lumbar flattening	Bilateral heel lifts
Fixed pelvic anterior tilt	Bilateral sole lifts or heel drops
Fixed pelvic posterior tilt	Bilateral heel lifts

[a] From Panzer DM, Fechtel SG, Gatterman MI. Postural complex. In: Gatterman MI, ed. Chiropractic management of spine related disorders. Baltimore: Williams & Wilkins, 1990:282, with permission.

have a number of causes relating to the spine, pelvis, knee, and foot. (The consensus is that LLI is most accurately measured from a standing comparative radiograph made at the level of the femoral heads.) LLI is a common cause of abnormal spinal curvature or scoliosis. The debate over when to use heel or sole lifts to correct LLI continues, although most researchers favor only lifting patients with ≥5 mm of inequality, when back or leg pain or discomfort with prolonged standing persists (88–92). Triano (89) points out that a 4 mm short leg may be important to an athlete but meaningless to the person who sits at a typewriter all day.

Sandoz (90) proposes that LLI be treated only when the following clinical criteria are met and according to the following procedures (based upon his own observations and the literature):

1. When a lift test shows palpatory and visual evidence for improved static posture upon lifting the short leg and worsening upon lifting the long leg. (A 1–1.5 cm thick board is first placed under the foot on the side of the suspected short leg, then under the contralateral foot.) The patient is not told beforehand what the doctor suspects. Only when static and visual inspection confirm the *blinded* patient's subjective impression that lifting the short leg feels better than lifting the long leg, should prescription of a shoe lift be considered.

2. When radiographs or visual inspection of the lumbar spine (standing and lying prone) reveal straightening in the non-weight-bearing position. The lumbar spine must be supple for adaptation to occur.

3. When the inclination of all vertebral plates and the sacral base conform to the same radius of incurvation. Hence, only when the short-leg side is the side of inferior sacral base height and convexity of lumbar curvature is the prescription for heel lift correction made.

4. Correction with heel lift is based upon a lift close or equivalent to the measured deficiency at the sacral base in adolescents or young adults; it seldom exceeds 50% of the measured deficiency at the sacral base in adults (when >7 mm, lifting is accomplished in two stages, for easier adaptation by the patient).

Even in the absence of lower back pain, patients with LLI >9 mm have architectural and degenerative changes in their lumbar spines, such as concavities in the endplates of vertebral bodies, wedging of the fifth lumbar vertebrae, and traction spurs (compared with control subjects without LLI) (93). However, Froh et al. (94) were unable to find an association between lumbar facet orientation and LLI in 40 consecutive patients seen at a back pain clinic, with pain severe enough to warrant a CT scan. Average LLI was 6.5 mm, with a range of 0.5 to 15.0 mm (94). While at least one chiropractic investigation (95) found correlation between x-ray examination of LLI and visual inspection using three anatomical points of reference (viz., iliac crest levelness, lumbar spine perpendicular to level sacral base, and levelness of posterosuperior iliac spine dimples), most researchers favor an x-ray taken at the level of the femur heads, to reduce the distortion inherent in radiography (88, 90, 93, 94, 96).

Giles and Taylor (97) used this method and found a mean error of 1.12 mm (±0.92 mm) in their investigation of LLI treatment with shoe lift. Of 195 chronic LBP patients with LLI >9 mm but without sacral anomalies or spondylolysis, 89 agreed to participate in the research. While no control group was used, 94% of these patients suffering chronic LBP for more than 6 months had been to at least one health care practitioner (medical practitioners, chiropractors, and physiotherapists), and most had received multiple treatments without lasting relief. None had been treated with a shoe raise. Follow-up assessments at 4 and 12 months revealed an age-related response of scoliosis. Patients aged 19 to 30 ($n = 17$) had their scoliosis angles reduced from a mean of 7° pretreatment to 1° after shoe lift therapy. In the 31–50 age group ($n = 25$), mean curvatures were 7° pretreatment and 3° post–heel lift. However, patients over 50 years old ($n = 8$) had a mean prelift curvature of 5°, and there was little change in postlift radiographs (mean = 4°). Some patients accepted the heel lift therapy but would not allow x-ray reassessment because of the "invasive" nature of radiography.

The authors also noted clinically significant reduction in the number of attacks of LBP in the 12 months after shoe-raise prescription, when compared with the previous 12 months, and improvement in time loss from work as well (97). Although this study has significant limitations, it should spark interest in better-controlled research.

Hypolordosis, Cervical

Borden et al. (98) took radiographs of the right lateral cervical spines of 90 men and 90 women with no history of neck pain, who entered a hospital for routine chest x-rays. At a target-to-film distance of 72 inches, 98% of the subjects had a cervical curvature of 12 mm average depth (measured from a line from the superior aspect of the odontoid to the most posteroinferior aspect of the body of the 7th cervical vertebra). Only 13 subjects had hypolordosis, and osteoarthritis was observed in those individuals, which was generally proportional to the degree of hypolordosis. Women over the age of 50 generally had greater than average lordosis; men over 50, and especially over age 70, generally had less than average lordosis. These medical radiologists concluded that a loss of the cervical lordosis is abnormal, especially when there is no loss of dorsolumbar curvatures.

Norris and Watt (99) were the first to relate the cervical lordotic radiographic appearance after motor vehicle trauma to the postinjury prognosis. While others had observed a relationship between loss of lordosis and cervical trauma (10, 34), these researchers compared symptoms, neurolog-

ical signs, and radiographic appearance immediately after injury with findings after final insurance settlement. Patients with motor vehicle trauma were divided into three groups at presentation: group 1, symptoms but no physical findings; group 2, symptoms and minimal clinical signs, including reduced range of motion; group 3, symptoms, reduced range of motion, and signs of neurological loss. Lordosis visualized on the lateral cervical spine was classified as normal, straight, or kyphotic.

Onset of symptoms was delayed in 6 of 27 patients in group 1, in 6 of 24 in group 2, and in 2 of 10 patients in group 3. Assessment revealed that 74% of group 1 patients had normal cervical lordosis; only 42% and 30% of groups 2 and 3, respectively, had normal curvatures. Conversely, straight cervical spines (hypolordosis) were found in 60% of group 3, 45.5% of group 2, and only 18.6% of group 1. Generally, patients in groups 2 and 3 were more likely to file claims seeking injury compensation, and after settlement assessments, their complaints remained or worsened over time.

Based on their findings, Norris and Watt proposed that a simple classification based primarily on presenting symptoms and signs can predict the short-term prognosis for neck injuries after motor vehicle trauma. The prognosis may be modified by the presence of degenerative joint disease (which was more common in groups 2 and 3), by loss of the cervical lordosis on entrance radiographs, or by both. Chiropractic authors Foreman and Croft (39) used these and similar findings from other studies to devise just such a prognostic scale.

The first observations on chiropractic reduction of cervical hypolordosis in the scientific literature were made by Leach (100), who retrospectively evaluated treatment results of 35 patients who presented with cervical hypolordosis or kyphosis with or without recent trauma. Based upon criticisms of radiographic technique in the medical literature, suggesting that even minor variations in head tilt affect the appearance of the cervical curvature on the neutral lateral film, he

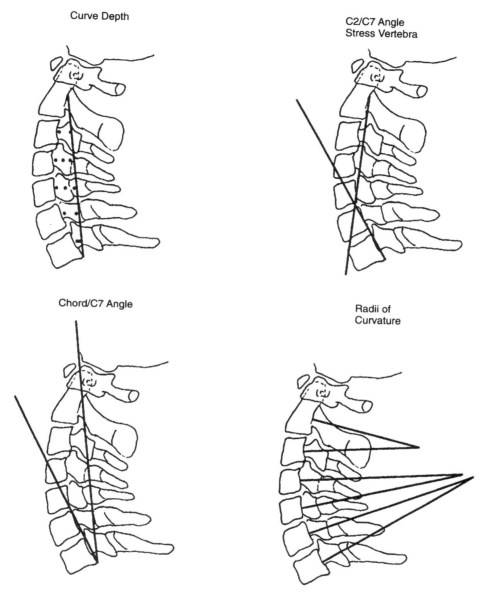

Figure 10.4. Mensuration techniques for assessment of cervical lordosis used by Owens and Leach (102), Leach (100), and Pederson (101). While Leach (100) found that the chord/C7 angle method (*bottom left*) revealed postmanipulative improvement in 29 primarily chronic cases, Pederson (101) was unable to detect improvement in hypolordosis after adjustments with 9 acute mild trauma cases using the same method. In contrast, in a follow-up investigation Owens and Leach (102) studied 35 sets of films in a blinded investigation and used a sonic digitizer with computer analysis. They found that the curve depth and C2/C7 angle stress vertebra methods demonstrated more postadjustive improvement than chord/C7 angle and radii of curvature methods. The curve depth method was also used in original landmark work by Borden and co-workers (98), which established the normal curve depth of 12 mm in the cervical spine.

developed a method for determining the effect of head tilt on lordosis and applied the calculation to the analysis. He used a modification of Hildebrandt's technique for mensuration of the cervical lordosis (the degree of cervical curve depth (CCD) is developed by measuring the angle created by the odontoid/C7 line, and a line drawn along the posterior border of the vertebral C7 body) (Fig. 10.4; bottom left). He found 4.5° of improvement (P <.01) in 20 patients receiving chiropractic diversified adjustments only, applied bilaterally at the level of greatest posterior angulation, while the patients were supine. Nine patients who received a cervical pillow for additional in-home correction and support had 2.2° of improvement (P <.05), also compared with a control group of 6 subjects who had manipulation not intended to correct their cervical hypolordosis. (Follow-up assessments up to 1 year later revealed −0.83° worsening of the cervical hypolordosis in the control group).

Patients with chronic brachial symptomatology had more significant postradiographic improvement than patients presenting immediately after motor vehicle trauma, suggesting that improvement in the hypolordosis was not simply "natural remission" secondary to acute muscle spasms. The author was unable to establish a correlation between the number of adjustment sessions and the degree of correction after care, but he suggested that variables that could not be addressed in this study could explain this outcome and proposed that such a relationship probably exists.

Analysis of variables revealed that with increasing age, use of a cervical pillow in addition to CMT promotes cervical hypolordosis correction (r = .66). The author concluded that most improvement is generally seen in the first 3–4 weeks of thrice-weekly sessions, with reexamination made at that time. Adjustments continue less often when initial care yields results, but reexaminations are made generally at 10-visit intervals until no further improvement is evidenced. Follow-up maintenance adjustments are recommended monthly—more or less according to associated symptomatic, clinical orthopaedic, and neurological findings—to help stabilize the correction, while the patient follows a program of strengthening exercises to aid in rehabilitation. Follow-up examinations annually, biannually, and/or as needed are recommended to assure that any reduction is permanently maintained (100).

Pederson (101), however, found no significant changes in the appearance of the cervical lordosis before and after chiropractic manipulation. Using Leach's method in a prospective trial with 9 patients after minor cervical trauma and 17 controls without cervical trauma, there were more hypolordotic curvatures (7 of 15) and fewer normal curvatures (3 of 15) in the control group prior to treatment. In the treated group prior to CMT, 3 of 9 had significant hypolordosis and 3 of 9 had normal curvatures. After treatment, ll of 17 control subjects clearly continued to have hypolordosis, while only 1 of the 9 treated subjects had the most obvious form of hypolordosis after CMT (viz., cervical curve depth 0–10°).

Statistical analysis failed to discriminate a clear treatment effect, however, and based upon his findings and review of literature, Pederson concluded that Leach's method was not desirable, that cervical hypolordosis may be a variant of normal, and that only S-shaped cervical hypolordosis is related to a poor long-term prognosis. Further, he concluded that the shape of cervical hypolordosis does not appear to change with CMT in cases of minor trauma. Using Leach's method, his findings on correlation of CCD with patient age did agree with those of Borden and co-workers (98); CCD increased in older female patients and decreased in older males.

Plaugher, Cremata, and Phillips (110) also took issue with the findings of Leach, after comparing 25 films before and after 6.5 chiropractic adjustments with 25 films of control subjects. They obtained excellent inter- and intraexaminer reliability (r = 0.89–0.97, P <.001), and films were analyzed from C1 to C7 and from C2 to C7 by measuring the angles formed by lines drawn horizontal to the articulating surfaces. This methodology showed no significant improvement in cervical hypolordosis after CMT.

In a follow-up investigation, Owens and Leach (102) retrospectively studied 33 sets of pre- and postadjustment films meeting preset inclusion criteria, from a pool of 45 sets. Twenty-three females and 10 males, aged 9–69 years (av., 31.5) had reported symptomatology for an average of more than 3 years. Treatment time averaged slightly more than 4 months and included an average of almost 18 sessions of adjustments.

To improve the study design, four blinded assessors (doctors on the research staff of Life Chiropractic College, experienced in radiographic analysis and in the use of the computer digitizer) marked landmarks (hard palate, posterior aspects cervical vertebrae, etc.) and used a sonic digitizer to enter the points into a computer, which then used 20 analyzed factors. The study examined four primary methods of x-ray mensuration and determined that two—C2/C7 angle and the curve depth method (Fig. 10.4)—were superior in documenting improvement (P <.05) in cervical lordosis after chiropractic. The number of adjustments correlated with improvement in curve depth determined by both the C2/C7 angle (r = .64) and the curve depth (r = .78) methods. Since the average length of pain associated with the cervical lesion was over 3 years in these patients, the authors concluded that it was unlikely that reduction in hypolordosis after CMT was due to natural remission.

Interestingly, the method previously described by Leach (100) was ineffective in demonstrating statistically significant improvement, and in a separate cohort of normal college students, variation between pre- and posttreatment measures was greatest using this method (102). In this regard, the study was in agreement with Pederson's (101) findings of lack of discriminability with this procedure; however, while Pederson's data did not reveal statistically significant improvement in hypolordosis after CMT, they did reflect a trend toward reduction in hypolordosis after care.

There are several possible explanations for the lack of statistically significant improvement in hypolordosis after CMT in Pederson's (101) trial, primarily the lack of sufficient treatment sessions/time (14 days as opposed to 1–4 months, and 6 (?) sessions as opposed to 10–18). Similarly, Plaugher et al. (110) may have failed to see changes after CMT for any of a number of reasons, including a lack of sufficient treatment sessions (6.5 as opposed to 10–18) and a lack of mensuration technique sensitive to subtle improvement in the midcervical spine (although they did find significant improvement in retrolisthesis, which may indeed have revealed midcervical improvement in their study—see comments under "Retrolisthesis" below). Moreover, both Pederson (101) and Plaugher et al. (110) may have failed to discriminate changes in cervical lordosis after CMT due to type II error, since they reviewed fewer sets of x-rays (9 and 25 patients, respectively) than did Leach (100) and Owens and Leach (102)(29 and 35, respectively). Probably the explanation involves some combination of the above differences.

Improvement in cervical hypolordosis may represent a classic example of reduction of radiographically demonstrable intervertebral subluxation after CMT. In addition to the published trials of Leach (100) and Owens and Leach (102), numerous chiropractic trade publications have anecdotally reported similar findings, using chiropractic techniques such as those of Donald Harrison, D.C. (Chiropractic Biophysics), W. V. Pierce, D.C. (Pierce-Stillwagon), and others (e.g., Pettibon technique). At least one of these technique founders has begun exploring the interexaminer reliability of using videofluoroscopy to measure cervical spine kinematics, with a hoped-for application of dynamically measuring cervical hypolordosis correction (103).

Idiopathic Scoliosis

A number of claims of cure of idiopathic scoliosis have been made in chiropractic trade journals and self-published chiropractic books and pamphlets. Unfortunately, few reports appear in refereed, chiropractic science journals for treatment of either idiopathic or adult scoliosis (see also Chapter 9).

Nykoliation et al. (104) reviewed the literature, presented four case histories, and presented an algorithm for the chiropractic management of scoliosis. Nonstructural scoliosis (viz., normal mobility on side bending without appearance of a rib hump during trunk flexion) may be due to LLI or other factors (e.g., muscle spasm) and may be corrected conservatively; structural scoliosis (viz., during full trunk flexion a rib hump is observed on the side of convexity) cannot be actively corrected, and conservative management is aimed primarily at preventing progression by the use of CMT, bracing, and transcutaneous neuromuscular stimulation.

Danbert (105) reviewed the current literature to assess a role for CMT in the management of idiopathic scoliosis. The etiology of idiopathic scoliosis may involve genetic, neuromuscular, hormonal, biochemical, or other abnormalities. Some form of collagen abnormality may underlie a decrease in the passive connective tissue component. There is good evidence for a genetic basis for this change in most cases of idiopathic scoliosis. Asymmetry of trunk muscle myoelectric activity is seen in curvatures >25°, and activity is generally elevated on the side of convexity. However, left/right asymmetry is not significantly different in minor curvatures <25°, suggesting that myoelectric activity is not responsible for scoliosis but is responsive to it.

Based on these and similar findings, researchers believe that it is unlikely that adjusting the apices of scoliotic curvatures—a common practice in chiropractic—can halt or reduce idiopathic scoliosis. Indeed, without bracing or other intervention, adjustments alone may even contribute to progression by promoting motion in spinal regions already suffering from instability (104, 105). However, the combination of CMT (to improve mobility) and neuromuscular stimulation has been reported to halt progression and may prove beneficial (106).

Focarile and co-workers (107) analyzed the results of 17 trials meeting their preset criteria for acceptance, and concluded that the effectiveness of nonsurgical treatment for idiopathic scoliosis has not been established. Patients treated by the Boston brace did not have significantly less progression than did wearers of the Milwaukee brace; nor did brace wearers fare any better than patients receiving lateral electrical surface stimulation. Posture training had no significant effect over the other therapies as well. Generally, 30% of subjects were impaired at the end of care regardless of the intervention, and brace failures (i.e., curves progress to 45° or patient undergoes surgery) were five times higher if the curve had progressed to 30° by the start of bracing. These researchers called for randomized prospective comparative trials to determine whether these interventions are effective.

A prospective study of 896 children without curvature at age 11 (average) revealed that by age 14 (average) scoliosis had developed in 24 boys and 41 girls (viz., Cobb angle ≥10° in a posteroanterior standing radiograph) (108). Rib hump was the most powerful predictor of future scoliosis in both boys and girls. Hence, boys with humps of 6 mm had a fivefold risk of developing scoliosis, compared with boys having a symmetric trunk (hump = 0 mm) at the age of 10.8 years. Regression analysis revealed that increased kyphosis predicted future scoliosis in girls, while increased lumbar lordosis predicted future scoliosis in boys.

Any chiropractic treatment approach should focus on prevention of progression, so an understanding of risk factors for progression is imperative (104–108). For example, the risk of progression is greatest during growth years, especially during the onset of puberty. Claims of "cure" of idiopathic scoliosis after CMT based on uncontrolled case reports must be rejected because many minor curves self-correct or halt with or without intervention, and controlled investigations of chiropractic adjustive intervention are necessary before further claims are made.

Kyphosis

Sandoz (109) holds that adjustments to the dorsal spine in cases of hyperkyphosis may reduce the disorder by mobilizing the posterior joints, allowing the erector muscles to actively diminish the degree of kyphosis. However, he cautions that beneficial effects may be short lived if extensor muscle exercises are not used to improve the muscular deficiencies that may have originally caused the disorder. He acknowledges the difficulty of erector muscle exercise for the elderly, who are particularly prone to the condition because of osteoporotic and degenerative events. In his unblinded observational study of 10 women (av. age 62) and untreated control subjects (av. age 64), adjustments were more effective in increasing vital lung capacities and in reducing kyphosis (109). Certainly, further research on this is warranted.

Retrolisthesis

Intra- and interexaminer reliability for measurement of retrolisthesis was excellent, with a low standard error (r = .74–.90, P <.001), in an investigation by chiropractic researchers Plaugher, Cremata, and Phillips (110). When compared with films of 25 control subjects who did not receive chiropractic intervention, 25 films made on patients before and after CMT revealed significant postadjustive improvement in retrolisthesis. No similar pre/post changes were observed with sacral base angle, lumbar lordosis angle, scapular angle or Cobb's angle. This statistically significant improvement in radiographically demonstrable retrolisthesis occurred after an average of 6.5 adjustments (probably Gonstead technique; viz., high-velocity, short-lever, high-amplitude manipulation, and a "nonspecific, bilateral lumbar roll").

Innominate Tilt

Cibulka, Delitto, and Koldehoff (111) found significant changes in innominate tilt after side-posture lumbosacral-type manipulation (P <.05), with excellent intratester reliability for inclinometric assessments before and after the intervention (r = .84). Inclino-metric measurements did reveal altered innominate tilt of the same side and an equal and opposite tilt of the opposite side. While these findings were not measured radiographically, one might assume that static pelvic films would have confirmed these measurements.

Spondylolisthesis

Much is known about the clinical course of spondylolisthesis and the role of conservative care in its management (reviewed above) (57–59). Chiropractors have claimed a role in its treatment using manipulative therapy at spinal segments adjacent to the lesion for amelioration of SDF that appears to develop secondary to the instability (60).

Cox and Trier (112) were the first to investigate improvement in symptoms related to spondylolisthesis with regard to radiographic grading of instability. Films of 10 consecutive chiropractic patients with this lesion (9 involving L5, 1 involving L3) were reviewed for the presence of <3 mm of translatory movement during trunk flexion (compared with the neutral standing postural film; <3 mm = stable, >3 mm = instability). Cox technique (flexion-distraction with a small roll placed under the spondylolisthesis segment with the patient prone—thenar contact of the spinous process above the listhesis gives a cephalic lift during the distraction—applied three times for 20 seconds) resulted in 75% or greater relief for the five stable listhesis patients and <50% relief for the other five patients, whose films demonstrated instability of the lesion. These researchers concluded that suspension radiography to test for unstable spondylolisthesis might be useful in predicting the manipulative efficacy of flexion-distraction.

In addition, after reviewing the literature on manipulation and spondylolisthesis, RAND researchers concluded that spinal manipulation is somewhat appropriate for grades 1 and 2 spondylolisthesis but somewhat inappropriate for grades 3 and 4 (113).

Upper Cervical Subluxation

A great deal has been written about specific correction of upper cervical misalignments and subluxation in the chiropractic literature. Indeed, B. J. Palmer, considered to be the "Developer of Chiropractic," used upper cervical technique exclusively during most of his career and championed its use with research and philosophy (see Chapter 4). (Unfortunately, Palmer did not publish in peer-reviewed science journals, and did not publish studies of reliability nor of validity.)

Many or most advocates of the upper cervical techniques today hold that upper cervical corrective adjustments are critically important, regardless of the patient's symptomatology, when upper cervical misalignment is found. For example, The Upper Cervical Monograph is published by the National Upper Cervical Chiropractic Association, whose members specialize in upper cervical chiropractic adjustments, usually to the exclusion of other adjustive techniques (114). (Another organization, the International Upper Cervical Chiropractic Association, Redwood City, California, promotes upper cervical research and education as well.)

An initial retrospective investigation of atlas laterality and rotation before and after upper cervical adjustive technique indicated that of 523 cases, mean deviation from 0° misalignment was 2.75 for rotation and 2.63 for laterality (115). Grostic and DeBoer (115) found that after upper cervical manipulation, values had improved to 1.43 and 1.40°, respectively. However, no data on reliability, precision, or validity were given in their research, and therefore only tentative conclusions could be reached. The authors stated that a blinded evaluation of variability, replicability, and reliability of Grostic method of upper cervical analysis should be undertaken.

Sigler and Howe (116) challenged the reliability of upper cervical marking systems by using three experienced upper cervical practitioners (Grostic technique). Twenty films were marked by three examiners, and 60 inter- and 20 intraobserver comparisons were made. The average atlas laterality measurement for the 60 markings was 1.83°, and the average difference between the doctors

was 1.05°. At the point where all three doctors agree 80% of the time, the range of error is 2°. These chiropractic authors concluded that with ranges of error of such magnitude, any measured differences found with this system are just as likely to be from marking error as from actual atlas position change.

Jackson et al. (117) used a different measure of atlas laterality used in Pettibon technique diagnosis (viz., the upper angle, between the center skull line and the atlas plane line, and the lower angle, formed by the bisection of C2 and C5). In contrast with the findings on Grostic analysis by Sigler and Howe (116), with this method, six chiropractic practitioners had very good inter- and intraexaminer reliability for marking x-rays. Scattergrams revealed no nonlinear data. Further, for intraobserver measures, there were no statistically significant differences between the first and second readings for any of the experts. Thirty sets of nasium films were read, then reread 3–4 weeks later, after being reblinded and cleaned by the research coordinator. Hence, confidence for the appropriateness of the Pearson correlations for estimating reliability for each chiropractor was deemed good. Correlations for intraobserver reliability ranged from 0.93 to 0.98 (standard error 0.33–0.5° for upper angle, 0.5–0.75° for the lower angle). In both cases, measurement error is less than the 1° claimed by the founder of the technique. Similarly, intraclass correlation coefficients for all experts was 0.90 for the upper angle and 0.93 for the lower angle, representing very good interexaminer reliability (analysis of variance (ANOVA) α 0.98 upper angle, α 0.99 lower angle). The authors concluded that while the investigation did not address the issue of reliability of patient positioning, it did provide strong support for the Pettibon technique x-ray marking system, when used by trained chiropractic professionals. They suggested that future studies were needed of patient positioning reliability and then of validity as an assessment procedure.

Further studies of reliability of upper cervical x-ray marking systems have been published in the non-peer-reviewed chiropractic literature, but these must be questioned until they are published in acceptable format in a science journal (114). After the reliability of x-ray examinations is established, more can be learned of the value of precise upper cervical analytic techniques to measure minute vertebral misalignments that may be a type of VSC. These x-ray techniques require more precision than chiropractic x-ray assessments such as those used by Owens and Leach (102), which ostensibly measure grosser misalignment patterns (see "Hypolordosis," above).

Discussion

There are two themes central to this chapter. We must first understand that the original chiropractic model of "bone out of place" or "misalignment" is essentially related to 19th century medical models (see Chapter 4), is simplistic at best, and should be used only when quantified and qualified using current radiologic terminology. This lesion, termed subluxation in this chapter, suffers from conflicting evidence about our ability to reliably detect and report it.

Second, we must separate the concept of *phases of vertebral subluxation complex* from the concept of misalignment. Based upon research presented in this chapter and in the prior section of this text, *phases of VSC may occur with or without concomitant changes in vertebral alignment as viewed on static radiographs. Indeed, it may be that only the worst forms of VSC ever result in radiographically demonstrable intervertebral subluxation.*

Zengel and Davis (118) investigated projectional distortion of an x-ray image by means of a stereotaxic positioning device. To identify distortion in the image of a third lumbar vertebra, they varied object-film distance, vertical and horizontal off-centering, rotation, and lateral flexion. Mathematical analysis of the results revealed that for object-film distances of 35.64 and 19.48 cm, the vertebra displayed 1 mm of apparent rota-

tion for every 2–3 cm of lateral off-centering, regardless of whether the vertebra was rotated or laterally flexed. Moreover, as long as a given segment is compared with its adjacent segment, they concluded that apparent vertebral rotation on an x-ray may approximate true rotation closely enough. Panjabi, Chang, and Dvoràk (119) found large errors when remarking radiographs to be digitized; however, only minimal differences between digitizers were found when redigitizing the same radiographic pair. When marking certain landmarks from L1 to L5, the authors concluded that poor radiographic film quality promotes errors in kinematic parameters as well.

Award winning research by Shaffer and co-workers (120) revealed that even when good inter- and intra-examiner reliability for an x-ray marking system is found, unacceptable rates of false-positive and false-negative examinations may occur, with respect to actual changes expressed by a model. Of seven different methods used to evaluate translation (retrolisthesis) based on roentgenograms of an experimental model, several had excellent inter- and intraexaminer reliability using either high- or low-quality film (r = .955–.995); however, when measurements of translation were used to assess whether instability had occurred (i.e., −3.0 to +3.0 mm translation), one method (line marked on the anterior margin of the inferior vertebral body; during flexion and extension the anterior, inferior corner of the vertebra above is measured with relation to this line) produced the lowest false-positive (18%) and false-negative (10%) rates. When compared with trials using clinical films, however, poor-quality films adversely affected reliability.

Issues of inter- and intraexaminer reliability for the Gonstead technique pelvic marking system were addressed by Plaugher and Hendricks (121), who found high concordance and significant agreement (p <.001) for two examiners marking 71 full spine films twice. In every case, intraexaminer agreement was superior to interexaminer concordance. These and similar efforts are needed to determine which analytic techniques are reliable and which should be discarded. Researchers hoping to establish CMT as an effective approach to reducing intervertebral subluxation must first determine which chiropractic radiographic methods are reliable.

The problem of congenital asymmetry must be considered as well, especially when using precision upper cervical marking systems that consider 1 or 2 mm offsets to be significantly abnormal. Febbo, Morrison, and Bartlett (122) found differences in occipital condyle longitudinal diameter, transverse diameter, and convergence angles in dried specimens from 24 skulls that were x-rayed and digitized with computer assistance. Based on the base-vertex x-rays—used in upper cervical specific and some other chiropractic techniques—measurements were always different between left and right. Such findings challenge the basis for some x-ray line-marking systems in chiropractic, and further research is warranted.

Another issue confronting the profession concerns the validity of using x-ray as a screening procedure prior to CMT; the potential hazards associated with radiation must be weighed against the potential benefits (26). These concerns are especially warranted if chiropractic researchers cannot establish the reliability of using x-ray marking systems, as well as the validity of their use both in planning chiropractic care and in assessing the results of adjustive intervention.

While Phillips (26) argues that only 44 of 400 cases of LBP demonstrated posterior osteophytes and that there was no evidence these contributed to pain, disability, or extended care, perhaps a better question is would that radiographic finding cause a chiropractor to alter his technique of administering an adjustment? And would that alteration in adjustive technique (e.g., lighter adjustive thrust or adjustment administered instead to adjacent hypomobile segments) provide safer intervention? These questions have yet to be asked, let alone answered, but I speculate that most chiropractors would indeed alter their delivery of chiropractic manipulation in an area of degenerative joint disease, spondylolisthesis, or other biomechanical instability.

Moreover, a wide variety of acknowledged causes and types of intervertebral subluxations have been cited in the medical literature. Subluxations may occur from postural, nontraumatic, traumatic, degenerative, infectious, developmental, and congenital faults. As humans, we are probably susceptible structurally to low back subluxation by our very evolution.

There is interplay between the causative factors cited in this chapter, and more than one factor may be precipitating the intervertebral subluxation. Turek (44) points out that excessive imposed weight, an acute lumbosacral angle, degenerative changes associated with advancing age, loss of the intervertebral disc, chronic occupational postural strains, and a vertical disposition of the articular facets are predisposing factors that may encourage tearing of the capsular ligaments and lumbar intervertebral subluxation.

If it is argued that intervertebral subluxation by medical criteria occurs infrequently, there is comparatively little question that SDF occurs more commonly (see Section 2, especially Chapters 5 and 9); this lesion also is the most likely explanation for chiropractic effectiveness, considering the good results of randomized trials of CMT for acute low back and neck pain. As SDF is—by our definition—a VSC phase 1 lesion, the next question to be addressed with regard to our stated hypothesis involves the ability of SDF to promote instability within the spine.

SDF has been characterized by fixation and hypomobility primarily, and a large body of research on immobilization degeneration supports the idea that spinal hypomobility leads to degenerative events as well (see "Immobilization Degeneration," above). It is quite probable—given the purported higher incidence of SDF than of radiographically demonstrable intervertebral subluxation in the population—that VSC phase 1 more commonly proceeds directly to a milder form of VSC phase 3. Probably the worst cases of spinal degeneration are VSC phase 1 that proceed first to VSC phase 2 (phase of instability) or that begin at VSC phase 2 after major trauma (e.g., posttrauma angular deformity associated with ligamentous instability). VSC phase 2 must be dealt with sternly by the body's adaptive mechanisms, producing significant osteoarthritis (viz., VSC phase 3, the phase of stabilization) (10, 34, 79, 80).

The wide variety of causative factors of both SDF and intervertebral subluxation—from subluxations following traumatic birth, major trauma, and twisting during sleep and from SDF due to abnormal postures and minor trauma—and the fact that the general population deals with one or more of these stresses daily, suggest that the vertebral subluxation complex hypothesis is plausible as broadly presented. However, while SDF may commonly lead to facilitation and spinal degeneration by the process of fixation and immobilization degeneration, true intervertebral subluxation probably occurs only with instability associated with more serious traumatic and other pathophysiological events.

Other researchers looking at chiropractic technique systems are addressing another issue central to the idea of reduction of intervertebral subluxation using chiropractic adjustment. In a follow-up to prior work, Smith, Fuhr, and Davis (123) investigated bone movement in response to percussive thrusts created by a mechanical adjusting device (Activator technique), using piezo-electric accelerometers attached to bone in an anesthetized dog. Bone movement up to 1 mm of translation was established in this model. Hessell et al. (124) have measured force exerted during spinal manipulation using the Thompson technique, by measuring preloading force, peak force, duration of manipulation, impulse of manipulation, and application of peak force (see Chapter 5 and Fig. 9.4). Such investigations should help tell us how much of which type of CMT is needed to achieve a desired response, whether bone movement to reduce a purported in-

tervertebral subluxation (VSC phase 2) or joint movement to improve its dynamic function (VSC phase 1).

However, until more is known about the manipulable lesion and researchers have operationally defined it in prospective randomized trials showing improvement in dependent variables (outcome measures) with which it is associated, our understanding will be aided by following Sandoz's (79) advice. The terms VSC phase 1, VSC phase 2, and VSC phase 3 should be used only as broad categorizations. Clinicians and researchers should use acceptable medical radiographic criteria for intervertebral subluxation, when indicated, and further descriptors that will promote inter- and intraprofessional dialogue and provide more qualification and quantification necessary for competent clinical records. This might at least temporarily settle some arguments within the profession about VSC terminology (125–128); although philosophical and theoretical differences probably will remain until research provides greater knowledge of VSC and its effects and cure.

A few examples of acceptable chiropractic diagnoses using the unified model for phases of vertebral subluxation complex follow:

1. VSC phase 1 lesion: C2/C3 SDF with right rotation restriction and cervicogenic headache.
2. VSC phase 2 lesion: grade 2 spondylolisthesis of L5 (unstable on flexion of the trunk) with mild degenerative joint disease at L5/S1 (explain particulars of DJD in a separate radiology report) and sciatic neuritis.
3. VSC phase 3 lesion: C5/C6 spondylosis (explain particulars of DJD in a separate radiology report) with right lateral bending restriction and cervicalgia.

With appropriate descriptors based on what we do know about SDF, RDF, and intervertebral subluxation, chiropractic researchers can even more aggressively pursue knowledge of VSC, and its correction by chiropractic techniques. The reader should consult Appendix B for an alternative model of VSC prepared by Charles Lantz, Ph.D., D.C.

Summary

The vertebral subluxation complex hypothesis is probably correct in that a wide variety of causative or predisposing factors may commonly promote the onset of SDF and intervertebral subluxation—precursors to spinal degenerative lesions—in the general population. Since postural, nontraumatic, and traumatic factors cause SDF and intervertebral subluxations, the entire population is susceptible to the VSC (6–10, 17, 35–43).

Certain occupations, activities (e.g., gymnastics), and habits (e.g. smoking) promote disc degeneration, which promotes the lesion (72–74). Disc degeneration especially predisposes the elderly (10, 41, 44–49, 69, 70). Infections induce the lesion in children, and erosive arthritides may cause subluxations in yet another group of individuals (10–14, 19, 54–55). Congenital and developmental causes have also been implicated (10, 34, 46, 57–63).

A unified model for phases of vertebral subluxation complex (VSC), based upon a synthesis of the literature, includes: VSC phase 1, the phase of SDF; VSC phase 2, the phase of instability, and VSC phase 3, the final phase of stabilization (79, 80). Research on immobilization degeneration, in addition to other biomedical research, lends strong support for this model to predict progression of spinal degenerative lesions (10, 81–87). However, it is most likely that SDF leads to spinal degeneration without true intervertebral subluxation. Indeed, this progression of VSC phase 1 to VSC phase 3 is probably the most common course for a spinal lesion; VSC phase 2 appears to be associated with more traumatic and other pathophysiological events that occur less often.

Correction of intervertebral subluxation (VSC phase 2 lesions) was reviewed in this chapter, including abnormal curvatures, cervical hypolordosis, idiopathic scoliosis, kyphosis, retrolisthesis, innominate tilt, spondylolisthesis, and upper cervical subluxation (88–117). Chiropractors who use the unified model for phases of VSC should adopt radiographic and other descriptors commonly used in the medical professions, to promote more accurate inter- and intraprofessional dialogue and clinical record keeping.

REFERENCES

1. Palmer DD. The science, art and philosophy of chiropractic. Portland, Ore.: Portland Printing House, 1910.
2. Palmer BJ. The science of chiropractic. Davenport, Ia.: Palmer School of Chiropractic, 1908.
3. Dintenfass J. Chiropractic: a modern way to health. New York: Pyramid, 1970.
4. Verner JR. The science and logic of chiropractic. Brooklyn: Cerasoli, 1941.
5. Pharoah DO. Chiropractic orthopody. Davenport, Ia.: Palmer School of Chiropractic, 1956.
6. Seletz E. Whiplash injuries. JAMA 1958;168:1750–1755.
7. Jacobson G, Adler DC. Examination of the atlantoaxial joint following injury with particular emphasis on rotational subluxation. Am J Roentgenol 1956;76:1081–1094.
8. Hughes JT. Spinal cord trauma. In: Greenfield's neuropathology. London: Edward Arnold, 1976:665–666.
9. Braakman R, Penning L. Injuries to the cervical spine. In Vinken PJ, Bruyn GW, eds. Handbook of clinical neurology. Injuries to the spinal cord part 1. New York: Elsevier, 1976;25:341–345.
10. Hadley LA. Anatomico roentgenographic studies of the spine. Springfield, Ill.: Charles C Thomas, 1964.

11. Grogono BJS. Injuries of the atlas and axis. Br J Bone Joint Surg 1954;36B:397–410.

12. Hess JH, Bronstein IP, Abelson SM. Atlanto-axial dislocations unassociated with trauma and secondary to inflammatory foci in the neck. Am J Dis Child 1935;49:137.

13. Sullivan AW. Subluxation of the atlanto-axial joint. J Pediatr 1949;35:451–464.

14. Mathern GW, Batzdorf U. Grisel's syndrome. Clin Orthop 1989;18:131–146.

15. Hopla DM, Mazur JM, Bass RM. Cervical vertebrae subluxation. Laryngoscope 1983;93:1155–1159.

16. Robinson PH, DeBoer A. La maladie de Grisel: a rare occurrence of "spontaneous" atlanto-axial subluxation after pharyngoplasty. Br J Plast Surg 1981;34:319–321.

17. Sunderland S. Anatomical perivertebral influences on the intervertebral foramen. In: Goldstein M, ed. The research status of spinal manipulative therapy. Washington, D.C.: Government Printing Office, 1975:129–140.

18. Davidson RC, Horn JR, Herndon JH, Grin OD. Brain stem compression in rheumatoid arthritis. JAMA 1977;238:2633–2634.

19. Rana NA, Hancock DO, Taylor AR, Hill AGS. Atlanto-axial subluxation and upward translocation of the odontoid process in rheumatoid arthritis. Am J Bone Joint Surg 1973;55A:1304.

20. Shapiro R. Discussion: comments on subluxation—pathophysiology and diagnosis. In: Goldstein M, ed. The research status of spinal manipulative therapy. Washington, D.C.: Government Printing Office, 1975:265–266.

21. Gibbons RW. The evolution of chiropractic: medical and social protest in America. In: Haldeman S, ed. Modern developments in the principles and practice of chiropractic. New York: Appleton-Century-Crofts, 1980:3–24.

22. MacRae J. Roentgenometrics in chiropractic. Toronto: published privately, 1974.

23. Howe JW. The role of x-ray findings in structural diagnosis. In: Goldstein M, ed. The research status of spinal manipulative therapy. Washington, D.C.: Government Printing Office, 1975:239–247.

24. Koentges A. Computerized axial tomography in the differential diagnosis of the vertebral subluxation. Ann Swiss Chiro Assoc 1985;8:25–45.

25. Ames RA. Posture in the assessment, diagnosis and treatment of chronic low back pain. J Aust Chiro Assoc 1985;15:21–31.

26. Phillips RB. Plain film radiology in chiropractic. J Manipulative Physiol Ther 1992;15:47–50.

27. Boden SD, Davis DO, Dina TS, et al. Abnormal magnetic resonance scans of the lumbar spine in asymptomatic subjects. J Bone Joint Surg 1990;72-A:403–408.

28. Phillips RB, Frymoyer JW, MacPherson BJ, Newberg AH. Low back pain: a radiographic enigma. J Manipulative Physiol Ther 1986;9:183–187.

29. Wiesel S. The reliability of imaging (computed tomography, magnetic resonance imaging, myelography) in documenting the cause of spinal pain. J Manipulative Physiol Ther 1992;15:51–53.

30. Wright HM. Perspectives in osteopathic medicine. Kirksville, Mo.: Kirksville College of Osteopathic Medicine, 1976.

31. Gregory WK. The bridge that walks. Natural Hist 1937;39:33–48.

32. Moore KL. Before we are born. Philadelphia: WB Saunders, 1974.

33. Krogman WM. The scars of human evolution. Sci Am 1951;185:54–57.

34. Jackson R: The cervical syndrome. Springfield, Ill.: Charles C Thomas, 1978.

35. Schleehauf K, Ross SE, Civil ID, Schwab CW. Computed tomography in the initial evaluation of the cervical spine. Ann Emerg Med 1989;18:815–817.

36. Maigne R. Orthopedic medicine, a new approach to vertebral manipulations. Springfield, Ill.: Charles C Thomas, 1972.

37. Birney TJ, Hanley EN Jr. Traumatic cervical spine injuries in childhood and adolescence. Spine 1989;14:1277–1282.

38. Kovacs A. Subluxation and deformation of the cervical apophyseal joints. Acta Radiol 1955;43:1–15.

39. Foreman SM, Croft AC. Whiplash injuries: the cervical acceleration/deceleration syndrome. Baltimore: Williams & Wilkins, 1988.

40. Dussault RG, Lander PH. Imaging of the facet joints. Radiol Clin North Am 1990;28:1033–1053.

41. Giles LGF. Anatomical basis of low back pain. Baltimore: Williams & Wilkins, 1989:6.

42. Warwick R, Williams PL, eds. Gray's anatomy. 35th ed (Br). Philadelphia: WB Saunders, 1973:412–413.

43. Lounavaara KI. Forward subluxation of atlas following birth trauma. Acta Pediatr 1949;37:341.

44. Turek SL. Orthopedics: principles and their application. Philadelphia: JB Lippincott, 1967.

45. Epstein JA, Epstein BS, Lavine LS, Carras R, Rosenthal AD, Sumner P. Sciatica caused by nerve root entrapment in the lateral recess: the superior facet syndrome. J Neurosurg 1972;36:584–589.

46. Kim YE, Goel VK, Weinstein JN, Lim T-H. Effect of disc degeneration at one level on the adjacent level in axial mode. Spine 1991;16:331–335.

47. Shirazi-Adl A. Finite-element evaluation of contact loads on facets of an L2-L3 lumbar segment in complex loads. Spine 1991;16:533–541.

48. Miller JAA, Schmatz C, Schultz AB. Lumbar disc degeneration: correlation with age, sex, and spine level in 600 autopsy specimens. Spine 1988;13:173–178.

49. Bernick S, Walker JM, Paule WJ. Age changes to the anulus fibrosus in human intervertebral discs. Spine 1991;16:520–524.

50. Vasan NS, Gutteling EW, Lee CK, Cibischino M, Parsons JR. A preliminary study of mechanically stress-induced changes in the extracellular matrix of the canine intervertebral disc. Spine 1991;16:317–320.

51. Bogduk N, Windsor M, Inglis A. The innervation of the cervical intervertebral discs. Spine 1988;13:2–8.

52. McCarthy PW, Carruthers B, Martin D, Petts P. Immunohistochemical demonstration of sensory nerve fibers and findings in lumbar intervertebral discs of the rat. Spine 1991;16:653–655.

53. Mendel T, Wink CS, Zimny ML. Neural elements in human cervical intervertebral discs. Spine 1992;17:132–135.

54. Hensyl WR, ed. Stedman's medical dictionary. Baltimore: Williams & Wilkins, 1990:135.

55. Aspergren DD. Brucellosis: a rare cause of the unstable spine. J Manipulative Physiol Ther 1990;13:165–168.

56. Leboeuf C, Kimber D, White K. Prevalence of spondylolisthesis, transitional anomalies and low intercrestal line in a chiropractic patient population. J Manipulative Physiol Ther 1989;12:200–204.

57. Seitsalo S, Osterman K, Hyvarinen H, Tallroth K, Schlenzka D, Poussa M. Progression of spondylolisthesis in children and adolescents: a long-term follow-up of 272 patients. Spine 1991;16:417–421.

58. Frennered AK, Danielson BI, Nachemson AL, Nordwall AB. Midterm follow-up of young patients fused in situ for spondylolisthesis. Spine 1991;16:409–416.

59. Apel DM, Lorenz MA, Zindrick MR. Symptomatic spondylolisthesis in adults: four decades later. Spine 1989;14:345–347.

60. Ventura JM, Justice BD. Need for multiple diagnosis in the presence of spondylolisthesis. J Manipulative Physiol Ther 1988;11:41–42.

61. Stein SM, Kirchner SG, Horev G, Hernanz-Schulman M. Atlanto-occipital subluxation in Down syndrome. Pediatr Radiol 1991;21:121–124.

62. Selby KA, Newton RW, Gupta S, Hunt L. Clinical predictors and radiological reliability in atlantoaxial subluxation in Down's syndrome. Arch Dis Child 1991;66:876–878.

63. La Francis ME. A chiropractic perspective on atlantoaxial instability in Down's syndrome. J Manipulative Physiol Ther 1990;13:157–160.

64. Ritterbusch JF, McGinty LD, Spar J, Orrison WW. Magnetic resonance imaging for stenosis and subluxation in Klippel-Feil syndrome. Spine 1991;16:S539-S541.

65. Zimmerman MC, Vuono-Hawkins M, Parsons JR, Carter FM, Gutteling E, et al. The mechanical properties of the canine lumbar disc and motion segment. Spine 1992;17:213–220.

66. Noren R, Trafimow J, Andersson GBJ, Huckman MS. The role of facet joint tropism and facet angle in disc degeneration. Spine 1991;16:530–532.

67. Singer KP, Giles LGF, Day RE. Influence of zygapophyseal joint orientation on hyaline cartilage at the thoracolumbar junction. J Manipulative Physiol Ther 1990;13:207–214.

68. Shirazi-Adl A. Finite-element simulation of changes in the fluid content of human lumbar discs: mechanical and clinical implications. Spine 1992;17:206–212.

69. Urban JPG, McMullin JF. Swelling pressure of the lumbar intervertebral discs: influence of age, spinal level composition, and degeneration. Spine 1988;13:179–187.

70. Stairmand JW, Holm S, Urban JPG. Factors influencing oxygen concentration gradients in the intervertebral disc: a theoretical analysis. Spine 1991;16:444–449.

71. Moore MR, Brown CW, Brugman JL, et al. Relationship between vertebral intraosseous pressure, pH, PO_2, pCO_2, and magnetic resonance imaging signal inhomogeneity in patients with back pain: an in vivo study. Spine 1991;16:S239-S242.

72. Swäard L, Hellsträom M, Jacobsson B, Nyman R, Peterson L. Disc degeneration and associated abnormalities of the spine in elite gymnasts: a magnetic resonance imaging study. Spine 1991;16:437–443.

73. Battié MC, Videman T, Gill K, et al. Smoking and lumbar intervertebral disc degeneration: an MRI study of identical twins. Spine 1991;16:1015–1021.

74. Andersson GBJ. Factors important in the genesis and prevention of occupational back pain and disability. J Manipulative Physiol Ther 1992;15:43–46.

75. Thelander U, Fagerlund M, Friberg S, Larsson S. Straight leg raising test versus radiologic size, shape, and position of lumbar disc hernias. Spine 1992;17:395–399.

76. Schneider MJ. The traction methods of Cox and Leander: the neglected role of the multifidus muscle in low back pain. Chiropractic Tech 1991;3:109–115.

77. Neault CC. Conservative management of an L4-L5 left nuclear disk prolapse with a sequestered segment. J Manipulative Physiol Ther 1992;15:318–322.

78. Siekerka JR. Nutrition and biochemistry of the intervertebral disc: a clinical approach. Chiro Technique 1991;3:116–121.

79. Sandoz RW. The natural history of a spinal degenerative lesion. Ann Swiss Chiro Assoc 1989;9:149–192.

80. Kirkaldy-Wills WH. The three phases of the spectrum of degenerative disease. In: Kirkaldy-Wills WH, ed. Managing low back pain. New York: Churchill Livingstone, 1983: 75–89.

81. Yoshida M. The effect of spinal distraction and immobilization on the facet joint cartilage—an experimental and clinical studies. J Jpn Orthop Assoc 1989;63:789–799.

82. Miyamoto S, Yonenobu K, Ono K. Experimental cervical spondylosis in the mouse. Spine 1991;16:S495-S500.

83. Appell H-J. Muscular atrophy following immobilisation: a review. Sports Med 1990;10: 42–58.

84. Videman T. The role of immobilization in the development of osteoarthritis. Clin Biomech 1987;2:223–229.

85. Waddell G. Bedrest—laid to rest. Spine 1987; 12:632–644.

86. Bergstrain EJ, Sinaki M, Offord KP, Wahner HW, Melton LJ. Effect of season on physical activity score, back extensor muscle strength, and lumbar bone mineral density. J Bone Miner Res 1990;5:371–377.

87. Snow-Harter C, Bouxsein M, Lewis B et al. Muscle strength as a predictor of bone mineral density in young women. J Bone Miner Res 1990;5:589–595.

88. Panzer DM, Fechtel SG, Gatterman MI. Postural complex. In: Chiropractic management of spine related disorders. Baltimore: Williams & Wilkins, 1990:256–284.

89. Triano JJ. Plenary session II: questions and answers. Chiro Technique 1990;2:151.

90. Sandoz RW. Principles underlying the prescription of shoe lifts. Ann Swiss Chiro Assoc 1989;9:49–90.

91. Soukka A, Alaranta H, Tallroth K. Heliövaara M. Leg-length inequality in people of working age: the association between mild inequality and low-back pain is questionable. Spine 1991;16:429–431.

92. Friberg O. Letter to the editor. Spine 1992;17: 458–459.

93. Giles LGF, Taylor JR. Lumbar spine structural changes associated with leg length inequality. Spine 1982;7:159–162.

94. Froh R, Yong-Hing K, Cassidy JD, Houston CS. The relationship between leg length discrepancy and lumbar facet orientation. Spine 1988;13:325–327.

95. Aspergren DD, Cox JM, Trier KK. Short leg correction: a clinical trial of radiographic vs. non-radiographic procedures. J Manipulative Physiol Ther 1987;10:232–238.

96. Lawrence DJ. Chiropractic concepts of the short leg: a critical review. J Manipulative Physiol Ther 1985;8:157–161.

97. Giles LGF, Taylor JR. Low-back pain associated with leg length inequality. Spine 1981;6:510–521.

98. Borden AGB, Rechtman AM, Gershon-Cohen I. The normal cervical lordosis. Radiology 1960;74:806–810.

99. Norris SH, Watt I. The prognosis of neck injuries resulting from rear-end vehicle collisions. J Bone Joint Surg 1983;65-B:608–611.

100. Leach RA. An evaluation of the effect of chiropractic manipulative therapy on hypolordosis of the cervical spine. J Manipulative Physiol Ther 1983;6:17–23.

101. Pederson PL. A prospective pilot study of the shape of cervical hypolordosis. Eur J Chiro 1990;38:148–161.

102. Owens EF Jr, Leach RA. Changes in cervical curvature determined radiographically following chiropractic adjustment. Proceedings of the 1990 International Conference on Spinal Manipulation, Washington, D.C., 1990:165–169.

103. Wallace HL, Wagnon RJ, Pierce WV. Inter-examiner reliability using videofluoroscope to measure cervical spine kinematics: a sagittal plane (lateral view). Proceedings of the 1992 International Conference on Spinal Manipulation, Chicago, 1992:7,8.

104. Nykoliation JW, Cassidy JD, Arthur BE, Wedge JH. An algorithm for the management of scoliosis. J Manipulative Physiol Ther 1986;9:1–14.

105. Danbert RJ. Scoliosis: biomechanics and rationale for manipulative treatment. J Manipulative Physiol Ther 1989;12:38–45.

106. Aspergren D, Cox J. Correction of progressive idiopathic scoliosis utilizing neuromuscular stimulation and manipulation: a case report. J Manipulative Physiol Ther 1987;10:147–156.

107. Focarile FA, Bonaldi A, Giarolo M-A, Ferrari U, Zilioli E, Ottaviani C. Effectiveness of nonsurgical treatment for idiopathic scoliosis: overview of available evidence. Spine 1991;16:395–401.

108. Nissinen M, Heliövaara M, Seitsamo J, Poussa M. Trunk asymmetry, posture, growth, and risk of scoliosis: a three-year follow-up of Finnish prepubertal school children. Spine 1993;18:8–13.

109. Sandoz R. Some physical mechanisms and effects of spinal adjustments. Ann Swiss Chiro Assoc 1976;6:91–141.

110. Plaugher G, Cremata EE, Phillips RB. A retrospective consecutive case analysis of pretreatment and comparative static radiological parameters following chiropractic adjustments. J Manipulative Physiol Ther 1990;13:498–506.

111. Cibulka MT, Delitto A, Koldehoff RM. Changes in innominate tilt after manipulation of the sacroiliac joint in patients with low back pain: an experimental study. Phys Ther 1988;68:1359–1363.

112. Cox J, Trier K. Chiropractic adjustment results correlated with spondylolisthesis instability. Proceedings of the 1991 International Conference on Spinal Manipulation, Arlington, Va., 1991:60–62.

113. Shekelle PG, Adams AH, Chassin MR, et al. The appropriateness of spinal manipulation for low-back pain: indications and ratings by a multidisciplinary expert panel. Santa Monica: RAND, 1991:90.

114. Palmer JF. Some comments on atlas laterality. Upper Cervical Monograph 1990;4:1,5–7.

115. Grostic JD, DeBoer KF. Roentgenographic measurement of atlas laterality and rotation: a retrospective pre- and post- manipulation study. J Manipulative Physiol Ther 1982;5:63–71.

116. Sigler DC, Howe JW. Inter- and intra-examiner reliability of the upper cervical x-ray marking system. J Manipulative Physiol Ther 1985;8:75–80.

117. Jackson BL, Barker W, Bentz J, Gambale AG. Inter- and intra-examiner reliability of the upper cervical x-ray marking system: a second look. J Manipulative Physiol Ther 1987;10:157–163.

118. Zengel F, Davis BP. Biomechanical analysis by chiropractic radiography: Part II. Effects of x-ray distortion on apparent vertebral rotation. J Manipulative Physiol Ther 1988;11:380–389.

119. Panjabi M, Chang D, Dvořák J. An analysis of errors in kinematic parameters associated with in vivo functional radiographs. Spine 1992;17:200–205.

120. Shaffer WO, Spratt KF, Weinstein J, Lehmann TR, Goel V. The consistency and accuracy of roentgenograms for measuring sagittal translation in the lumbar vertebral motion segment: an experimental model. Spine 1990;15:741–750.

121. Plaugher G, Hendricks AH. The inter- and intraexaminer reliability of the Gonstead pelvic marking system. J Manipulative Physiol Ther 1991;14:503–508.

122. Febbo T, Morrison R, Bartlett P. A preliminary study of occipital condyle asymmetry in dried specimens. Chiro Technique 1990;2:49–52.

123. Smith DB, Fuhr AW, Davis BP. Skin accelerometer displacement and relative bone movement of adjacent vertebrae in response to chiropractic percussion thrusts. J Manipulative Physiol Ther 1989;12:26–37.

124. Hessell BW, Herzog W, Conway PJW, McEwen MC. Experimental measurement of the force exerted during spinal manipulation using the Thompson technique. J Manipulative Physiol Ther 1990;13:448–453.

125. Dishman R. Review of the literature supporting a scientific basis for the chiropractic subluxation complex. J Manipulative Physiol Ther 1985;8:163–174.

126. Brantingham JW. A critical look at the subluxation hypothesis. J Manipulative Physiol Ther 1988;11:130–132.

127. Hubka MJ. Another critical look at the subluxation hypothesis. Chiro Technique 1990;2:27–29.

128. Cremata EE, Plaugher G, Cox WA. Technique system application: the Gonstead approach. Chiro Technique 1991;3:19–25.

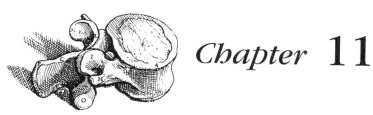

Chapter 11

Nerve Compression Hypothesis

*I*t was D. D. Palmer's (see Chapter 4) most important hypothesis: a bone out of place in the spine could press on a spinal nerve and thereby increase or decrease its flow of nerve energy (1).

Numerous other chiropractic authors have since commented on this idea, and it has become a source of dispute both within and outside the chiropractic profession (2–8). Although, according to the original Palmer thesis, this increased or decreased nerve energy constituted altered body tonus and therefore disease, the latter portion of his hypothesis is discussed in Chapter 14 as a component of the neurodystrophic hypothesis. For the purpose of discussion, the *nerve compression* hypothesis states that intervertebral subluxations may interfere with the normal transmission of nerve energy (i.e., action potentials and other associated neural phenomena) by irritating or compressing the spinal nerve roots.

Hadley (9, 10) and others (11–18) have shown that intervertebral subluxations are a cause of spinal nerve root compression. To our knowledge, Hadley is the only investigator to link a subluxation to specific nerve root pathology discovered during postmortem examination. Others (19–22) have linked disc herniation to nerve root pathology, and still other researchers (23, 24) have been working on an animal model for the subluxation, to study its effects in vivo. Luttges and his colleagues (25–28) at the University of Colorado presented studies of the local pathophysiology of nerve root compression and damage following various types of injury to animal nerves (see also Chapter 15).

Duncan's (29) work in 1948 represented a landmark in nerve studies. Since then, other investigators have detailed the pathophysiology of various types of nerve injury (28, 30–35). Gelfan and Tarlov (36) and Sharpless (37) have studied the susceptibility of nerve roots to compression. These studies and the work of Sunderland (17, 38–40) and others (9, 10, 41–44) tend to refute the suggestion by Crelin (8) that spinal nerve roots cannot be compressed in patients with subluxation. In light of these and other findings, this chapter considers the all-or-none law and reviews the contributions of those cited above.

Modern evidence is presented regarding biological events surrounding neurological dysfunction; lack of correlation between pain and MRI or CT findings of discal hernia, and between pain and plain film x-ray findings, support the argument that ischemia and edema are more critical in the pathophysiology of nerve root injury than are mechanical factors.

Clinical considerations of neurological dysfunction, primarily of nerve root lesions, are briefly reviewed. Both indications and contraindications for chiropractic adjustment or manipulation are considered.

Finally, from the literature, a pathophysiological and clinical picture is presented that includes demyelination, degeneration, muscle atrophy, flaccid weakness, diminished or absent superficial and deep tendon reflexes, and a decrease of the compound action potential (9, 10, 19–22, 27–37, 45–47).

Compression or Irritation?

As Triano and Luttges (48) pointed out at the Ninth Annual Biomechanics Conference on the Spine, the typical chiropractic patient shows signs of paresthesia or pain, which can be traced to cervical or lumbar spinal derangements. These patients are actually reporting increased neural activity. Spinal nerve root compression would be expected to result in effects quite the opposite of those seen in the practitioner's office (i.e., spinal nerve root compression would be expected to decrease nerve fiber function, which would result in decrements in the compound action potential as well as numbness or paralysis). Yet since the days of D. D. Palmer, some chiropractors have promulgated the nerve compression hypothesis to explain all of the many and varied effects of subluxations (2–6).

Palmer (1) was probably the first to suggest that there would be a clinically noticeable difference between mere "irritation" and "compression" of the spinal nerve roots. He stated that irritation of the nerves could result in hyperfunction and painful states and that intervertebral subluxations could squeeze, compress, or pinch the outgoing nerves within the intervertebral foramen. Hence, Palmer developed his hypothesis that disease resulted from either too much or not enough nerve energy.

Several important questions are raised by his assertion: Can intervertebral subluxations alter the shape of intervertebral foramina? Is it possible for spinal nerves to become irritated or compressed because of this change? Is it possible to irritate a spinal nerve without alteration of the intervertebral foramen? What might the clinical effects of this *subluxation pathophysiology* be? To an-

swer these questions, we first examine Crelin's study of the intervertebral foramen, as well as studies of the spinal nerve roots and some neurobiological events surrounding spinal injury.

Crelin's "Test of Chiropractic Theory"

Nature has developed an amazing protective mechanism to safeguard against nerve compression, even when subluxations cause foraminal encroachment. The first and second cervical nerve roots pass over the posterior arch of the atlas and behind the medial margin of the axial articulating facets, respectively (17), but the rest of the spinal nerve roots must pass through the intervertebral foramina located bilaterally at each intersegmental level. The posterior nerve roots are thicker than the anterior roots, especially in the cervical area, where the posterior nerve roots are three times as large. The nerve roots and their sheaths occupy between 35 and 50% of the total cross-sectional area of the intervertebral foramen, with the former figure pertaining especially to the dorsal foramina (40, 49). The remaining 50 to 65% of the foramen contains loose areolar connective and adipose tissue with the spinal artery, numerous veins, lymphatics, and the recurrent meningeal nerve (49). These latter contents cushion the nerve roots from the periosteal boundaries of the foramen.

This basic fact became the focus of attention when Crelin (8) studied the effects of gross rotational, compressive, and torsional forces on six fresh cadaver spines. Crelin, a well-recognized Yale anatomist, entitled the study, "The First Scientific Test of Chiropractic Theory." He used a Mura volt-ohm-microampere meter on the first vertebral column (from a 35-year-old man) (8):

> The meter was used to determine whether the border of the intervertebral foramen came into contact with the spinal nerve when compressive, bending, or twisting forces were applied to the vertebral column. The wire from the positive pole of the meter was wrapped around the spinal nerve that was placed against one side of the intervertebral foramen; the wire from the negative pole of the meter

was placed against the opposite side of the foramen. The meter was set at 1,000 ohms, and if the wires barely touched each other the recording needle would make a full swing across the face of the dial.

While the first spine was being tested, it became obvious that the nerve roots would never actually touch the bony foramen, according to Crelin, so the meter was disconnected. After testing the other spines, Crelin decided that the nerve compression hypothesis (which he called "chiropractic theory," although this is only one chiropractic theory) was false (8):

> This experimental study demonstrates conclusively that the subluxation of a vertebra as defined by chiropractic—the exertion of pressure on a spinal nerve which by interfering with the planned expression of Innate Intelligence produces pathology—does not occur.

More recently, Crelin (5) defended his investigation of chiropractic theory:

> In a living person there is a reflex response by the powerful spinal muscles to fight or resist any forces that would sublux a vertebra to the degree that it and/or spinal nerves could be damaged. In the spines I tested the only resistance to the displacement of the vertebrae were the attached passive ligaments.

Crelin obviously thought that his experiment duplicated the true conditions under which nerve root compression or irritation might occur. Several phenomena in real life, however, make the spinal nerve roots susceptible to such damage; an analysis of the spinal nerve roots is therefore in order.

Spinal Nerve Roots

Nerve complex has been defined as the nerve roots, posterior root ganglion, and the spinal nerve together with their connective tissue coverings (17). Each pair of anterior and posterior nerve roots invaginate the dura and arachnoid mater to pass through the intervertebral foramina. The dura mater becomes the strong perineurial sheath for the spinal nerve that is formed by the fusion of the two roots just past the dorsal nerve root ganglia. The perineurium is continuous

with the epineurium of the spinal nerve, and this combination increases the cross-sectional area of the spinal nerve, as opposed to the total cross-sectional area of the combined nerve roots. Thus, the nerve roots do not have the strong connective tissue sheaths (epineurial and perineurial) that support peripheral nerves (40).

Other factors indicate that the spinal nerve roots are more susceptible to irritation or compression than are the spinal nerves. For example, in humans, the nerve roots are placed in tension by traction on peripheral nerves (49). Thus head and neck movements place tension on cervical nerve roots (17):

> With ventroflexion, the nerve roots are tensed and the complex is drawn inward and upward toward the upper margin of the foramen; in dorsal extension, the complex is relaxed and returns to its original position. The nerve roots maximally involved in this way are the eighth cervical to the fifth thoracic, but ventroflexion of the cervical spine also tenses the lumbar and sacral nerve roots.

The elastic properties of the nerve roots allow them to accommodate such tension. Nerve roots do not display the tensile strength of their peripheral counterparts, however; nerve roots fail before peripheral nerves when nerve roots are tested under increasing tension (17, 39). Sunderland believes that this is due to structural differences; the nerve root fibers are arranged in parallel bundles with fewer enveloping collagen fibers than are found in peripheral nerve trunks. This is in addition to the fact that the nerve roots lack the connective tissue sheaths that support peripheral nerves.

The nerve roots of C4 to C7 are bound to the transverse processes of their respective vertebrae for protection against traction injury (17). For this reason, traction injuries that do not avulse the roots usually occur in the upper cervical spine, whereas traction injuries involving avulsion of nerve roots occur in the lower cervical spine where the nerve root is sheared from the transverse process (17). Hence, lower cervical traction injuries carry the added danger of spinal nerve root avulsion.

In examining the various postmortem and clinical studies concerning nerve root damage, Hadley (9) concluded:

> Any abnormal constriction in the size of a normal intervertebral foramen if not actually causing nerve root pressure, nevertheless decreases the reserve safety cushion space surrounding that nerve and may predispose to pressure. The subsequent development of radiculitis, edema, hemorrhage, additional disc pressure or movement of adjacent structures may be sufficient to produce radicular symptoms.

The significance of these postmortem findings is discussed below. It is noteworthy, however, that Hadley (9, 10) found evidence that cervical and lumbar subluxations could produce foraminal encroachment that would cause, or at least predispose the spinal nerve roots to, compression (Fig. 11.1). He also found that intervertebral sub-luxations could cause foraminal encroachment in the thoracic spine, but he determined that nerve root compression would be unlikely there because of the smaller diameters of the nerve roots (9, 10, 42, 43).

Other researchers have recognized the significance of foraminal encroachment in producing signs of nerve irritation or compression. Breig and Marions (41) studied 103 patients suspected of lumbosacral disc herniations and decided that nerve root compression would be likely at this site because of the anatomical and mechanical conditions. Rosomoff and Rossman (44) estimate that 75% of persons over 50 have some narrowing of the cervical intervertebral foramina.

In summary, there is a substantial amount of evidence to suggest that nerve roots are more mechanically predisposed to irritation or compression than are peripheral nerves.

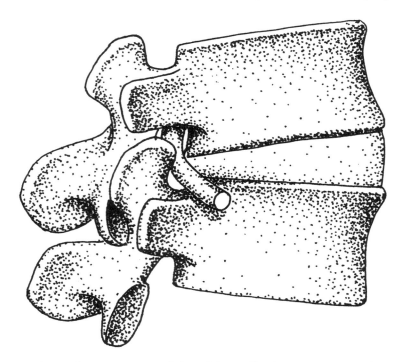

Figure 11.1. Schema illustrating susceptibility of the midlumbar nerve root to distortion (compression, stretch, deformation) after posterior subluxation of the articulating facets. Hadley (9, 10, 42, 43) was the first to demonstrate this phenomenon by postmortem research on human spines. Recent evidence suggests that biological events (viz., ischemia, edema, or venous obstruction of the intervertebral foramen) may be responsible for painful episodes when predisposed by subluxation or discal hernia after even trivial trauma or postural insult (see text).

Nerve roots have been reported to lack the tensile strength of peripheral nerves and to fail when deformed under increasing tension before their peripheral trunks (17, 39). It has also been reported that intervertebral subluxations may cause or at least predispose the nerve roots to irritation or compression in both cervical and lumbar levels (9, 10, 41–44). These weaknesses predispose the nerve roots to the very type of irritation or compression that might occur when subluxation results in foraminal encroachment.

These data contrast with the findings of Crelin (8), whose studies on cadaver spines—with their lifeless mechanics—provide little actual comparison to their living counterparts. Moreover, this chapter deals with the localized pathophysiology of the intervertebral subluxation, as determined by postmortem, operative, and experimental evidence, suggesting that Crelin's conclusions (although perhaps not his experiments) were highly inaccurate and misleading.

Neurological Dysfunction—A Biological Problem?

Perhaps the most damaging evidence for bone-out-of-place theorists, disc-hernia theorists, and other mechanists comes from modern neurophysiological research suggesting that bony and discal alignment may not be critical factors in pain production. For example, evidence that disc herniations exist in asymptomatic subjects abounds (50). And Quon et al. (51) demonstrated significant improvement in back and leg pain associated with an "enormous" CT-confirmed central disc herniation after only 2 weeks of chiropractic manipulation. Despite the improvement in objective and subjective findings, a follow-up CT scan 4 months later revealed no change in the size of the hernia. Moreover, after a review of the chiropractic literature, Phillips (52) argues that pretreatment lumbar x-ray findings do not predict the presence of low back pain and that biomechanical findings seen on plain films are not significantly different between back pain patients and control subjects.

Given these findings, researchers have been pressed to propose alternative hypotheses to explain pain and neurological dysfunction. In one such effort, Hoyland, Freemont and Jayson (53) studied 160 lumbar foramina in 46 cadaveric spines (age range 35–91 years) and determined that direct nerve compression by disc hernia or osteophytes was present in only eight cases. In contrast, age-related increase in fibrous tissue was noted in all cases, and there were significant correlations (r = 0.51–0.70, $p < .001$) between the area of the intervertebral foramina occupied by the venous anastomoses and the percentage area of the neural complex occupied by fibrous tissue (in the area of the nerve root and dorsal nerve root ganglion). Hence, neural fibrosis was associated with a reduced amount of neural tissue and with focal demyelination. For eight specimens, medical histories were available, confirming prior lower back pain. In these cases, direct neural compression was not found; however, all had at least one disc prolapse/protrusion (bulging), vascular compression, and neural fibrosis. These investigators concluded that vascular compression (associated with vascular spasm?) leads to reduced venous outflow and local tissue ischemia, periradicular fibrosis, nerve degeneration, and pain syndromes. Therefore, disc bulge or anatomical considerations may be factors in predisposing an individual to LBP, but vascular spasm and local tissue ischemia may be more important in triggering LBP and neural dysfunction.

Further evidence for a biological role for neural dysfunction comes from the work of Rydevik, Myers, and Powell (54), who examined tissue fluid pressure in the dorsal root ganglia (DRG) of five adult Sprague-Dawley rats before and after 10 light compressions with a 2-mm-wide forceps. Endoneurial fluid pressure in the ganglia rose to 9.6 cm ^{2} (precompression values were 3.7 cm^2; $p < .001$). Histological examination revealed edema and hemorrhage in the endoneurial space of the DRG. The authors speculated that pressure increase in the DRG (such as from a herniated disc), might reduce blood flow to the sensory nerve cell bodies, provoking root level pain.

Low, Lagerland, and McManis (55) at the Mayo Clinic Department of Neurology, summarized 10 years of their work on the physiology of nerve microvascular ischemia in a review article. Given the double blood supply of nerves (*extrinsic system* consists of regional nutritive arteries, arterioles, and venules together with the epineurial vessels; *intrinsic system* consists of longitudinal microvessels within the fascicular endoneurium (see also Chapter 15)) and the rich network of anastomotic vessels within and between each of these systems, some resistance to ischemia is implied. However, these authors concluded from their research that both systems are important in maintaining *nerve blood flow* (NBF) and that flow reductions associated with ischemia from either vascular bed will reduce total nerve perfusion. Due to a large safety margin in the resting NBF and because nerve energy requirements are relatively low, loss of perfusion through either system individually is not great enough to cause nerve infarction (55).

Several morphological differences in nerve capillaries affect NBF. Unusually large diameters make them susceptible to small changes in blood volume and perfusion pressure. Increased capillary distances make perfusion of the endoneurium inefficient (NBF is affected by changes in intercapillary distance) and predisposes nerve to edema, which further increases intercapillary distance. A third difference is in the poorly developed smooth muscle surrounding endoneurial arterioles (55). Measuring NBF during sympathectomy and after sympathetic stimulation should yield important information about potential autoregulation of NBF, especially given dense noradrenergic and peptidergic innervation of vasa nervorum and small arteries, although initial studies indicate that peripheral nerve has poor autoregulation (55).

This research confirmed that nerve edema is associated with chronic endoneurial hypoxia, apparently because of increased intercapillary distances associated with the edema (55). These and other factors associated with the *blood-nerve barrier* explain how ischemia may be more important to neurological dysfunction than would be actual mechanical deformation of a nerve by disc, osteophyte, or vertebral subluxation (see also Chapter 15).

Further, Christiansen and Meyer (56), at the National College of Chiropractic, suggest that induced sciatic neuropathy produces changes in muscle metabolism. Two and 4 weeks after silastic pellets were implanted transverse to the sciatic nerve of rats, decreased nerve conduction velocity was accompanied by decreased glycolytic enzyme activity in both fast and slow twitch muscle and increased malate dehydrogenase activity in the flexor digitorum longus. The fact that mildly neuropathic innervation produced such changes suggests that effects of local ischemia could combine with metabolic changes to effect a wide array of neurodystrophy (see also Chapter 14).

Collectively, these studies offer further, convincing evidence that subluxation complex must be considered from a dynamic perspective involving hemodynamic and biological events—events not studied in Crelin's work and not emphasized by prior chiropractic theorists. Additional evidence is presented below.

Postmortem Histological Examination

Postmortem examination of the spinal nerve roots following compression has been performed. Hadley (9, 10) studied the pathophysiology of nerve root compression from various causes, including subluxation. Lindblom and Rexed (30) dissected 17 cadaver spines to examine the nerve roots in cases of dorsolateral disc herniation. These studies are very significant because they directly link subluxation and disc lesions, respectively, to nerve root damage and pathology.

Hadley found that disc herniations, exostoses, or subluxations may produce pressure on the dorsal nerve root. He found in some cases a marked fibrosis and thickening of the epineurium that attached the root to the foramen walls. Such nerves were removed only by sharp dissection (normally nerves may be removed by blunt dissection). Histologic changes included stages of both nerve degeneration and regeneration (9):

> Certain nerve bundles and ganglion cells were found flattened. Many Schwann tubules outlined by the neurilemma were empty of myelin and axones where the macrophages had removed these degenerated elements. In other sections of the same nerve bundle, these tubules were seen already filled with multiple rods of Schwann protoplasm and nuclei . . . Some evidence of edema of the endoneurium was observed. Hemorrhage beneath the perineurium was found involving numerous roots in one specimen having adhesions about those structures. Sclerosis of arterioles within the nerve bundle was also observed.

Hadley believed that the disc lesion was blamed too often as the cause of the nerve root pressure. He documented evidence of subluxations in the cervical, thoracic, and lumbar areas but believed that only subluxation in the cervical and lumbar areas could cause nerve encroachment (9, 10, 42, 43). He preferred to use conservative care first and surgery only when the former had received a thorough trial run.

Lindblom (19) found 60 nerve root compressions in 160 cadavers from patients aged 14 to 87 years. Most of the compressions (in the lumbar spine) were caused by dorsolateral protrusions against the lateral border of the intervertebral canal. A follow-up study by Lindblom and Rexed (30) determined that compression of a spinal nerve root results in serious injury. Their findings, both macroscopically and microscopically, were generally in accord with those of Hadley. Lindblom and Rexed found cases in which the nerve roots were flattened or hollowed and cases in which the nerve and ganglion adhered to the protruding disc mass by dense connective tissue (separation required a knife). Of the 17 cadavers chosen for follow-up study, 44 segments were examined histologically by serial sectioning of the damaged nerves and of the corresponding normal nerves (30):

> The damage is most obvious in the ventral root bundles . . . The basic effect of the compression is degeneration of a greater or lesser number of the nerve fibers. The damage does not occur as a massive, single trauma to the nerves but as many, repeated small traumata. Furthermore, each trauma is not restricted to a sharply localized point but exerts its effect over a relatively large area. As a result the degenerating nerve fibers are usually diffusely strewn all over the cross section in smaller or greater numbers in proportion to the severity and duration of the compression. Also the standing of the degeneration varies from fiber to fiber, [with] some showing signs of a fresh [lesion], others of an earlier lesion.

Lindblom and Rexed were also in accord with Hadley on the clinical picture, with the characteristic feature being mixed degeneration and regeneration, depending on which fibers were most recently damaged. Degenerative fibers, when they were few, appeared as small patches with Schwann cell proliferation; large and small regenerated fibers were also present. With more degeneration, the damaged fibers formed a large "field" that surrounded isolated undamaged fibers. Lindblom and Rexed reported that damage to motor (ventral) roots was more severe than damage to sensory (dorsal) roots. In addition, damage to the spinal ganglion was even more prominent in cases of compression (30):

> Instead of showing the normal round cross section, it may sometimes appear as a crescent or sickle. This general deformation also influences the cells themselves, which become flattened and deformed, especially near the compressed margin of the ganglion. Some of these cells show definite signs of atrophy and changed staining reactions. In nearly every case there was a direct relationship between the degree of compression and the extent of damage to the nerve root.

Thus, the only postmortem studies (human) available indicate that subluxation is a factor in the compression of nerve roots and that the subsequent pathology depends on the severity of compression. Pathophysiological features at the site of subluxation might include demyelination and degeneration of an individual fiber or groups of fibers, edema of the endoneurium, sclerosis of arterioles within the nerve bundle, and damage to the spinal ganglion itself (9, 10, 30, 43).

Operative Confirmation

Various investigators have documented during surgery that nerve root compression may result in a variety of symptoms and clinical findings as well as damage to the nerve. In a classic study by Eaton (45), the diagnoses in 100 consecutive cases of nerve root pain were compared. Several important clinical aspects were documented. First, there was a characteristic distribution of the pain (segmental or dermatomal). Second, pain was intensified by increasing the intraabdominal and intrathoracic pressure (by coughing, sneezing, lifting, defecation, etc.). Third, stretching of the nerve roots (by bending the neck, stooping, straight leg raising, and the Lasègue test) produced or intensified the pain. These clinical findings were derived from this study that involved nerve compression lesions and diseases of known and unknown origin. Epstein et al. (46, 47) have shown that with L5 or S1 spinal nerve root compression, symptoms of pain, intermittent claudication (pain, tension, and weakness in limbs during walking) with increasing weakness or numbness, leg weakness, and sensory changes may occur. Furthermore, clinical findings might include sciatica, limitation of back mobility, paravertebral muscle spasm, scoliosis, depressed or absent ankle reflexes, diminished or absent patellar reflexes, weakness and atrophy of certain muscles (especially those affecting extensor hallucis longus and anterior tibial muscle groups), and paresis of the quadriceps and hamstrings (46, 47). According to Epstein et al., a positive Lasègue sign will be indicative of sciatica, and electromyography seems to be an accurate clinical tool for determination of nerve root entrapment. Frykholm (57) further documents findings of pain, numbness, paresthesias, and muscle weakness resulting from nerve

root compression. Breig and Marions (41) believe that disc herniation produces tension rather than compression on the nerves, but they recognize the subsequent damage that occurs. In their studies of 103 cases of suspected lumbosacral disc herniations, they reasoned that the neurological signs encountered were due to such tension or stretching of the nerve roots. Thus, the operative data suggest that a wide variety of subjective and clinical findings may result from nerve compression and hence, subluxation (41, 45–47, 57). Yet, postmortem and operative findings are only part of the pathophysiological picture.

Experimental Studies

A number of experimenters have studied the effects of nerve trunk and root compression in animals. Denny-Brown and Brenner (31) reviewed the literature and found references to paralysis resulting from even minimal mechanical trauma. They tried to establish this histologically and to determine the relationship between pressure on nerves and the onset and duration of subsequent paralysis. Two sets of experiments were carried out. In one set of experiments, it took direct pressure ranging from 160 to 1200 mm Hg, applied for "several" to 90 minutes, to block the conduction of cat sciatic nerve trunks. There were great variations in latency from case to case (i.e., the delay in failure of conduction). They concluded that at lower pressures the nerves continued to conduct impulses because adjacent vessels supplied the needed oxygen and that when higher pressures were applied to the nerve, conduction block occurred as these adjacent vessels and tissues became ischemic. Yet, no damage to the nerves was evident histologically, even in nerves that had not returned to normal conduction after 2 hours. In another set of experiments, the authors applied an infant's blood pressure cuff (folded to a width of 6 cm) to the thigh contralateral to the already operated-on thigh. This "tourniquet paralysis" resulted in definite histological changes, including early vacuolation and swelling of axis-cylinders and vacuolation of myelin. After 48 hours, myelin began disappearing at the nodes of Ranvier. The axis-cylinders no longer retained the *argentophil property* (i.e., having affinity for silver and chromium salts). Interestingly, repair continued long after normal nerve conduction had returned.

Duncan's (29) findings were in accord with those of Denny-Brown and Brenner. Yet, his research resulted in a more detailed picture of nerve compression pathophysiology. Duncan's objective was to mimic—by using the right sciatic nerve trunks of eight rats—the condition that is encountered with chronic nerve root compression in the intervertebral foramen. Ligatures were fitted loosely around the sciatic nerves of young rats (.40 cotton thread in four rats and .36 tantalum wire in the others). Additional experiments using tantalum sleeves with four kittens and with young rats proved largely unsuccessful. Six to 7 months later, the rats were sacrificed because of development of motor weakness in the affected limbs. Histological examination showed tremendous adaptability of the nerves to gradual compression. It was noted that this probably accounts for the discrepancies sometimes encountered at the intervertebral foramen (where one nerve root is distorted with little actual destruction, and another is barely distorted but markedly destroyed). Edema was present both proximal and distal to the ligation. This, too, was in accord with previous observations. Complete demyelination occurred at the zone of ligation, along with slight reduction in the axis-cylinder diameter. Distal to the ligation, up to 25% of the fibers became demyelinated without muscle impairment. Growth distal to the application of the ligature was retarded up to 50%. There was, in addition, reduction in the axis-cylinder diameter and thinning of the myelin sheaths both immediately proximal and distal to the ligature. These findings further detailed the pathophysiology of nerve compression.

One study of importance to the chiropractic profession was that of Dyck (32). For a century, researchers studied so-called hypertrophic interstitial neuropathy without understanding the cause. Dyck made repeated applications of a pressure cuff apparatus to rat sciatic nerve trunks for 1 to 2 1/2 hours each time. The intervals between application ranged from 11 to 63 days. A pressure of between 120 and 130 mm Hg was applied. In this way, demyelination and remyelination occurred repeatedly in the same axons. This is similar to the condition Hadley (9, 10) found in nerves following compression and associated with subluxation. Lindblom and Rexed (30) also noted degeneration of some fibers with regeneration of others in the same nerve following compression by disc herniation. Experimentally, Dyck produced the "onion-bulb" formations characteristic of hypertrophic neuropathy by forcing this continual demyelination and remyelination. The onion-bulb formation consists of myelinated fibers in the center, with an inner lamellae composed of circumferentially oriented Schwann cells separated by longitudinally oriented collagen fibrils and with an outer lamellae made up of fibroblasts. Dyck holds the view that the onion-bulbs of hypertrophic neuropathy are a response to repeated segmental demyelination and remyelination. From the studies already presented, it should be evident that subluxation plays a role in nerve compression and hence the degenerative and regenerative processes that would give rise to onion-bulb formation. A direct relationship between subluxation and hypertrophic neuropathy, however, has yet to be documented.

Using a modification of the Duncan (29) technique (which was largely unsuccessful), Aguayo et al. (33) applied siliconized rubber tubes to the medial popliteal branch of the sciatic nerve of young rabbits, which restricted the growth of the nerves. Gradual constriction of the nerves eventually resulted in slowing motor conduction across the constricted portion and in segmental demyelination in and around the area of compression. Histologic and electrophysiologic analysis revealed no indications of limb weakness, change in tonus, or muscle atrophy in the 17 animals included in the long-term studies. Leg lengths preconstriction and postconstriction were compared, and no appreciable difference between the control leg and the constricted leg was noted; thus the findings of Duncan (29) (retardation of growth in the leg with a restricted nerve) were questioned. Furthermore, there was no appreciable difference in the internodal distance between control and constricted nerves (nodes of Ranvier) except at the site of constriction. The characteristic demyelination and remyelination picture was noted, which is in accord with the findings of Hadley (9, 10), Lindblom and Rexed (30), and Dyck (32). Aguayo et al. (33) concluded that chronic compression changes are not simply the result of nerve thinning and displacement of substance in the area of constriction. Instead, they believed, the main factor in compression pathophysiology is the demyelination.

In an experiment similar to that of Denny-Brown and Brenner (31), Fowler et al. (34) blocked the conduction of sciatic nerves in baboons by applying an infant's sphygmomanometer cuff around the knee. Cuff pressures of 1000 or 500 mm Hg were maintained for 1–3 hours. Although most findings agreed with those of Denny-Brown and Brenner (31), several interesting findings were noted. Even after release of the cuff (within 24 hours), the conduction velocity of the nerve was reduced. This reduction occurred before the onset of demyelination and must be explained by other factors, such as occlusion of the nodes of Ranvier and the paranodal invaginations present for several days after compression. Perhaps even more importantly, the conduction velocity decreased through the compressed segment but became normal again after the zone of compression was passed. This was true both during and after compression with a pneumatic cuff, according to the experiments of both Denny-Brown and Brenner (31) and Fowler et al. (34).

Further experimentation on the effects of compression on nerve conduction velocity was completed by Rainer et al. (35). The ulnar nerves of 12 dogs were studied. Compression of the experimental nerves was obtained by the application of 500- and 900-gm weights. The nerve compression rarely exceeded 2 minutes—long enough to record stimulus and response. A significant drop in conduction velocities was recorded. Rainer et al. conjectured that the findings could be secondary to the effect of compression on various types of fibers within the trunk or could be due to transient ischemia secondary to compression, along with disturbed electrolyte balance.

Opponents of chiropractic theory have used these studies by neurophysiologists to support their position (7). The studies show that nerve conduction slows in a zone of compression but returns to normal after the zone (31, 34, 35). However, these are studies of peripheral nerve trunks, not of the roots, which have inherent weaknesses (38–40). Furthermore, modern studies of nerve root conduction suggest an entirely different picture (36, 37, 58).

Probably the first important study by neurophysiologists to implicate the susceptibility of nerve roots to compression was done by Gelfan and Tarlov (36). Mechanical compression of the dorsal nerve roots of dogs was used (36):

> The latency of inactivation by pressure, in contrast to the "all-or-nothing" character of the latency of complete anoxia, can be varied over a wide range. It is inversely related to the magnitude of the compressive force and can be graded continuously from intervals of minutes or hours to instantaneous, but reversible, blocking with higher pressures.

Gelfan and Tarlov agreed with others that larger fibers are more susceptible to compression than are smaller fibers. Since the dorsal spinal root fibers are relatively large, they obviously are clinically important to the chiropractor.

Following up on the work of Gelfan and Tarlov (36), Sharpless (37) used a technique designed to compress the nerve roots and trunks in graduations, which enabled him to determine the minimum pressure needed to achieve a conduction block. A miniature rubber balloon was lowered onto cat and rat nerve roots and trunks. The contact area increased as the pressure applied increased. Thus, at 10 mm Hg, an area of 2.5 mm was compressed, and at 50 mm Hg, an area of 4.5 mm was constricted. The A components of the action potentials were examined; the astonishing finding was that dorsal spinal roots are far more susceptible to compression than are peripheral nerve trunks (Fig. 11.2). He found that dorsal roots could withstand only minimal pressures, as opposed to the sciatic nerves, which could withstand far greater pressures. The compound action potentials (A components) were reduced to about half their initial values at pressures of only 20–25 mm Hg, an extraordinary sensitivity to compression. In the case of one rat (some cats yielded similar results), a pressure of only 10 mm Hg so affected conduction that the compound action potential fell to about 60% of its initial value in only 15 minutes and to 50% of its initial value in just 30 minutes. To illustrate this sensitivity, Sharpless pointed out that the most skilled surgeon could not touch his compression apparatus without recording at least 5 mm Hg. Sharpless believed that this conduction block of some fibers resulted from mechanical deformation rather than hypoxia or ischemia, since the large fibers are blocked first (anoxia is believed to influence small fibers first). Young and Sharpless (58) found that this sensitivity is altered at the point where the dura forms the epineurium, prior to entry of the roots into the foramina. At this point, the spinal nerves become resistant to compression block.

Rydevik et al. (59) took issue with these findings. Using 25 pigs as an animal model more anatomically correct in terms of the microvascular blood supply and surrounding cerebral spinal fluid, graded compression was applied to determine the effect upon sensory and motor nerve roots. A polyethylene balloon was inflated at constant, predetermined pressure levels adjacent to the lumbar spinal nerve roots studied. Specifically, the cauda equina was surgically exposed and compressed toward the ventral aspect of the canal to mimic a discal lesion. No significant changes in amplitudes of efferent or afferent recordings during 2 hours of either 0 or 50 mm Hg compression and 1.5 hours of recovery were observed. Significant changes were observed with 75, 100, and 200 mm Hg for 2 hours. For example, with 75 mm Hg compression, the amplitude of the EMG-P (efferent conduction) decreased to 64% of baseline after 2 hours and recovered to essentially precompression status within 30 minutes of decompression. With 100 mm Hg compression, EMG-P amplitude decreased to 46% of baseline after 2 hours ($p = .004$, compared with sham-treated pigs) and recovered to precompression status within 40 minutes of decompression. Similarly, afferent activity as monitored by compound nerve action potentials was assessed, and amplitude fell to 59.1% of baseline with 75 mm Hg after 2 hours, returning to baseline within 40 minutes of decompression. At 100 mm Hg, amplitude fell to 26.0% of baseline after two hours and incomplete recovery to only 57% of baseline ($p < .001$ and $p < .05$, respectively, compared with sham-treated pigs) occurred after decompression. Hence, these researchers found a critical pressure threshold of 50–75 mm Hg at which compression for 2 hours results in significant changes in both afferent and efferent nerve root conduction and after which recovery of sensory transmission is incomplete. Their findings differed somewhat from the findings of others (36, 37, 58), who held that nerve roots were more sensitive than peripheral trunks.

Prior research by Olmarker, Rydevik, and Holm (60) on 39 pigs revealed that rapid onset of compression (0.05–0.1 seconds) for 2 minutes at 50 mm Hg readily induced edema formation in the nerve roots. Edema formation occurred after slow onset of 50 mm Hg compression as well (15–20 seconds gradually increasing pressure), but it was less pronounced.

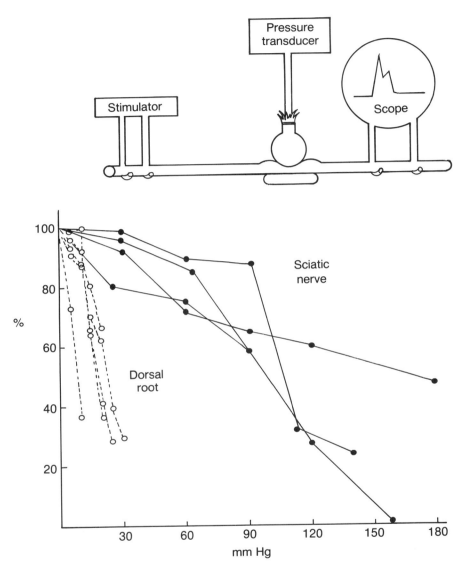

Figure 11.2. Using a variable pressure transducer, Sharpless (37) demonstrated that the A components of the compound action potentials of cat dorsal roots are extremely susceptible to compression block. The compound action potentials (volts × seconds) of the dorsal roots were reduced to half their initial values by a pressure of only 20 mm Hg. By comparison, much greater pressures were necessary to similarly affect the sciatic nerve trunks. However, more recently researchers have determined in pig nerve roots (that may more closely resemble the cauda equina of man) that the critical pressure required to block conduction lies between 50 and 75 mm Hg (59, 60).

Their most recent research verified that even applied for 4 hours, compressive forces of 0 and 50 mm Hg did not significantly reduce the amplitudes of afferent and efferent conduction (61). However, 100 and 200 mm Hg applied to the spinal nerve roots of 20 Yorkshire minipigs for 4 hours provoked sustained conduction block that was not recoverable after 1.5 hours. They suggested that an interaction between biomechanical and microvascular mechanisms is the most likely explanation for the nerve root conduction deficits seen in their research.

These findings generally agree with those of MacGregor et al. (27) who, using a pressure vessel model, determined that large fibers would be compressed the most and thus blocked first (Fig. 11.3). A pressure vessel model also accounts for the gradient character of nerve root conduction block. The longer the pressure is applied, the more viscous displacement occurs in the fibers.

Triano and Luttges (62) demonstrated changes in mouse sciatic nerve consistent with what would be expected in human nerve compression states. Using Silastic plugs affixed adjacent to mouse sciatic nerve in vivo, they found a 31–40% increase in weight (from accumulation of inflammatory edema), which persisted throughout the test period. Increased nerve weight from edema was responsible for conduction velocity decreases, progressive facilitation in the early (5–25 msec) delay periods of nerve refractory sensitivity (by double-pulse studies), and second responses of significantly increased facilitation of refractory recovery that reached maximal levels at 6 days. They believed that such responses to a soft mechanical irritant mimicked neurological disorders faced by the clinician, involving minimal nerve irritation or compression, such as sciatic neuritis. Gait disturbances and other behavioral changes in the test mice showed that although gross degenerative changes had not occurred morphologically, some irritation and pain was present. Hence, ischemic events play a key role, according to their findings.

Luttges and Gerren (63) describe 12 consequences of nerve injury that are not yet fully understood and which include modification of receptor sensitivity, altered fiber projection into the cord, altered sensory input with subsequent changes in cord cells, altered function of Schwann and other supporting cells, sprouting that favors neuromas and single fiber sizes, abnormal reinnervation of tissue by an appropriate type of nerve, abnormal reinnervation by an inappropriate type of nerve, afferent neural activity arising from nonreceptor mechanisms, altered axon dimension and temporal patterning of input, sensory fiber activity initiated chemically or electrically by sympathetic afferents, and differential sensory inputs from selective loss of certain fibers or cells.

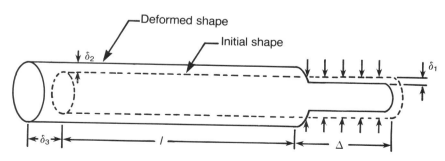

Figure 11.3. MacGregor et al. (27) determined that large nerve fibers should be compressed the most and should be blocked first. According to their model, displaced fluid forces radial distention of the membrane, δ_2, along the length, l, and forces longitudinal displacement, δ_3, at the "end" of the cylinder.

After a comprehensive literature review, they concluded that the lack of information regarding nerve root morphology following experimental compression, as well as regarding quantification or characterization of adaptation of dynamic tissue physiology after prolonged compression, has made it difficult at best to corroborate clinical findings with experimental research. Anatomical and physiological considerations of dorsal nerve root and dorsal root ganglion sensitivity to injury include the 12 items cited above (Fig. 11.4).

Various researchers have studied in detail these degenerative and regenerative phenomena and axoplasmic flow and its relationship to nerve crush (25–28). Because axoplasmic flow may be altered by nerve compression, it should be considered as a component of nerve compression pathophysiology. We discuss axoplasmic aberrations in Chapter 15 and regard it as a tertiary hypothesis.

A review of the literature on experimental studies of nerve root and trunk compression thus reveals many findings of great interest to the chiropractic profession and of great importance to chiropractic theory. In summary, compression injuries cause degenerative and regenerative events that result in aberrant levels of certain nerve proteins along the course of the nerve (27–29, 31–37). Although it appears that changes in the velocity and amplitude of the compound action potential occur at the site of compression, the changes in velocity are only temporary (31, 34–37). The amplitude of the compound action potential, however, appears to be severely and permanently affected by dorsal nerve root compression, although the spinal nerve that exits through the intevertebral foramen is resistant to such compression (36, 37, 58). These effects of nerve root compression appear to be due to some combination of biomechanical distortion of the nerve and focal ischemia, as

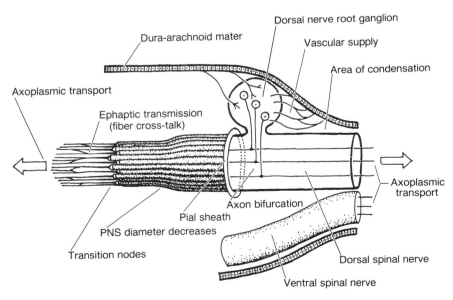

Figure 11.4. The dorsal nerve root and dorsal nerve root ganglion are susceptible to injury and aberrant function physiologically via a number of mechanisms. This schema illustrates these anatomical and physiological components of dorsal nerve root susceptibility. (Adapted from Luttges MW, Gerren RA. Compression physiology: nerves and roots. In: Haldeman S, ed. Modern developments in the principles and practice in chiropractic. New York: Appleton-Century-Crofts, 1980:65–92.)

hypothesized by previous authors (31, 35–37, 51–63).

All-or-None Law

Since the subject of the all-or-none law seems to surface frequently among students and chiropractors, a brief explanation is in order. The *all-or-none* law refers to the fact (discovered by Bowditch in 1871) that heart muscle—regardless of strength of stimulus—responds completely or not at all (64, 65). Studies have confirmed that this principle is valid in other muscles and nerves throughout the body. However, occasionally the action potential reaches a point on a membrane where it cannot generate enough voltage to stimulate the next area of the membrane (65).

Moreover, the law applies only to individual nerve fibers (64, 65). Gelfan and Tarlov (36) and Sharpless (37) have demonstrated that in nerve compression, block of only some fibers in the nerve is possible. The remaining fibers respond to the stimulus normally (36, 37). Thus, some fibers are blocked while others respond by firing, thereby varying the amplitude of the compound action potential of the nerve. In this way, a subluxation could conceivably affect total nerve output. Hence, there is no disagreement between the all-or-none law and the nerve compression hypothesis.

Clinical Considerations

Nerve root compression or irritation may result in several manifestations that can be clinically confusing to the chiropractor as well as to the orthopedist, neurologist, or specialist in physical medicine (45, 65).

Clinical considerations include tests to increase the intensity of pain (coughing, lifting, etc.), which would indicate nerve root compression or a space-occupying lesion (45). Any test that stretches the involved nerve root (e.g., Lasègue, straight leg raiser, foraminal compression) and produces or intensifies pain—especially distal pain—also

indicates nerve root compression or a space-occupying lesion (45).

Other clinical findings that have been demonstrated in cases of nerve root compression and/or irritation include intermittent claudication with increasing weakness or numbness, leg weakness, sensory changes, limitation of mobility of the involved joint, paravertebral muscle spasm, scoliosis, depressed or absent reflexes in the area of cutaneous innervation, and weakness, paresis, or atrophy of muscles in the involved area of cutaneous innervation (45–47, 57). Benchmark tests used generally in chiropractic practice today center around four signs: (*a*) mechanical maneuvers (e.g., foraminal compression test for cervical nerve roots, straight leg raise for lumbar nerve roots) increase pain distally (arm to fingers or leg to toes) more so than proximally, (*b*) loss of deep tendon reflexes segmentally related to, (*c*) numbness or hypesthesia, especially in the hands or feet with a dermatomal distribution, and in more chronic or severe cases, (*d*) weakness and even atrophy of muscles that correlate segmentally with other neurological signs.

Laboratory investigation includes infrared thermography (a positive thermogram is a fairly reliable noninvasive method of evaluating compression nerve injury; see Chapters 7 and 9) and electromyography to determine and differentiate nerve compression (conduction velocity test) from such disorders as descending pathway lesions (H and F reflex tests) (67).

Somatosensory evoked potentials (SEPs) are widely used to demonstrate the level of nerve root lesion, and research indicates good specificity and sensitivity when compared with operative confirmation (68), although its use is more established for peripheral nerve disorders and evaluation of long tracts of the spinal cord (69).

INDICATIONS FOR CHIROPRACTIC

RAND researchers recently rated the appropriateness of spinal manipulation with regard to 1550 indications (70). Generally, the multidisciplinary panel of experts—after reviewing the scientific literature—rated spinal manipulation as extremely appropriate for LBP syndromes with no neurological signs of nerve root lesion; a slightly appropriate rating was given for LBP without sciatica but with minor neurological signs and imaging evidence of posterolateral herniated nucleus palposus. For sciatica without neurological signs and negative imaging, the researchers rated the indication for spinal manipulation as equivocal (70). In addition, numerous case studies and investigations are beginning to favor chiropractic adjustment for a number of conditions involving nerve root or neurological dysfunction (see Chapter 9 for details).

CONTRAINDICATIONS FOR CHIROPRACTIC

RAND researchers concluded that for sciaticas with even minor neurological signs and imaging confirming posterolateral herniated nucleus palposus, spinal manipulation was deemed inappropriate (70). Moreover, in most cases of central herniation without stenosis confirmed by imaging with sciatica and even minor neurological signs, the researchers rated spinal manipulation as extremely inappropriate.

Some of us in private practice have regularly treated such cases (this author has observed that as long as neurological signs are mild and unless a free fragment is documented with imaging, the vast majority of sciaticas respond to chiropractic intervention; See also Chapter 9). Their conclusions—while discouraging—should compel us to demand that chiropractic researchers move away from examining chiropractic for uncomplicated low back pain and toward more complicated sciaticas with neurological and positive findings of discal hernia on imaging.

Based on a review of cases of cauda equina after manipulation of the lumbar spine from 1911 to 1989, Haldeman and Rubinstein (71) found 10 reported cases after manipulation without anesthesia and an ad-

ditional 16 cases after the more vigorous manipulation with anesthesia. They reported three new cases from 88 malpractice suits brought against chiropractors. In the cases reported, both the chiropractor and the emergency room physician failed to comprehend the nature of the problem and take appropriate action. Since the patients were subsequently untreated for this complication for several days, residual symptomatology occurred which might have been prevented with appropriate intervention.

Haldeman and Rubinstein hold that given the estimated 124 million-plus office visits to chiropractors annually and even factoring in unreported cases, this complication occurs only rarely. While concluding that this complication should not make disc hernia a contraindication for chiropractic manipulative intervention, they state that an awareness of the syndrome is needed by all providers. Of the three additional cases reported, two patients presented to the chiropractor with back and leg pain suggestive of disc hernia; one had final progression of symptoms when his back "locked up" in the shower, and the other had an increase in symptoms after she developed a progressive cough. Certainly, these two cases do not present unequivocal evidence that the manipulation caused or aggravated the disc herniation. The third case was more dramatic; immediately upon standing up after chiropractic manipulation, the patient could not support his weight, and progressive neurological deficits were noted. However, this patient was an achondroplastic dwarf, and congenital spinal stenosis in these patients is known to predispose to neural compression after even minor injuries (72). These investigations do raise the question of achondroplastic dwarfism as a contraindication for forceful spinal manipulation, especially in the presence of disc hernia. In these cases, bowel and bladder disturbance, leg weakness, and rectal and genital sensory changes after manipulation should have alerted both chiropractor and physician that immediate surgical decompression for cauda equina syndrome was indicated (69, 70). Instead, neurological deficits continued to progress, some of which were not reversible later even with surgery.

Discussion

Modern research increasingly points to biological events—more so than to mechanical events—as initiators of neurological dysfunction in the typical patient. Generally, nerve root lesions are not ascribed to intervertebral subluxation in the literature. Whether ischemia associated with severe facet syndrome can provoke root level signs is doubtful, and indeed researchers classify facet syndrome (most analogous to chiropractic vertebral subluxation complex (VSC)) by absence of referral of pain past the knee (see Chapters 6 and 10). However, since there is no benchmark or operational definition of VSC, no one can rule out a role for this lesion in producing radicular signs. Nonetheless, it is probably inappropriate to think of bone-out-of-place as viable except in limited cases (e.g., cervical or lumbar hypolordosis in the presence of spinal stenosis? See Chapter 10). In a more likely scenario, some combination of VSC/discal lesion has combined with a recent trauma or a final postural insult, to trigger ischemia-inducing neurological dysfunction with clinical signs of neurological deficits.

Hadley's (9) assertion that abnormal constriction of the intervertebral foramen may predispose to further effects of edema and additional disc pressure has been further supported by recent research. The fact that imaging-verifiable discal hernia occurs with or without pain (50), that radiographically demonstrable intervertebral subluxation occurs with or without pain (52), and that biological models confirm experimental findings supporting a role for ischemia-induced neurological dysfunction, suggests a role for *mechanical predisposition and biological initiation of neurological dysfunction* (53–63).

Certainly, simplistic hypotheses such as bone pressing on nerve, whether proposed by chiropractors or dismissed by anatomists, do little to advance the theory of chiropractic. Only further research can increase our knowledge of this area of clinical practice, and in the interim, patient communication should be updated to reflect our current understanding of these lesions. In the interim, it is not unreasonable to suppose that VSC may predispose patients to discal hernia and aging (see also Chapter 10), as well as subsequent ischemia, edema, and neurological dysfunction.

Some conclusions based on this survey of relevant literature will help answer the questions posed earlier in this chapter. A significant amount of evidence appears to document the following conclusions:

1. Intervertebral subluxations may cause foraminal encroachment throughout the spine, especially in the thoracic and lumbar areas (9–18, 38, 39, 46, 47, 49).
2. It is unlikely that neural involvement would occur with thoracic foraminal encroachment (9, 10, 17, 42, 43).
3. It appears probable that some type of traction could expose the highly sensitive nerve roots to the compressive action of the constricted foramen, and it is possible that the roots extend to the intervertebral foramen in some cases (17, 37–40, 49).
4. In many instances, the nerve roots combine to form the spinal nerve before they enter the foramen; the spinal nerve is not very susceptible to compression block but is relatively susceptible to block or derangement of axoplasmic transport (31, 34, 35, 55, 56).
5. Nerves affected by foraminal encroachment may undergo degenerative and regenerative processes that impair their function while compressed and until complete regeneration occurs (Table 11.1) (19–22, 25–41, 45–47).

A study by Wall et al. (73) confirmed that local pressure applied to the dorsal nerve

Table 11.1.
Pathophysiology of Various Types of Nerve Compression

Types of Compression	Electrophysiology	Pathophysiology
Mild, brief (37, 76, 80 54, 59, 60)	Decreased compound action potential, immediate recovery; with increasing pressures recovery is incomplete	Demyelination; edema and hemorrhage in the endoneurial space of the DRG; more pronounced edema after rapid onset of compression
Mild, chronic (62)	Velocity decreased, facilitation of refractory recovery	Edema
Moderate (31, 34, 77)	Conduction block, recovery takes several weeks	Demyelination
Slow, progressive, chronic (29, 33, 60)	Conduction block occurs after 2 hrs at 50 mm Hg, and after 2 min at 200 mm Hg	Demyelination; edema formation less pronounced
Severe, transient (19, 77)		Proximal edema with fiber disarray; distally, wallerian degeneration
Severe, chronic (78–79)		Edema; nerves escape perineurium to develop new pathways and/or to remyelinate

roots may result in injury discharge lasting up to 18 seconds before conduction block. The many and varied clinical phenomena that have been associated with nerve root involvement are reviewed in this chapter under "Clinical Considerations." Although the data show the distinct possibility that nerve root compression or irritation may result from certain intervertebral subluxations, they do not prove that this relationship is a common clinical occurrence.

Finally, we should not forget the myriad of other potential confounding factors that may predispose nerve roots to inflammatory and degenerative changes in some persons, such as ligamentous entrapment by the mamilloaccessory and other lumbosacral ligaments (74,75). In 11% of 51 geriatric-age cadavers, ligaments extending from the transverse process and body of L5 to the ala (97%) or promontory (3%) of the sacrum were observed to be compressing the anterior primary rami of the fifth lumbar spinal nerve (74). This information is especially important to the clinician because extraforaminal compression of this type would not be revealed by normal imaging procedures (myelogram, discogram, CT).

Summary

Palmer (1) proposed the first *nerve compression* hypothesis when he stated that intervertebral subluxations can interfere with the normal transmission of nerve energy. *Subluxation pathophysiology* includes various stages of degenerative and regenerative processes that impair the function of the involved nerve roots, as well as clinical signs and symptoms of intermittent claudication, leg weakness, sensory changes, limitation of mobility of the involved joint, paravertebral muscle spasm, scoliosis, and depressed or absent reflexes in the area of cutaneous innervation (9–22, 25–43, 45–49, 57). Although there is a definite possibility that nerve root compression or irritation may be caused by intervertebral subluxations, especially in the cervical and the lumbar spine, it has not been proven that this relationship is a common clinical occurrence (9–18, 38, 42, 43, 46-49). Moreover, modern neurophysiological investigations suggest that biological events including ischemia and edema are at least as important to the pathophysiology of spinal nerve dysfunction as are mechanical factors such as discal hernia or intervertebral subluxation (53–63). It is perhaps most likely that intervertebral subluxation predisposes one to both discal hernia and aging as well as to trauma or posture-induced ischemia that causes pain. However, long-term controlled epidemiological studies will be necessary to validate or reject this hypothesis (9,10,39–43,53–63).

REFERENCES

1. Palmer DD. The science, art and philosophy of chiropractic. Portland, Ore.: Portland Printing House, 1910.

2. Haldeman S, Drum D. The compression subluxation. J Clin Chiropractic (archive ed) 1971;1:10–21.

3. Hviid H. A consideration of contemporary chiropractic theory. J Natl Chiropractic Assoc 1955;25:17–18, 68.

4. Janse J. Basic concepts of chiropractic theory. In: Janse J, ed. Principles and practice of chiropractic. Lombard, Ill.,: National College of Chiropractic, 1976:43–50.

5. Crelin ES. Chiropractic. In: Stalker D, Glymour C, eds. Examining holistic medicine. Buffalo: Prometheus Books, 1989:197–220.

6. Schreiber T. Chiropractic—founded on tone. J Natl Chiropractic Assoc 1949;19:15–16.

7. Botta JR, ed. Chiropractors healers or quacks? Part 1: the 80-year war with science. Consumer Reports 1975;40:542–547.

8. Crelin ES. A scientific test of the chiropractic theory. Am Sci 1973;61:574–580.

9. Hadley LA. Anatomico-roentgenographic studies of the spine. Springfield, Ill.: Charles C Thomas, 1964:172–183 and 477.

10. Hadley LA. Intervertebral joint subluxation, bony impingement and foramen encroachment with nerve root changes. Am J Roentgenol Rad Ther 1951;65:377–402.

11. Braakman R, Penning L. Injuries to the cervical spine. In: Vinken PJ, Bruyn GW, eds. Handbook of clinical neurology. Injuries to the spinal cord part 1. New York: Elsevier, 1976;25:341–345.

12. Epstein JA, Epstein BS, Lavine LS, Carras R, Rosenthal AD, Sumner P. Sciatica caused by nerve root entrapment in the lateral recess: the superior facet syndrome. J Neurosurg 1972;36:584–589.

13. Grogono BJS. Injuries of the atlas and axis. Br J Bone Joint Surg 1954;36:397–410.

14. Chesterman JT. Spontaneous subluxation of the atlantoaxial joint. Lancet 1936;1:539.

15. Schlessinger PT. Incarceration of the 1st sacral nerve in a lateral bony recess of the spinal canal as a cause of sciatica: anatomy—two case reports. J Bone Joint Surg 1955;37A:115-124.

16. Sullivan AW. Subluxation of the atlanto-axial joint. J Pediatr 1949;35:451–464.

17. Sunderland S. Anatomical perivertebral influences on the intervertebral foramen. In: Goldstein M, ed. The research status of spinal manipulative therapy. Washington, D.C.: Government Printing Office, 1975:129–140.

18. Kovacs A. Subluxation and deformation of the cervical apophyseal joints. Acta Radiol 1955;43:1–15.

19. Lindblom K. Protrusions of discs and nerve compression in the lumbar region. Acta Radiol 1944;25:195–212.

20. Schaumburg HH, Spencer PS. Pathology of spinal root compression. In: Goldstein M, ed. The research status of spinal manipulative therapy. Washington, D.C.: Government Printing Office, 1975:141–148.

21. Von Reis G. Pain in the distribution area of the 4th lumbar root. Acta Psychiatr Neurol 1945;36[suppl]:1–135.

22. Frykholm R. Cervical nerve root compression resulting from disc degeneration and root-sleeve fibrosis. Acta Chir Scand [suppl] 1951;160:1–149.

23. DeBoer KF, McKnight ME. Surgical model of a chronic subluxation in rabbits. J Manipulative Physiol Ther 1988;11:366–372.

24. Lin H-L, Fujii A, Rebechini-Zasadny H, Hartz DL. Experimental induction of vertebral subluxation in laboratory animals. J Manipulative Physiol Ther 1978;1:63–66.

25. Luttges MW, Kelly PT, Gerren RA. Degenerative changes in mouse sciatic nerves: electrophoretic and electrophysiologic characterizations. Exp Neurol 1976;50:706–733.

26. Kelly PT, Luttges MW. Electrophoretic separation of nervous system proteins on exponential gradient polyacrylamide gels. J Neurochem 1975;24:1077–1079.

27. MacGregor RJ, Sharpless SK, Luttges MW. A pressure vessel model for nerve compression. J Neurol Sci 1975;24:299–304.

28. Luttges MW, Groswald DE. Degenerative and regenerative characterizations in the proteins of mouse sciatic nerves. In: Suh CH, ed. Proceedings of the 7th Annual Biomechanics Conference on the Spine. Boulder: University of Colorado, 1976:71–81.

29. Duncan D. Alterations in the structure of nerves caused by restricting their growth with ligatures. J Neuropathol Exp Neurol 1948;7:261–273.

30. Lindblom K, Rexed B. Spinal nerve injury in dorsolateral protrusions of lumbar discs. J Neurosurg 1948;5:413–432.

31. Denny-Brown D, Brenner C. Paralysis of nerve induced by direct pressure and by tourniquet. Arch Neurol Psychiatry 1944;51:1–26.

32. Dyck PJ. Experimental hypertrophic neuropathy. Arch Neurol 1969;21:73–95.

33. Aguayo A, Nair CPV, Midgley R. Experimental progressive compression neuropathy in the rabbit. Arch Neurol 1971;24:358–364.

34. Fowler TJ, Danta G, Gilliatt RW. Recovery of nerve conduction after a pneumatic tourniquet: observations on the hind-limb of the baboon. J Neurol Neurosurg Psychiatry 1972;35:638–647.

35. Rainer GW, Mayer J, Sadler TR, Dirks D. Effect of graded compression on nerve conduction velocity. Arch Surg 1973;107:719–721.

36. Gelfan S, Tarlov IM. Physiology of spinal cord, nerve root and peripheral nerve compression. Am J Physiol 1956;185:217–229.

37. Sharpless SK. Susceptibility of spinal roots to compression block. In: Goldstein M, ed. The research status of spinal manipulative therapy. Washington, D.C.: Government Printing Office, 1975:155–161.

38. Sunderland S. Mechanisms of cervical nerve root avulsion in injuries of the neck and shoulder. J Neurosurg 1974;41:705–714.

39. Sunderland S, Bradley KC. Stress-strain phenomena in human spinal nerve roots. Brain 1961;84:120–124.

40. Sunderland S. The anatomy of the intervertebral foramen and the mechanisms of compression and stretch of nerve roots. In: Haldeman S, ed. Modern developments in the principles and practice in chiropractic. New York: Appleton-Century-Crofts, 1980:45–64.

41. Breig A, Marions O. Biomechanics of the lumbosacral nerve roots. Acta Radiol 1962;1:1141–1160.

42. Hadley LA. Constriction of the intervertebral foramen. JAMA 1949;140:473–476.

43. Hadley LA. Roentgenographic studies of the cervical spine. Am J Roentgenol 1944;52:173–195.

44. Rosomoff HL, Rossman F. Treatment of cervical spondylosis by anterior cervical diskectomy and fusion. Arch Neurol 1966;14:392.

45. Eaton LM. Pain caused by disease involving the sensory roots (root pain). JAMA 1941;177:1435–1439.

46. Epstein JA, Epstein BS, Lavine LS, Carras R, Rosenthal AD, Sumner P. Sciatica caused by nerve root entrapment in the lateral recess: the superior facet syndrome. J Neurosurg 1972;36:584–589.

47. Epstein JA, Epstein BS, Lavine LS, Carras R, Rosenthal AD, Sumner P. Lumbar nerve root compression at the intervertebral foramina caused by arthritis of the posterior facets. J Neurosurg 1973;39:362–369.

48. Triano J, Luttges MW. Subtle, intermittent mechanical irritation of sciatic nerves of mice. In: Suh CH, ed. Proceedings of the 9th Annual Biomechanics Conference on the Spine. Boulder: University of Colorado, 1978.

49. Sunderland S. Meningeal-neural relations in the intervertebral foramen. J Neurosurg 1974;40:756–763.

50. Nachemson A. Editorial comment: lumbar discography—where are we today? Spine 1989;14:555–557.

51. Quon JA, Cassidy JD, O'Connor SM, Kirkaldy-Willis WH. Lumbar intervertebral disc herniation: treatment by rotational manipulation. J Manipulative Physiol Ther 1989;12:220–227.

52. Phillips RB. Plain film radiology in chiropractic. J Manipulative Physiol Ther 1992;1:47–50.

53. Hoyland JA, Freemont AJ, Jayson MIV. Intervertebral foramen venous obstruction: a cause of periradicular fibrosis? Spine 1989; 14:558–568.

54. Rydevik BL, Myers RR, Powell HC. Pressure increase in the dorsal root ganglion following mechanical compression. Spine 1989;14: 574–576.

55. Low PA, Lagerlund TD, McManis PG. Nerve blood flow and oxygen delivery in normal, diabetic, and ischemic neuropathy. Int Rev Neurobiol 1989;31:355–348.

56. Christiansen JA, Meyer JJ. Altered metabolic enzyme activities in fast and slow twitch muscles due to induced sciatic neuropathy in the rat. J Manipulative Physiol Ther 1987;10:227–231.

57. Frykholm R. Deformities of dural pouches and strictures of dural sheaths in the cervical region producing nerve-root compression. J Neurosurg 1947;4:403–413.

58. Young S, Sharpless SK. Mechanisms protecting nerve against compression block. In: Suh CH, ed. Proceedings of the 9th Annual Biomechanics Conference on the Spine. Boulder: University of Colorado, 1978.

59. Rydevik BL, Pedowitz RA, Hargens AR, Swenson MR, Myers RR, Garvin SR. Effects of acute, graded compression on spinal nerve root function and structure. Spine 1991;16:487–493.

60. Olmarker K, Rydevik B, Holm S. Edema formation in spinal nerve roots induced by experimental, graded compression: an experimental study on the pig cauda equina with special reference to differences in effects between rapid and slow onset of compression. Spine 1989;14:569–573.

61. Olmarker K, Holm S, Rosenqvist A-L, Rydevik B. Experimental nerve root compression: a model of acute, graded compression of the porcine cauda equina and an analysis of neural and vascular anatomy. Spine 1991;16: 61–69.

62. Triano JJ, Luttges MW. Nerve irritation: a possible model of sciatic neuritis. Spine 1982;7:129–136.

63. Luttges MW, Gerren RA. Compression physiology: nerves and roots. In: Haldeman S, ed. Modern developments in the principles and practice of chiropractic. New York: Appleton-Century-Crofts, 1980:65–92.

64. Hensyl WR, ed. Stedman's medical dictionary. Baltimore: Williams & Wilkins, 1990: 844.

65. Guyton AC. Textbook of medical physiology. Philadelphia: WB Saunders, 1991:60.

66. Watkins RJ. Slipped disc? sprain? or syndrome? Dig Chiropractic Econ 1975;17: 20–23.

67. Triano JJ. The use of instrumentation and laboratory examination procedures by the chiropractor. In: Haldeman S, ed. Modern developments in the principles and practice of chiropractic. New York: Appleton-Century-Crofts, 1980:231-268.

68. Owen JH, Padberg AM, Spahr-Holland L, Bridwell KH, Keppler L, Steffee AD. Clinical correlation between degenerative spine disease and dermatomal somatosensory-evoked potentials in humans. Spine 1991;16: S201–205.

69. Haldeman S, Chapman-Smith D, Peterson DM Jr, eds. Guidelines for chiropractic quality assurance and practice parameters. Proceedings of the Mercy Center consensus conference. Gaithersburg, Md.: Aspen, 1993: 47,134–135.

70. Shekelle PG, Adams AH, Chassin MR, et al. The appropriateness of spinal manipulation for low-back pain. Indications and ratings by a multidisciplinary expert panel. Santa Monica, Calif.: RAND, 1991.

71. Haldeman S, Rubinstein SM. Cauda equina syndrome in patients undergoing manipulation of the lumbar spine. Spine 1992;17: 1469–1473.

72. Woo CC. Postmyelographic cauda equina syndrome in an asymptomatic acquired spinal stenosis of a young acromegalic. J Manipulative Physiol Ther 1988;11:118–123.

73. Wall PD, Waxman S, Basbaum AL. Ongoing activity in peripheral nerve: injury discharge. Exp Neurol 1974;45:576–589.

74. Olsewski JM, Simmons EH, Kallen FC, Mendel FC. Evidence from cadavers suggestive of entrapment of fifth lumbar spinal nerves by lumbosacral ligaments. Spine 1991;16:336-347.

75. Giles LGF. The relationship between the medial branch of the lumbar posterior ramus and the mamillo-accessory ligament. J Manipulative Physiol Ther 1991;14:189–192.

76. Gilliatt RW. The cause of nerve damage in acute compression. Trans Am Neurol Assn 1974;99:71–74.

77. Spinner M, Spencer PS. Nerve compression lesions of the upper extremity. Clin Orthop 1974;104:46–67.

78. Weiss P, Hiscoe HB. Experiments on the mechanism of nerve growth. J Exp Zool 1948;107:315–395.

79. Sunderland S. The effect of rupture of the perineurium on the contained nerve fibres. Brain 1940;69:149–152.

80. Pedowitz RA, Garfin SR, Massie JB, et al. Effects of magnitude and duration of compression on spinal nerve root conduction. Spine 1992;17:194–199.

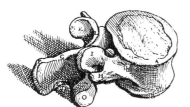

Chapter 12

Compressive Myelopathy Hypothesis

Compressive myelopathy was suggested in the hypothesis first forwarded by B. J. Palmer, who originated the *Hole-In-One technique* (HIO) after years of clinical research (1):

> Spinal cord is an accumulation and assembling of all efferent and afferent fibers that go to or come from all the body. As they gather, they more nearly, in ratio, fill neural canal . . . These facts, plus absence of osseous locking of vertebral motion, make constricted pressure a reality and of paramount and vital importance.

Compressive myelopathy refers to destruction of spinal cord tissue typically caused by pressure from neoplasms, hematomas, and other masses (2). Of course the "developer of chiropractic" (see Chapter 4) had another etiology in mind. He believed that of all the spinal bones, the occipito-atlantal-axial relationship was most important (1). Misalignments here— according to Palmer—could affect any and all functions of the body because of direct compression of the spinal cord, or what we now term compressive myelopathy (1). These "subluxations" were identified by positive radiographic findings (misalignments identified on upper cervical x-ray views) and positive thermographic findings (an abrupt change in skin tempera-

ture detected by an instrument with thermocouples carefully pushed along the spine (1).

Today, the chiropractic scientific literature has given relatively little attention to the pathophysiology of compressive myelopathy as it relates to spinal lesions (a search of the *Index to Chiropractic Literature* for the years 1985–1990 found only one original paper). Haldeman (3), in a comprehensive review of the compression subluxation, did not mention the possibility of this arthrosis adversely affecting spinal cord function by direct compression. Moreover, the medical literature has commonly reported that fracture/dislocation of vertebrae may result in compressive myelopathy; the possibility that severe subluxations could do the same, however, at times has been ignored (4, 5).

Nevertheless, since Palmer's original observations, a number of medical authors (7–20) have recognized that marked subluxations may play a role in compression and displacement of the spinal cord. These investigators have documented case after case in which severe subluxations may (even in the absence of a complicating fracture) cause paresthesias, numbness, transient paraplegia, quadriplegia, and even death. The fascinating and serious finding that crib death, or sudden infant death syndrome (SIDS), may be the result of birth trauma and subsequent brainstem involvement after cervical subluxation is reviewed (21–26), and a recent blinded chiropractic investigation of upper cervical radiographic findings in SIDS cases is discussed (44).

In light of these findings, we will define the *compressive myelopathy* hypothesis: intervertebral subluxation may, in some severe cases (and even in the absence of fracture/dislocation), irritate, compress, or destroy the spinal cord. This hypothesis raises several important questions. Is the lesion that Palmer described really analogous to the medical lesion termed *intervertebral subluxation?* For Palmer's hypothesis to be valid, the x-ray and thermographic analytic techniques he used must stand up to current standards of inter- and intraexaminer reliability, or conclusions drawn from their use are rendered worthless. Have issues of reliability and discriminability been addressed or resolved? Despite widespread continued use of Palmer's hypothesis and technique among adherents today (a national association of upper cervical chiropractic specialists is attempting to refine his technique; viz., National Upper Cervical Chiropractic Research Association [NUCCRA], Monroe, Michigan), few controlled studies have been published in peer-reviewed journals in support of the method; however, at least one initial study was promising (some studies of inter- and intraexaminer reliability of upper cervical x-ray marking systems were presented in Chapter 10).

Still another chiropractic technique system focuses on the entire cerebrospinal fluid (CSF) system from the cranium to the sacrum, and is termed *Sacro-Occipital technique* (SOT). We will briefly explore the relationship between fluid dynamics in the neural canal and cranial vault, and how they may interact with the axial skeleton; these concepts underscore the hypotheses that SOT and other *craniosacral* adjusting techniques are based upon. Some good research by osteopaths on this subject has been published in science journals, but little research is available from referreed journals regarding clinical applications of this data, including diagnosis and treatment. What is available will be discussed in this chapter (64–72). There is plausible evidence indicating effectiveness of these techniques in some studies. However, our questions about inter- and intraexaminer reliability of the diagnostic protocols underpinning these procedures again must be addressed. We discuss these considerations later in this chapter.

In addition to subluxations and fracture/dislocations, spondylosis is recognized as a common cause of compressive or ischemia-induced myelopathy when those events occur (27–30) and is reviewed in this chapter. Other causes of compressive myelopathy including tumors are briefly discussed in this chapter as well, along with pertinent experimental studies (31–37).

Subluxations and Compressive Myelopathy

Various authors (6–15) have reported that severe trauma may cause marked subluxations that compress or otherwise adversely affect the spinal cord. Subluxations associated with arthritides have also been reported to produce brainstem compression (16–20, 38). Lax ligamentous structure has been cited by at least one author as a cause of subluxation that compresses spinal cord structure (8). Nearly all of these cases occur when the articular facets are clearly not overriding (which would be a luxation according to most authors) and there is no evidence of fracture.

In 1911, Ely (11) reported a case in which the atlas was subluxated forward, following a 9-foot fall down an elevator shaft. Aside from a cut on the skull, which was dressed, a persistent headache was the only subjective complaint for the next 4 weeks. Shortly thereafter, numbness, tingling, and marked sweating heralded the onset of gradual paralysis of all four extremities, and the patient was admitted to a nearby hospital. On examination, the rectus lateralis and right and left recti postici obliqui superior and inferior muscles were reported to be rigid. Cranial nerve testing was essentially negative. Knee jerks were greatly exaggerated, however, and a positive right Babinski sign and ankle clonus indicated neurological dysfunction. At this time, an atlas-axis subluxation was identified on a "skiagram" (x-ray). An exasperating course of treatment followed in which plaster cervical collars were repeatedly applied and removed over a period of months. Each time a collar was applied, the objective and subjective findings (including paralysis) were relieved and remissions ensued. Each time a collar was removed, however, the paralysis returned, to the dismay of patient and doctors alike. Finally, the doctors operated, tying the posterior arches of atlas and axis together, while an anesthesiologist attempted to reduce the subluxation with manipulation, *through the mouth*! Nearly complete paralysis of the limbs, bladder, and rectum immediately followed the operation, but within 3 months, the patient was walking again. Six months after the operation, the patient had recovered fully from the subluxation. (Without being too facetious, we cannot help but quote one of the doctors involved, who summarized the course of treatment by saying, "It is a great case.") This was perhaps the first radiographically and operatively documented case of subluxation causing spinal cord compression.

A host of modern neurosurgeons, orthopedists, and radiologists have documented the role subluxation may play in cord compression. Braakman and Penning (7) have identified anterior atlas subluxations as a cause of spinal cord lesions. Guttmann (12) states that spinal cord compression occurs more commonly following subluxation of the cervical spine than of the thoracolumbar spine. Jackson (14), Seletz (19), and Brodsky (9) have recognized the possibility of cord or cauda equina compression following subluxation.

Eismont, Arena, and Green (6) reported a bilateral facet dislocation at C6 and C7 after a 33-year-old woman fell and struck her occiput. She had pain in her neck, paresthesias in the left arm to fingers, a positive Lhermitte sign in both upper and lower extremities,

and motor weakness (4+ of 5) of the left triceps. Otherwise, she was neurologically intact and had no up-going toes (viz., negative Babinski). Fifty pounds of traction with skull tongs was unsuccessful after 36 hours; imaging other than x-ray was not done because the authors thought the pain was due to the dislocations. Open surgical reduction, wiring, and arthrodesis was accomplished by a posterior approach; however, motor and sensory function below the C6 level was absent immediately after the procedure. An emergency myelogram revealed a large extruded disc behind the body of the C6 vertebra; during subsequent surgery, the fragment extruded from the spinal canal was larger than what remained between the vertebrae. Unfortunately, she never regained neurological function and remained quadriplegic during 5 years of follow-up. These clinicians presented five additional cases: a 32-year-old man with severe neck pain after a motor vehicle accident, a 19-year-old college linebacker paralyzed after a tackle, a 65-year-old woman who fell and struck her head at home after fainting, a 32-year-old man with severe neck pain after a motor vehicle accident, and a 15-year-old high school football player quadriplegic after a tackle. A few regained some or all neurological function after surgery; others did not, and the 15-year-old football player died 19 days after the game, of ascending necrosis of the cord with involvement of the cord, medulla, and lower brainstem. All had one clinical finding in common: marked herniation of a cervical disc that in some cases was forced further into the spinal canal upon reduction of facet dislocation or subluxation. The authors recommend that magnetic resonance imaging (MRI) be used for any patient with increasing symptoms or any neurological deficit after injury, especially during attempted reduction of the subluxation or dislocation.

Brain (8) acknowledged that the transverse ligament may become lax, which allows forward atlas subluxation and, with forward flexion of the neck, results in brainstem compression (39).

Following certain accidents, a transient paraplegia (intermittent) and the onset of neurological signs may be delayed from days to as long as 40 years (9, 14). Hughes (13) acknowledged both operative and postmortem demonstration of subluxations as a cause of spinal cord lesions. He suggested that immediately following a traumatic accident, there may not appear to be any gross abnormality of the spine. Instead, he proposed, a large number of fibers are affected but only to a minor degree (most are recoverable). Jacobson and Adler (15) reported a case that is in accord with this description. Following an accident, their patient reported loss of sensation in both legs and difficulty in moving all four extremities. Radiologic examination revealed rotational subluxation with probable upper cervical cord compression. An anteroposterior film revealed a 3.5-mm offset of the left articular mass of the atlas. Yet within days, the neurological and subjective findings disappeared. Although there was no delay in onset of neurological and subjective findings, there was indication that a large number of fibers were slightly affected.

Wollin and Botterell (20) have found neurological signs indicating spinal cord involvement in many of their patients with forward dislocations of the atlas on the axis.

However, there is a difference of opinion about the relative frequency of the subluxation and/or cord lesion. Although some authors have implied or suggested that subluxation and/or cord lesion is a relatively common cause of compressive myelopathy (10, 12, 13, 16–18), others believe it to be rare (19, 39).

One of the syndromes more commonly associated with subluxation and brainstem compression involves the various arthritides. A number of investigators (10, 16–18) have clearly linked subluxations to arthritides, but it is commonly accepted that the arthritides cause the subluxations. Subsequent spinal cord involvement has been reported by Davidson et al. (10), Rana et al. (16), Matthews (17), and Robinson (18). Rana et al. (16) found atlas-axis subluxation with

translocation of the odontoid upward into the medulla oblongata in fully 25% of their patients with rheumatoid arthritis. The extent of neurological involvement did not correspond to the degree of subluxation. They noted objective CNS signs and a subsequent narrowing of the spinal canal to 13–52% of its normal size in 27 of 41 patients with subluxations. Matthews (17) identified subluxations in 7% of his rheumatoid outpatients. Davidson et al. (10) reported on atlas-axis subluxation causing dysphagia and other neurological indications in a woman with rheumatoid arthritis; the subluxation was causing brainstem compression. Robinson (18) suggested that atlas-axis subluxation with subsequent spinal cord compression can lead to development of not only various neurological signs but also quadriplegia and even sudden death. He noted occipital headaches, paresthesias, and objective signs of compressive myelopathy with sensory and/or pyramidal signs in 14 of 22 patients with atlas-axis subluxation and rheumatoid arthritis. Latchaw and Mayer (38) suggested that subluxation may also occur frequently in Reiter's disease (arthritis, nongonococcal urethritis, and conjunctivitis).

Thus, subluxations have been implicated in a wide variety of cases as the direct and indirect cause of compressive myelopathy (7–18, 38, 39).

Cervical Subluxation with Myelopathy Associated with Sudden Infant Death

Sudden infant death syndrome (SIDS) has long been an enigma in pediatric practice. Although current mechanisms and hypotheses suggest that sleep apnea involving chronic or recurring hypoxia is the most likely cause of the great majority of cases of SIDS, a number of other hypotheses have been tested and may be applicable (24–26). The mechanism for sleep apnea is under study and may involve predisposing chemical and anatomical factors; several recognized researchers, however, have identified normal and traumatic birthing as a cause of cervical subluxation with a resultant myelopathy as the underlying cause of a significant number of SIDS cases (21–23).

TRAUMATIC BIRTH

Alexander et al. (21) reported on a case of atlas subluxation following traumatic birth. The subluxation was complicated by fracture of the odontoid. Other than initial signs of cerebral palsy, there appeared to be no warning of imminent danger for months after the birth. Yet the infant died following nearly complete paralysis. Postmortem examination revealed that the cord at the first cervical level was one-fifth its normal size (Fig. 12.1). The authors believed that had the displacement been identified even 1 month prior to death, surgical intervention could have restored the cord to near-normal function.

Schmorl and Junghanns (22) reviewed European medical research regarding SIDS and cervical spine injury. Noting that there was increased incidence of disruption of the spine, especially with breech deliveries, the authors concluded that subarachnoid hemorrhage, hematomyelia, and cervical subluxation are frequently observed (22):

> Even very severe injuries of the spinal cord have occurred without demonstrable spinal damage. In the case of forceps deliveries, spinal cord damages are found predominantly along the cervicothoracic transition. Normal deliveries are frequently associated with injuries to the upper area of the cervical spine. Therefore, [the] possibility of distortions and subluxations of the skull articulations should be kept in mind.

In reviewing his classical work on the subject of SIDS and neonatal injury, Towbin (23) found spinal cord injury in 30 of 170 cases and varying degrees of brainstem injury in 13 of 430 cases. He cited an extensive review of the literature, which indicated that

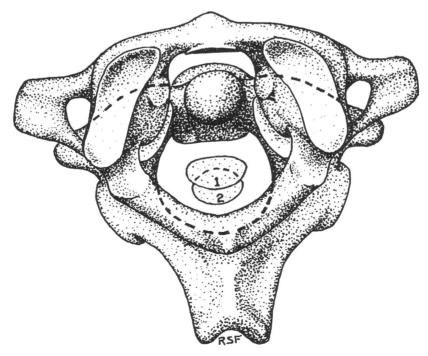

Figure 12.1. Superior view of the atlas-axis shows subluxation of the atlas anteriorly, with resultant flattening of the spinal cord (1) at the first cervical level. According to Schmorl and Junghanns (22), even normal deliveries can result in injuries to the upper area of the cervical spine of the newborn.

significant spinal cord or brainstem injury was found in 10–33% of cases of neonatal death at autopsy. In his study, prior difficulties of histological preparation of the friable newborn brainstem were overcome by using whole-brain embedding and serial histological sectioning. He grouped neonatal deaths from spinal cord or brainstem injury into three classifications: deaths occurring at or shortly after birth, caused by intolerable stress or injury to brainstem or cord structures; deaths occurring several days after birth, in patients with strong cardiac function but with respiratory depression at birth, later complicated by pneumonia or hyaline membrane disease; and deaths in infants who may live for months or years but who show initial significant reversible or persistent neurological defects as the only signs of imminent danger. He concluded that "there must exist a large number of instances with mild injury, with minimal neurological symptoms, going unnoticed clinically or being relegated to the category of cerebral palsy."

Towbin suggested that the cerebral hypoxic damage found after many brainstem and cord injuries leads to widespread neuronal devastation, especially in the forebrain; cerebral palsy, mental retardation, epilepsy, and other nervous system disorders may be the ultimate result.

SLEEP APNEA AND HYPOXIA

The role of spinal cord and brainstem injury in causing hypoxia and eventually resulting in crib death has been enhanced by modern research on SIDS. In an exhaustive review of literally hundreds of SIDS research projects worldwide, Valdes-Dapena (24) concluded that hypoventilation and altered cardiac function are significant risks for near-miss infants, since they predispose infants to sudden death. Analyzing conclusions reached by researchers of other hypotheses regarding etiology of SIDS (including prolonged Q-T interval, viral infection, botulism, postmortem vitreous humor, toxic agents, thiamine metabolism, infanticide, allergic response to house dust mites, and DPT immunizations), she found evidence that could explain only a few causes of SIDS. Considerable weight, however, was placed on the finding that tissue markers for hypoxia and hypoxemia have been identified in SIDS victims at postmortem examination. As a group, SIDS infants are morphologically different from normal infants at autopsy. Chronic hypoxia (hypoventilation) resulted in increased medial muscle mass in walls of small pulmonary arteries and in increased weight of the right cardiac ventricle; chronic hypoxemia resulted in, among other things, abnormal gliosis in the respiratory centers of the brainstem. In one study, the posterior arch of the atlas in 10 of 17 infants inverted through the foramen magnum on extension of the head, which resulted in the potential for bilateral vertebral artery compression (and brainstem hypoperfusion, which leads to SIDS).

Other researchers support a hypoxia mechanism for SIDS as well. Kahn and Blum (25) rejected the hypothesis that SIDS is the result of overheating and an abnormal thermoregulatory system. Kinney and colleagues (26) have reaffirmed the finding of brainstem gliosis after chronic hypoxemia. In five areas of the medulla oblongata which are related to involuntary respiration, significantly more reactive astrocytes were found at postmortem examination in SIDS victims than in normal infants. This supports the theory of a mechanism of SIDS that involves a sleep apnea, which is precipitated by defective control of involuntary respiration. Spinal cord injury in adults has been associated with sleep apnea because of loss of intercostal muscle function and loss of spinal muscle function (41).

Other risk factors for SIDS include low maternal age, multiparity, maternal smoking, male infants, and twins (42, 43). Maternal smoking doubled the risk of SIDS among 279,938 infants in Sweden during the first week after birth; indeed, a clear dose-response effect was seen (42). Maternal smoking also influenced the time of death; infants of smokers died at an earlier age than other SIDS babies (42).

CHIROPRACTIC IMPLICATIONS

Chiropractic investigators Schneier and Burns (44) made a blinded roentgenological evaluation of the upper cervical segments in 40 SIDS and 10 non-SIDS infants taken to the county coroner's office in Philadelphia, Pennsylvania. To follow up on the work of Gilles (45)—the first to associate atlantoaxial instability with SIDS—they and x-ray company personnel trained the assistant coroner's staff in the use of x-ray equipment, and Gilles' procedures were used. Special equipment included an infant "hugger," and the relationship of the tubestand to the bucky was constant, as they were bolted together. They made duplicate 14 × 17 films (to visualize as much of the spine as possible), with the central ray focused on the atlas; four sets included A-P, lateral, flexion, and extension views, made as soon after death as was practical. The coroner kept all records and a set of films on all infants. Blinded x-rays were sent to the investigators, marked only by number. Of 74 sets of films, only 50 met preset criteria for analysis (during neutral, flexion, and extension, certain reference points could be clearly visualized).

Results revealed no significant differences between SIDS and non-SIDS infants with regard to most measures made, except that all cases of atlas inversion occurred in SIDS cases. Moreover, the standard deviation for the SIDS data was typically more than twice that for the non-SIDS data. Indeed, the differences between variances were significant for every measure ($p = .005$ to $p = .01$) except maximum motion, where the difference was borderline ($p = .09$).

However, there was a significant ($p = 0.02$) difference between SIDS and non-SIDS infants in one of the four measures. The absolute value of atlantooccipital angle during flexion minus the atlantooccipital angle during extension (Abs DF-DE) was 7.4° in SIDS babies and 3.1° in control infants. Confounding the analysis, however, the atlas neutral angle fell outside the flexed and extended angle measurements in 84% of all the infants. This paradoxical movement prevented conclusions based upon traditional atlantoaxial movement patterns. The authors noted that while paradoxical inverse atlas tilt occurs in many clinical cases, it has not been established that the same mechanism would not continue after death. Possibly due to the lack of more control subjects, a significant relationship of atlas inversion with SIDS could not be demonstrated ($p = .19$), although it was suspected (44).

All cases where the atlas inverted into the foramen magnum were SIDS cases, supporting similar findings by Gilles and co-workers (45). Perhaps more importantly, significant variances in SIDS cases (over controls) may implicate atlantooccipital hypermobility in sudden infant death. The authors advocated follow-up investigation using a larger cohort of control infants (44).

Probably the only medical practitioner to openly advocate chiropractic manipulation as a treatment for birth trauma and postnatal damage to the occiput/atlas/axis is Gutmann (46). Since 1953 he has advocated and written in such journals as *Manuelle Medizin* about manipulative treatment of cervical-diencephalic-static syndrome (CDS). According to Gutmann (46), the clinical picture has three characteristic groups of symptoms: disturbance of motor responses (both postural-tonic and kinesiological-phasic), central disturbance of negative regulatory systems (the brainstem component), and inclination to infections in the throat, nose, and ear region.

Gutmann (46) considers children suffering pre-, con-, and postnatal primary immediate cerebral damage to be primarily at risk for SIDS. Others at risk include those suffering indirect reflexogenic brainstem disturbance during pre-, con-, or postnatal traumatization of atlantooccipital joints with persistant disturbances of relation and coordination. Typically, a disturbance in central motor responses follows suction-belljar delivery, a fall from a diaper table, or other early childhood or birth trauma. Skull and facial asymmetries, retarded mental and linguistic development, and other signs of disturbance within the reticular structure of the brainstem ensue. Subsequently, the most common clinical finding suggesting an underlying manipulable lesion is torticollis with a one-sided compulsive position and increasing asymmetry of the skull. Delayed postural development and upright position, disturbed and asymmetrical kinesiological motor response, infantile scoliosis, functional impairment of the hip joints, low- to high-grade hip dysplasia, iliosacral distortions, and so-called growing pains are associated with CDS as well. Due to its role in normal growth and maturation, other effects of brainstem involvement include overall poor thriving, loss of appetite, circulatory disturbances, indigestion, loss of equilibrium, nausea and vomiting, swift exhaustibility, restlessness to the point of psychomotor attacks, disturbance of concentration initiative, loss of ability to learn, speech disturbance, unexplained fever paroxysms, cerebral spasms, and head and upper neck aches.

The susceptibility of children with CDS to recurrent infection in the bronchi, ear, nose, and throat has been reported by Guttman (46), Lewit (47), and Mohn (48). Lewit (47) holds that among young children with chronic tonsillitis, 92% had cervical blockage, primarily at the atlantooccipital joint. (In the European literature, "blockage" generally refers to fixation during motion palpation; often the term "fixation" is used in the English manual therapy literature instead.) Often first triggered by the tonsillitis, it is felt that blockage maintains a noxious reflex that predisposes to further infection, which further maintains the blockage by reflex spasms (viz., viscerosomatic and somatovisceral reflexes; see also *Pediatric Disorders* in Chapter 9).

In case histories presented, blocked atlantoaxial joints and cervical kyphosis or atlantoaxial dislocation observed by x-ray were primary diagnostic findings. Specifically, the diagnosis is based upon (46):

1. Massive pain and avoidance during palpation of the atlantooccipital region;

2. Muscular fixation and blockage between the atlantooccipital joints (with young infants, the youngest were 4 weeks old), blockage is almost impossible to palpate, and x-ray is only diagnostic tool available);
3. X-ray to determine point of contact and direction of manual "impulse" (i.e., light fingertip thrust without audible release).

Guttman (46) states that his experiences are based on treatment of over 1000 cases, and that in one cohort of 180 adults, 21 of 45 without problems had C1 lateralization ($n = 6$) or C2 rotational ($n = 15$) blockages; 35 of 38 with "fleeting problems" had some occipital-atlantal-axial blockage, and in the remaining 97—who received manual treatment (manipulation)—blockages were found at C1 (lateralization, $n = 32$; C1 rotation, $n = 48$) and C2 ($n = 54$). By comparison, of 100 sick children with CDS, atlas lateralization was the most common blockage ($n = 88$), and all 75 infants with CDS had atlas lateralization.

Therapy, almost exclusively applied to the atlantooccipital region, consists of a "directed manual impulse application at the cross continuation of the atlas in reclining position with the head fixed in place" (46). The most gentle application, reserved for the youngest infants, is a light "tap" with the index finger, gradually repeated and "uninterrupted." The length of time for this treatment is not specified. The only complication cited is a transient crisis-like worsening in infants who present with cerebral spasms; parents and family physicians should be forewarned accordingly, according to Guttman (46). He reports excellent success with this light manual therapy in the vast majority of cases and recommends a manual treatment for diagnostic purposes when diagnostic inadequacies result in inconclusive physical findings. He performs an extensive review of medical literature in foreign-language science journals and indicates that there are other proponents of his hypothesis regarding CDS.

Unfortunately, his are uncontrolled observations, and natural remission may be expected to account for some or many of the results he attributes to the light manipulative thrust. Studies that adequately control, or at least assess, the dependent variables he describes are necessary before conclusions can be reached about his diagnostic and treatment methods. Certainly, his observations should spur interest in serious controlled chiropractic research in this important area of postnatal and infant care.

Although the role that spinal cord and brainstem injury with subluxation plays in causing the hypoxia or chronic hypoxemia that leads to crib death—or in central motor disturbances as described in the literature—is unknown, strong evidence from the literature suggests such a role in a significant number of cases (21–26). Chiropractic investigators Banks et al. (49) point out, however, that the current literature suggests that SIDS is probably due to a multiplicity of factors.

Spondylosis and Compressive Myelopathy

Spondylosis, with its degenerative and arthritic events, can lead to spinal cord compression (27–30). Several authors (27–29) have implicated osteophytic bars growing out from the ventral wall of the spinal canal as the mechanism for compression in cases of spondylosis of the cervical vertebrae. Osteoarthroses associated with trauma have been identified in the etiology of subluxated lateral facet joints by Brodsky (9).

Denno and Meadows (29) have described a new sign helpful for the early diagnosis of cervical spondylotic myelopathy. *Dynamic Hoffmann's sign* involves repeated use of Hoffman's sign (viz., with hand and wrist at rest, the terminal phalanx of the middle finger is snapped between the examiner's thumb and index finger, which extends the patient's middle finger suddenly and elicits a flexion stretch reflex) while the patient flexes and extends his neck. Normally, with a positive Hoffman's sign, the patient's thumb and index terminal phalanx

flick simultaneously in response, indicating possible corticospinal tract dysfunction. However, cervical stenosis (as assessed by cervical radiography and myelography) was indicated by a negative Hoffman's sign but a positive dynamic Hoffman's sign. The authors concluded that a positive dynamic Hoffman's sign could be used successfully for the early diagnosis of cervical spondylotic myelopathy.

Gooding (30) has provided a more elaborate mechanism that may explain cord involvement and the neurological signs that are noted. He proposes that the spondylotic degenerative events produce spinal nerve root fibrosis and that this fibrosis induces a general spasm of the lateral spinal arteries, which subsequently produces spinal cord ischemia in the cervical region. Interestingly, spondylosis is associated with subluxations in many instances by some authors (27).

Experimental Studies of Compressive Myelopathy

Studies by several researchers tend to support the Gooding (30) concept that the spinal nerves may play an important role in production of cervical cord symptoms. For instance, Hukuda and Wilson (31), in experiments on the spinal cords of dogs, determined that the effects of vascular insufficiency and mechanical compression are additive. Even a slight degree of nerve root fibrosis, when combined with osteophytic growth in the spinal canal, could produce subjective and objective findings. Tarlov and Klinger (32) found that light compression of the canine spinal cord for 15–120 minutes resulted in instantaneous sensory/motor paralysis that was completely reversible. In further studies, Gelfan and Tarlov (33) determined that dorsal column fibers were the most sensitive to mechanical compression and were the slowest to recover after the pressure was released.

More recently, Hukuda and co-workers (28) produced cervical spondylotic myelopathy in 44 mongrel dogs; spinal cord pathology was characteristically different and depended upon the type of load. The study suggested that cervical spondylotic myelopathy might progress stepwise rather than linearly when aggravating factors such as hypotension, hypertension, and occluded anterior spinal artery were combined. In this regard their findings continue to agree with Gooding's earlier hypothesis (30).

Clinical Considerations

This section briefly reviews some clinical considerations in the diagnosis of compressive myelopathy, etiologies of compressive myelopathy other than subluxation/spondylosis, and some aspects of chiropractic techniques with regard to this lesion.

DIAGNOSIS

Compressive myelopathy results in damage to the sensory and motor fiber systems of the CNS. Upper motor neuron lesions result in spastic paralysis, and lower motor neuron lesions result in flaccid paralysis. Increased deep tendon reflexes and a positive Babinski sign are noted in the former. If there is a brainstem or brain lesion, mental status and cranial nerve function may be altered. The level of the offending lesion may be determined by checking deep tendon and stretch reflexes and by observation of flaccid weakness and sensation (50).

Some chiropractic researchers and practitioners now use somatosensory evoked potentials (SSEPs), which aids in evaluating cord function (51). For example, when 18 controls and 37 patients with a cervical lesion were examined with SSEPs, abnormal N_2 (80%) and abnormal N_3 (100%) waves were observed in cervical myelopathy. However, abnormal N_2 was only seen in patients with radiculopathy, thus permitting the differential diagnosis between these two types of lesions. Moreover, preoperative and postoperative SSEPs improved proportionately with clinical symptoms (52).

Moreover, advanced imaging techniques are now increasingly available to doctors of chiropractic; hence a patient who sought the help of the author of this textbook had recently received an MRI examination of his cervical spine to rule out discal hernia (Fig. 12.2). Such tests greatly aid in the diagnosis of compressive myelopathy.

OTHER ETIOLOGIES OF COMPRESSIVE MYELOPATHY

Besides the more common causes of spinal cord compression—fracture/dislocations, discal hernia, subluxations, and osteophytes and ischemia associated with spondylosis—there are some lesser known clinical entities.

Down's Syndrome

Stein et al. (60) documented five new cases of atlantooccipital subluxation in individuals with Down's syndrome. Posterior movement of the occiput with respect to C1 occurred on extension and reduced on flexion in all but one individual who demonstrated anterior subluxation of the atlas. Only two had significant neurological problems (see also Chapter 9).

Grisel's Syndrome

Infectious processes resulting in ligamentous laxity and atlantoaxial subluxation (AAS) are referred to as *Grisel's syndrome* (see also Chapter 10). Patients generally seek treatment for progressive unrelenting throat and neck pain followed by torticollis and AAS (61). Neurological complications are less common (15% of cases) but can range from radiculopathy to myelopathy and may be fatal. The authors describe an adult who had AAS since childhood; early recognition and differential diagnosis of upper cervical instability is essential for any child complaining of upper cervical pain after an infectious process (61).

Juvenile Onset Diabetes Mellitus

In one report, spastic paraplegia appeared to have been caused by an extradural mass of lipid that was symmetrically compressing the subarachnoid space and the cord (37). Operatively, it was seen that

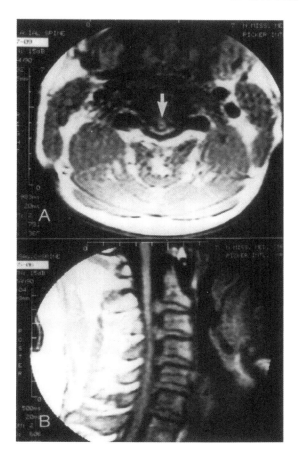

Figure 12.2. A & B. Magnetic resonance imaging of the patient who presented to the author's practice. **A**, A moderately large central herniation of the C3–C4 disc appears to indent the thecal sac (*arrow* points to hernia). **B**, Bulging appears at other levels as well. Clinically, numbness and weakness of the hands bilaterally had not responded satisfactorily to physical therapy prior to presentation, nor to a subsequent trial of chiropractic, although light chiropractic diversified adjustments and in-home use of cryotherapy did resolve most of the patient's neck pains. His progress remained unchanged over the next years after dismissal, and he declined neurosurgery before and after chiropractic.

the cord compression was due instead to dural constriction that had completely obliterated the subarachnoid space and shut off the flow of CSF. This lesion was associated with the juvenile onset of diabetes mellitus, according to the authors (37).

Mucopolysaccharidosis Type VII

Mucopolysaccharidosis type VII (MPS VII) was associated with AAS in a 15-year-old boy who first had difficulty with walking by age 12 (62). By age 14 he was wheelchair-dependent, with severe bilateral dysplastic changes of the femoral head and acetabulum. Lateral spine films revealed vertebra plana throughout, with central beaking. The neurological compromise was associated with displacement of the odontoid forward on the body of the axis through a defect at its base. Despite posterior spinal fusion from occiput to C3, with stabilization by a halo cast, and initial

improvement in neurological findings, he died 3 months postsurgery. The authors strongly urge upper cervical assessment of all patients with this disease (62).

Os Odontoideum

Pediatric AAS (an atlantodental interval (ADI) of 10 mm during flexion and extension) has been associated with cerebral and cerebellar infarcts and angiographically documented stenosis of the vertebral arteries (58).

Reiter's Syndrome

From 1978 to 1988, only 6 cases of AAS were associated with the arthritis, conjunctivitis, and urethritis that form the triad known as *Reiter's syndrome* (63). AAS has been detected as early as one year and as late as 11 years after the initial diagnosis of Reiter's syndrome has been made. The authors recommend a cervical flexion/

extension x-ray series to assess the ADI in all cases of Reiter's syndrome with cervical symptoms.

Rheumatoid Arthritis

Development of widespread rheumatoid arthritis has been associated with atlantoaxial subluxation (AAS) by a number of authors (35, 36, 53–57). Using regression analysis to ascertain risk factors for development of AAS in 145 cases of rheumatoid arthritis, researchers determined that a high joint score index (viz., summing the number of certain affected joints such as the hips, knees, elbows, wrists, and metacarpophalangeal and proximal interphalangeal joints) and a low blood hemoglobin level were independent risk factors (35). Hence, development of AAS is associated with widespread rheumatoid arthritis. The regression model showed that erosions of the dens, ulnar deviations, and length of hydroxychloroquine treatment predicted AAS development (35). Glew et al. (36), in agreement with these findings, reported erosion of the dens only in patients with rheumatoid arthritis (65% of 26 rheumatoid patients). Compression myelopathy in rheumatoid arthritis associated with 8 mm AAS can result in sudden death; myocardial infarction (MI) associated with upper cervical cord lesion was initiated while a patient received Advanced Cardiac Life Support (ACLS) (53). The extreme instability of the atlantoaxial joint was underscored in this case by the fact that hyperextending the patient's neck during intubation caused MI (53). Normally, 8 mm AAS would not interfere with usual household activity, but subjected to the stresses involved in intubation, the instability proved fatal (53).

Kawaida et al. (54) used plain x-ray films to predict compressive myelopathy in 55 cases of rheumatoid arthritis. AAS was considered to be anteriorly subluxated when the ADI was greater than 3 mm in flexion, neutral, and extension cervical lateral films. The space available for the spinal cord (SAC) was also determined in each position. MRI examination showed compressive myelopathy in 7 of the 18 patients, including all those with an ADI greater than 8 mm (a retrodental pannus caused myelopathy in another case with an ADI of only 4 mm and an SAC of 16 mm). The most frequent clinical symptom was pain of the occipital and neck regions, limited motion of the neck, crepitus, and torticollis; sphincter disturbance was present in four, three reported episodes of transient loss of consciousness, and none had nystagmus or cerebral nerve palsy. The diagnosis of myelopathy could not always be made neurologically because of longstanding arthralgias and advanced articular extremity lesions associated with advanced rheumatoid arthritis, which make muscle strength and tendon reflexes difficult to test.

Halla and Hardin (55) evaluated 650 patients with rheumatoid arthritis in a 7-year period and determined that 9% ($n = 61$) had C1-C2 involvement. These patients were generally younger, female, and seropositive; they had significantly more nodules and erosions and a longer disease duration. Main findings were lateral mass collapse ($n = 28$; more likely to have myelopathy and, when severe, was associated with nonreducible rotational tilt of the patient's head), lateral facet joint sclerosis and erosion ($n = 27$), and lateral subluxation without bone or cartilage change ($n = 6$).

In a study of 250 rheumatoid patients, researchers found that indicators for surgery were intractable pain, cervical myelopathy, and severe AAS; early neurological deficit was a poor indicator for surgery in this group (56).

While the presence of rheumatoid arthritis poses risks for the chiropractic clinician with regard to the potential for AAS, it is not a contraindication to chiropractic intervention. A case report of a 51-year-old hospital-based registered nurse who sought chiropractic care underscores the potential benefit of this intervention. She had pains and tissue swelling conforming to the criteria for the classification of rheumatoid arthritis (viz., morning stiffness, soft tissue swelling, swelling of wrist joints, and presence of rheumatoid factor) that were of six months' duration. At that time she had been diagnosed as having early-onset rheumatoid arthritis. Despite excellent health and normal weight and blood pressure, she had severe migrating joint pains and had failed to respond to aspirin, Naprosyn, Tolectin, digoxin, Dolobid, Clinoril, and Plaquenil, as well as to an elimination diet prescribed by an allergist. Subsequent chiropractic intervention using Bennett technique (viz., manual stretching of long muscles, and massage or stimulation of areas of hypertonicity thought to correspond with certain internal organs; thought to affect the autonomics via vasomotor reflex action) and a diet (eliminate fried and fatty foods, soups, alcohol, dairy products except cottage cheese, raw fruits, commercial bakery products, nuts, candy, condiments, and the cabbage family of vegetables) was implemented. Within 4 weeks, hand spasms had eased; within 6 weeks, she discontinued antiinflammatory drugs. By 8 weeks, she denied pain and could go dancing. Thrice-weekly treatments sessions were reduced in frequency, and by 4 months she tolerated stress better and experienced less pain when under stress. Except for stress or a poor diet initiating minor irritation, she was discharged after 4 years of remission with the admonition to listen to her body and keep up her threshold of resistance (viz., through watching her diet, rest?) (57).

Tumors

Tumors, although rare, are obviously given attention (34–36). Boyd (34) classifies spinal cord tumors as either extramedullary or intramedullary. Extramedullary tumors, frequently benign, are of two types: extradural, which is the more severe and is commonly a metastatic carcinoma or lymphoma; and intradural, which is the more common, is usually benign, and may persist for some time before signs of cord or nerve root involvement appear. Although the cord may be severely compressed by a tumor, it still has a remarkable ability to recover (34). Operative removal of the lesion often results in positive recovery (34). In addition to tu-

mors, other lesions have been associated with compressive myelopathy.

CRANIOSACRAL RESEARCH

Nephi Cottam, a Morman chiropractor who graduated from Palmer in 1915 and practiced in Utah, may have been the first chiropractor to claim cranial bones could move and be adjusted (8; Harrington M, unpublished manuscript). His collaboration with an osteopathic pioneer in craniopathy, William Garner Sutherland (64), apparently laid the foundation for Drs. Major Bertrand DeJarnette (SOT), and George Goodheart (Applied Kinesiology), whose present-day chiropractic techniques use the concept of craniosacral adjusting. Central to DeJarnette's technique is identification of subluxation by palpation of occipital and trapezius fibers, for the detection of "nodules and fibers," which are associated with specific spinal segments and somatosomatic and somatovisceral reflexes (5; Windham SE, unpublished manuscript).

These techniques attempt to affect CSF dynamics via skeletal manipulation. For example, SOT attempts to manipulate fluid dynamics of the neural canal and vault (65). In a review of literature, Flanagan (65) points out that spinal stenosis, discopathy, space-occupying lesions, and cord injury can increase pressure in the neural canal and affect its contents. Concussion, skull fracture, stroke, tumor, hydrocephalus, hypertension, and endocrine dysfunction can increase intracranial pressure and affect contents of the vault as well (65). Chiropractic techniques attempting to manipulate this system would have to consider such potential sources of increased intracranial and intraneural pressure, which are generally beyond the help of adjustive intervention. In addition to SOT and Applied Kinesiology, other chiropractic techniques such as upper cervical specific (viz., H.I.O., B. J. Palmer's, and Grostic technique), Logan Basic technique, and others (see Chapters 4 and 10) attempt to affect cerebrospinal flow by reducing pressure at the upper cervical spine level, the sacrum, cranial vault, or elsewhere

(65). Even some techniques involving flexion-distraction of the lumbar spine purport to reduce lumbar canal pressures or otherwise rehabilitate the spine.

Unfortunately for users of these techniques, Flanagan (65) concludes that while these hypotheses are plausible, there is no scientific evidence that manipulation of the axial skeleton can affect fluid dynamics in the spinal canal and cranial vault. Even if it can, there is no scientific literature showing clinical usefulness of the techniques in the treatment of disease or dysfunction (65). He does acknowledge that axial skeletal improprieties can affect neural canal pressures without totally blocking the veins, so although the CSF pressure gradient is small, it is critical to absorption rates. If it can be established that manipulation can affect changes within this system, potentially serious conditions associated with disturbed fluid dynamics could be amenable to certain chiropractic adjustments.

In this regard, Adams and co-workers (66) executed a well-designed controlled trial with specially designed equipment to measure parietal bone mobility with reference to the medial sagittal suture in the surgically exposed skull of anesthetized adult cats. Confirming the hypotheses of both osteopathic and chiropractic theorists and rejecting commonly held notions that cranial sutures are solid and that the cranium is a rigid enclosure, they demonstrated the viscoelastic nature of suture lines in most of these animals. Their data provided direct quantitative evidence that the parietal bones in the anesthetized cat move both laterally and rotationally in reference to the medial sagittal suture that separates them on the dorsal surface of the skull. Indeed, they demonstrated that these movements can be initiated by external forces applied to the head and by internal ones associated with peripheral pulse and respiratory movements. For instance, inward forces directed on the sides of the head caused the parietal bones to move laterally closer and to rotate inwardly. This caused intracranial pressure increases and transient changes in heart rate and respiratory rate

and depth. Release of the force was accompanied by return of the bones to their nearest positions, CSF pressure lowering, and stabilization of the animal's cardiovascular and respiratory responses. In contrast, downward force applied to the sagittal suture elicited no cardiovascular or respiratory effects. Movements occur because of changes in intracranial pressure produced by induced hypercapnia and by controlled injections of artificial CSF into a lateral cerebral ventricle. Hence, bolus intravenous administration of norepinephrine transiently elevated intracranial pressure and altered cranial bone alignments. They concluded that compliance of the sutures must be considered in defining total cranial compliance (66). Such provocative findings challenge traditional concepts of rigidity of cranial sutures, and provide *hypothetical* support for the use of chiropractic and osteopathic craniosacral techniques.

In an annotated bibliography of research in the field of craniosacral adjusting, Retzlaff (67) cited well over 250 papers published in science and osteopathic journals. Most of the papers dealt with hypothetical and experimental aspects of craniosacral mechanisms, however, and few related to the reliability of diagnostic methods. Indeed, papers by Frymann (68) (techniques for clinical mensuration of mobility of the cranium), by Mitchell et al. (69) (studies of the ability of clinicians to detect small-amplitude, low-velocity movements of a plastic appliance simulating human parietal bones), and by Upledger et al. (70) (reliability and reproducibility of craniosacral examination findings of children) were the only studies addressing the reliability of craniosacral diagnostic procedures (67). Some of the work in this field appears to have serious implications, given the breadth of citations covering use of craniosacral techniques ostensibly to benefit such diverse conditions in children as learning, behavioral, and developmental disturbances as well as head injury (67). Given such enormous potential, serious research on the reliability of craniosacral technique diagnosis and analysis is warranted.

CONTRAINDICATIONS TO CHIROPRACTIC

There is evidence that with increasing neurological loss, the prognosis for remission using conservative care such as chiropractic is poorer (71). In cases of discal hernia, for example, researchers concluded for RAND that chiropractic adjustments are rarely indicated in the presence of a neurological deficit, even when adjustments for a similar episode had proved to be efficacious (72). Moreover, cauda equina has occurred after chiropractic adjustments, although rarely (73). Unfortunately, clear evidence about the predilection for such complications remains elusive, and all that we seem to know is that—given the tens of millions receiving manipulations annually—these complications are indeed rare (74).

A case of Brown-Séquard syndrome after chiropractic adjustment was attributed to the "sudden forced manipulation of the neck involved in a chiropractic 'adjustment,' superimposed on the presence of advanced cervical spondylosis" (75), which occurred on the previous day. An epidural hematoma was relieved with surgical decompression, resulting in immediate return of motor function in the right upper and lower extremities. The immediate postmanipulative period was uneventful, but the next day, the 86-year-old man suddenly could not move his right leg while driving, resulting in an automobile accident. The lack of an established causal relationship and lack of any description of the manipulative intervention or of contact with the doctor of chiropractic make such reports suspect; it is known that spinal arthritides, hypertension, and anticoagulant medication are predisposing factors to epidural hematoma (75). Despite these limitations, in the presence of such risk factors, careful adjustment or manipulation is recommended (see Chapter 13) to prevent such complications.

Although some medical researchers believe manipulation should not be accomplished in the presence of neurological signs, evidence continues to mount that discal hernia-related pain resolves with chiropractic adjustments, whether or not the hernia itself resolves (76). Cassidy, Thiel, and Kirkaldy-Willis reported that 13 of 14 patients with discal hernia presenting to a back pain clinic at the Royal University Hospital in Saskatoon, Saskatchewan, Canada, had significant improvement in clinical symptoms and neurological signs after 2–3 weeks of daily side-posture lumbar chiropractic adjustments. However, only 6 of 14 had significant reduction in hernia at follow-up CT examination 3 months later. (Pain associated with discal hernia is thought to result more from inflammation than from the hernia itself.) They conclude that patients should be reassured that significant pain relief will occur in 4 to 6 weeks, with decreased signs of dural tension at 6 weeks. Foot drop and altered sensations in the lower extremity can take several months to recover, while an absent ankle jerk will more than likely remain absent. Instead of arguing against chiropractic in patients with mild neurological signs, they claim that surgery is indicated only when severe leg pain has failed to respond to conservative measures or in the presence of cauda equina syndrome (76) (see also Chapter 9). Clearly, in the absence of definitive randomized comparative trials of chiropractic adjustments as opposed to surgery and percutaneous discectomy, we do not know which approach holds the most promise with the least risk.

Discussion

It seems most likely that a combination of factors results in spinal cord compression or insufficiency. Subluxations can affect the second cervical nerve adversely, and by the pathway described by Gooding (30), the resultant spasm of spinal arteries could, conceivably, render the cord ischemic (6, 19). This would selectively block multisynaptic responses first, according to some investigators (33). In addition, more severe subluxations—especially with upward translocation of the odontoid—have directly caused cord compression (7, 8, 10–18). Mechanical compression appears to affect the dorsal column fibers (kinesthetic sensations, fine pressure, fine touch, and vibratory sense) more quickly and for longer (longer recovery time necessary) than other fibers (33). Spondylotic events commonly occur with subluxations, and osteophytes could combine with less severe subluxations to produce mechanical cord compression in many unrecognized, subclinical cases (27–30). Even adults with low anteroposterior diameters of the spinal canal have significantly increased myelopathy after trauma (40).

Similarly, anatomical and physiological variations in the cervical spine of the neonate may predispose it to the traction and extension forces used during even normal delivery and cause subluxation, brainstem or cord damage, chronic hypoxia or hypoxemia, and crib death (21–26). However, even though chiropractic investigators Schneier and Burns (44) found inversion of the atlas in SIDS cases, most likely these cases resulted from a multiplicity of factors, not just birth trauma (49). Controlled trials of assessment and treatment protocols in chiropractic pediatrics must be completed before the anecdotal observations by Guttman (46) (regarding successes of chiropractic adjustments for infants after birth trauma) or others can be given serious weight (see also Chapter 9).

While more strictly controlled research by osteopathic investigators has established parietal bone movement—with regard to the medial sagittal suture—in the anesthetized cat as a result of inward forces applied to the cranium, this and similar research provides hypothetical support for some craniosacral adjusting techniques but not clinical empirical validation of these methods (66). Much more research is needed on reliability, reproducibility, and discriminability of craniosacral methods to fully validate their use in diagnosis and treatment (67–70).

This is true as well for upper cervical techniques. While at least one initial study favors inter- and intraexaminer reliability of one upper cervical x-ray marking technique

(see Chapter 10), a number of such techniques await even initial studies of reliability. Then the natural variance of such measures in human subjects must be addressed; even if line-marking analysis of plain film x-rays by chiropractic upper cervical technique systems is deemed to be reliable, is it reproducible over time in human subjects? Even if reliability and reproducibility are established, it will be necessary to demonstrate that chiropractic methods of adjusting improve the subsequent analyzed findings in blinded investigations and that improvement in such parameters improves some aspect of health or otherwise improves wellness (even if adjustments are not aimed at eliminating some disease or symptom).

Finally, we asked if the lesion Palmer described really was analogous to the medical lesion *intervertebral subluxation*. More than likely it was not. Generally, the mild misalignments chiropractic technique systems term subluxation are 1, 2, or 3 mm deviations; in contrast, medical radiographic criteria for atlantodental subluxation, for example, generally require >3 mm displacement before the diagnosis of atlantoaxial subluxation is made (54), and compressive myelopathy is not commonly associated with this lesion until more than 8 mm of ADI displacement occurs, probably "severe" misalignment by any chiropractic standards. Until the advent of SSEPs, brain mapping, MRI, and other imaging systems, we really did not have the tools necessary to begin to test the effects of the "milder" purported chiropractic lesions on CNS or cerebrovascular relationships. Judging by the difficulty in establishing craniosacral techniques—despite some serious efforts by some osteopathic researchers (67)—it will be some time before we know whether Palmer's hypothesis (viz., that the chiropractic type of atlantoaxial subluxation caused constriction of the spinal cord which interfered with its function and that H.I.O. adjustments could restore cord function) has any merit whatsoever.

Alternatively, upper cervical adjustment may simply stimulate a neuroendocrine or neuromuscular response that contributes to health, or it may remove upper cervical fixations or segmental dysfunction (see Section 2). Even if the *hypotheses* underpinning upper cervical and craniosacral techniques are disproved, the methods may still prove efficacious and have clinical merit. Perhaps rather than spending precious resources researching hypothetical aspects of these techniques, researchers should begin reliability and outcome assessments in clinical trials. In this way the patient will be served first, and hypothetical constructs can be argued later. In the interim, the *compressive myelopathy* hypothesis—that intervertebral subluxation may, in severe cases (and even in the absence of fracture/dislocation) irritate, compress, or destroy the spinal cord—certainly has merit (7–20, 27–37, 51–61). However, this lesion is usually associated with severe ligamentous instability secondary to severe trauma, spondylosis, infections, or other processes, and any relationship to the "milder" chiropractic subluxations identified by x-ray line-marking analyses remains to be established.

Perhaps an exception to this is found in a recent example of posttraumatic myelopathy associated with milder anterior subluxation at C4 (viz., angular deformity associated with significant cervical kyphosis) cited by Woo (77). An 11-year-old boy with early posttraumatic incomplete spastic tetraplegia below C7 presented to the chiropractor's office after steroid therapy and 3 months of nonsurgical medical treatment failed to alter his clinical condition. Originally injured after "flopping high jumps," he began to develop iatrogenic Cushing's syndrome in the course of steroid treatment. Unable to stand or walk, he had bowel and bladder dysfunction, triceps hyperreflexia, spasticity with hyperreflexia in the lower limbs, crossed reflex, and significant ankle clonus. Weakened grip and atrophy of thenar and hypothenar was observed. Spinal manipulation of the lower cervical and upper thoracic spine was performed, and cryotherapy and analgesic balm was applied for 2 weeks. Home exercises were begun immediately, and swimming was encouraged. After 2 months of in-

tensive treatment and rehabilitation he was able to walk with axillary crutches and became almost independent. By 3 months, bowel and bladder function had returned, along with motor and sensory function, yet hyperreflexia, clonus, and flexion reflex persisted. X-rays revealed reduction in C5 and T1 rotary subluxations but persistent angular deformity at C4. The patient was discharged but seen regularly for 9 years; his neurological recovery remained stable.

Certainly this case demonstrates that milder nonsurgical subluxations may result in serious neurological impairment, which can be effectively managed by a careful chiropractic apprach. More research on these milder cases of compressive myelopathy should be pursued with regard to the chiropractic treatment approach.

Other evidence presented by Radanov et al. (78), who found evidence of cervicoencephalic syndrome (headache, fatigue, dizziness, poor concentration, disturbed accommodation, and impaired adaptation to light intensity) in 51 patients after cervical trauma, suggests that functional brainstem disturbance can occur without neurological signs (see also Chapter 13). Hence, there may indeed be an entire class of milder forms of compressive myelopathy for which chiropractic care is indicated.

Anatomical and physiological variance plays an important role in the development of myelopathy. What role subluxation of the apophyseal joints may play remains to be fully explored, but it is suggested that myelopathy after subluxation may be more likely if the spine is anatomically or physiologically predisposed to such an event.

Summary

Severe subluxations have been shown to cause spinal cord compression (7, 8, 10–18, 53–62). Cervical spine injury and, specifically, subluxation have been associated with brainstem and cord injury that leads to hypoxia, hypoxemia, and crib death (SIDS), even after "normal" delivery (21–26). And while chiropractic investigators have confirmed prior research indicating atlas inversion occurs in some SIDS deaths but not in non-SIDS cases (44), it is likely that SIDS results from a multiplicity of factors and not from birth trauma alone (24–26, 41–43). This finding is consistent with the compressive myelopathy hypothesis. Spondylosis, other arthritides and syndromes, fracture/dislocations, and tumors can also cause compressive myelopathy (3–5, 27–30, 34–36, 53–62). Experimental research indicates that the effects of these lesions could be additive (28–32). Possible effects of cord compression include headache, numbness, tingling, paresthesias, quadriplegia, transient paraplegia, practically any combination of neurological findings, and even death (7, 10, 11, 13, 15, 16–19).

A number of chiropractic methods hypothetically address cerebrovascular and cranial vault fluid dynamics, collectively termed craniosacral adjustive techniques (65). In addition, upper cervical specific chiropractic adjustive techniques address purported mechanical upper cervical lesions that hypothetically interfere with brainstem and CNS function (1, 65) (see also Chapter 10).

While some clinical research is hopeful (67), the reliability, reproducibility, and discriminability of these methods remain to be performed, and some of these hypotheses involve mechanisms difficult to measure even in the most controlled environments (66, 68–70). Alternative explanations of the apparent clinical effectiveness of these procedures should not be dismissed out-of-hand by practitioners of these methods, as scientific inquiry continues to yield new knowledge. For example, if line-marking analysis of upper cervical subluxation by chiropractic methods fails to be validated as reliable or clinically useful, it may be that upper cervical techniques restore motion to fixed upper cervical joints (viz., SDF) or stimulate neuroendocrine or neuromuscular responses that contribute to wellness or health. At any rate, while the *compressive myelopathy* hypothesis as defined here is a satisfactory explanation of the effects of radiographically demonstrable (by medical criteria) subluxation, the "milder" chiropractic subluxation remains to be established as a similar model for compressive myelopathy.

REFERENCES

1. Palmer BJ. The subluxation specific—The adjustment specific. Davenport, Ia.: Palmer School of Chiropractic, 1934:205.

2. Hensyl WR, ed. Stedman's medical dictionary. 25th ed. Baltimore: Williams & Wilkins, 1990:1013.

3. Haldeman S. The compression subluxation. J Clin Chiro (arch ed) 1971;1:10–21.

4. Vick N. Grinker's neurology. 7th ed. Springfield, Ill.: Charles C Thomas, 1976.

5. Eliasson SG, et al. Neurological pathophysiology. New York: Oxford University Press, 1974.

6. Eismont FJ, Arena MJ, Green BA. Extrusion of an intervertebral disc associated with traumatic subluxation or dislocation of cervical facets. J Bone Joint Surg 1991;73-A:1555–1560.

7. Braakman R, Penning L. Injuries to the cervical spine. In: Vinken PJ, Bruyn GW, eds. Handbook of clinical neurology. Injuries to the spinal cord part 1. New York: Elsevier, 1976;25:341–345.

8. Brain R. Some aspects of the neurology of the cervical spine. J Fac Radiol Lond 1956;8: 74–91.

9. Brodsky AE. Low back pain syndromes due to spinal stenosis and posterior cauda equina compression. Bull Hosp Joint Dis 1975;36:66–79.

10. Davidson RC, Horn JR, Herndon JH, Grin OD. Brian stem compression in rheumatoid arthritis. JAMA 1977;238:2633–2634.

11. Ely LW. Subluxation of the atlas. Ann Surg 1911;54:20–29.

12. Guttman L. Conservative management. In: Vinken PJ, Bruyn GW, eds. Handbook of clinical neurology. Injuries to the spinal cord part 2. New York: Elsevier, 1976;26:289–306.

13. Hughes JT. Spinal cord trauma. In: Greenfield's neuropathology. London: Edward Arnold, 1976:665–666.

14. Jackson R. The cervical syndrome. Springfield, Ill.: Charles C Thomas, 1978.

15. Jacobson G, Adler DC. Examination of the atlanto-axial joint following injury. Am J Roentgenol 1956;76:1081–1094.

16. Rana NA, Hancock DO, Taylor AR, Hill AGS. Atlanto-axial subluxation and upward translocation of the odontoid process in rheumatoid arthritis. Am J Bone Joint Surg 1973; 55A:1304.

17. Matthews JA. Atlanto-axial subluxation in rheumatoid arthritis: a five-year follow-up study. Ann Rheum Dis 1974;33:526–531.

18. Robinson HS. Rheumatoid arthritis—atlanto-axial subluxation and its clinical presentation. Can Med Assoc J 1966;94:470–477.

19. Seletz E. Trauma and the cervical portion of the spine. J Int Coll Surg 1963;40:47–62.

20. Wollin DG, Botterell EH. Symmetrical forward luxation of the atlas. Am J Roentgenol 1958;79:575–583.

21. Alexander E, Masland R, Harris C. Anterior dislocation of first cervical vertebra simulating cerebral birth injury in infancy. Am J Dis Child 1953;85:173–181.

22. Schmorl G, Junghanns H. Human spine in health and disease. 2nd ed. New York: Grune & Stratton, 1972:272.

23. Towbin A. Latent spinal cord and brain stem injury in newborn infants. Dev Med Child Neurol 1969;11:54–68.

24. Valdes-Dapena MA. Sudden infant death syndrome: a review of the medical literature 1974–1979. Pediatrics 1980;66:597–614.

25. Kahn A, Blum D. Letter to the editor (in reply). Pediatrics 1983;71:987.

26. Kinney HC, Burger PC, Harrell FE, Hudson RP. `Reactive gliosis' in the medulla oblongata of victims of the sudden infant death syndrome. Pediatrics 1983;72:181–187.

27. Sandler B. Cervical spondylosis as a cause of spinal cord pathology. Arch Phys Med Rehabil 1961;42:650–659.

28. Hukuda S, Ogata M, Katsuura A. Experimental study on acute aggravating factors of cervical spondylotic myelopathy. Spine 1988; 13:15–20.

29. Denno JJ, Meadows GR. Early diagnosis of cervical spondylotic myelopathy: a useful clinical sign. Spine 1991;16:1353–1355.

30. Gooding MR. Pathogenesis of myelopathy in cervical spondylosis. Lancet 1974;2:1180–1181.

31. Hukuda S, Wilson CB. Experimental cervical myelopathy: effects of compression and ischemia on the canine cervical cord. J Neurosurg 1972;37:631–652.

32. Tarlov IM, Klinger H. Arch Neurol Psychiatr 1954:71:271.

33. Gelfan S, Tarlov IM. Physiology of spinal cord, nerve root and peripheral nerve compression. Am J Physiol 1956;185:217–229.

34. Boyd W. A textbook of pathology. 8th ed. Philadelphia: Lea & Febiger, 1970:1281–1282.

35. Kauppi M, Konttinen YT, Honkanen V, Sakaguchi M, Hamalainen M, Santavirta S. A multivariate analysis of risk factors for anterior atlantoaxial subluxation and an evaluation of the effect of glucocorticoid treatment on the upper rheumatoid cervical spine. Clin Rheumatol 1991;10:413–418.

36. Glew D, Watt I, Dieppe A, Goddard PR. MRI of the cervical spine: rheumatoid arthritis compared with cervical spondylosis. Clin Radiol 1991;44:71–76.

37. Heilbrun MP, Davis DO. Spastic paraplegia secondary to cord constriction by the dura. J Neurosurg 1973;39:645–647.

38. Latchaw RE, Mayer GW. Reiter disease with atlantoaxial subluxation. Radiology 1978; 126:303–304.

39. Hess JH, Bronstein IP, Abelson SM. Atlantoaxial dislocation. Am J Dis Child 1935;49: 1137–1147.

40. Epstein N, Epstein JA, Benjamin V, Ransohoff J. Traumatic myelopathy in patients with cervical spinal stenosis without fracture or dislocation; methods of diagnosis, management, and prognosis. Spine 1980;5: 489–496.

41. Star AM, Osterman AL. Sleep apnea syndrome after spinal cord injury. Spine 1988; 13:116–117.

42. Haglund B, Cnattingius S. Cigarette smoking as a risk factor for sudden infant death syndrome: a population-based study. Am J Public Health 1990;80:29–32.

43. Beal S. Sudden infant death syndrome in twins. Pediatrics 1989;84:1038–44.

44. Schneier M, Burns RE. Atlanto-occipital hypermobility in sudden infant death syndrome. Chiropractic: J Chiro Res Clin Invest 1991;7:33–38.

45. Gilles FH, Bina M, Sotrel A. Infantile atlanto-occipital instability. Am J Dis Child 1979; 133:30.

46. Gutmann G. Blocked atlantal nerve syndrome in infants and small children. ICA Int Rev Chiro 1990:37–43.

47. Lewit K. Kopfgelenkblockierungen und chronische tonsillitis. Manuelle Medizin 1976;14:106–109.

48. Mohn U. Kopfgelenkblockierungen biem keinkind (cervical-diencephal-statistches syndrom nach Gutmann). Manuelle Medizin 1977;15:45.

49. Banks BD, Beck RW, Columbus M, Gold PM, Kinsinger FS, Lalonde MA. Sudden infant death syndrome: a literature review with chiropractic implications. J Manipulative Physiol Ther 1987;10:246–252.

50. Berkow R, ed. The Merck manual. 16th ed. Rahway, N.J.: Merck & Co, 1992:1464–1465.

51. Burke E, Glick D, Grostic J, Sheres B. Interpeak latency relationships between nerves using a new evoked potential protocol for the identification of neurologic insult. Proceedings of the 1992 International Conference on Spinal Manipulation, Chicago, Ill., 1992:26.

52. Kotani H, Senzoku F, Hattori S, Moritake Z, Hara T, Omote K. Evaluation of cervical cord function using spinal evoked potentials from surface electrode. Spine 1992;17:339–344.

53. Yaszemski MJ, Shepler TR. Sudden death from cord compression associated with atlanto-axial instability in rheumatoid arthritis: a case report. Spine 1990;15:338–341.

54. Kawaida H, Sakou T, Morizono Y, Yoshikuni N. Magnetic resonance imaging of upper cervical disorders in rheumatoid arthritis. Spine 1989;14:1144–1148.

55. Halla JT, Hardin JG. The spectrum of atlantoaxial facet joint involvement in rheumatoid arthritis. Arthritis Rheum 1990;33: 325–329.

56. Floyd AS, Learmonth ID, Mody G, Meyers OL. Atlantoaxial instability and neurologic indicators in rheumatoid arthritis. Clin Orthop 1989;14:177–182.

57. Nelson WA. Rheumatoid arthritis a case report. Chiro Tech 1990;2:17–19.

58. Bhatnagar M, Sponseller PD, Carroll C, Tolo VT. Pediatric atlantoaxial instability presenting as cerebral and cerebellar infarcts. J Pediatr Orthop 1991;11:103–107.

59. Macaya A, Roig M, Gili J. Mielopatia cervical en la luxación atlantoaxoidea: evaluación de dos casos mediante resonancia nuclear magnética. Arch Neurobiol 1989;52:239–242.

60. Stein SM, Kirchner SG, Horev G, Hernanz-Shulman M. Atlanto-occipital subluxation in Down syndrome. Pediatr Radiol 1991;21: 121–124.

61. Mathern GW, Batzdorf U. Grisel's syndrome. Clin Orthop 1989;18:131–146.

62. Pizzutillo PD, Osterkamp JA, Scott CI, Lee MS. Atlantoaxial instability in mucopolysaccharidosis. J Pediatr Orthop 1989;9:76–78.

63. Kransdorf MJ, Wehrle PA, Moser RP. Atlantoaxial subluxation in Reiter's syndrome: a report of three cases and a review of the literature. Spine 1988;13:12–14.

64. Wales A. The work of William G. Sutherland, D.O. J Am Osteopath Assoc 1972;71: 788–793.

65. Flanagan MF. Relationship between CSF and fluid dynamics in the neural canal. J Manipulative Physiol Ther 1988;11:489–492.

66. Adams T, Heisey RS, Smith MC, Briner BJ. Parietal bone mobility in the anesthetized cat. J Am Osteopath Assoc 1992;92:599–622.

67. Retzlaff EW. Annotated bibliography of research in the cranial field. In: Retzlaff EW, Mitchell FC Jr, eds. The cranium and its sutures. New York: Springer Verlag, 1987: 68–89.

68. Frymann VM. A study of the rhythmic motions of the living cranium. J Am Osteopath Assoc 1971;70:1–18.

69. Mitchell FL Jr, Roppel RM, St Pierre N. Accuracy and perceptual decisional delay in motion perception. J Am Osteopath Assoc 1978;78:149.

70. Upledger JE, et al. The reproducibility of craniosacral examination findings: a statistical analysis. J Am Osteopath Assoc 1977;76: 67–76.

71. Kirkaldy-Willis WH, Cassidy JD. Spinal manipulation in the treatment of low-back pain. Can Fam Physician 1985;31:535–540.

72. Shekelle PG, Adams AH, Chassin MR, et al. The appropriateness of spinal manipulation for low-back pain: indications and ratings by a multidisciplinary expert panel. Santa Monica, Calif.: RAND, 1991:70–73.

73. Haldeman S, Rubinstein SM. The precipitation or aggravation of musculoskeletal pain in patients receiving spinal manipulative therapy. J Manipulative Physiol Ther 1993; 16:47–50.

74. Shekelle PG, Adams AH, Chassin MR, Hurwitz EL, Phillips RB, Brook RH. The appropriateness of spinal manipulation for low-back pain: project overview and literature review. Santa Monica, Calif.: RAND 1991:4, 5.

75. Zupruk GM, Mehta Z. Brown-Séquard syndrome associated with posttraumatic cervical epidural hematoma: case report and review of the literature. Neurosurgery 1989; 25:278–280.

76. Cassidy JD, Thiel HW, Kirkaldy-Willis WH. Side posture manipulation for lumbar intervertebral disk herniation. J Manipulative Physiol Ther 1993;16:96–103.

77. Woo C-C. Post-traumatic myelopathy following flopping high jump: a pilot case of spinal manipulation. J Manipulative Physiol Ther 1993;16:336–341.

78. Radanov BP, Dvořák J, Valach L. Cognitive deficits in patients after soft tissue injury of the cervical spine. Spine 1992;17:127–131.

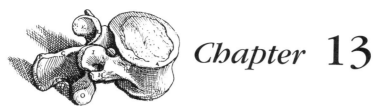

Chapter *13*

Hypothesis of Vertebrobasilar Arterial Insufficiency

*M*any patients apparently seek and obtain relief, through chiropractic care, from conditions such as migraine, dizziness, and other complaints localized to the cranial region, but the mechanism for such relief is disputed (1–4). Palmer (4) stated that racking the bones of the spine into their proper alignment had restored a man's hearing. He believed that distortion of the intervertebral foramen had compressed nerves at their root, resulting in the hearing loss (see Chapter 4). Christensen (5) cited work by medical specialists in Denmark, including one series of seven patients with hearing deficits who were successfully treated by cervical manipulation. Haldeman (6) extensively reviewed the literature concerning the influence of the autonomic nervous system (ANS) on cerebral blood flow. He concluded that the ANS appears to affect cerebral blood flow to some degree, but not enough to seriously compromise the nutrient supply to nervous system tissue. Haldeman has, therefore, indicated that there is no proof that chiropractic adjustment can affect the innervation to the blood vessels of the cranium enough to give rise to symptoms there. There is, however, another mechanism whereby adjustment of the cervical vertebrae directly affects a considerable portion of cerebral blood flow.

Various medical researchers have determined that injury to the cervical spine, congenital anomalies, spondylosis (atherosclerosis, arteriosclerosis of vertebral arteries), and subluxation of the cervical vertebrae may result in deflection or compression of the vertebral arteries (7–20). These studies are presented in this chapter. In some rare cases, embolism within the higher cerebral vessels may result in stroke, other neurological deficit(s), and death (21–32). Chiropractors have noticed that this vertebrobasilar arterial insufficiency syndrome may be caused by cervical disrelationships (33–35). The hypothesis that cervical intervertebral subluxations may cause deflection or compression of the vertebral arteries, thereby altering cerebral circulation, is termed the hypothesis of *vertebrobasilar arterial insufficiency* (VBAI). Medical doctors have suggested that manipulation may initiate the syndrome, and chiropractic researchers agree that the presence of the syndrome is a contraindication for adjustment or manipulation (21–32, 36).

We suggested that when vertebral subluxation complex (VSC) caused this syndrome, chiropractic adjustments might be useful in correction of it (37), and recent information from chiropractic researchers who apparently share this viewpoint is presented in this chapter (39, 40). Fitz-Ritson (40) devised a useful test for distinguishing cervicogenic vertigo that is apparently responsive to chiropractic adjustive intervention (see also Chapter 9). However, under certain conditions adjustment is contraindicated, and issues relating to predilection for this injury after adjustments are discussed below (41–44). As more is known of chiropractic manipulative therapy (CMT) and risk factors for accidents associated with this intervention, greater awareness by practitioners should translate into safer applications of adjustments (45, 46). Finally, we review some current research on head movements and the vertebral arteries (47–50).

Characteristics of VBAI

Typically, an osteophyte, subluxation, or fracture/dislocation of a cervical vertebra (usually atlantoaxial) initiates a peculiar complex of symptoms by compressing or deflecting a vertebral artery as it passes through the involved foramen transversarium (7–12) (Fig. 13.1).

Congenital bony anomalies and anomalies in the origin of the vertebral artery have also been associated with this syndrome (15, 20). The vertebral arteries comprise a very considerable portion of the blood supply to the cranium (17, 18) and the major blood supply to the brainstem (9). Symptoms have been previously described as the Barré-Lieau syndrome and include headache, nausea, vomiting, nystagmus, and suboccipital tenderness (12). A more complete picture includes dizziness and "drop attacks" (instantaneous and temporary quadriplegia on rotation and extension of the neck) (9, 13–16). Arteriosclerotic involvement may result in hemorrhage of the tunica media and cause a dissecting aneurysm, effectively shutting off the lumen of the vertebral artery (11, 16). Whether atheromatous changes develop in compressed vessels following chronic subluxation, etc. (12, 16) or develop incidentally, further trau-

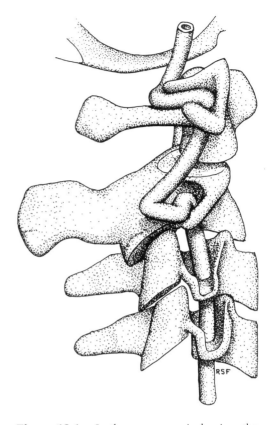

Figure 13.1. In the upper cervical spine, the vertebral arteries are most susceptible to deflection and obstruction by subluxation (including, especially, atlas laterality as well as articular process slippage to below the level of the transverse process), osteophytic spurring, increased tortuosity from lower cervical degenerative joint disease, and even cervical spine manipulation itself.

ma may induce enough subintimal hemorrhage to complete the occlusion (11).

ROLE OF INTERVERTEBRAL SUBLUXATION IN ETIOLOGY OF VBAI

Various researchers have documented the role of intervertebral subluxation in causing VBAI. For the most part this is the vertebral subluxation complex phase 2 (phase of instability) that is defined by medical radiographic criteria and was discussed in some detail in Chapter 10. Jackson (7) associates lateral atlas subluxation with constriction of the vertebral arteries as they course through the transverse foramina (7):

> Relaxation or stretching of the guy ligaments may allow lateral subluxation of the head of the atlas on the axis and excessive rotation of the axis in its relationship to the head of the atlas, and may be responsible for irritation of the vertebral arteries as they wind around the atlanto-axial joints and the superior facets of the atlas.

Jackson believed that constriction of these vessels most often occurs in the upper cervical spine (atlas, axis, third cervical), where they are most susceptible to trauma (whiplash, sporting injuries, etc.). She recognized that such constriction produces vascular insufficiency to the brain, with subsequent dysfunction, and stated that the sympathetic nerve supply to these vessels, following trauma, may initiate a persistent vasoconstriction that may develop into permanent narrowing and complete constriction. Further vascular insufficiency of the spinal cord may result if vasoconstriction or narrowing of the anterior and posterior spinal arteries (cranial branches of the vertebral arteries) occurs in addition to vertebral artery involvement.

Kovacs (8) has determined from clinical and cadaver studies that subluxation in the cervical spine may be a common factor in the etiology of VBAI. He has associated the syndrome with chronic and other forms of headaches (8):

> We believe that headache radiating from the top of the skull and the nuchal region as well as the upper cervical sympathetic syndrome described by Barré-Lieau, is more frequently produced by pressure exerted on the vertebral artery and nerve by the superior articular process than by other conditions.

Kovacs found slippage of the articular process to below the level of the transverse process in 22 of 40 chronic headache sufferers. For 20 of these 22, anteflexion-traction relieved the headache and was found radiographically to have corrected the subluxation. Kovacs also studied 54 postmortem cases. He demonstrated chronic subluxa-

tions by radiography and found bony excavation within the transverse foramina, where the pulsating vertebral arteries had actually etched into the bones. These studies document dramatically the role of subluxation in causing headaches.

Schneider and Schemm (9) have recognized the role of atlas-axis and atlas-occiput dislocation in producing the vertebral artery compression syndrome. They believed that either the aforementioned dislocations or direct contusion of the spinal cord results in spinal cord and neurological involvement. They explained that compressing the vertebral arteries within the transverse foramen of a dislocated or fractured atlas inhibits the blood supply to the circle of Willis (circulus arteriosus cerebri) and hence the anterior spinal artery. Hypoxia of the spinal cord results, with increased motor activity to the lower extremities (relative to the upper extremities) and varied sensory findings. They noted paralysis lasting from minutes to days.

Seletz (10) described the brief posterior subluxation that occurs in whiplash cases. He believed that symptoms of vertigo, ataxia, diplopia, severe attacks of migraine headache, hemicrania with nausea and vomiting, and transient disturbance of speech and swallowing were due to compromised circulation of the vertebral arteries following neck sprain or whiplash.

Gurdjian et al. (11) described five cases of carotid and vertebral artery involvement following various types of accidents. Fracture/dislocation of cervical vertebrae was found to be associated with vertebral artery involvement. One patient with vertebral artery compression showed no signs of brainstem or cerebellar involvement. The authors believed that in this case, the artery being compressed was already congenitally small, so further occlusion of it did not sufficiently inhibit blood flow to the circle of Willis.

Hadley (12) has implicated grossly hyperplastic arthrotic posterior vertebral joints as a cause of vertebral artery compression. Such subluxations are, according to Kovacs (8), chronic and irreparable.

OTHER ETIOLOGIES OF VBAI

Husni et al. (13) found basilar artery insufficiency in 20 patients reporting dizziness. The dizziness was traced to vertebral artery occlusion at the fifth and sixth cerebral vertebrae. Only patients in whom lateral rotation of the neck resulted in vertebral artery occlusion were included in this study. In 18 of the patients, the vertebral artery on one side was congenitally smaller than that on the other side; in every patient in whom unilateral blockage of the vessel produced symptoms, it was the larger artery that was blocked.

Disparity between vertebral artery diameters in the same person is quite common. Stein et al. (14) found that 45 of 130 cadavers had a right vertebral artery smaller than the left. Only in 59 cadavers were the arteries of equal diameter. A chiropractic researcher, Thiel (47), examined 16 cadaver spines (mean age: male, 73; female, 71) and also found larger-diameter left vertebral arteries (left, 4.28 mm; right, 3.83 mm).

Husni et al. (13) found that during surgery, tension on certain interdigitations of tendons (the tendinous slips of origin of the longus colli and scalenus medius muscles) resulted in compression of the involved vertebral artery. Sectioning the tendons and interposing a pedicle to prevent regrowth yielded dramatic symptomatic and objective improvement in nearly all patients. These patients had suffered dizziness, vertigo, headaches, and loss of consciousness, as well as gait and visual disturbance, nausea, numbness, and scalenus anticus before the operations. The authors concluded that when VBAI syndrome occurs with simple rotation and extension of the neck, it is caused by mechanical obstruction by tendons and can be corrected with surgery.

Anderson et al. (15), however, reported on a 37-year-old man with marked occlusion of the left vertebral artery after simple rotation of the neck to the right side and upward (no dislocations or osteophytes observable). His right vertebral artery was hypoplastic, and the left vessel was of anomalous origin (from the aortic arch medially to the origin of the subclavian artery). He suffered headaches, vertigo, and nystagmus, which were markedly aggravated by the previously described neck movement.

In a comprehensive study, Sheehan et al. (16) concluded that cervical spondylosis was the primary cause of vertebrobasilar arterial compression syndrome. They found that a common form of the syndrome occurs when spondylosis (with osteophytic encroachment of the vertebral artery) and cerebrovascular atherosclerosis are combined. They also found vertebral artery occlusion in 26 of 46 patients with recurrent cerebrovascular symptoms and/or cervical spondylosis. Rotation of the neck resulted in further narrowing or complete occlusion of the vessel on the side on which the osteophyte was compressing the artery. In addition to osteophytes, it was found angiographically that atheromatous plaques (3 patients) and arteriosclerotic tortuosity (10 patients) were associated with this syndrome. A significantly greater occurrence of spondylotic vertebral artery compression was found in men than in women. A special complaint of some patients was sudden, transient quadriparesis with subsequent falling to the ground (no loss of consciousness). This "drop attack" was believed to be pathognomonic for the syndrome. Interestingly, these authors were in accord with Kovacs (6) who found signs of nerve root and cord compression in some patients with subluxation as well as VBAI.

Tatlow and Bammer (17) cited three cases in which rotation of the neck resulted in neurological signs and symptoms referable to VBAI. In this early study, postmortem examination showed that rotation and extension of the neck on the involved side, when combined with vascular abnormalities or the presence of osteophytes, resulted in occlusion of the vertebral artery. Anticoagulant therapy was successful in clinical cases when trauma in the presence of arteriosclerosis had resulted in thrombus formation higher up in the cerebral arteries. This mechanism was hypothesized to explain certain cases of stroke and death following cervical manipulation.

Other authors (14, 18, 19) have documented atheromatous plaques as one of the most common causes of VBAI syndrome. Barton and Margolis (20) documented two other cases of VBAI syndrome caused by rotational obstruction at the atlantoaxial joint. They found that rotational obstruction only initiates this syndrome when the contralateral vertebral artery is already compromised (congenitally).

CONTRAINDICATION FOR CHIROPRACTIC ADJUSTMENT

Medical (21–30) and chiropractic (31, 32, 36) researchers acknowledge that in the presence of certain predisposing factors, cervical manipulation may result in thrombus formation, ischemia, stroke, and death.

Terrett (41, 42) reports that there have been 113 documented cases of vascular accidents following cervical spine manipulation, most of which apparently occurred after chiropractic ($n = 66$), medical ($n = 18$), or osteopathic ($n = 9$) rotary procedures. Of these, covering the years 1934 through 1987, at least six resulted in tetraplegia ("locked-in" syndrome), 36 resulted in permanent neurological deficit, 10 had incomplete neurological recovery, 11 had complete recovery, and 28 died (27, 31). Terrett's literature review concludes that there is no age predilection for manipulative accidents; most injuries occurred in the 31-to-35 age group (also the age group most commonly presenting to chiropractors in the survey sample)(41). Often no clear premanipulative indicator of VBAI is present, but, frequently, the most serious accidents have occurred when a second manipulation was performed on a patient who showed signs of brainstem ischemia immediately after a prior manipulation. Hence, if a spinal manipulation initiates signs or symptoms of brainstem ischemia, Terrett (42) warns that:

It is negligent for a practitioner to ignore warning signs such as vertigo or dizziness and continue with SMT [spinal manipulative therapy] (42).

According to this chiropractic researcher, at least 27% of the documented chiropractic cases (including at least 38% of the deaths attributed to CMT) occurred in this manner, after the practitioner failed to be alerted by signs of brainstem ischemia (Table 13.1) occurring after chiropractic, or to respond to same (42). He advises that when signs of brainstem ischemia occur after chiropractic intervention, the practitioner instead should immediately: (*a*) *cease manipulation* (do not remanipulate and retraumatize an artery undergoing pathological change), (*b*) *observe the patient* (symptoms may spontaneously resolve within a short period of time), and (*c*) *refer if symptoms do not subside* (the referral should include contact with the emergency room or physician to describe treatment rendered and the possible need for immediate anticoagulant medication) (42). Clearly, the chiropractor must not panic and remanipulate the spine under any circumstances, according to this review of literature (41–42). According to Terrett, biased reporting of manipulative accidents is suggested by reviewing this literature, and

Table 13.1.
Signs and Symptoms of Vertebrobasilar Arterial Insufficiency[a]

Ataxia
Diplopia
Dizziness
Drop Attacks
Dysarthria
Dysphagia
Falling to one side
Nausea
Numbness
Nystagmus
Visual disturbance
Vomiting

[a]Adapted from Kamrath KR. Deciding when to use cervical spinal manipulative therapy in treating patients with symptoms of vertebrobasilar ischemia: a diagnostic rationale. Chiro Technique 1991;3:122–125 and Terrett AGJ. Vascular accidents from cervical spine manipulation: report on 107 cases. J Aust Chiro Assoc 1987;17:15–24.

it is not surprising to find most cases occurring after CMT. If anything, the relative safety of CMT is suggested by considering that 41% of all accidents occur at the hands of nonchiropractors (generally less experienced at the art of manipulative therapy), who probably administer a disproportionately small percentage of all manipulations performed annually (37, 41, 42).

According to the medical literature, the typical case involves a patient who receives a standard rotary cervical adjustment or manipulation. Indeed, according to Martienssen and Nilsson (43), 45 of 49 cases of cerebrovascular accidents in which the type of manipulation was reported occurred after rotary manipulation applied to the cervical spine. They considered this to represent a contraindication to this type of manipulation (43), but it may also occur because this is perhaps the most common type of cervical manipulation utilized. However, evidence continues to mount that with the head in hyperextension coupled with rotation (viz., typical setup for cervical rotational manipulation) the vertebral arteries are predisposed to unusual stresses that impair brainstem circulation.

Danek (49) investigated this position, using a Doppler ultrasonic flowmeter, in 25 young persons (aged 16 to 26) sent to a diagnostic center, complaining of headache, vertigo, hearing disorders, and collapses, without any organic blood-vessel illness. The rheoencephalographic (REG) examinations revealed that with the head hyperextended and rotated to the right, 80% of these subjects had decreased REG amplitude affecting the right half of the head, and 16% of the subjects had reduced REG amplitude affecting the left half of the head. A similar preponderantly ipsilateral response was found with hyperextension and left rotation. In addition, the pulse-wave time lengthened more than 15 ms on the ipsilateral half of the head with hyperextension and rotation to the right (60% of cases) and to the left (44% of cases). As flow asymmetry between the vertebral arteries occurred significantly in 48% of the subjects, they concluded that

even more serious disorders of blood flow might be expected with a failing spine and in the presence of vessel anomalies.

An alternative mechanism to explain disturbance of the brainstem and vertebrobasilar system might occur via the effect of spinal manipulation, for example, on blood flow within the internal carotid arteries. To investigate this hypothesis, Opala and Arkuszewski (48) made arteriograms in 1638 patients with transient ischemic attacks, cerebral infarcts, or other signs of CNS involvement from 1970 to 1974. Arteriograms made in the frontal plane showed coilings of the internal carotid in 0.55% of patients with signs of insufficient blood flow and in about 9% of those with tortuous internal carotid arteries (48).

Factors predisposing to brainstem ischemia after rotational manipulation, based on this literature, include:

1. Unilateral vertebral artery obstruction by congenital or developmental factors. When the contralateral artery is then diminished by the rotary and extension movements found in cervical spine manipulation, both arteries become obstructed. Such factors include arteriosclerosis, vascular anomaly, and unilateral vertebral artery occlusion.
2. Degenerative joint disease, even in the lower cervical spine, can result in a loss of disc height, which shortens the cervical spine and allows the vertebral arteries to become more tortuous. This condition may effectively reduce the lumen of these vessels, predisposing them to further occlusion by cervical spine manipulation.
3. Osteophytic outgrowths, especially from the zygapophyses, can obstruct the course of the vertebral arteries. In this case, cervical spine manipulation on the side of the osteophytic outgrowths reduces the flow through the artery on the same side.

Manipulation of a patient who has one or more of these or other predisposing factors

(Table 13.2) may result in thrombus formation, ischemia, and stroke, especially in the presence of vascular disease (21–30, 32).

Giles (36) contends that a differential diagnosis of VBAI syndrome contraindicates regular chiropractic adjustment. He believed that the Cyriax method of careful manipulation during strong traction is a better form of treatment for these predisposed individuals. He stated that bed rest, limitation of neck movement, and possibly intervention with anticoagulants or surgical procedures (depending on the severity of the condition) are the treatments of choice for patients with VBAI syndrome. This puts him basically in accord with Sheehan et al. (16) on the course of treatment.

A case of cerebrovascular infarction in a 16-year-old boy who fell asleep with his head rotated to the left and extended is noteworthy (29). In this patient with congenitally anomalous vertebral artery distribution, the entire blood supply to the left occipital cortex was derived from the right vertebral artery. That normal physiologic head movements can result in cerebrovascular infarction in predisposed individuals underscores the necessity of identifying these individuals before introduction of chiropractic manipulative therapy.

Table 13.2.
Risk Factors for Vertebrobasilar Arterial Insufficiency[a]

Amaurosis fugax
Anticoagulants
Arteriosclerosis
Bruits of the carotid arteries
Cervical spondylosis
Cigarette smoking
Contraceptives
Diabetes
Family history of strokes
Headaches resistent to drug therapy
Hypertension
Rotational manipulation
Sudden fainting related to a turning of the head
Transient ischemic attacks
Transient paresthesias or palsy

[a]Information from (39, 42, 43, 48).

Clinical Considerations

Researchers have stated that VBAI is a relatively common syndrome (7–13). From their point of view, it causes a bizarre group of symptoms including dizziness; vertigo; nystagmus; ataxia; "drop attacks" considered pathognomonic of the syndrome; chronic, acute, and migraine headache; acute quadraparesis; hemicrania; nausea; vomiting; and disturbances of speech, swallowing, and possibly, balance. Although some investigators (7–12) have directly associated this syndrome with cervical subluxation, all recognize a host of other causes, including osteophytes, abnormal presence of only one vertebral artery or one congenitally stenotic vessel, abnormal tortuosity of one or both vertebral arteries (as occurs in arteriosclerosis), other vascular disease such as atherosclerosis, congenital bony anomalies, and anomalies in origin of the vessels (7–20). Any combination of these symptoms or clinical signs, especially when initiated or aggravated by hyperextension and rotation of the neck, indicated the possible presence of the VBAI syndrome (7–17).

The differential diagnosis includes Ménière's disease, certain brain tumors, and other disease and functional states causing dizziness or vertigo (36, 50). In a literature review, Douglas (50) stated that patients with nonvestibular disorders (and hence the best candidates for chiropractic?) are likely to present with nonspecific symptoms of faintness, giddiness, or lightheadedness. Conversely, the three best predictors of serious causes of "dizziness" were age over 69 years, lack of true vertigo, and neurological deficit (50).

A test useful in determining the presence of this syndrome has been described (36). It involves having the patient stand with eyes closed and arms stretched forward (horizontally); the patient is asked to rotate the head fully to one side and hold that position for 1 minute. This is repeated for the other side. Sway of the outstretched arms suggests cerebral ischemia caused by cervical rotation (36).

Fitz-Ritson (40) describes a test used prospectively in one trial to discriminate cervicogenic vertigo responsive to CMT that was described earlier in this text (see Chapter 9). Other chiropractic investigators advocate categorization of VBAI to rate potential risks and modify treatment approach (viz., more careful manipulation?) (39). In contrast with the opinions of Giles (36) and Sheehan and colleagues (16), even in the presence of VBAI some chiropractors insist that more episodes of neural ischemia may be prevented by cervical manipulation than are caused by it (37, 39). However, a tentative diagnosis of VBAI suggests careful chiropractic management, and in the presence of atherosclerotic or arteriosclerotic phenomena or other risk factors that are not yet fully defined, standard adjustment may be contraindicated (19–32, 36, 41, 42).

Discussion

Conflicting ideas are prevalent among the researchers involved in the study of this syndrome. Some investigators are critical of the chiropractic profession because cases of stroke and death following chiropractic adjustment of the neck have been reported (21–30). These cases are extremely rare, however (13 deaths attributed to CMT in over 50 years) (42), and a survey among the members of the Swiss Society for Manual Medicine revealed slight neurological complications occurred secondary to cervical manipulation in one of 40,000 cases, while serious complications occurred in one of 400,000 neck manipulations (44).

In fact, other researchers have associated this syndrome with subluxations of cervical vertebrae (7–12). This implies that subluxation may be associated with a wide variety of symptoms referable to the cranium. The hypothesis of VBAI becomes important in light of the position held by Haldeman (6) and others who have shown that sympathetic tone plays a minor role in cerebral blood flow and, hence, that mechanisms based on a neurovascular connection are question-

able (38). (Although Fitz-Ritson (51) demonstrated direct connections between the C2 dorsal root ganglia and the medullary nucleus X of the vestibular system (by labeling the right ganglion in each of three *Macaca irus* monkeys with ^{3}H-leucine and using autoradiographic techniques with light and dark-field microscopes), descending inhibition and other "dampening" processes may insulate the vestibular apparatus from facilitative spinal lesions as well.) Since chiropractors make their prime objective the correction of subluxations, they are probably playing a role in correcting this condition.

At any rate, there appears to be conclusive evidence to suggest that cervical intervertebral subluxations may indeed cause VBAI, especially in the presence of spondylosis (7–20). Of course these represent lesions diagnosed radiographically by medical criteria and associated with instability. The correction of these lesions—with significant translations and listhesis—using CMT has not been fully evaluated (see Chapter 10). The hypothesis of VBAI is worthy of study as a mechanism that may explain the role of chiropractic in correcting certain conditions of cervicocranial origin, yet there is good evidence that manipulation or adjustment should be administered carefully—if at all—in such cases (37–45). Finally, we should remember the advice of Haldeman and Rubinstein (46) and explain the purpose of a particular treatment approach to patients, keep records that reflect a logical approach in treatment, and be careful when using levers that place stress on areas already compromised by prior injury.

Summary

The vertebrobasilar arterial insufficiency (VBAI) syndrome results from a variety of conditions including subluxation (7–20). The rotation and extension movements of the neck may initiate or aggravate the syndrome and result in "drop attacks" and symptoms including, typically, dizziness (13–16). Chiropractic adjustments or other manipulations appear to initiate the syndrome in some rare cases (21–30, 41–44). A test is described to identify the syndrome (in addition to neck movements of rotation and extension) (36). It is hypothesized that chiropractors may be inadvertently correcting this condition in many individuals, by correcting subluxations (37, 39, 40). Understanding risk factors and signs of brainstem ischemia may help prevent some accidents and promote safer application of CMT in cases of dizziness and vertigo (39, 40).

REFERENCES

1. Watkins RJ. The neurological first aid kit. Chiro Econ May/June 1970.

2. Janse J. History of the development of chiropractic concepts; chiropractic terminology. In: Goldstein M, ed. The research status of spinal manipulative therapy. Washington, D.C., Government Printing Office, 1975: 25–42.

3. Parker GB, Tupling H, Pryor DS. Proceedings of the Australian Association of Manipulative Medicine. Aust NZ J Med 1976;8:589.

4. Palmer DD. The science, art and philosophy of chiropractic. Portland, Ore.: Portland Printing House, 1910:18.

5. Christensen F. An updated study of chiropractic in Danish medicine. Eur J Chiro 1983; 31:86–99.

6. Haldeman S. The influence of the autonomic nervous system on cerebral blood flow. J Can Chiro Assoc 1974;19:6–12, and 14.

7. Jackson R. The cervical syndrome. Springfield, Ill.: Charles C Thomas, 1978.

8. Kovacs A. Subluxation and deformation of the cervical apophyseal joints. Acta Radiol 1955;43:1–15.

9. Schneider RC, Schemm GW. Vertebral artery insufficiency in acute and chronic spinal trauma. J Neurosurg 1961;18:348–360.

10. Seletz E. Whiplash injuries—neurophysiological basis for pain and methods used for rehabilitation. JAMA 1958;168:1750–1755.

11. Gurdjian EX, Hardy WG, Lindner DW, Thomas LM. Closed cervical cranial trauma associated with involvement of carotid and vertebral arteries. J Neurosurg 1963;20: 418–427.

12. Hadley LA. Anatomico-roentgenographic studies of the spine. Springfield, Ill.: Charles C Thomas, 1964:158–171.

13. Husni EA, Bell HS, Storer J. Mechanical occlusion of the vertebral artery. JAMA 1966; 196:475–478.

14. Stein BM, McCormick WF, Rodriguez JN, Taveras JM. Postmortem angiography of cerebral vascular system. Arch Neurol 1962; 7:545–559.

15. Anderson R, Carleson R, Nylen O. Vertebral artery insufficiency and rotational obstruction. Acta Med Scand 1970;188:475–477.

16. Sheehan S, Bauer RB, Meyer JS. Vertebral artery compression in cervical spondylosis. Neurology (Minneap) 1960;10:968–986.

17. Tatlow WFT, Bammer HG. Syndrome of vertebral artery compression. Neurology (Minneap) 1957;7:331–340.

18. Bauer RB, Sheehan S, Meyer JS. Arteriographic study of cerebrovascular disease. Arch Neurol 1961;4:119–131.

19. Faris AA, Poser CM, Wilmore DW, Agnew CH. Radiological visualization of neck vessels in healthy men. Neurology (Minneap) 1963;13:386–396.

20. Barton JW, Margolis JW. Rotational obstruction of the vertebral artery at the atlantoaxial joint. Neuroradiology 1975;9:117–120.

21. Green D, Joynt RJ. Vascular accidents to the brain stem associated with neck manipulation. JAMA 1959;170:522–524.

22. Miller RG, Burton R. Stroke following chiropractic manipulation of the spine. JAMA 1974;229:189–190.

23. Mueller S, Sahs AL. Brain stem dysfunction related to cervical manipulation. Neurology (Minneap) 1976;26:547–550.

24. Pratt-Thomas HR, Berger KE. Cerebellar and spinal injuries after chiropractic manipulation. JAMA 1947;133:600–603.

25. Schwartz GA. Posterior inferior cerebellar artery syndrome of Wallenberg after chiropractic manipulation. Arch Intern Med 1956; 97:352–354.

26. Smith RA, Estridge MN. Neurologic complications of head and neck manipulations. JAMA 1962;182:528–531.

27. Braun IF, Pinto RS, DeFilipp GJ, Lieberman A, Pasternack P, Zimmerman RD. Brain stem infarction due to chiropractic manipulation of the cervical spine. South Med J 1983;76: 1507–1510.

28. Horn SW. The locked-in syndrome following chiropractic manipulation of the cervical spine. Ann Emerg Med 1983;12:648–650.

29. Hope EE, Bodensteiner JB, Barnes P. Cerebral infarction related to neck position in an adolescent. Pediatrics 1983;72:335–337.

30. Okawara S, Nibbelink D. Vertebral artery occlusion following hyperextension and rotation of the head. Stroke 1974;5:640–642.

31. Jaskoviak PA. Complications arising from manipulation of the cervical spine. J Manipulative Physiol Ther 1980;3:213–220.

32. Kleynhans AM. Complications of and contraindications to spinal manipulative therapy. In: Haldeman S, ed. Modern developments in the principles and practice of chiropractic. New York: Appleton-Century-Crofts, 1980:359–384.

33. Kleynhans AM. Vascular changes occurring in the cervical musculocutaneous system. J Can Chiro Assoc 1970;15:19–21.

34. Palmateer DC. Greater occipital-trigeminal syndrome. J Clin Chiro (arch ed), 1972: 46–48.

35. Zeoli NJ. Anatomical and pathological considerations of the circle of Willis. Dig Chiro Econ 1971;13:44–45.

36. Giles LGF. Vertebra-basilar artery insufficiency. J Can Chiro Assoc 1977;22:112–117.

37. Leach RA. The chiropractic theories: a synopsis of scientific research. 2nd ed. Baltimore: Williams & Wilkins, 1986:117–118.

38. Heistad DD, Marcus ML, Gross PM. Effects of sympathetic nerves on cerebral vessels in dog, cat and monkey. Am J Physiol 1978; 235:544–552.

39. Kamrath KR. Deciding when to use cervical spinal manipulative therapy in treating patients with symptoms of vertebrobasilar ischemia: a diagnostic rationale. Chiro Technique 1991;3:122–125.

40. Fitz-Ritson D. Assessment of cervicogenic vertigo. J Manipulative Physiol Ther 1991;14: 193–198.

41. Terrett AGJ. Vascular accidents from cervical spine manipulation: report on 107 cases. J Aust Chiro Assoc 1987;17:15–24.

42. Terrett AGJ. It is more important to know when not to adjust. Chiropr Technique 1990; 2:1–9.

43. Martienssen J, Nilsson N. Cerebrovascular accidents following upper cervical manipulation: the importance of age, gender and technique. Am J Chiro Med 1989;2:160–163.

44. Dvorak J, Orelli Fv. How dangerous is manipulation to the cervical spine? Case report and results of a survey. Manual Med 1985;2: 1–4.

45. Lädermann J-P. Accidents of spinal manipulations. Ann Swiss Chiro Assoc 1981;7:161–208.

46. Haldeman S, Rubinstein SM. The precipitation or aggravation of musculoskeletal pain in patients receiving spinal manipulative therapy. J Manipulative Physiol Ther 1993; 16:47–50.

47. Thiel HW. Gross morphology and pathoanatomy of the vertebral arteries. J Manipulative Physiol Ther 1991;14:133–141.

48. Opala G, Arkuszewski Z. Rotation of the cervical spine and angiographic picture of the internal carotid artery. Manual Med 1989;4: 47–48.

49. Danek V. Haemodynamic disorders within the vertebrobasilar arterial system following extreme positions of the head. Manual Med 1989;4:127–129.

50. Douglas F. The dizzy patient: strategic approach to history, examination, diagnosis, and treatment. Chiro Technique 1993;5:5–14.

51. Fitz-Ritson D. The direct connections of the C2 dorsal root ganglia in the *Macaca irus* monkey: relevance to the chiropractic profession. J Manipulative Physiol Ther 1985;8: 147–156.

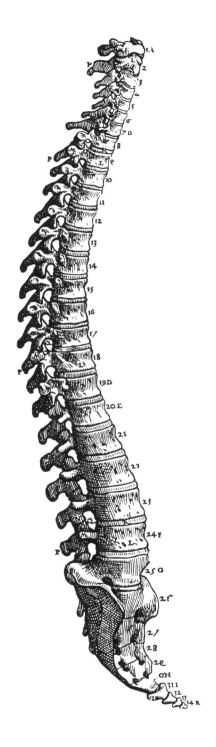

Spinal Pathophysiology and Neurodystrophy

The microbe is nothing,
the soil is everything.

Louis Pasteur

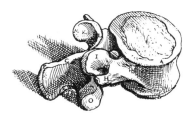

Chapter 14

Neurodystrophic Hypothesis

*C*hiropractic was founded on the idea of body tone. Palmer (1) writes:

> The amount of nerve tension determines health or disease. In health there is normal tension, known as tone, the normal activity, strength and excitability of the various organs and functions as observed in a state of health. The kind of disease depends upon what nerves are too tense or too slack.

This idea of body tone has been considered sheer quackery by most medical investigators throughout this century and for plausible reasons (2–4). Medical researchers have determined the causes of many diseases, most of which responded well to antibiotic and other therapies (5). Moreover, North American immunologists determined that a variety of factors (including genetic, cell-mediated, lymphoid, thymic, and hormonal) are involved in the defense of the human body to disease (6–24).

Immunologists have demonstrated specific primary and secondary responses to antigens in vitro and ways to inhibit such responses in vitro (5–9). The results of immunizing the peoples of the world to a number of diseases have been mixed, however (25–33). Although smallpox has apparently been wiped out, other less encouraging mass immunization programs, such as for the supposed "swine flu" epidemic in 1976, have met with disaster, cost lives, and

wasted millions of dollars (29, 33). Nevertheless, according to much of the literature, there appears to be little reason for immunologists, medical doctors, scientists, or anyone else to believe in the chiropractic tenet that intervertebral subluxations (or facilitation associated with the initial phase of VSC) are involved in the genesis of organic disease.

However, since the first edition of this text, psychoneuroimmunology has emerged as a field of scientific study. A theme central to the research in this field is that there is interaction between central nervous system function and immunity (34–41). This contradicts traditional medical and scientific thought that there is no relationship between the nervous system and immunity, and therefore, chiropractic manipulation cannot affect immune function (3, 4).

These researchers and previous investigators in the former U.S.S.R., Germany, and North America have made discoveries that appear to substantiate the chiropractic *neurodystrophic* hypothesis (42–66): neural dysfunction is stressful to the visceral and other body structures, and this "lowered tissue resistance" can modify the nonspecific and specific immune responses and alter the trophic function of the involved nerves (1, 67–74). Some of these researchers (39–41, 56–66, 75–86) have concluded that the nervous system is intimately involved in specific and nonspecific body defenses. For instance, the classic works of Selye (42–43) and others (49–51) in North America have demonstrated neuroendocrine-immune connections in experiments and clinical investigations. Moreover, psychoneuroimmunologists have now documented a connection between immunologic competence and the anterior hypothalamus (36–38, 44–48). Indeed, modulation of the immune response by norepinephrine has been linked to a specific hypothalamic nucleus (98).

An important new contribution to this hypothesis comes from Patricia Brennan, Ph.D., an immunologist at National College of Chiropractic. Brennan and co-workers (101, 102) significantly advanced our understanding of chiropractic adjustment by identifying biological effects of adjustment on immunity that are not present after placebo intervention. The major emphasis of this chapter is on clarifying these mechanisms and providing an answer to the questions: What role does the nervous system play in specific and nonspecific body defenses? and, To what degree might the spinal lesion act as a neuroendocrine-immune stressor?

Theories of Immunity: Clonal Selection, Network, and Systemic

According to current North American immunologic concepts, the specific immune response in humans appears to be based on the classical precipitin reaction (5–9). Hence, when an *antigen* (Ag) (i.e., any foreign substance capable of eliciting an antibody response) is mixed with its corresponding antiserum (i.e., one containing antibodies specific for the administered Ag) in vitro, a precipitate is formed.

The reaction depends on the valency of the antigen, which varies according to its size and the species synthesizing the antibody. Included among the factors regulating the binding of antigen to antibody are the normal intermolecular forces that regulate binding between any two unrelated proteins (i.e., *coulombic*, or the attraction between

oppositely charged ionic groups; *hydrogen bonding*; *hydrophobic bonding*; and *Van der Waals'* bonding, or the interaction between the external "electron clouds").

Antibodies that react with antigen to form a precipitate are known as *precipitins*. What is important, however, is that the actual attraction of antibody to antigen is thought to be totally independent of direct neural regulation. In thousands of experiments, immunologists have shown that the primary and secondary immune responses can not only be demonstrated in vitro but also be inhibited in vitro (5–9).

Experiments on rats and guinea pigs have demonstrated that the actual "memory" for any given antigen is coded into the DNA of small lymphocytes and macrophages; again the nervous system is not directly involved (5–7, 10). In one series of experiments (5), immunologists injected specific antigens into "virgin" rats (animals that had not been previously exposed to any specific antigen). Small lymphocytes were taken from these "primed" animals and injected into other, unprimed, genetically identical recipients. The unprimed animals produced strong secondary antibody responses. Hence, the small lymphocytes carried "sensitization" to the antigen from the first to the second group of animals, which proves that the actual memory for the secondary antibody response was coded into the small lymphocytes (6).

Further experiments have demonstrated that two types of lymphocytes (viz., "bursa equivalent," or *B cells*, which are thymus-independent, and thymus-dependent, or *T cells*) appear to work with macrophages to stimulate antibody synthesis (5–7, 14–19). Several theories appear in the literature which attempt to explain how these defenses work in humans.

CLONAL SELECTION THEORY OF BURNET

A current model based on *The Clonal Selection Theory of Acquired Immunity* by Burnet (11) holds that antigen inside the body is processed either (*a*) within a viral-infected or malignant cell and joined by a class I MHC (major histocompatibility gene complex) molecule in a vesicle, and then transported to the cell surface for display to a *cytotoxic T cell* for destruction, or (*b*) extracellularly by antigen-presenting cells (APCs: accessory cells that chemically process antigen, such as macrophages, dendritic cells of the spleen and lymph, B cells, and/or virtually any nucleated cell in the body), which break down the material in an intracellular compartment and link it to class II MHC molecules, after which they are transported together to the cell surface and displayed to *helper T cells* (27). Apparently, the MHC molecule acts as a receptor site for T and B cells; even a fragment of viral or malignant gene combined with class II MHC enables a cytotoxic T cell to identify and destroy entire cells that have "gone bad" (27).

This linkage stimulates helper T cells (which secrete substances that mobilize other cells) to send three "messages" (Fig. 14.1). One message occurs when the T cell releases "receptor" protein molecules, which have been coded for the antigen, throughout the area of invasion. Monocytes that pick up these proteins are immediately

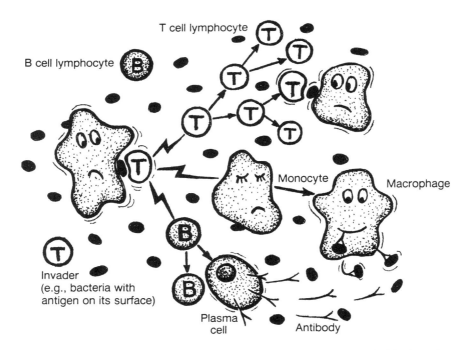

Figure 14.1. One well-known model of antigen-antibody interaction holds that after processing by antigen processing cells such as macrophages, antigen is bound to an MHC molecule and transported to the cell surface. There, one of the two types of MHC acts as a receptor site for adherence with either (*a*) cytotoxic T cell lymphocytes, which will destroy a viral or malignant cell (not shown), or (*b*) helper T cell lymphocytes, which secrete substances that mobilize other elements of the immune system in the presence of bacteria or other extracellular invaders (27).

Shown here is the subsequent threefold helper T cell response: (*a*) call for increased T cell production; (*b*) cause monocytes to become active macrophages; and (*c*) call for B cells to proliferate and become plasma cells that synthesize antibodies. Antibodies are Y-shaped proteins that attach to antigens on invading bacteria, etc. The shaft of the antibody attaches to macrophages, which may then more quickly engulf and destroy the invader. (Adapted from Gore R. The awesome worlds within a cell. Nat Geog Mag 1976;150:355–395.)

activated to become aggressive macrophages. Other "messages" go out to produce more T cells and to signal B cells to proliferate and become plasma cells (which in turn produce and release antibodies specific for the invading antigen). Much evidence supports this and similar models based on Burnet's theory, which may be the most widely accepted theory of immunity in North America today (5–7, 14–19, 22, 27).

NETWORK THEORY

Perelson (22) describes immune *network theory* as a system providing for both stability and responsiveness. B cell networks may be arranged so that one side of the transition networks has small localized structures much as might be predicted by clonal selection and circuit models; on the other side, profound idiotypic networks become possible, with signals moving about and antigen stimulation affecting large portions of the network:

> Whether signals actually have such profound effects or just stimulate local portions of the network depends crucially on antibody affinities and concentrations, molecules such as lymphokines . . . and the dynamical laws governing the interactions among the cells and molecules of the immune system. These dynamical laws still need to be uncovered and provide a challenge to both experimentalists and theorists (22).

SYSTEMIC IMMUNITY

Coutinho (23) speaks of moving beyond clonal selection and network, and looking instead to systemic immunology, since properties such as tolerance and self-nonself distinctions are distributed and cannot be simply reduced to individual components. He writes that while we can manipulate genes, engineer molecules, and control cellular behaviors, immunologists are at a loss when trying to manipulate the system:

> Surprisingly, perhaps, we continue to treat allergy as we did before IgE was known, we have no specific therapy for autoimmune diseases, we are unable to tolerize the recipient of an organ to the tissues of the donor, and we seem incompetent to derive vaccines to protect the larger part of the world population from parasite infections (23).

As if responding to his plea, immunologists have performed a wide variety of experiments that indicate that other factors may play important roles in the immune response. Cell-mediated, humoral, lymphoid, thymic, genetic, nutritional, endocrine, neural, and stress-related factors have been positively identified as modifying and at least partially controlling both the specific and the nonspecific immune response to disease. The latter three are discussed in detail in the next few sections, as they are probably the most important chiropractically.

Cell-Mediated Immunity

Cell-mediated immunity (CMI) plays a prominent role in protecting the body from a variety of pathogens. A classic series of experiments showed that certain organisms may not respond to an attack when antibodies are the lone defenders but will readily succumb when lymphocytes are actively involved (6). Donor rats injected with moderate doses of *Mycobacterium tuberculosis* overcame this infection and became immune to further injections. Later injections into these sensitized animals resulted in vigorous secondary immune responses. Amazingly, if a different organism (e.g., *Listeria monocytogenes*) is simultaneously injected during a second challenge with *M. tuberculosis*, the animals respond by killing both invaders (normally, the *Listeria* infection alone would overcome the animals). These experiments suggested that initiation of a specific secondary immune response enhanced a simultaneous nonspecific response to other unrelated organisms with similar growth habits (both *Listeria* and tubercle bacilli may live and grow inside macrophages, even following ingestion by phagocytosis).

Further experiments showed that this nonspecific response was cell-mediated by

T cell lymphocytes. This was demonstrated by first infecting a series of rats with *M. tuberculosis*. Specific immune sera, macrophages, and lymphocytes were taken from these initial donor rats and independently injected into three other groups of rats. Rats that received only the specific immune sera (containing specific antibodies for *M. tuberculosis*) were challenged with injections of *L. monocytogenes* and *M. tuberculosis*. They became infected. The second group received macrophages from the donor rats; following injection with *L. monocytogenes* and *M. tuberculosis*, they too became infected. The third group received lymphocytes from the donor animals; they became immune to further challenge with both *Listeria* and tubercle bacilli (6) (Fig. 14.2).

Recent experimentation has conclusively confirmed these findings and has suggested that CMI, as opposed to humoral immunity (viz., specific immune sera, specific antibody response) is crucial to the control of human leprosy (6). Other bacteria and viruses are similarly overcome by cell-mediated rather than humoral immunity. (Note that lymphocytes are considered part of both humoral and cell-mediated responses to disease.)

Humoral Immunity

Humoral immunity is fundamental to any specific defense response to bacteria, viruses, protozoa, and possibly, helminths (5–7). The immunoglobulins function as the specific antibodies that fight antigens entering the body (i.e., the *humoral response*). The precipitin reaction (considered a classic humoral response) is used primarily to determine the antibody content of the immune serum or the valency of the antigen.

The thymus gland has been implicated in aging and in the immune response (5–7, 12, 49, 50). T cells must pass through or be acted on by the thymus before they are activat-

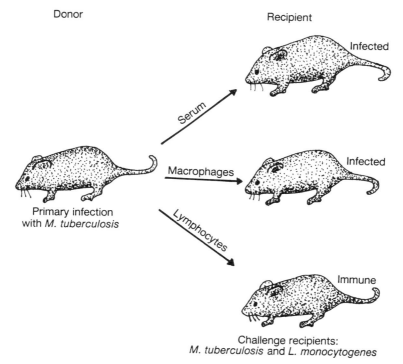

Donor

Recipient

Serum

Infected

Macrophages

Infected

Lymphocytes

Immune

Primary infection
with *M. tuberculosis*

Challenge recipients:
M. tuberculosis and *L. monocytogenes*

Figure 14.2. After injection of rates with immune sera, macrophages, and lymphocytes from rats infected with *M. tuberculosis*, only the animals receiving lymphocytes are immune to further challenge by *L. monocytogenes* and *M. tuberculosis*. (Adapted from (6).)

ed, to participate properly in the immune response. Since T cells are central to the clonal selection model, it is easy to see why the thymus is now viewed as a primary organ of immunity.

Many experiments have shown that the thymus is crucial to the immune response, but two classic experiments have primarily established the thymic role in immunologic competence. In one study, thymectomy of mice at birth resulted in decreased circulating lymphocyte counts, impairment of graft rejection, decreased normal humoral antibody response to many antigens, and general wasting due to the inability of the mice to fight infections (6).

In the other study, adult mice were irradiated to destroy their immunologic competence. One subgroup of irradiated mice was injected with bone marrow cells; the other subgroups were given injections of adult spleen and lymph node cells. Injections of bone marrow cells did not restore immunologic competence to previously irradiated mice. Immunologic competence was restored, however, in the groups of irradiated mice receiving injections of adult spleen and adult lymph node cells (6). These and other authors concluded that the thymus acts on blood marrow cells to make them immunologically competent (5–7, 12, 49, 50). Although it was once thought that thymus gland activity was independent of neural regulation, there is now evidence that the CNS regulates thymic activity (87).

Genetic Influence

Genetic factors are fundamental to the immune response. Not only is the resistance of different species highly variable, but the actual memory for the secondary response is coded into at least the DNA of T cell lymphocytes and probably that of macrophages (5–7, 10). Chandra (13) has shown that malnutrition in young rats not only can greatly impair their immune response (by causing reduced growth, involution of lymphoid organs, and lymphopenia) but also can impair antibody formation in the next two generations of animals (i.e., their progeny).

Comparing these findings with clinical findings suggested that impaired immunocompetence following intrauterine malnutrition may endure for a long time. Further, immunodeficiency diseases such as autoimmunity, neoplasias, and frequent infections may appear in the human mother as well as in her offspring as a result of this malnutrition. Thus, malnutrition may interfere with the immune response, and the effects are passed down to future generations, apparently by genetic code (13).

In addition to cell-mediated, humoral, lymphoid, thymic, genetic, and nutritional factors affecting or participating in the immune response, which appear to be independent of neural influence, other factors would appear to lend credibility to the neurodystrophic hypothesis.

Selye's General Adaptation Syndrome

The classic works of Selye (42, 43), which summarized thousands of studies by other scientists, demonstrated for the first time that exposure to stress can cause "diseases of adaptation." Selye ultimately was credited with defining and revising the theories surrounding stress into one comprehensive model that has since been praised around the world. The "general adaptation syndrome" (GAS) is a model for stress that can explain the many diverse physiological reactions to various stressors.

ALARM REACTION

The GAS begins with the "alarm reaction" (AR). When the human is first exposed to stress (either a *systemic* stressor or a *topical* stressor), the AR begins, which may include any or all of the following:

1. Adrenocortical enlargement with histologic signs of hyperactivity. This systemic nonspecific reaction includes secretion of increased amounts of cortisone and adrenocorticotropic hormone (ACTH).

2. Thymicolymphatic involution, including eosinopenia, lymphopenia, and polynucleosis.
3. Gastrointestinal tract ulcers.
4. Miscellaneous signs of damage or shock.

STAGE OF RESISTANCE

Following the initial response of AR, the human physiological response shifts to the "stage of resistance" (SR), which will be functional as long as the endocrine, and other, systems can respond normally. Various "conditioning factors" can modify the hormonal actions and hence the SR, however. These include:

1. Hereditary, nutritional, and age factors;
2. Increased protein diet resulting in increased production of corticotropic hormone;
3. Increased sodium ion concentration augmenting the action of mineralocorticoids (MCs);
4. Stress itself.

Stress itself is probably the most effective and common factor in conditioning the actions of adaptive hormones. *Systemic* stressors (which stimulate the GAS response) increase the antiphlogistic, lympholytic, catabolic, and hyperglycemic actions of antiphlogistic corticoids (ACs), while *topical* stressors increase the salient effects of adaptive hormones. Topical stressors modify the course of inflammation by eliciting a phlo-

gistic response that actually facilitates inflammation. A topical stressor stimulates a local adaptation syndrome (LAS) response.

DISEASES OF ADAPTATION

These conditioning factors determine whether the stress will be manifest by the so-called diseases of adaptation (including such experimentally and clinically verified diseases as hypertensive and inflammatory rheumatic diseases, nephrosis, nephritis, nephrosclerosis, hypertension, vascular lesions, rheumatic fever, rheumatoid arthritis, gastrointestinal ulcers, aldosteronism, periarteritis nodosa, hyperthyroidism, thyroiditis, certain types of liver disease, Von Gierke's disease, and certain tumors) or by the "physiologic adaptation syndrome," which is the response that allows our bodies to adapt to stress rather than to succumb to it (Fig. 14.3).

Other events that inhibit the GAS and may result in a disease (or diseases) of adaptation include:

1. Any absolute increase or decrease in the amount of adaptive hormones (e.g., corticoids, ACTH, somatotropic hormone (STH), and aldosterone) that are produced during stress.
2. Any absolute increase or decrease in the amount of adaptive hormones that become retained in their respective peripheral target organs during stress.
3. Any disproportion in the relative secretion of various antagonistic adap-

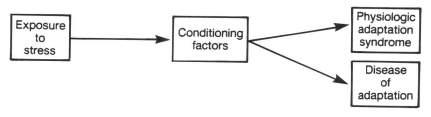

Figure 14.3. According to the Selye model (42, 43), the stage of resistance will be functional unless it is modified by the various conditioning factors, which may result in physiologic adaptation or disease of adaptation.

tive hormones (the actions of ACTH and other ACs are antagonistic to the actions of STH and the prophlogistic corticoids or PCs) during stress.

4. The production of metabolic derangements that alter the target organ's normal response to adaptive hormones. Stress can produce such metabolic derangements through the previously mentioned "conditioning factors."

5. Any abnormal neural, renal, hepatic, and/or other responses.

The entire GAS is based on the idea that under optimum conditions the body can respond to various stressors by adapting to them. When the hypophyseoadrenocortical system is not functioning correctly, however, the relative pathogenicity of many systemic and local stressor agents increases. It is thus easy to see why diseases caused by inability of the body to adapt to stressors are termed diseases of adaptation. Other body systems are involved in adaptation; hence, according to researchers, an abnormal response by the nervous system—or by other major systems—may play an important role in the etiology of diseases of adaptation.

Selye (42, 43) and these investigators determined that the nervous system is involved in the hypophyseoadrenocortical response to stress by a number of pathways. Frustration, for example, may act as a neurogenic stressor to greatly stimulate ACTH secretion. Experiments with animals showed that such a "neurogenic stressor" follows a path through the hypothalamus to the anterior lobe of the pituitary (adenohypophysis), where ACTH is secreted into the systemic circulation. By another pathway, autonomic nervous system stimuli causing vasoconstriction actually prepare the tissues of the body (extrarenal) for the antiphlogistic effects of cortisol and cortisone. Further connections between the neuroendocrine systems also were demonstrated. Thus, the hypophyseoadrenocortical system affects the central nervous system (e.g., corticoids may cause anesthesia, euphoria, depression, and even transient paralysis).

Calabrese (20) argues that modern research supports the concept that the AR is a potent immunomodulator, since chronic sympathetic-mediated arousal simulates a glucocorticoid and catecholamine response. Prolactin and luteinizing hormone responsiveness to stress habituates after 10 days of a daily stressor, and responsiveness to a subsequent unfamiliar stressor is attenuated (21). Cameron and Nesse (96) demonstrated that while normal stress and abnormal anxiety both evoke adrenergic and adrenal hyperactivity responses, an increase in epinephrine is found during a panic attack with normal stress, while epinephrine is not elevated with anxiety. These studies offer continuing evidence that the host may adapt to stressors but may, under certain circumstances, be predisposed to abnormal responsiveness to further stressors.

These findings, based on more than 30,000 scientific studies, have become extremely important to the chiropractic profession. For the first time ever, pathways (Fig. 14.4) have been scientifically demonstrated which verified that the nervous system participates in the response to stress and may therefore be a factor in any of the so-called diseases of adaptation.

Neuroendocrine-Immune Connection

The studies of Selye (42, 43) demonstrated for the first time that the response to stress was coordinated by a neuroendocrine mechanism. Yet during the 1950s, there was little evidence from the North American literature to demonstrate any connections between this neuroendocrine response and immunologic competence. Denckla (50) and others (47–49, 51–53) have shown that there is such a connection.

At Harvard Medical School, Denckla (50) thoroughly reviewed the literature and noted various interactions between age and the neuroendocrine and immune systems. Various studies showed that the pituitary was connected with the immune system; two hormones controlled by the pituitary—growth hormone and thyroid-stimulating

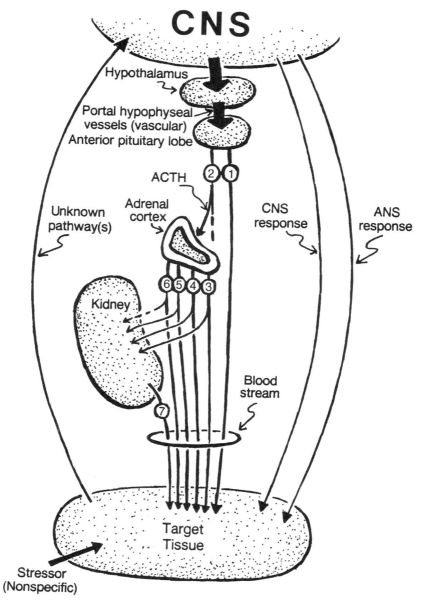

Figure 14.4. Pathways of the stress response showing that the CNS is an important mediator of stress in humans. Endocrine glands secrete the following hormones needed for this response: (*1*) somatotrophic hormone (STH), (*2*) adrenocorticotrophic hormone (ACTH), (*3*) prophlogistic corticoid, (*4*) noradrenaline, (*5*) adrenaline, (*6*) antiphlogistic corticoid, and (*7*) renal pressor substance. In some cases, according to Selye, the unknown pathways that alert the CNS to the presence of a nonspecific stressor could be the nervous impulse(s). (Adapted from (42, 43).)

hormone—were shown to be beneficial to immunologic competence.

Xenograft rejection (i.e., rejection of a graft transplanted from another species) is considered a valid monitor of immune system competence. Bilder and Denckla (51) showed that xenograft rejection in young and old intact rats took place in 6.0 and 13.8 days, respectively. After removal of the pituitary gland and later injection of thyroxine (T_4) and growth hormone, however, the older (64 weeks) rats rejected xenografts in approximately 6.5 days, a rejection time that was not significantly different from that for younger (4 weeks) rats. This demonstrated that the pituitary was a significant factor in certain aspects of maturation and senescence within the immune system.

These researchers and others showed that the decline in sensitivity of target tissues to pituitary hormones (measured by minimal O_2 consumption) with age was not due to a decrease in hormonal levels. Instead, they suggested that with advancing age, the pituitary releases a factor that is increasingly detrimental to the immune response (51). Physiologists have determined that pituitary secretions are under humoral and neural influences; this implies connections between the neuroendocrine system and aging of certain components of the immune system (49–51).

Selye may have opened the door to neuroendocrine and/or stress research, but psychiatrists in the mid-1970s appear to have walked through that door. Stein et al. (44) reviewed the literature (including their own studies) that convincingly demonstrated psychosocial and neural influences on the immune system. In their experiments, the central nervous system and, specifically, the hypothalamus had direct effects on the humoral immune response (see also "Anterior Hypothalamus and Immunologic Competence" in this chapter) (44, 45).

Various experimental studies in mice have shown that psychosocial factors can modify host resistance to infection with herpes simplex virus, poliomyelitis virus, Coxsackie B virus, polyoma virus, and vesicular stomatitis virus by increasing their relative pathogenicity. Clinical findings have verified these observations, according to the authors (44, 45). Other psychosocial factors increased the susceptibility of these animals to infection by other agents but were not factors that necessarily involved the nervous system; in contrast, the previously named agents all increased in relative pathogenicity when psychological stressors did not necessarily involve the nervous system.

Even more astonishing, psychosocial factors mediated through the nervous system were conclusively shown to affect the development, course, and outcome of neoplastic disorders (44). Stein et al. cited studies showing that infantile stimulation affects the development, course, and outcome of cancer (Walker 256 sarcoma) injected into rats. In mice, the survival time after transplantation with lymphoid leukemia was significantly decreased with previous infantile stimulation. Mammary carcinomas and survival time following injections of various subcellular fractions into experimental animals also were modified by psychosocial factors mediated through the nervous system (44).

Research along similar lines by Monjan and Collector (54) has demonstrated not only that stress in clinical animals sometimes can depress immune responsiveness but also that other environmental stressors may enhance immune responsiveness.

Murphy et al. (55) have shown that hippocampal lesions promote increased plasma corticosterone levels and gastric ulcers in animals confronted with stress. When various groups of rats were restrained (a psychological stress), all animals with hippocampal lesions developed ulcers in the glandular portion of the stomach (mean total length of ulcer was 3.78 mm). Only one animal in the cortical control group (animals with the portion of the cortex above the hippocampus removed bilaterally by aspiration) developed an ulcer (length, 0.50 mm). Only two animals in the normal group developed ulcers with simple restraint (mean total length, 0.37 mm). Among animals stressed by simple restraint, those with hippocampal lesions had significantly more ulceration (p = .001) than control animals (55).

Riley (41), after research and an extensive literature review, concluded that animal housing, unnecessary handling of laboratory rats and animals, and other variables may be responsible for the often conflicting results regarding stress and the immune system. He distinguishes between direct stress-induced pathologies and stress-induced modulation of immune responsiveness. With acute or chronic stress, an incipient or latent neoplasm or infection, either preexistent or introduced during the stress state, can be induced into overt pathology.

Viral and neoplastic pathologies that are under partial or complete control by cell-mediated immunologic defenses may be clearly enhanced by stress. In the case of neoplastic pathologies, stress enhances disease as a result of the adverse effects of stress on specific immunologic elements of the host, which suggests an indirect role of stress on pathology. Riley (41) suggested:

1. If there is no underlying disease, stress-associated infectious or neoplastic pathologies will not be observed.
2. The effects of stress will not be observed even if there are latent pathologies, unless the unimpaired immunologic system is in partial or complete control of the disease.
3. The adverse effects of stress will be observed only when the host immune defenses and the resident pathology are in a state of equilibrium, which thus permits stress to modify and impair the host's immunologic competence.

Keller et al. (38) showed that stress can impair immunity in direct proportion to the intensity of the stressor. They measured the number of circulating lymphocytes by phytohemagglutinin stimulation of lymphocytes in whole blood and isolated cultures and found that a series of graded stresses (home cage controls, apparatus controls restrained by tape and electrodes attached but with no current delivered, and low- and high-shock animals) progressively suppressed lymphocytic function (38).

In an extensive review of human studies on the relationship of stress to immune function, Locke (39) identified three important factors: duration and proximity of the stressor, adaptive capacity of the individual, and differential effects of various stressors on various immunologic components.

It appears that a wide variety of psychosocial factors, when mediated through the central nervous system, can decrease the level of immunologic competence and increase the relative pathogenicity of infectious agents and neoplastic disorders (44–54).

Reflex Mechanism of Immunologic Competence

While Selye and his many colleagues were documenting the role of the nervous system in the response to stress throughout the 1950s, other researchers in the U.S.S.R., Germany, and North America were finding evidence that appears to conflict with the previously mentioned model of antigen-antibody interaction. Several of these investigators who used radioactive isotopes in classic pulse-chase experiments appear to have demonstrated that antibody formation may be initiated by some nervous system reflex.

Speransky (56, 57) performed a series of experiments at the All-Union Institute of Experimental Medicine in Leningrad throughout the 1920s and the 1930s. In early experimentation on epilepsy, Speransky found that introduction of any of a variety of substances into the nervous system resulted in epileptic attacks. Neither the substance nor the nerve were found to vary the course of the disease. Moreover, intravenous injection of the same substances (croton oil, phenol, formalin, acids, bile, etc.) was not accompanied by the development of convulsive attacks. In this way it was shown that epilepsy was of reflex origin.

Speransky's research began with study of the role of the nervous system in various disease processes but progressed quickly. It was known that antitoxin introduced into the sciatic nerve of a dog would act as a chemical barrier to tetanus toxoid injected into the leg, blocking passage of the tetanus antigen. In one classic series of experiments, Speransky injected normal serum into the sciatic nerve to achieve the same blockade against the tetanus antigen. Incredibly, Speransky found that injection of tetanus toxoid into the nerve blocked passage of the previous tetanus toxoid inoculation. In fact, when injected into canine sciatic nerve to block intramuscular injection of tetanus toxoid, tetanus toxoid was a more efficient barrier than tetanus antitoxin.

Further experimentation with other diseases and animals led Speransky and his associates to conclude that the nervous system reacted to various noxious stimuli more directly than had previously been suspected (56):

> The appraisal of these data led so often to a conflict with the many existing views that very soon we perceived the necessity of giving up the study of isolated questions. By the force of circumstances, we were compelled to pass to a revision of the conceptions of the basic processes of general physiology, from the point of view of the nervous component in their origin and history.

Discoveries made by Speransky were not totally unique. In North America, Kuntz (58–60) reviewed the literature, including many studies recorded in German, and found studies by Reitler (1924), Bogendorfer (1927, 1932), Belak (1939), Illenyi and Borzsak (1938), Frei (1939), and Hoff (1942) that appeared to substantiate a role for the nervous system in regulating immune reactions. For example, he reports that Reitler initiated antibody formation in rabbits by injecting antigen into an ear following ligation of its vessels, then amputated the ear within 3 seconds of injection. This demonstrated that antibody titer increased reflexly and in the absence of antigen in the circulating blood.

According to Kuntz (60), the data showed "that the production of immune substances represents specific reflex secretory reactions to specific stimuli . . . [and] that an immune reaction once initiated may continue in the absence of nervous influences." However, several important questions were raised by this experiment, which was subsequently performed by Speransky (56) and others (61) with similar results. Other scientists suggested that perhaps even in that short time, the antigen had diffused into the proximal tissues and hence into the systemic circulation. It was also suggested that perhaps the operation was not sterile. If this were true, substances other than antigen could have stimulated a polyclonal response (a nonspecific increase in antibody). An immunologist at a major medical school pointed out that an endotoxin, lipopolysaccharide, or gram-negative microorganism could stimulate such a response and thereby invalidate the study.

Because of these and similar criticisms of this research, most North American scientists (notable exceptions included Kuntz and Selye) did not accept the conclusions, but others in Russia actively reviewed these data. From preliminary studies by Gordienko et al. (61) at the Rostov-on-Don State Medical Institute, it was concluded that the reflex theory of antibody formation proposed by Speransky, Reitler, Freidberger, and others was credible.

The success of their preliminary studies led Gordienko et al. to try to determine more accurately the possibility of reflex antibody formation. They performed 98 experiments on rabbits, divided into three groups (62) (Fig. 14.5). To determine the rate of absorption of antigen, rabbits in group 1 were injected with the highly radioactive phosphorus isotope (^{32}P). A vaccine containing 800 million to 1 billion microorganisms was injected intracutaneously into the tip of the other ear in these animals and group 2 controls. Since antigen was in a colloidal suspension, it was said to have been absorbed into the tissues more slowly than the radioactive phosphorus.

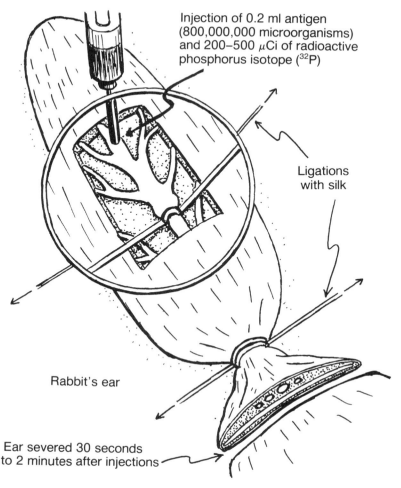

Injection of 0.2 ml antigen
(800,000,000 microorganisms)
and 200–500 μCi of radioactive
phosphorus isotope (^{32}P)

Ligations
with silk

Rabbit's ear

Ear severed 30 seconds
to 2 minutes after injections

Figure 14.5. In Gordienko's experiments on rabbits, one group of animals were injected with radioactive isotope (^{32}P) and 800 million microorganisms in typhoid vaccine solution. The absence of the isotope in the carotid artery following ear severance and the increase in agglutinin titer 7 days later strongly imply a neural reflex involvement in immunity.

The phosphorus was injected into the auricular nerve at the distal end of the rabbit's ear (the auricular nerve had been isolated, raised, and ligated). The entire ear was tightly constricted at its base with a silken ligature. In this series, as in all of Gordienko's experiments using ^{32}P, massive amounts of the isotope were injected into the nerve (200–500 microcuries). Two minutes after ^{32}P and antigen injection, the ear was severed at its base. Cessation of absorption of ^{32}P was determined by blood radioactivity (carotid artery) before the introduction of

radioactive phosphorus isotope, immediately after, and several minutes after ear sectioning. Agglutinin titers before and 7 days after the injection were compared. Results (Table 14.1) showed that the variations in blood radioactivity after introduction of the isotope are negligible and fall within normal limits.

They concluded that the ear ligation technique guaranteed negligible or minimal (less than 10,000 microorganisms/kg animal weight) absorption of antigen introduced into the skin distal to the base, when the ear

Table 14.1.
Carotid Artery Radioactivity before and after ^{32}P Injection into Ligated and Severed Rabbit Ear[a]

Rabbit No.	^{32}P Introduced (μCi)	Impulses/min/ml Blood before Introduction of ^{32}P	Cpm/ml Blood Introduction Immediately after of ^{32}P and Severance of Ear
2	200	39–41	37–44
3	180	32–35	35–37
4	200	32–35	32–35
5	200	40–42	38–43
6	200	36–40	36–41
7	200	35–35	45–45
8	200	38–42	38–45
9	200	40–41	40–44

[a]From Gordienko AN, Kiseleva VI, Saakov BA, Bondarev IM, Zhigalini LI. The possibility of a reflex mechanism producing antibodies when antigen acts on skin receptors. In Gordenko AN, ed. Control of immunogenesis by the nervous system. Washington D.C., National Technical Information Service, 1958:44–52.

is severed at its base within 2 minutes. They estimated that total antigen resorption under such conditions could not exceed 1–2%. Yet the agglutinin titers (Table 14.2) increased significantly in 12 of 15 animals (62). These increases could not be explained by accidental resorption of small amounts (under 10,000 microorganisms/kg animal weight) of antigen, since according to Gordienko et al. (62), others had previously shown that at least 100,000 microorganisms/kg animal weight must enter the blood before agglutinin titers rise to the levels shown in these experiments.

To establish that the increased agglutinin titer was specific (not simply a polyclonal response, etc.), they duplicated this experiment in another series of rabbits (group 3), using paratyphoid B vaccine; as a control, agglutinin titers were determined on paratyphoid A vaccine that was not injected. Had the agglutinin responses previously seen been due to some polyclonal response from infection of the rabbit ears, agglutinin titers to both paratyphoid B and paratyphoid A would be expected to rise. Data showed, however, that the reaction was specific only for the paratyphoid B antigen that had been introduced into the rabbit ear (62) (Table 14.3).

In another series of experiments, Gordienko et al. (63) determined that when various antigens contact nervous system receptors in the skin and blood vessels, they create specific bioelectric potentials that vary according to the antigen. These changes in the normal neural discharge were monitored electrophysiologically (Table 14.4). Control animals were injected with physiologic solution, and except for some minute changes in oscillations, there were no visible bioelectric aberrations. In contrast, when typhoid, paratyphoid B, or dysentery vaccine or staphylococci were injected near the lateral femoral cutaneous or auricular nerves, specific and dramatic changes in the normal bioelectric frequencies and amplitudes of the action potentials were recorded.

These findings offered dramatic and visible proof that the nervous system is capable of differentiating between various antigenic stimuli and lent further credibility to the hypothesis that antibody formation may be mediated by the nervous system. After years of research, Gordienko (64) concluded:

1. As foreign microorganisms pass receptors, the irritation results in specific changes in bioelectric potentials from the involved afferent nerve. The body reacts to these stimuli by mobilizing leukocytes and synthesizing antibody.
2. Endless possibilities for the kind of "warning" that the nervous system

Table 14.2.
Agglutinin Titers to Typhoid Vaccine before and after Severance of Rabbit Ear[a]

Rabbit No.	Initial Agglutinin Titer	Agglutinin Titer after 7 Days
2	1:20	1:160
3	1:80	1:320
4	1:20	1:80
5	1:10	1:80
6	1:20	1:80
7	1:10	1:160
8	1:40	1:160
9	1:40	1:160
457	1:00	1:40
430	1:00	1:00
644	1:00	1:00
235	1:00	1:640
213	1:00	1:00
230	1:00	1:2560
151	1:00	1:1280

[a]From Gordienko AN, Kiseleva VI, Saakov BA, Bondarev IM, Zhigatini LI. The possibility of a reflex mechanism producing antibodies when antigen acts on skin receptors. In Gordienko AN, ed. Control of immunogenesis by the nervous system Washington, D.C., National Technical Information Service 1958:44–52.

Table 14.3.
Alterations in Agglutinin Titers before and after Injection of Paratyphoid B Vaccine and Subsequent Severance of Rabbit Ear with Antigen Depot[a]

Rabbit No.	Initial Titer Paratyphoid		Titer after 7 Days Paratyphoid	
	A	B	A	B
46	0	0	0	640
449	0	0	20	320
485	0	0	0	320
464	0	0	0	20
524	0	0	0	80
547	0	0	20	20
663	0	20	20	0
479	0	0	20	80
240	0	0		0
336	20	20	20	80

[a]From Gordienko AN, Kiseleva VI, Saakov BA, Bondarev IM, Ahigalini LI. The possibility of a reflex mechanism producing antibodies when antigen acts on skin receptors. In Fordienko AN, ed. Control of immunogenesis by the nervous system. Washington, D.C., National Technical Information Service, 1958:44–52.

may receive are effected by utilization of conduction velocities of various fiber types in combination with the rate of stimulation of fibers.

3. The action of receptors, afferent fibers, and the central nervous system is specific with regard to control of immunogenesis.

The possibility that the nervous system influences leukocyte distribution and/or mobilization also has been explored by Gordi-

Table 14.4.
Effects of Various Antigens and Control Solution on Amplitude and Velocity of Nerve Conduction
(Auricular and Lateral Femoral Cutaneous Nerves)[a]

Antigen[b]	Conduction Velocity (oscillations/sec)	Amplitude (mV)
Typhoid	5–6	10–12
Phase I	14–16	15
Phase II	18–20	25
Paratyphoid B vaccine	Uninterrupted (peak outbursts lasting up to 10 sec)	30–35–40 90–100
Dysentery	10–15 (single and group outbursts)	10–15
Staphylococci	Reaction lasts 5–8 min (similar to other antigens)	
Type A	Fast or in single groups	Low
Type B	Slow oscillations	High
Control solution	(Only negligible alterations)	No change

[a]From Gordienko AN, Kiseleva VI, Saakov BA, Let'en AV. Electrophysiological phenomena in the nerve following action of antigens on the skin receptors. In Gordienko AN, ed. Control of immunogenesis by the nervous system. Washington, D.C., National Technical Information Service, 1958:22–27.
[b]Injected intradermally after hexanol narcosis (isolation) of the nerve.

enko et al. (64) and others. In a study of splanchnoperipheral balance during chill and fever, Peterson and Müller (65) demonstrated the possibility that the nervous system influences leukocyte distribution. They continuously injected unanesthetized normal dogs with small amounts of living colibacilli suspensions, using the Woodyatt pump. Approximately 4–5 million organisms/ml were injected every minute. Lymph, muscle, and rectal temperatures were monitored; constant monitoring of leukocyte counts and control of blood chemistry was observed.

They hypothesized that the chill produced in dogs by the continuous injection of colibacilli was associated with increased splanchnic activity and temperatures. They hypothesized, but could not demonstrate conclusively, a mechanism whereby bacteria entering the bloodstream are fixed by reticuloendothelial elements (the concept of a reticuloendothelial system is no longer considered valid (14)) in the splanchnic area. According to these authors, this mechanism stimulates these cells and the organs nearby (i.e., the liver, spleen, stomach, etc.) via the sympathetic nervous system. They further hypothesized that sympathetic stimulation throughout the periphery gave rise to the muscle tremor, blood vessel constriction, and refocus of circulation to the

splanchnic area involved, which is seen in chill and fever.

As early as 1927, their findings indicated that the autonomic nervous system may play a role in maintaining splanchnoperipheral balance during the course of infectious diseases, particularly during chill and fever. Their findings were not considered conclusive, however. If radioactive tracer had been available to them, they could have determined whether or not the bacteria were indeed fixed in the splanchnic area.

In a similar study, Arquin (66) studied the leukocyte counts in dogs and humans throughout active hunger contractions. He determined that stomach tonus is directly related to specific fluctuations in the peripheral leukocyte counts. He believed that dilatation of the stomach following intramuscular injection of a nonspecific milk preparation was only part of a larger splanchnic response. In his experiments, such dilatation was accompanied by peripheral leukopenia, while gastric contraction was associated with peripheral leukocytosis.

His study was thus in accord with the findings of Peterson and Müller. One immunologist I questioned about this and other studies suggested that the "chemistry" that causes hunger contractions also may affect the balance of peripheral leukocytes. If this were true, stomach tonus and peripheral leukocyte balance may not necessarily be linked in a cause-effect relationship. Physiologists believe, however, that "hunger contractions" result from a decrease in blood glucose circulating through the lateral hypothalamus (i.e., the so-called *hunger center*). In addition, the amygdala and cortical areas of the limbic system (including infraorbital regions, the hippocampal gyrus, and the cingulate gyrus) have been implicated in regulation of the hunger response. The only "chemistry" that could possibly mediate this balance would have to be blood glucose. It certainly appears more credible that the nervous system participates in this response by some unknown pathways (neuroendocrine? hypothalamic?). Kuntz (59, 60) held that the nervous system probably regulates leukocyte distribution.

Hypothalamus and Immunity

A number of more recent articles tend to support a hypothalamic-immune connection and suggest that the central nervous system functions in antibody formation, hypersensitivity, and anaphylactic responses.

Lowered histamine sensitivity following spinal cord section was shown by Cooper (76). Stein et al. (44) suggested, however, that this was more likely a secondary effect of peripheral disturbances in blood circulation and temperature control. Stanton et al. (77) showed that spinal cord sectioning in rats depressed the hemolysin response, but the depression was prevented by maintaining the animals at correct body temperature.

CONNECTIONS WITH THE ANTERIOR HYPOTHALAMUS

The hypothalamus has been connected with the anaphylactic reaction by a number of researchers (44, 45, 78, 83). Recently, Stein et al. (44) demonstrated lowered titers of circulating antibody (P <.01), significant protection against lethal anaphylaxis (P <.001), and depressed delayed hypersensitivity reactions in male Hartley guinea pigs

with electrolytic lesions in the anterior basal hypothalamus. Bilateral electrolytic lesions were induced in the anterior, median, or posterior basal hypothalamus of guinea pigs. Other guinea pigs were operated on but not lesioned (sham operated) or were not operated on at all (controls). Each group was initially sensitized to picryl chloride (a hapten), which acted as an antigenic stimulus, 1 week after the operation. Delayed cutaneous reactions to picryl chloride and tuberculin (purified protein derivative) were studied, agglutinin titers to picryl chloride hapten were determined to detect the level of circulating antibodies, and anaphylaxis reactions were recorded for each group.

Anaphylaxis occurred in 71% of the control animals and only 18% of the guinea pigs with anterior hypothalamic lesions; this was taken as strong evidence that this brain center plays an important role in the reaction (44). Agglutinin titers for antibody to picryl chloride were four times higher in the control guinea pigs than in the hypothalamically lesioned guinea pigs. Skin test reactions to picryl chloride and tuberculin were significantly diminished in animals with anterior hypothalamic lesions. These delayed hypersensitivity reactions were more intense in the nonoperated and sham-operated control groups. Median and posterior hypothalamic lesions, however, had no significant effect on lethal anaphylaxis, circulating antibody to the picryl chloride hapten, or delayed hypersensitivity reactions.

In vitro studies of the anterior hypothalamic-immune connection by Schiavi et al. (78) suggested that anterior hypothalamic lesions may reduce antibody titer via interference with antibody binding to host tissue, via modification of the antigen-antibody reaction, or via alteration of the content and release of histamine and other vasoactive substances. It was suggested that this lesion may alter the normal responsiveness of target tissues to the substances released by the antigen-antibody union (78).

Thus, this hypothalamic-immune connection is the most likely explanation for the effects of psychosocial factors in decreasing the immune response in animals (see "Neuroendocrine-Immune Connection" in this chapter) and thereby increasing the susceptibility of these animals to various viruses and bacteria as well as neoplasias, leukemias, and cancers (44).

In an extensive literature review in 1981, Solomon and Amkraut (37) discussed the history of psychoimmunology and detailed specific studies, including Soviet work, that identified a specific portion of the rabbit dorsal hypothalamus, whose ablation completely suppressed the primary antibody response. Prolonged retention of antigen in the blood, inability to induce streptococcal antigen myocarditis, and prolonged graft retention also were effected by dorsal hypothalamic destruction (of specific nuclei), while an enhanced antibody response was seen with electrical stimulation of the same nuclei. They cited other Soviet work that suggested direct hypothalamic regulation of immune responsivity. Specifically, the firing rates of neurons (as determined by implanted electrodes) of specific hypothalamic nuclei significantly increased after immunization; this suggested a feedback loop between the immune and nervous systems.

Brooks et al. (36) found that bilateral electrolytic lesions of specific limbic nuclei show alterations in lymphoid cell number and changes in lymphocyte activation in rats. Induced by concanavalin A, splenocytes decreased in number after anterior hypothalamic, ventromedial hypothalamic, and mamillary body lesioning. The number of thymocytes decreased after anterior hypothalamic lesioning but increased after hippocampal lesioning. Spleen cell responsiveness to concanavalin A decreased after anterior hypothalamic lesioning but was enhanced after mamillary body, hippocampal, and amygdaloid lesioning. Thymocyte mitogen reactivity was enhanced by lesions of the hippocampus and amygdaloid complex.

The authors concluded that the neuroendocrine system was most likely responsible for the effects, which were greatest 4 days after lesioning; thymocyte mitogen reactivity

and spleen cell responsiveness returned to normal levels within 14 days. They suggested that neuroimmunomodulation is mediated by the interaction of specific hormones with specific surface receptors, which alters intrinsic lymphocyte function. They raised the question, however, of a functional anatomical link between the CNS and the immune system.

Other evidence suggests that this is a valid conclusion. Nayar et al. (84) have shown that transection of sympathetic nerve can induce tumor-like growths in the salivary glands, reservoirs, gastric ceca, and midgut of the cockroach. Stein-Werblowsky (47) demonstrated that chemical sympathectomy increases the receptivity of tissues to tumor grafts and/or phosphorylcholine conjugates. Injections of 0.5 ml tumor suspension intraperitoneally resulted in tumors in 24 of 38 sympathectomized (0.7 ml of 50% ethanol injected into the left paravertebral region) rats; only 1 of 30 intact rats developed tumor. In animals sacrificed as soon as the tumor became palpable, the growths appeared to be confined to the left side, which would normally be innervated by the left sympathetic chain.

Another set of experiments showed that chemical sympathectomy had no effect on tumor "take" in immune rats (47). Stein-Werblowsky (47) concluded that the sympathetic nerves are concerned only with *initiation* of the immune or inflammatory reaction and that they set off a series of reactions leading to cell-mediated homograft immunity. In his experiment, the secondary immune response appeared to be independent of sympathetic influence.

Sympathetic influence on mild, nonlethal bile-induced pancreatitis has been demonstrated by Gilsdorf et al. (85). Increased sympathetic nervous system activity (viz., electrical stimulation of celiac ganglion) in the presence of nonlethal bile reflux pancreatitis (viz., 1 ml 10% bile infused into the pancreatic duct) induced severe pancreatitis in 13 of 20 animals and mild pancreatitis in 2 more. In contrast, only 2 of the 12 animals without the sympathetic stimulation developed severe pancreatitis; the other 10 did not develop pancreatitis. Another series demonstrated that ablation of the anterior hypothalamus induced severe lethal necrotizing pancreatitis from a mild, nonlethal bile-induced form.

Exactly how sympathetic influences alter immune responses remains to be seen. Stein-Werblowsky (47) appeared to favor a two-stage mechanism in which an initiating agent such as a neurotropic substance precedes the promoting agent. He predicted that the high incidence of lung cancer in cigarette smokers might be due to such a mechanism; the initiating agent may be the nicotine (which blocks the sympathetic ganglia) and the promoting agent may be the benzopyrene found in tobacco tar.

The stimulatory effect of caffeine on α-adrenoreceptors and its blocking effect on β-adrenoreceptors and cholinoreceptors is thought to stimulate proliferative activity; an increase in hepatocarcinogenesis was documented in mice after caffeine consumption, while low-dose ethanol reduced NDEA carcinogenesis, presumably via slackened α-adrenoreceptor and enhanced β-adrenoreceptor and cholinoreceptor activity (97).

It has been much more difficult to explain the role of the anterior hypothalamus in immunologic competence and, specifically, in the humoral immune response. Numerous investigators (44, 45, 47, 48, 54, 78, 83) have shown that the lesions to this brain center provide protection against lethal anaphylaxis, cause depressed delayed hypersensitivity, and result in lower titers of circulating antibody.

In view of modern immunologic research, some neuroendocrine mechanism(s) may be involved (9–19, 42, 43, 49–53, 75). Stein et al. (44) have proposed several mechanisms. The anterior hypothalamus is involved in regulation of secretion of thyroid-stimulating hormone (TSH), and it is known that this hormone is beneficial to the immune response (44, 50). A functional anatomical link between the CNS and the immune system was also considered possible, and evidence that the CNS regulates thymic activity strongly supports this view (36, 37, 86–90).

Psychoneuroimmunologists made several breakthrough discoveries in the 1980s, which greatly added to our understanding of neuroimmune function.

NORADRENERGIC INTERACTIONS WITH IMMUNITY

Felten and co-workers (98) extensively reviewed their research and that of others on noradrenergic sympathetic interactions with the immune system. Some of this research is provocative and has direct implications for our *neurodystrophic hypothesis*. They found that (98):

1. T helper cells are particularly sensitive to loss of noradrenergic innervation.
2. Cells other than T or B lymphocytes may be targets for norepinephrine (NE) action. Several macrophage functions, such as synthesis of complement components and activation to a cytocidal state, are inhibited by NE or α-agonists. Ag processing or presentation and interleukin-1 (IL-1) secretion and synthesis may be affected.
3. Adrenergic and cholinergic receptors in various tissues add incredibly to the potential matrix of ligand-receptor-transduction combinations, since these activate or inhibit adenylate cyclase and cAMP generation, activate guanylate cyclase, generating cGMP, and stimulate inositol phosphate turnover and elevate intracellular free calcium.
4. Cytokines from cells of the immune system are most likely acting as neuroregulatory signals, affecting both the electrical activity of neurons in the hypothalamus and the metabolism of central neurotransmitters such as NE. Immunization lowered NE levels in the hypothalamus during peak turnover of NE in the spleen, suggesting classic long and short hormone loops, respectively.

5. Specifically, the paraventricular nucleus (PVN) of the hypothalamus appears to be the key regulator for both neuroendocrine and autonomic outflow from the CNS. PVN contains oxytocin- and vasopressin-secreting magnocellular neurons (as does its counterpart, the supraoptic nucleus); however, PVN has corticotrophin releasing factor–secreting neurons that regulate the adrenocorticotrophic hormone–glucocorticoid axis. In addition, PVN sends descending projections that regulate preganglionic nerves of both the sympathetic and parasympathetic nervous systems. In experiments after immunization, coincident with the peak of splenic response, PVN NE levels were decreased significantly— indicating turnover—while other nuclei were unaffected.

6. The immune system must provide specific signals, such as IL-1 or leukocyte-derived pituitary-like hormones bearing "sensory" information to the nervous system, for an integrated response to occur.

7. NE may affect other events in the organs of the immune system such as blood flow, vascular permeability, and/or lymphocyte traffic.

These researchers stated that PVN probably provides an important chemical/anatomical feedback circuit between the immune system and the brain (98). They conclude:

> The neurotransmitter could influence activation, maturation, proliferation, differentiation, migration, receptor expression, and synthesis and secretion of lymphokines, monokines, or other mediators. At the very least, neurotransmitters represent yet another class of immunoregulatory molecules in an already complex system of intercellular communication. The links between the nervous and immune systems, established by our and other laboratories, provide the anatomical, physiological, and chemical basis for an integration of responsiveness of the whole organism, not only to "simple" molecular or cellular signals from the internal and external milieu, but also to "complex" psychosocial signals from the outside environment (98).

The anterior hypothalamus has been reported to play an important role in immunologic competence (98), which may explain neural mediation of psychosocial stress in humans. By this route, environmental and social stresses can reduce a person's resistance to disease, leukemias, infections, and even cancer (37, 44).

A similar pathway has been found for the effects of psychosocial stress on atherosclerosis. Gutstein et al. (91) demonstrated that electrical stimulation of the lateral hypothalamus resulted in atherosclerotic lesions in rats. Their findings suggested that a neural mechanism may be involved, even in the absence of coexisting hypercholesterolemia or hypertension, either by direct neural transmission affecting the vascular wall or by elaboration of arteriopathic substances (e.g., angiotensin II) in extravascular sites. However, in a study of 491 patients acute and chronic life events stress did not correlate with the presence of coronary atherosclerosis as assessed by coronary angiography (99). Clearly, more research on this is needed.

Spinal Lesions and Immunity

Early evidence that spinal lesions could be directly linked to immunologic competence in humans was presented by Speransky (57), who studied experimental and clinical cases of lobar pneumonia. Patients with viral pneumonia complaining of interscapular pain were treated by accepted medical procedures or by antibiotic therapy and injection of procaine into the interscapular paravertebral musculature. Patients who received the additional procaine injections were found to have significantly decreased morbidity and mortality.

EARLY OSTEOPATHIC INVESTIGATIONS

Osteopathic research on this question was performed early in this century by Deason (79), in an experimental study of filariasis. The study actually began by accident, when a number of rhesus monkeys showed signs of the disease after being received for study at the A. T. Still Research Institute in Chicago. The infectious microfilaria were found in the blood, lymph, cerebrospinal fluid, nasal discharges, urine, and fecal discharges of the affected monkeys. Clinical signs included diarrhea, loss of weight, and stupor. Body temperature in the infected animals ranged from subnormal to 104°F. The blood and urine pictures were considered diagnostic.

Seven monkeys were treated by drug therapy alone, including magnesium sulfate and thymol (then considered to be an anthelmintic) (0.1 g every 2 hours), and all failed to recover. Seven of 14 animals treated by correction of vertebral lesions by osteopathic manipulation in addition to drug therapy made complete recoveries, and another 6 showed signs of partial recovery before they died (3 of the deaths were probably due to secondary complications of pneumonia or tuberculosis).

In addition to correcting spinal lesions, osteopaths stimulate lymphatic drainage as well as venous and arterial circulation in patients with various infections (80). According to osteopathic records, during the pandemic of 1918, of 100,000 patients with influenza treated by osteopathic methods, the mortality rate was 0.25% (10% if deaths due to the complication of pneumonia are included), while the overall mortality rate at that time was 5% (30–60% if deaths due to the complication of pneumonia are included) (80).

Modern osteopathic treatment includes the use of Chapman's reflexes (i.e., viscerosomatic reflexes from the liver, spleen, and adrenal cortex) to evaluate and/or stimulate certain viscera (80). (Certain points anterior and posterior to these organs may display overreaction or underreaction of the corresponding organ.) These points are stimulated by circular friction massage for 20–40 seconds; according to osteopathic literature, these points correspond highly to acupuncture meridians (80).

MODERN CHIROPRACTIC INVESTIGATIONS

Modern chiropractic research began with case studies of three pain patients whose pain abated after chiropractic adjustments, and who showed increases in immunoglobulins A, G, and M (IgA, IgG, and IgM) by radial immunodiffusion assays 14 days after initiation of care. Conversely, in one patient that had no improvement in pain after CMT, serum values dropped markedly. Of the antibodies tested, IgG values seemed most sensitive to manipulative effectiveness (100).

Vora and Bates (94), at Northwestern College of Chiropractic, demonstrated significant increases in B cell lymphocytes following 4 weeks of twice-weekly spinal manipulations in patients known to have radiographically demonstrable spinal lesions. Unfortunately, the number of patients studied was small.

Provocative research by Brennan and coworkers (101) at the National College of Chiropractic demonstrated significant increases in zymosan-stimulated chemoluminescence (CL) of both polymorphonuclear neutrophils (PMNs) and monocytes from 42 subjects who received thoracic spine manipulation at T1 through T6 at the level of greatest motion restriction, based on passive motion palpation. These responses were significantly higher than pretreatment measures and were higher than measures obtained after sham manipulation ($n = 38$) and after soft tissue manipulation ($n = 19$) to volunteers randomly assigned to those control groups (101). Measurement of forces required to adjust the dorsal spine suggested a force threshold for enhancement of the CL response. Plasma levels of substance P (SP) were elevated in both treated and sham-control groups.

In a follow-up to this investigation, Brennan et al. (102) found that the mean manipulation force associated with priming effects of mononuclear cells for enhanced endotoxin-stimulated tumor necrosis factor (TNF) production by chiropractic manipulation was 878 ± 99 N. A small but significant ($\text{P} =$

.009) increase in SP was also noted after upper dorsal adjustment. They speculated that manipulation at a certain force causes release of SP by proprioceptive function and that both SP and TNF may have primed neutrophils for enhanced respiratory burst. They further speculated that it is not unreasonable that a positive feedback loop between TNF, SP, and possibly other cytokines such as IL-1, IL-6, γ-interferon, or prostaglandins might be involved. They advocated use of these immunologic responses as biological markers for true versus sham manipulation. Since these effects diminished toward pretreatment levels by 45 minutes posttreatment in asymptomatic students, they did not speculate further about the viscerosomatic implications of their research (102).

Few studies directly link vertebral lesions with immunologic competence. The work of Gordienko, Selye, Stein, Schiavi, Cooper, Felten and others, as presented in this chapter, appears to suggest that such a connection is likely. This connection should be an important area for future research, especially for chiropractors and osteopaths.

Discussion

The concept of immunity in humans is multifaceted and not easily understood. The variety of viewpoints involved and the limitations on our understanding of the subject make dogmatic positions untenable. We may simplify the problem, however, by separating the various positions into two principal groups.

Traditional medical thought held that immunity was completely independent of neural influence, direct or indirect. In this model, the thymus (previously thought to be independent of neural regulation) was given an important role, and in vitro suppression and enhancement of classical precipitin and other immunologic reactions led investigators to believe that immune function was largely the result of complicated but random chemical reactions. In this model, the anti-

gen of invading microorganisms was matched up to receptor sites on certain T cell lymphocytes that triggered an immune response (3, 5–24, 55, 92, 93).

Even the lowly earthworm, sea star, and sea urchin (*Lytechinus pictus*), which are invertebrates, have adaptive immunity (93). In fact, *L. pictus* has a highly sensitive immune system capable of rejecting allografts from unrelated sea urchins in only 30 days. This rejection time is even more amazing when one considers the low metabolic temperature of these animals (15–20°C). The experiments on *Lytechinus* support the theory of transplantation (viz., that graft tissues are recognized as antigenically foreign by the host and subsequently are rejected) and demonstrate that complicated immune responses can occur in the absence of a nervous system similar to that of *Homo sapiens*.

If complicated immunologic responses can occur in the absence of a nervous system, however, it must also be acknowledged that complicated immune reactions can be suppressed in the presence of a nervous system. Moreover, immunosuppression clearly can result from direct, or at least indirect, neural influence. Hypnotic-induced inhibition of an allergic reaction (urticarial skin test) as well as enhancement can be demonstrated despite the presence of antibodies in the sera (IgE), as documented by the allergic reaction in nonallergic volunteers who received sera from the hypnotized patients (34).

Present medical thought, however, holds that immunity is indirectly influenced by neuroendocrine factors and, indeed, by direct neural modulation. A growing number of researchers (20–23, 36–38, 44–48, 54, 56–66, 78–85, 96–102) now hold that the nervous system plays an important role in signaling the onset of invasion by microorganisms, by participating in some way with at least the primary immune response and, principally, by participating in the humoral immune response. Their research is supported to some degree by an overwhelming amount of evidence that now links the nervous system to immunity by way of its control of endocrine function (34–43, 49–53, 75–77, 86–89, 94, 96–98). Even the thymus, once thought to be free of neural influence, has now been shown to be influenced directly by CNS activity (87, 98).

In fact, it is probably fair to say that nearly all immunologists now recognize some role for the nervous system in modulating immune system function, if not a primary role. Evidence for direct involvement of the hypothalamic periventricular nucleus in norepinephrine-mediated immunomodulation is substantial (98). This provocative finding may yet support the older studies by Speransky, Kuntz, and Gordienko, which presupposed that immunity was directly influenced by neural signals, somehow triggered by antigen. Even barring such a role—which any chiropractor would love to embrace—the potential for interaction between neurotransmitters and clonal networks is almost beyond comprehension (98). Such an understanding helps explain how the nervous system may modify immunologic function in the presence of psychosocial stresses, and there is now clearly convincing evidence for such an effect.

Measures of stress and family environment, for example, were important predictors of atopic dermatitis severity after controlling for age and other variables (103). *Combat stress reaction* (CSR), also known as battle fatigue, battle shock, and war neurosis, and its long-term sequel, *posttraumatic stress disorder* (PTSD), cause absenteeism, increased medication usage, alcoholism, and increased cigarette consumption, as well as diarrhea, vomiting, nausea, enuresis, chest pains, and other somatic complaints (104). In yet another example of cellular immune function influenced by stress, Halvorsen and Vassend (105) demonstrated an increase in the number of monocytes during college examination stress, but significantly fewer large (probably activated) CD4 and CD8 cells and cells expressing the IL-2 receptor. Moreover, the proliferative response of T cells to antigens, mitogens, and allogeneic cells decreased from 6 weeks preexamination to 14 days postexamination.

However, just when we believe we have a handle on how the nervous system influences such dread reactions as myocardial infarction (e.g., through type A behaviors), new studies fail to verify such connections (106). Vernon et al. (107) presented preliminary evidence that chiropractic manipulative therapy stimulated a plasma β-endorphin response, which could not be independently substantiated (108). So too, findings by Koren and Rosenwinkel (109) that a number of spinal misalignment patterns identified by x-ray predict MMPI-generated personality profiles—providing almost ideal support for the chiropractic hypothesis that correction of subluxation leads to improvement in mental function (110)—must be considered preliminary until confirmed by other investigators working independently of one another.

What is important for the chiropractic profession is that regardless of the specific mechanisms involved, there are pathways for neural modulation of immunologic competence. If psychosocial stresses can influence immunologic competence by acting through neuroendocrine or direct neural mechanisms, why couldn't the intervertebral subluxation or vertebral subluxation complex (VSC)? Reviews of medical studies throughout this book have shown that the effects of the segmental dysfunction (SDF; VSC phase 1), facilitation, and intervertebral subluxation (VSC phase 2) are wide ranging, in some cases possibly altering neural transmission, vertebral artery supply, axoplasmic transport, and somatoautonomic neural traffic. One or more of these effects may alter hypothalamic function (e.g., vertebral arteries provide most of the blood supply to the brainstem and hypothalamus; see also Chapter 13). In this way endocrine and immune function might possibly be affected by facilitation and/or intervertebral subluxations.

It is particularly gratifying that our profession's much maligned founders (D. D. Palmer has been called a "grocer and magnetic healer" by our detractors) were 95 years ahead of the time with regard to the basic emphasis they placed on neural influence on all body functions, including immunity. Of course, we now recognize other factors and their roles in health and disease, but then to a lesser degree so did the Palmers. D. D. Palmer spoke of altered tonus, and B. J. Palmer spoke of "dis-ease" or the lack of organized function or relative health (1, 67, 95).

If there is any doubt that the chiropractic *neurodystrophic hypothesis*, "that neural dysfunction is stressful to the visceral and other body structures, and this "lowered tissue resistance" can modify the nonspecific and specific immune responses, and alter the trophic function of the involved nerves," is not a valid clinical research hypothesis, then it also remains to be demonstrated how neuroendocrine function can alter immunologic competence. There simply can be no question that the autonomic nervous system regulates directly and indirectly the functions of all organs and tissues and influences even biochemical processes at the cellular and subcellular level (35, 40).

That this trophic influence can affect "innate resistance" in humans, as the Palmers stated, is no longer purely speculative. Moreover, the issue now is more a chiropractic clinical one: finding proof that VSC or intervertebral subluxations in humans affect immune system function, or that adjustments enhance immunity regardless of whether a spinal lesion is operationally defined or found, and that adjustments can exert enough of a clinical effect to play a role in protection from or recovery after infectious processes, or all of these.

In light of a preliminary case study suggesting that an enhanced immunologic response is seen even 14 days after adjustments in previously symptomatic subjects (100), it appears that a follow-up to Dr. Brennan's (101, 102) work should include symptomatic subjects evaluated for longer periods. Perhaps there is even enough evidence to justify a trial using perhaps patients with chronic infections who are undergoing antibiotic intervention without success (such as chronic otitis media?).

Such studies should draw the profession together, because if the immunity boost after CMT is truly nonconsequential and not clinically useful, then stronger arguments may be made against chiropractors who use such applications of chiropractic even on an experimental basis, and together we can all go down the musculoskeletal road that some would argue is our only justifiable domain. However, if research in this key area of chiropractic theory is fruitful in the above context and should adjustments prove to be either preventive or curative, then we can all move together toward broader-based applications of chiropractic that are truly wellness-oriented and not solely symptom-based, as is the current fashion in both medicine and chiropractic, despite the protestations of some (70, 74).

Despite our best efforts to answer the query, the question remains: To what degree might the spinal lesion act as a neuroendocrine-immune stressor? Whether or not this mechanism plays a significant role or merely a modest or negligible role in health remains to be determined. Nevertheless, the human nervous system does appear to play an important functional role in immunologic competence. It seems reasonable to assume that postural and musculoskeletal abnormalities can affect this neural role in much the same way as psychic stressors (high-pitched tones) caused mice to become more susceptible to tumor "take" and viral and bacterial infections (44).

Moreover, given an initial case study that suggested a long-term boost in antibodies after chiropractic adjustments concomitant with pain relief (100) and in light of more scholarly controlled trials revealing even a temporary increase in respiratory burst in polymorphonuclear neutrophils, in priming of mononuclear cells for enhanced endotoxin-stimulating tumor necrosis factor production, and in increased substance P release after chiropractic manipulation (101, 102), it would seem that we are finally poised to begin to ask, and answer, some of the most important questions raised by the founder. Indeed, as we approach the chiropractic centennial and we ponder whether chiropractic will turn to the limited musculoskeletal specialty or to a wellness/wholistic provider model—a question that may well be influenced by how we address investigating the neurodystrophic hypothesis—we would do well to consider one of the many quips of the founder's son, B. J. Palmer:

> The world's progress is held back by just one thing—our universal unwillingness to grow (111).

Summary

This chapter has focused on the role of the nervous system in immunologic competence and on the possibility of its derangement in the presence of SDF, facilitation, and intervertebral subluxation. Primary and secondary immune responses can be demonstrated and inhibited in vitro (5–9). This fact and most traditional immunologic research suggested that the human immune response was largely independent of neural influence (3, 5–24, 92, 93).

The founder of chiropractic, however, believed that irritated nerves would result in "lowered tissue resistance" (1). The *neurodystrophic hypothesis*—that neural dysfunction is stressful to the visceral and other body structures, and this "lowered tissue resistance" can modify the nonspecific and specific immune responses, and alter the trophic function of the involved nerves" (1, 67–74)—was developed from his early writings.

Psychoneuroimmunologic research in the past decade has identified a strong relationship between CNS function and immunologic competence (34–41). Some of these researchers and others (39–41, 56–66, 75–86) have concluded that the nervous system is intimately involved in specific and nonspecific body defenses. Not only has a connection between portions of the hypothalamus and immune responses been established, but also a functional anatomical link between the thymus and the CNS has been identified (36, 37, 86–90). Other researchers have identified what they believe is a mechanism whereby the nervous system signals, guides, and directs the immune response (37, 56–64). Current evidence supports a role for norepinephrine-immunomodulation by a specific hypothalamic nuclei, the paraventricular nucleus (98).

There is overwhelming evidence to support the chiropractic *neurodystrophic hypothesis*, but there is scant evidence to directly link the spinal lesion with immunologic competence in human clinical studies. However, initial chiropractic investigations suggesting short- (94, 101, 102) and long-term (100) enhancement of certain immune functions after adjustments suggests a biological effect of chiropractic, although the clinical implications remain obscure and await further investigation.

REFERENCES

1. Palmer DD. The science, art and philosophy of chiropractic. Portland, Ore.: Portland Printing House, 1910:19.
2. Editors. Chiropractic: the unscientific cult. Chicago: AMA Department of Investigation, 1966.
3. Botta JR, ed. Chiropractors healers or quacks? Part 1: the 80-year war with science. Consumer Reports 1975;40:542–547.
4. Botta JR, ed. Chiropractor healers or quacks? Part 2: how chiropractors can help-or harm. Consumer Reports 1975;40:606–610.
5. Frobisher M, Fuerst R. Microbiology in health and disease. Philadelphia: WB Saunders, 1973:275–309.
6. Roitt IM. Essential immunology. Oxford: Blackwell, 1974:1–19, 43–82, 86–94, and 166.
7. Freedman SO, Gold P. Clinical immunology. Hagerstown, Md.: Harper & Row, 1976.
8. Hobart MJ, McConnell I. The immune system. Oxford: Blackwell, 1975.
9. Frelinger JA, Niederhuber JE, Schreffler DC. Inhibition of immune responses in vitro by

specific antiserums to Ia antigens. Science 1975;188:268–270.

10. Editors. Spotting invaders: Which cells decide? Sci News 1977;111:358.

11. Burnet FM. The clonal selection theory of acquired immunity. Nashville: Vanderbilt University Press, 1959:49–68.

12. Volpe EP, Turpen JB. Thymus: central role in the immune system of the frog. Science 1975;190:1101–1103.

13. Chandra RK. Antibody formation in first and second generation offspring of nutritionally deprived rats. Science 1975;190:289–290.

14. Mogensen S. Role of macrophages in natural resistance to virus infections. Microbiol Rev 1979;43:1–26.

15. Romagnani S, Maggi E, Lorenzini M, Giudizi GM, Biagiotti R, Ricci M. Study of some properties of the receptor for IgM on human lymphocytes. Clin Exp Immunol 1979;36:502–510.

16. Yodoi J, et al. Lymphocytes bearing Fc receptors for IgE. J Immunol 1979;123:455–460.

17. Fundenberg HH, ed. Basic and clinical immunology. Los Altos, Calif.: Lange, 1976.

18. Gell PGH, et al. Clinical aspects of immunology. Oxford: Blackwell, 1975.

19. Roberts NJ, Douglas RG, Simons RM, Diamond ME. Virus-induced interferon production by human macrophages. J Immunol 1979;123:365–369.

20. Calabrese JR. Dr. Calabrese replies. Am J Psychiatry 1988;145:537.

21. Briski KP, Sylvester PW. Effects of repetitive daily acute stress on pituitary LH and prolactin release during exposure to the same stressor or a second novel stress. Psychoneuroendocrinology 1987;12:429–437.

22. Perelson AS. Immune network theory. Immunol Rev 1989;110:5–36.

23. Coutinho A. Beyond clonal selection and network. Immunol Rev 1989;110:63–87.

24. Editors. Antibody construction. Science Digest, 16–17 Dec 1975.

25. Illich I. Medical nemesis. New York: Bantam, 1977.

26. Grant M. Handbook of community health. Philadelphia: Lea & Febiger, 1975.

27. Grey HM, Sette A, Buus S. How T cells see antigen. Sci Am 1989;257:56–64.

28. Wilson G. The hazards of immunization. London: Athlone Press, 1967.

29. Mendelsohn R. To immunize or not? It's a puzzler (nationally syndicated column). Des Moines Sunday Register, 4E, 1 Jan 1978.

30. Kotulak R. Dormant antiviral vaccines may be trouble years later. Chicago Tribune, 31 March 1975.

31. De Long R. Genetic manipulation. Science News, 31 July 1976.

32. Restak R. Meat cleaver or scalpel. Saturday Review, 26 Nov 1976.

33. Editors. Government using deception to sell vaccination program. Caveat Emptor 1976; 6:264.

34. Hall HR. Hypnosis and the immune system: a review with implications for cancer and the psychology of healing. Am J Clin Hypn 1983;25:92–103.

35. Gurkalo VK, Zabezhinski MA. On participation of the autonomic nervous system in the mechanisms of chemical carcinogenesis. Neoplasma 1982;29:301–307.

36. Brooks WH, Cross RJ, Roszman TL, Markesbery WR. Neuroimmunomodulation: neural anatomical basis for impairment and facilitation. Ann Neurol 1982;12:56–61.

37. Solomon GF, Amkraut AA. Psychoneuroendocrinological effects on the immune response. Annu Rev Microbiol 1981;35:155–184.

38. Keller SE, Weiss JM, Schleifer SJ, Miller NE, Stein M. Suppression of immunity by stress: effect of a graded series of stressors on lymphocyte stimulation in the rat. Science 1981;213:1397–1400.

39. Locke SE. Stress, adaptation, and immunity: studies in humans. Gen Hosp Psychiatry 1982;4:49–58.

40. Guth L. "Trophic" influences of nerve on muscle. Physiol Rev 1968;48:645–687.

41. Riley V. Psychoneuroendocrine influences on immunocompetence and neoplasia. Science 1981;212:1100–1109.

42. Selye H, Heuser G eds. Fifth annual report on stress. New York: MD Publications, 1956: 25–63.

43. Selye H. Stress and disease. New York: McGraw-Hill, 1956.

44. Stein M, Schiavi RC, Camerino M. Influence of brain and behavior on the immune system. Science 1976;191:435–440.

45. Macris MT, Schiavi RC, Camerino MS, Stein M. Effect of hypothalamic lesions on immune processes in the guinea pig. Am J Physiol 1970;219:1205–1209.

46. Greenspan J, Melchior J. The effect of osteopathic manipulative treatment on the resistance of rats to stressful situations. J Am Osteopath Assoc 1966;65:87–91.

47. Stein-Werblowsky R. The sympathetic nervous system and cancer. Exp Neurol 1974;42:97–100.

48. Editors. Social stress and the immune system. Sci News 1975;107:68–69.

49. Fabris N, Pierpaoli W, Sorkin E. Lymphocytes, hormones and ageing. Nature 1972; 240:557–559.

50. Denckla WD. Interactions between age and the neuroendocrine and immune systems. Fed Proc 1978;37:1263–1267.

51. Bilder GE, Denckla WD. Restoration of ability to reject xenografts and clear carbon after hypophysectomy of adult rats. Mech Ageing Dev 1977;6:153–163.

52. Van Dijk H, Jacobse-Geels H. Evidence for the involvement of corticosterone in the ontogeny of the cellular immune apparatus of the mouse. Immunology 1978;35:637–642.

53. Settipane GA, Pudupakkam RK, McGowan JH. Corticosteriod effect on immunoglobulins. J Allergy Clin Immunol 1978;62: 162–166.

54. Monjan AA, Collector MI. Stress-induced modulation of the immune response. Science 1977;196:307–308.

55. Murphy HM, Wideman CH, Brown TS. Plasma corticosterone levels and ulcer formation in rats with hippocampal lesion. Neuroendocrinology 1979;28:123–130.

56. Speransky AD. A basis for the theory of medicine. Leningrad: International Publications, 1943:144–160.

57. Speransky AD. Experimental and lobar pneumonia. Am Rev Soviet Med 1944; 2:22–27.

58. Kruntz A. Anatomic and physiologic properties of the cutaneo-visceral vasomotor reflex arc. J Neurophysiol 1945.

59. Kuntz A, Haselwood LA. Circulatory reactions in the gastrointestinal tract elicited by local cutaneous stimulation. Am Heart J 1940;20:743–749.

60. Kruntz A. Autonomic nervous system. Philadelphia: Lea & Febiger, 1945.

61. Gordienko AN, Tsynkalovskii RB, Saakov BA, Karnitskaya NV. Reflex mechanism of antibody production following intracutaneous administration of antigen with subsequent removal of antigen depot. In: Gordienko AN, ed. Control of immunogenesis by the nervous system. Washington, D.C.: National Technical Information Service, 1958: 38–43.

62. Gordienko AN, Kiseleva VI, Saakov BA, Bondarev IM, Zhigalini LI. The possibility of a reflex mechanism producing antibodies when antigen acts on skin receptors. In: Gordienko AN, ed. Control of immunogenesis by the nervous system. Washington, D.C.: National Technical Information Service, 1958:44–52.

63. Gordienko AN, Kiseleva VI, Saakov BA, Let'en AV. Electrophysiological phenomena in the nerve following action of antigens on the skin receptors. In: Gordienko An, ed. Control of immunogenesis by the nervous system. Washington, D.C.: National Technical Information Service, 1958:22–27.

64. Gordienko AN, ed. Control of immunogenesis by the nervous System. Washington, D.C.: National Technical Information Service, 1958:1–21.

65. Peterson WF, Müller EF. The splanchnoperipheral balance during chill and fever. Arch Intern Med 1927;40:573–593.

66. Arquin S. Stomach tonus and peripheral leukocyte count (splanchnoperipheral balance). Arch Intern Med 1928;41:913–923.

67. Palmer BJ. The subluxation specific—the adjustment specific. Davenport, Ia.: Palmer School of Chiropractic, 1934:95–99.

68. Verner JR, Weiant CW, Watkins RJ. Rational bacteriology. New York: published privately, 1953:204.

69. Watkins RJ. The neurology of immunization. Ohio Chiro Phys Assoc, 1–12, 1959.

70. Homewood AE. The neurodynamics of the vertebral subluxation. 3rd ed. St Petersburg, Fla.: Valkyrie Press, 1979.

71. Carver W. Carver's chiropractic analysis. Oklahoma City: Carver Chiropractic College, 1921.

72. Watkins RJ. Principles of nerve activity. Unpublished, 1978.

73. Janse J. History of the development of chiropractic concepts; chiropractic terminology. In: Goldstein M, ed. The research status of spinal manipulative therapy. Washington, D.C.: Government Printing Office, 1975: 25–42.

74. Gillet H, Ward L. A discussion on spinal stress. J Clin Chiro 1978;2:36–46.

75. Hoyrup E. Impaired adrenal function as a contributory factor in constitutional asthenia. Acta Psychiatr Neurol 1956;107[suppl]: 185–196.

76. Cooper IS. A neurologic evaluation of the cutaneous histamine reaction. J Clin Invest 1950;29:465–469.

77. Stanton A, Muenning L, Kopeloff LM, Kopeloff N. Spinal cord section and hemolysin production in the rat. J Immunol 1942; 44:237–246.

78. Schiavi RC, Macris NT, Camerino M, Stein M. Effect of hypothalamic lesions on immediate hypersensitivity. Am J Physiol 1975;228: 596–601.

79. Deason J. An experimental study of filariasis. Still Res Inst Bull 1916;2:191–215.

80. Rumney I. Osteopathic manipulative treatment of infectious diseases. In: Stark EH, ed. Osteopathic medicine. Acton, Mass.: Publication Sciences Group, 1975:165–169.

81. Korr IM. The spinal cord as organizer of disease processes: some preliminary perspectives. J Am Osteopath Assoc 1976;76:89–99.

82. Korr IM. Sustained sympathicotonia as a factor in disease. In: Korr IM, ed. The neurobiologic mechanisms in manipulative therapy. New York: Plenum, 1978:229–268.

83. Luparello TJ, Stein M, Park CD. Effect of hypothalamic lesions on rat anaphylaxis. Am J Physiol 1964;207:911–914.

84. Nayar KK, Arthur E, Balls M. The transmission of tumors induced in cockroaches by nerve severance. Experientia 1971;27: 183–184.

85. Gilsdorf RB, Long D, Moberg A, Leonard AS. Central nervous system influence on experimentally induced pancreatitis. JAMA 1965; 192:134–137.

86. Kaneko M, Hiroshige T. Fast, rate-sensitive corticosteriod negative feedback during stress. Am J Physiol 1978;234:R39–45.

87. Bulloch K, Moore RY. Innervation of the thymus gland by brain stem and spinal cord in mouse and rat. Am J Anat 1981;162:157–166.

88. Radford HM. The effect of hypothalamic lesions on estradiol-induced changes in LH release in the ewe. Neuroendocrinology 1979;28:307–312.

89. Gray GD, Smith ER, Damassa DA, Ehrenkranz JRC, Davidson JM. Neuroendocrine mechanisms mediating the suppression of circulating testosterone levels associated with chronic stress in male rats. Neuroendocrinology 1978;25:247–256.

90. Follenius E, Dubois MP. Distribution of fibres reacting with an α-endorphin antiserum in the neurohypophysis of Carassius auratus and Cyprinus carpio. Cell Tissue Res 1978;189:251–256.

91. Gutstein WH, Harrison J, Parl F, Kiu B, Avitable M. Neural factors contribute to atherogenesis. Science 1978;199:449–451.

92. Bleier R, Albrecht R, Cruce JAF. Suprapendymal cells of hypothalamic third ventricle: Identification as resident phagocytes of the brain. Science 1975;189:299–301.

93. Coffaro KA, Hinegardner RT. Immune response in the sea urchin Lytechinus pictus. Science 1977;197:1389–1390.

94. Vora GS, Bates HA. The effects of spinal manipulation on the immune system (a preliminary report). ACA J Chiro 1980;14:S103-S105.

95. Gold RR. The triune of life. Davenport, Ia.: International Chiropractic Association, 1966.

96. Cameron OG, Nesse RM. Review: systemic hormonal and physiological abnormalities in anxiety disorders. Psychoneuroendocrinology 1988;13:287–307.

97. Gurkalo VK, Zabezhinski MA. On participation of the autonomic nervous system in the mechanisms of chemical carcinogenesis. Neoplasma 1982;29:301–307.

98. Felton DL, Felton SY, Bellinger DL, et al. Noradrenergic sympathetic neural interactions with the immune system: structure and function. Immunol Rev 1987;100:225–260.

99. Tennant CC, Langeluddecke PM, Fulcher G, Wilby J. Acute and chronic life event stress in coronary atherosclerosis. J Psychosom Res 1988;32:13–20.

100. Alcorn SM. Antibodies and antigens—their definition, source and relevant function. J Aust Chiro Assoc 1978;11:18–37.

101. Brennan PC, Kokjohn K, Kaltinger CJ, et al. Enhanced phagocytic cell respiratory burst induced by spinal manipulation: potential role of substance P. J Manipulative Physiol Ther 1991;14:399–408.

102. Brennan PC, Triano JJ, McGregor M, Kokjohn K, Hondras M, Brennan DC. Enhanced neutrophil respiratory burst as a biological marker for manipulation forces: duration of the effect and association with substance P and tumor necrosis factor. J Manipulative Physiol Ther 1992;15:83–89.

103. Gil KM, Keefe FJ, Sampson HA, McCaskill CC, Rodin J, Crisson JE. The relation of stress and family environment to atopic dermatitis symptoms in children. J Psychosom Res 1987;31:673–684.

104. Solomon Z, Mikulincer M, Kotler M. A two year follow-up of somatic complaints among Israeli combat stress reaction casualties. J Psychosom Res 1987;31:463–469.

105. Halvorsen R, Vassend O. Effects of examination stress on some cellular immunity functions. J Psychosom Res 1987;31:693–701.

106. Mann AH, Brennan PJ. Type A behavior score and the incidence of cardiovascular disease: a failure to replicate the claimed associations. J Psychosom Res 1987;31:685–692.

107. Vernon HT, Dhami MSI, Howley TP, Annett R. Spinal manipulation and beta-endorphin: a controlled study of the effect of a spinal manipulation on plasma beta-endorphin levels in normal males. J Manipulative Physiol Ther 1986;9:115–123.

108. Christian GF, Stanton GJ, Sissons D, et al. Immunoreactive ACTH, β-endorphin and cortisol levels in plasma following spinal manipulative therapy. Spine 1988;13:1411–1417.

109. Koren T, Rosenwinkel E. Spinal patterns as predictors of personality profiles: a pilot study. Int J Psychosom 1992;39:10–17.

110. Dannenbring GL. Health psychology: implications for chiropractic research. J Manipulative Physiol Ther 1993;16:19–24.

111. Palmer BJ. As a man thinketh. Davenport, Ia.: Palmer School of Chiropractic, undated.

Chapter **15**

Axoplasmic Aberration Hypothesis

*F*irst noted by osteopathic researchers in 1962, chiropractic researchers at the University of Colorado have made great strides in documenting and quantifying the effects of trauma on the neural mechanism of axoplasmic transport (AXT) (1–6). One of the few studies by chiropractic researchers not at the University of Colorado was conducted by Fernandez (7).

Mechanisms of AXT have received much attention (8–19). There are fast and slow, or "bulk," AXT mechanisms, and AXT occurs in opposite directions along the nerve fiber (9–13, 18–25). In addition to proteins, glycoproteins, and neurotransmitters, constituents that are required for proper nerve growth and maintenance are mobilized by AXT (11, 20–25).

Triano and Luttges (1) and others at the University of Colorado have shown that even moderate compression or intermittent irritation can significantly block or alter AXT in spinal nerves (2–4, 43). Sjostrand et al. (26) have demonstrated vagal sensitivity to AXT block. The *axoplasmic aberration* hypothesis (i.e., that AXT may be altered in certain cases in which the spinal nerve roots or spinal nerves are compressed or irritated by intervertebral subluxation or facilitation) is discussed below in light of these and similar studies.

Unifying Transport Mechanism

The transport of axoplasmic components has been investigated frequently in the past decade. Weiss and Hiscoe (8) first noted that nerve growth might be influenced by axoplasm constituents. Later studies confirmed their observations and showed rapid or *fast axoplasmic transport* (FAXT) as well as "bulk flow," or slow, AXT mechanisms, which simultaneously carry a variety of constituents through nerves in probably all mammalian species (9, 10). Because the transport of these elements in neurons is not limited to the axon, Samson (9) has suggested that a more proper term would be neuroplasmic transport.

In addition to FAXT and slow AXT, there is transport of constituents in both directions inside nerve fibers. *Anterograde* or forward-moving products include those deemed important for nerve growth (11). *Retrograde*, or backward-moving, materials are transported from the nerve terminals to the cell bodies (11). Various researchers (14–17) have demonstrated chemicals that block AXT, in an attempt to develop a unifying concept to explain its mechanism.

Intracellular movement in neurons appears to be similar to that in all eukaryotic cells (9). Three primary areas have been ex-

323

plored with the electron microscope, AXT-blocking chemicals, and radioactive tracers (e.g., pulse-chase experiments): the plasma membrane, tubular organelles (endoplasmic reticulum and microtubular channels), and fibrillar elements (actomyosin, microfilaments, neurofilaments, and microtubules)(9).

One proposed mechanism for AXT is based on the fact that actomyosin is found universally in eukaryotic cells (10), and the actomyosin complex is responsible for nearly all of the intracellular and cellular movements. Because these units, known especially for their role in muscle fiber contraction, are also found in neurons, Allen (10) has suggested that they may perform a functional role in AXT. This is considered a unifying concept because it would explain why the movement seen in AXT is found throughout the animal kingdom. Probably, at least the intracellular movements involving bulk cytoplasmic transport (slow AXT) are motivated by actomyosin (9).

A similar proposal was based on the extensive studies of Ochs (12, 13, 18). Injection of ^{3}H-leucine or ^{3}H-lysine into L7 dorsal nerve root ganglion or into the motoneuron region of the spinal cord resulted in a characteristic crest, followed by a plateau, of transported labeled axoplasmic constituents (12). The rate for FAXT was constant, 410 ± 50 mm/day, regardless of nerve fiber size, diameter, and presence or absence of myelination. A wide variety of constituents, independent of their molecular weight, were found to move in this manner. Ochs (12, 13, 18) proposed a *sliding filament* hypothesis in which constituents bind to a transport filament that is transported by connecting cross-bridges (similar to actin/myosin) along the microtubules (MTs) and/or neurofilaments of the nerve fiber. Slow AXT actually involves materials exported into the nerve fibers later, from some storage space or compartment within the cell body, at a rate of 1 to 3 mm/day. Hence, slow AXT occurs because these constituents are released from the compartment over time, which explains the plateau seen in these studies (12, 13, 18).

Samson (19) agreed with the microtubule hypothesis, although he suggests direct binding to constituents with actomyosin cross-bridges. This is a unifying mechanism because MTs are found universally in the motile processes of flagella, sperm tails, and elsewhere in the cell. According to Samson, their intracellular location shows that they at least act as "guides" for AXT. Drugs that disrupt or have an affinity for MT protein subunits also stop AXT, which is further proof of their involvement (19).

Other mechanisms for AXT have been proposed, but these should suffice to indicate the complexity and specificity of AXT (9–13, 18, 19). We next consider the fact that both retrograde transport and anterograde transport occur, to determine the implications of nerve compression.

Anterograde and Retrograde AXT

As previously mentioned, both anterograde and retrograde AXT occurs. Anterograde movement involves greater numbers of constituents and is faster than retrograde AXT (anterograde FAXT occurs at 410 ± 50 mm/day; retrograde FAXT at 110–220 mm/day) (12, 13).

Anterograde movement of axoplasmic constituents involves the transport of products important for nerve growth mechanisms (11). These constituents are apparently synthesized in the nerve cell bodies and moved by AXT to the neuron terminals proximodistally (11). Embryonic sensory neurons depend on nerve growth factor (NGF) not only for growth but also for survival, at least in vitro (20). Anterograde AXT is also essential for transport of proteins and glycoproteins that maintain synaptic membranes and of other constituents of functional significance to the nerve endings (21). The role of AXT in supplying the *trophic* needs of tissue, even if only neural tissue, cannot be overemphasized.

Bjoerklund et al. (22) have shown that transplants preincubated in a medium containing NGF are more densely and more rapidly innervated by adrenergic fibers.

Moreover, preincubation of these transplants in media containing antibodies to NGF markedly impairs the reinnervation of the transplant with adrenergic nerve fibers (22). Similarly, sectioning the peripheral processes of rat sciatic nerve affects the substance P (a neurotransmitter) content of dorsal horns (23), which was attributed to neural degeneration and subsequent arrest of AXT (anterograde) (23). There is evidence that substance P is a transmitter for primary afferent fibers, specifically for nociceptive afferents in the substantia gelatinosa of the spinal cord (27, 28). These studies verify that anterograde AXT is an important, if not an essential, factor in the maintenance of the neuromuscular system.

Retrograde AXT involves materials that are transported from nerve terminals to the cell bodies, including NGF (24, 25). NGF is taken up selectively into sympathetic neurons and is transported to the cell body, where it apparently regulates the production of enzymes involved in transmitter synthesis; nerve activity does not affect the AXT of NGF (29). NGF acts only on the neurons that transport it, and there is no evidence that NGF is released to act on extracellular sites (30). Treatment of newborn animals with antibodies to NGF causes widespread sympathetic nervous system destruction (25). The retrograde transport of NGF is probably necessary for the development and maintenance of innervating adrenergic neurons (25). Thus both retrograde and anterograde AXT are important to neuromuscular development and maintenance.

Nerve Compression and AXT

Nerve compression may play a significant role in aberrant AXT. Although Ochs (31) has shown that compressive forces of 300 mm Hg block FAXT in sciatic nerve, lesser pressures can produce that result. Using ^{3}H-leucine, Sjostrand et al. (26) demonstrated FAXT block in sensory vagus nerve after only 50 mm Hg pressure maintained for 2 hours (32), demonstrating the extreme susceptibility of AXT to compression trauma.

This block was reversed within 1 day; greater pressures required longer recovery times (26, 32). In contrast, much greater pressures are required to block nerve conduction (33–35). Apparently, among the most probable explanations for FAXT block by nerve compression is the possibility that local ischemia or changes in the ionic environment dramatically alter the normal AXT mechanism (31). This is consistent with the fact that alteration of the ionic balance within neurons can block FAXT (12, 13, 31).

Studies at the University of Colorado, under the direction of Suh (1–4, 36–38), have thoroughly documented the protein composition of peripheral nerves in health and disease. Using modern electrophoretic and electrophysiologic techniques, Luttges et al. (2) more specifically analyzed degenerative and regenerative events within the neuron, using sodium dodecyl sulfate polyacrylamide gel electrophoresis (SDS-PAGE) of subcellular fractions. They identified more than 40 major protein bands with this system (2, 3) (Fig. 15.1). These proteins were analyzed during nerve degeneration following various types of experimentally induced traumata, including nerve crush, ligation, and section. In comparison with those in control nerves, some proteins exhibited increased composition and others exhibited decreased composition. One early study indicated that nerve conduction capacity varied in proportion to the apparent deterioration of nerve proteins (2); cut and ligation-type injuries produced more severe damage than crush injuries.

To determine more precisely the damage involved with crush injuries, Luttges and Groswold (4) used fine forceps to crush a 2-mm area of mouse sciatic nerve. After 10 days, electrophoretic and histologic examinations revealed only minimal discoloration and swelling in the sciatic nerve proximal to the zone of injury. Distal to the injury, however, large decreases were noted in some proteins (myelin, glycoprotein, and slow- and fast-migrating basic proteins (BP_{S1}, BP_{S2}, BP_{F1}, and BP_{F2}; S1 and F1 indicate slow and fast AXT, respectively), along with obvious swelling and discoloration (Table 15.1). For

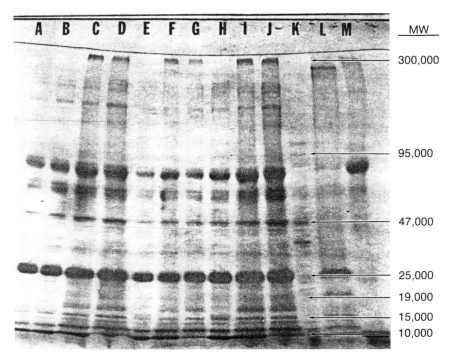

Figure 15.1. Samples of proximal (*A* and *B*), distal (*C*), and control (*D*) sciatic nerve proteins following midthigh sciatic nerve ligation. Estimates of molecular weight (*MW*) are based on T_3 bacteriophage proteins (*K*) and autoradiographic techniques. Other samples involve variations in extraction and centrifugation procedures, as well as in the amount of protein being analyzed. Using an SDS-PAGE system, Luttges and co-workers (2–4) identified more than 40 major protein bands in mouse sciatic nerve (see text). (From Suh CH. Researching the fundamentals of chiropractic. In: Suh CH, ed. Proceedings of the 5th Annual Biomechanics Conference on the Spine. Boulder, Colo.: University of Colorado, 1974:1–52.)

every 4 glycoprotein molecules, there were 2 BP_F and 1 BP_S, which appeared to migrate as a unit. Luttges et al. believed that this might be some type of axoplasmic functional unit.

Finally, Luttges, Stodieck, and Beel (6) studied the biomechanical characteristics of sciatic nerve and associated spinal roots of mice after crush injuries and determined that both nerve and roots differ considerably in sustained force before failure and in other biomechanical properties. A 1-mm longitudinal section of the sciatic nerve in adult mice was crushed with mosquito forceps covered with tape; the nerve was inspected and the wound closed. Although antibiotics were not administered, infections were rare. Animals were sacrificed 0–21 days after crush and nerves were quickly removed and

coated with mineral oil. Spinal column containing lumbar segments was similarly dissected. Both the sciatic nerves and their corresponding roots were tested for stretch, and after mechanical testing, nerve and root materials were collected, and PAGE analysis (with Coomassie brilliant blue stain) for type and amount of protein was made.

Two-tailed *t* tests and ANOVA revealed significant alterations in postcrush nerves and roots. For example, the average load required to bring roots to their proportional limit was 2.73 g, a value that was 30 times less than that needed to bring the nerves to the proportional limit. Moreover, while the elasticity of roots was comparable to that of nerves, stiffness was five times lower than in nerves. Finally, by structural protein analysis,

Table 15.1
Characteristics of Mouse Protein following Crush Injury to Sciatic Nerve[a]

Degenerative Characteristics	Regenerative Characteristics
Proximal to midthigh crush By the tenth day, slight discoloration and slight edema; slight decrements of myelin glycoprotein and certain fast-migrating basic proteins	*Proximal and distal to midthigh crush* A. Decreased levels of certain slow-migrating basic proteins B. At 21 days, increments in some basic proteins distal to nerve crush and decrements in some proteins proximal to crush; myelin increases and concentrations of nuclear histones are evident at 35 days C. Between 40 and 50 days, protein characteristics return to normal
Proximal and distal to midthigh crush A. By 10 days, nuclear histones are discernible B. By the thirtieth day, migration of certain fast-migrating basic proteins and histones C. Histones increase, then decrease in quantity D. Increases of certain proteins during degeneration	*Distal to midthigh crush* A. By 21 days, increased slow- and fast-migrating proteins and myelin glycoprotein B. At 21 days, protein of high molecular weight increases in quantity; other proteins show increments at this point also
Distal to midthigh crush By the tenth day, discoloration and edema; decrements of myelin glycoprotein and slow- and fast-migrating basic proteins	

[a]From Luttges MW, Groswald DE. Degenerative and regenerative characterizations in the proteins of mouse sciatic nerves. In Suh CH, ed. Proceedings of the 7th Annual Biomechanics Conference on the Spine. Boulder, Colo.: University of Colorado, 1976:71–81.

regenerating nerve contains many more cells, especially Schwann cells. The authors note that damaged nerve does not regain normal internodal spacing (nodes of Ranvier), which remains about one-half that of undamaged nerves; this may be associated with the continuing decreased nerve conduction velocities noted by researchers (6).

These scientists appear to be well on the way to characterizing degenerative and regenerative events; however, Hart (39) points out that this research should lead to further investigation, which has not been forthcoming. A search of the *Index to Chiropractic Literature* and the *Journal of Manipulative and Physiologic Therapeutics* failed to reveal any further citations from 1987 to 1992.

Discussion

As seen in Chapter 10, intervertebral subluxations may result in foraminal encroach-ment in all areas of the human spine, and the likelihood of subsequent neural involvement is greatest in the cervical and lumbar regions where the diameter of spinal nerve in comparison with the intervertebral foramen is largest. Neurophysiologists have determined that nerve roots are highly susceptible to compression block but that spinal nerves are very resistant to block (33–35). This chapter has shown that delivery of constituents to various locations in the nerve cell by AXT is a highly important aspect of neuronal function. The vagus nerve is susceptible to AXT block when even minimal pressures are applied (50 mm Hg for 2 hours) (26, 32).

The possibility of damaging the blood-nerve barrier (40) has not been discussed in this chapter. However, even pressures of 600 mm Hg applied for 4 hours do not affect the blood-nerve barrier; consequently, this aspect of neuronal function has been given little attention (41).

Several important points should be kept in mind with regard to the effect of compression on neuronal function. Nerve conduction, axonal transport, and blood-nerve barrier are all affected by trauma. They differ, however, in susceptibility and reversibility and may be differentially affected (42). Although some researchers have found a correlation between regeneration and AXT, others have not (2, 4, 12, 43–45). Cuenod (44) reported that AXT can recover in the absence of nerve regeneration and that block of AXT by colchicine does not cause nerve degeneration, even after 6 weeks.

In their classical study of the effect of mild, intermittent irritation of mouse sciatic nerves (by a Silastic implant) on conduction velocity and chemical composition (via electrophoretic analysis), Triano and Luttges (1) found altered vascular composition of albumin and red blood cells. It may be assumed that these changes were due to alterations in AXT. The clinical implications of this finding include the possibility that many of the varied and diffuse descriptions of sciatic distributed pain, numbness, etc. may be the result of altered AXT and subsequent toxic levels of proteins in various portions of the nerve. The patient who proudly proclaims, "Doctor, you must be helping; that pain is moving on down my leg," may be describing reversal of AXT block. Obviously, it is too soon to make accurate predictions, but the evidence clearly demonstrates the relative susceptibility of nerve to AXT block or irritation, and this may indeed be one chemical basis for pain in many neuromuscular pain syndromes treated by the chiropractor.

These studies indicate that AXT is a specific and important mechanism for the maintenance, repair, and growth of the nervous system. They suggest that the clinical evaluation of damage to this mechanism may be currently impossible, since damage to AXT may occur with or without damage to nerve conduction and blood-nerve barrier.

Early work by Korr (5) and other osteopathic investigators yielded much information: (a) spikes or waves of axoplasmic transport were observed and (b) each of four waves carries different types of proteins; (c) transfer of protein from nerve to muscle varies from nerve-to-nerve transport; (d) transfer of proteins across the junction is selective; (e) the neuron supplies protein for muscle that is not found in the muscle, and hence, (f) some proteins synthesized in nerve are destined for muscle, others for nerve. Further, based on numerous studies, they concluded that spinal segmental facilitation would alter AXT. (This may be expected since facilitation is thought to be associated with ischemic events that certainly affect adjacent neuromuscular junctions; see Chapter 8.) More recent evidence continues to support the concept that neuropathy proceeds as a direct result of accumulated decrements in retrograde axon transport, at least in some cases. These studies appear to confirm the axoplasmic aberration hypothesis, since in those cases in which intervertebral subluxation or facilitation (preceded by the most common form of VSC, the segmental dysfunction of phase 1) does affect the spinal nerves or roots, AXT may certainly be altered with significant consequences.

Summary

Axoplasmic transport (AXT) mechanisms have been studied in some detail, and microtubules, actomyosin, and some transport filament may be involved (8–19). AXT is an important mechanism for the transfer of specific proteins, glycoproteins, other constituents, and NGF in the neuron (12, 13, 21–24). Although nerve conduction, AXT, and the blood-nerve barrier respond differently to various insults, AXT is more susceptible to compression trauma (26, 31). The axoplasmic aberration hypothesis appears to be valid, in that when spinal nerves or roots are compressed or irritated by intervertebral subluxation or segmental facilitation, AXT may certainly be altered with significant consequences.

REFERENCES

1. Triano JJ, Luttges MW. Nerve irritation: a possible model of sciatic neuritis. Spine 1982;7:129–136.

2. Luttges MW, Kelly PT, Gerren RA. Degenerative changes in mouse sciatic nerves: electrophoretic and electrophysiologic characterization. Exp Neurol 1976;50:706–733.

3. Kelly PT, Luttges MW. Electrophoretic separation of nervous system proteins on exponential gradient polyacrylamide gels. J Neurochem 1975;24:1077–1079.

4. Luttges MW, Groswald DE. Degenerative and regenerative characterizations in the proteins of mouse sciatic nerves. In: Suh CH, ed. Proceedings of the 7th Annual Biomechanics Conference on the Spine. Boulder, Colo.: University of Colorado, 1976:71–81.

5. Korr IM. The spinal cord as organizer of disease processes: IV. Axonal transport and neurotrophic function in relation to somatic dysfunction. J Am Osteopath Assoc 1981; 80:451–459.

6. Luttges MW, Stodieck LS, Beel JA. Postinjury changes in the biomechanics of nerves and roots in mice. J Manipulative Physiol Ther 1986;9:89–98.

7. Fernandez JL. The transport of protein in nerves. ACA J Chiro 1972;10:17–24.

8. Weiss P, Hiscoe HB. Experiments on the mechanism of nerve growth. J Exp Zool 1948;107:315–395.

9. Samson F. Axonal transport: the mechanisms and their susceptibility to derangement; anterograde transport. In: Korr IM, ed. The neurobiologic mechanisms in manipulative therapy. New York: Plenum, 1978:291–309.

10. Allen RD. Some new insights concerning cytoplasmic transport. Symp Soc Exp Biol 1974;8:15–26.

11. Warwick R, Williams P, eds. Gray's anatomy. 35th ed. Philadelphia: WB Saunders, 1973: 773.

12. Ochs S. A brief review of material transport in nerve fibers. In: Goldstein M, ed. The research status of spinal manipulative therapy. Washington, D.C.: Government Printing Office, 1975:189–196.

13. Ochs S, Chan SY, Worth R. Calcium and the mechanism of axoplasmic transport. In: Korr IM, ed. The neurobiologic mechanisms in manipulative therapy. New York: Plenum, 1978:359–367.

14. Bunt AH, Lund RD. Vinblastine induced blockage of orthograde and retrograde axonal transport of protein in retinal ganglion cells. Exp Neurol 1974;45:288–297.

15. Shelanski ML, Taylor EW. Isolation of a protein subunit from microtubules. J Cell Biol 1967;34:549–554.

16. Wilson L, Bamburg JR, Mizel SB, Grisham LM, Creswell KM. Interaction of drugs with microtubular proteins. Fed Proc 1974;33: 158–166.

17. Zweig MH, Chignell CF. Interaction of some colchicine analogs, vinblastine and podophyllotoxin with rat brain microtubular protein. J Biochem Pharmacol 1973;22:2141–2150.

18. Ochs S. Characteristics and a model for fast axoplasmic transport in nerve. J Neurobiol 1971;2:331–345.

19. Samson FE. Mechanism of axoplasmic transport. J Neurobiol 1971;2:347–360.

20. Stach RW, Stach BM, West NR. Nerve fiber outgrowth from dorsal root ganglia: ion dependency of nerve growth factor action. J Neurochem 1979;33:845–855.

21. Goodrum JF. Axonal transport and metabolism of ^{3}H fucose- and ^{35}S sulfate-labeled macromolecules in the rat visual system. Brain Res 1979;176:255–272.

22. Bjoerklund A, Bjerre B, Steneri U. Has nerve growth factor a role in the regeneration of central and peripheral catecholamine neurons? In: Fuxe K, Olson L, Zotterman Y, eds. Dynamics of regeneration and growth in neurons. New York: Pergamon, 1974:389–409.

23. Jessell T, Tsunoo A, Kanazawa I, Otsuka M. Substance P: depletion in the dorsal horn of rat spinal cord after section of the peripheral processes of primary sensory neurons. Brain 1979;Res 168:247–259.

24. Johnson EM, Blumberg HM, Costrini NV, Bradshaw RA. Reduction by reserpine of the accumulation of retrogradely transported 125 nerve growth factor in sympathetic neurons. Brain Res 1979;178:389–401.

25. Stoeckel K, Paravicini U, Thoenen H. Specificity of the retrograde axonal transport of nerve growth factor. Brain Res 1974;76:413–421.

26. Sjostrand J, Rydevik B, Lundborg G, McLean WG. Impairment of intraneural microcirculation, blood nerve barrier and axonal transport in experimental nerve ischemia and compression. In: Korr IM, ed. The neurobiologic mechanisms in manipulative therapy. New York: Plenum, 1978:337–355.

27. Nakata Y, Kusaka Y, Segawa T. Supersensitivity to substance P after dorsal root section. Life Sci 1979;24:1651–1654.

28. Piercey MF, Dobry PJK, Schroeder LA, Einspahr FJ. Behavioral evidence that substance P may be a spinal cord sensory neurotransmitter. Brain Res 1981;210:407–412.

29. Lees G, Chubb I, Freeman C, Geffen L, Rush R. Effect of nerve activity on transport of nerve growth factor and dopamine β-hydroxylase antibodies in sympathetic neurones. Brain Res 1981;214:186–189.

30. Hendry IA, Bonyhady R. Retrogradely transported nerve growth factor increases ornithine decarboxylase activity in rat superior cervical ganglia. Brain Res 1980;200:39–45.

31. Ochs S. Energy metabolism and supply of P to the fast axoplasmic transport mechanism in nerve. Fed Proc 1974;33:1049–1058.

32. Rydevik B, McLean WG, Sjostrand J, Lundborg G. Blockage of axonal transport induced by acute, graded compression of the rabbit vagus nerve. J Neurol Neurosurg Psychiatry 1980;43:690–698.

33. Aguayo A, Nair CPV, Midgley R. Experimental progressive compression neuropathy in the rabbit. Arch Neurol 1971;24:358–364.

34. Rainer GW, Mayer J, Sadler TR, Dirks D. Effect of graded compression on nerve conduction velocity. Arch Surg 1973;107:719–721.

35. Sharpless SK. Susceptibility of spinal roots to compression block. In: Goldstein M, ed. The research status of spinal manipulative therapy. Washington, D.C.: Government Printing Office, 1975:155–161.

36. Suh CH. Researching the fundamentals of chiropractic. In: Suh CH, ed. Proceedings of the 5th Annual Biomechanics Conference on the Spine. Boulder, Colo.: University of Colorado, 1974:1–52.

37. MacGregor RJ. A model for reticular-like networks: ladder nets, recruitment fuses, and sustained responses. Brain Res 1972;41:345–363.

38. MacGregor RJ, Oliver RM. A general-purpose electronic model for arbitrary configurations of neurons. J Theor Biol 1973;38:527–538.

39. Hart RE. Letter to the editor. J Manipulative Physiol Ther 1987;10:135.

40. Kolber AR, Bagnell CR, Krigman MR, Hayward J, Morell P. Transport of sugars into microvessels isolated from rat brain: a model for the blood-brain barrier. J Neurochem 1979;33:419–432.

41. Sjostrand J. Discussion. In: Korr IM, ed. The neurobiologic mechanisms in manipulative therapy. New York: Plenum, 1978:369–373.

42. Sjostrand J. Discussion. In: Korr IM, ed. The neurobiologic mechanisms in manipulative therapy. New York: Plenum, 1978: 357–358.

43. Spencer PS. Reappraisal of the model for `bulk axoplasmic flow.' Nature New Biol 1972;240:283–285.

44. Cuenod M. Contributions of axoplasmic transport to synaptic structures and functions. Int J Neurosci 1972;4:77–87.

45. Moretto A, Sabri MI. Progressive deficits in retrograde axon transport precede degeneration of motor axons in acrylamide neuropathy. Brain Res 1988;440:18–24.

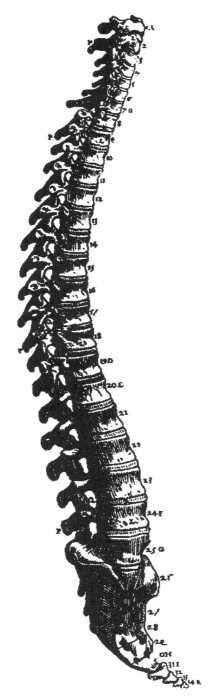

Section **5**

Approaches to Developing Chiropractic Science

The quality of a person's life is in direct proportion to their commitment to excellence, regardless of their chosen field of endeavor.

Vincent T. Lombardi

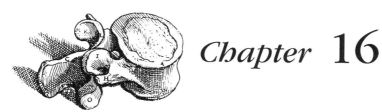

Chapter **16**

Developing Chiropractic Scientist-Practitioners

*T*hree approaches to a theory of science and scientific knowledge have been presented: the subjective, the consensual, and the objective (1). The subjective approach considers the individual scientist's beliefs about evidentiary support to be supremely important, with those of the scientific community holding secondary status (1). The consensual approach holds that every aspect of science depends primarily upon social consensus of the particular scientific group (1). Some believe that reliable standards of care are best determined by those who provide that care, through the consensual approach (2). The objective approach posits that science, the practice of science, scientific methods, and scientific knowledge exist whether or not a particular group adopts them (1).

Perhaps the best argument for adopting a new method for developing scientific knowledge about chiropractic is found in the experiences of clinical psychologists, who attended a consensus conference in August 1949 in Boulder, Colorado:

> The manifest lack of dependable knowledge in clinical psychology and personality demands that research be considered a vital part of the field of clinical psychology (3).

Out of that conference a process was developed to orient new graduates toward becoming scientist practitioners. A *scientific practitioner* adopts the principles and methods of science in clinical practice. A *scientist/practitioner* (S/P) contributes to the advancement of science in the profession, through clinical research and publication (3).

A critical thinker reading this text must conclude that a number of testable hypotheses in chiropractic need clinical research before serious clinical applications can be fully explored. The S/P model offers hope that a large body of scientific research can be developed within chiropractic—as it was within psychology—to help meet the research needs of clinicians. This research can only be developed relatively soon if a large number of S/Ps regularly contribute to chiropractic *scientific literature* (i.e., peer-reviewed, preferably indexed, journals; Table 16.1).

Another argument for adoption of the S/P model for chiropractic clinicians is that currently an effort is under way to define chiropractic science *and practice* not by subjective or objective approaches, but by consensus. *Recently*, RAND researchers (4) and Mercy Conference (5) attendees used variations of consensual processes to define chiropractic practice standards. Only when large numbers of chiropractic clinicians adopt principles and practices of science and regularly contribute to the chiropractic science literature, can they expect to meaningfully contribute to the consensus process. This is because consensus conference atten-

Table 16.1.
Peer-reviewed, Chiropractic Science Journals in 1994

Chiropractic History Journal[a]
Chiropractic Research Journal
Chiropractic Sports Medicine
Chiropractic Technique
European Journal of Chiropractic
Journal of the Australian Chiropractic Association
Journal of the Canadian Chiropractic Association
Journal of Chiropractic Education[a]
Journal of Chiropractic Research
Journal of the Neuromusculoskeletal System
Journal of Manipulative and Physiological Therapeutics[b]

[a] Not a journal of applied clinical science but is peer-reviewed.
[b] Only chiropractic science journal indexed by *Index Medicus* and available on-line through the National Library of Medicine's literature search and retrieval system, *Medline*.

dees—by choice—must base their arguments for or against a procedure or protocol on literature appearing in peer-reviewed, science journals (5). *Clinicians in practice cannot contribute to the consensus process effectively by merely sitting on such panels; instead, they must contribute to the literature that future Mercy-style consensus conference attendees will debate.*

One of the early advocates for chiropractic research, C. O. Watkins, D.C., perhaps explained most simply why we need chiropractic S/Ps(6):

the science of chiropractic is the responsibility of chiropractors.

Clinicians can team up with university and chiropractic college–based professional researchers in a sort of "buddy system" to help prioritize the research needs of practitioners (6). This is especially important when a small profession such as chiropractic lacks the federal funding for research that other even smaller professions such as osteopathy have at their disposal.

In 1985, the Foundation for Chiropractic Education and Research (FCER)—the primary funding agency for research in chiropractic—was distributing less than a third of a million dollars for clinical research, while the American Osteopathic Association's board of trustees funded 33 of 45 proposals worth a similar amount, $316,997 (7, 8). In 1985, federal and outside source funding for

chiropractic research was zero dollars, while total federal and outside source funding for osteopathic research was in excess of $15 million (8). Even by 1993, projected FCER and proposed meager federal funding does not approach a tenth of that figure (FCER funding for education and research in 1992/1993 was $945,826; E. Reichel, personal communication).

Clearly, chiropractic continues to be locked out of federal help for our research efforts, despite convincing evidence for the superiority and cost-effectiveness of chiropractic care, at least for certain back pain syndromes, and despite the fact that chiropractors probably treat many more patients annually than do osteopaths (see Section II and especially Chapter 9).

A polarizing influence within the chiropractic community, regarding development of attitudes of science, was aided by the influence of political medicine (9). In creating a "Catch-22" by condemning chiropractic education as inadequate, while simultaneously denying D.C. faculty and students access to hospital environments that could help overcome the deficiencies in chiropractic clinical training, organized medicine has—wittingly or unwittingly—helped solidify antimedical and antiscience attitudes within some chiropractors (9). Even today, these sentiments run so deeply within the profession that only a groundswell of new S/Ps, whose goal is to advance the science and clinical effectiveness of chiropractic, may be able to finally overcome these remaining effects of the medical boycott of the 1960s and 1970s (10).

By one account, only 0.6% of the profession has contributed to the chiropractic scientific literature in North America and Australia, and only 0.1% contributes to the literature regularly (11). And while some argue that we need theories that provide testable hypotheses, others point out that our theories currently lack practical applications, owing to a lack of clinical research (12, 13). These arguments underscore the need to adopt the S/P model within chiropractic, but other, more practical considerations point in this direction as well. For example, studies continue to confirm that patients attending chiropractic college teaching clinics have less intense pain, report less worker time loss, and report less disability than those presenting to private chiropractic offices (14). Chiropractic S/Ps can help meet critical research needs by pooling their patients who have more robust pain levels with patients from college outpatient settings in multicenter trials and by using single subject and other novel research methodologies whenever applicable (see Chapter 17).

This chapter explores approaches to philosophy, attitudes, and issues related to the development of scientist/practitioners within our ranks and briefly addresses related issues in chiropractic education, in development of standards of care, and in the fostering of advances in chiropractic research by individual chiropractors. These issues are at the core of the continued development of the science of chiropractic and perhaps are at the core of our very survival in the coming 21st century.

Which Philosophy of Chiropractic?

Universally, modern clinical psychologists trace dysfunction in an adult to the roots established in childhood. Perhaps that is why it took a clinical psychologist, Dr. Joseph Keating, to help the chiropractic pro-

fession focus our attention on our current and past philosophies and the role of our history in creating some of the antiscience dysfunction that is within us today (1, 6, 9). An astute therapist gently works with his patient to gain confidence and trust before the necessary confrontations with the past that are so unsettling yet necessary for growth beyond dysfunction, so Keating (15) endears us by his histories of the philosophies of "Old Dad Chiro" (the founder, D. D. Palmer; see Chapter 4) while he confronts us with the reality that some of our early theosophical roots appear to confound the development of our science—and of S/Ps—today (16).

This section briefly explores arguments regarding which philosophy chiropractic should adopt.

SHOULD THEOSOPHY HAVE A ROLE IN CHIROPRACTIC PHILOSOPHY?

Despite Ian Coulter's (17) plea that critical rationalism is the only philosophy the chiropractic profession must adopt, others continue to argue that Universal Intelligence (i.e., God) has a place in chiropractic philosophy and that this "theosophy" is what makes chiropractic so special:

> Trying to mix mysticism with metaphor, theology with theory, religion with science is exactly what makes chiropractic dynamic, unique, and controversial. This process offers a hint of still to be discovered paradigms of human health and illness that may be too complex for our present scientific rationale (18).

While the branch of philosophy dealing with *metaphysics* (i.e., beyond the physical world; religion, ghosts, magic, the transcendental, and anything that we cannot physically measure, see, touch, or define) may not be essential for chiropractic science, nor for any science (19), there are chiropractic philosophers who believe it need not be abandoned:

> Chiropractic philosophy must be freed from its primitive catechismal chains and be allowed to flower within and beyond metaphysics, into epistemology, logic and ethics (20).

CHIROPRACTIC PHILOSOPHY: DYNAMIC OR STATIC?

However, if Charlton (20) allows a role for metaphysics in the philosophy of chiropractic, he emphasizes its role must be dynamic, debatable, and not based on dogmatic adherence to the initial philosophies espoused by the founders of chiropractic:

Unfortunately, much of what some of us have called chiropractic philosophy has been a rehash of DD, BJ, Stephenson and others [see Chapter 4] as if it were a catechism passed on by apostolic chant. Our forebearers began chiropractic philosophy, they did not end it! There was no formal closure of the cask! We can, in fact, we must aggressively promote philosophical discourse in chiropractic (20).

In line with this thinking, the philosopher W. Randall Albury, Ph.D., (21) holds that chiropractic should make a serious attempt to develop a current chiropractic philosophy, much as a mature person makes an effort to develop an awareness of self. However, rather than being noncritical of chiropractic philosophy and rather than holding to initial chiropractic Palmeran philosophy as if it were a religion, Albury states:

The examination and development of chiropractic philosophy is chiefly a matter for the profession itself to pursue or not, as it judges best. It may even wish to disown its philosophy or let it die quietly from neglect. But if as a group the profession does intend to have a chiropractic philosophy, my plea as an outsider is: please make it a questioning chiropractic philosophy (21).

Instead Barge (22) seems to argue that chiropractors should cling to original Palmeran philosophy:

We are a God in Man philosophy, a hands on healing art, rather than deny our philosophical concepts we should cherish and ameliorate our concepts of Cause and Cure. Let those who would follow the medical model "become part of medicine, they are more akin to it than chiropractic."

Yet even within the so-called straight chiropractic philosophical camp, others such as Richards (23) and Strang (24) agree with Albury (21) that chiropractic philosophy should be "alive, ever ready to accommodate new, relevant discoveries in science" (24).

Perhaps Donahue (25) summarizes the problem best in his paper proposing the development of a contemporary philosophy of chiropractic. Stating that we must use philosophy to define who we are as chiropractors as well as what we do and that this in turn defines our research priorities, he laments the current state of purported "philosophical" discourse within the profession:

Chiropractic philosophy, on the other hand has been nothing more than the espousing of dogmatic, doctrinaire tenets which have served to stagnate the intellectual process of those who "believe" and polarize those who disbelieve. A few of the "believers" of the chiropractic profession are very involved at college homecomings, conventions or practice building seminars. As a result, their voice is far out of proportion to their professional importance. Since the rank and file majority of the profession do not object or passively participate, they lend them tacit support. The result is that chiropractors are beginning to lose their sense of who and what they are, and where they are going. Therefore a new—contemporary—kind of chiropractic philosophy needs to be developed to replace the inadequate old. It has been suggested in this paper that such a philosophy may be as important to future research as is the research itself (25).

INFLUENCE OF CHIROPRACTIC PHILOSOPHY ON RESEARCH ADVOCACY

Keating (26) and others (7, 27) hold that adherence to original chiropractic Palmeran philosophy (theosophy?) has hindered development of the science of chiropractic (see also Chapter 4). If Palmeran theosophy (viz., belief that adjustive correction of upper cervical subluxation unites man with God) is taken to the extreme, since one cannot absolutely prove or disprove the presence or absence of God in man, why perform research? Indeed, "chiropractic works—our patients prove it everyday" (7).

Probably only a very small percentage of chiropractors today hold such rigid beliefs, but they are vocal and politically active. Barriers to research production in chiropractic have included—in addition to dogmatic adherence to Palmeran theosophy—a number of misinformed and antiscientific attitudes (Table 16.2). Only when such attitudes are systematically debated and overturned will a broader base of support for research advocacy and production be developed (7). Each individual chiropractor is responsible for the lack of progress in the development of science in chiropractic, and by developing an attitude of advocacy for scientific method, by reading and supporting chiropractic science journals, and by supporting chiropractic research with financial contributions, the individual clinician—as a scientific practitioner or as an S/P—can influence others and help promote advances in chiropractic science and practice (7, 29).

Instead of the philosophy of chiropractic being the rationale for abandoning research or an explanation for a dogma that is not debatable (in which context *research* may be advocated for public relations purposes rather than as a natural extension of gaining

new knowledge to enhance patient care through critical rationalism), Donahue (25) holds that philosophy should guide research priorities.

Issues in Chiropractic Education

Despite a long struggle against limited funding and organized medicine, chiropractic education has made almost incredible advances—by almost any measure—since 1974, when the U.S. Office of Education recognized the Council on Chiropractic Education as the sole accrediting agency for chiropractic colleges (30). Yet education of chiropractic doctors as S/Ps has apparently not been a consistent goal of the colleges.

Jamison (31) studied practitioners in Australia and noted that largely they failed to understand the power of various research designs to provide clinically useful data. Apparently chiropractic students at most colleges are not taught the nuances of critical rationalism, and field practitioners do not typically read science journals but instead rely on trade journals for most of their infor-

Table 16.2.
Chiropractic Practitioner Attitudes That Hinder the Development of Science and the Scientist/Practitioner Model

Attitude/Belief	Response
Medicine will "steal" adjustment if we publish research	Organized medicine will only "steal" adjustments if medical instead of chiropractic researchers establish its effectiveness
It is unethical to withhold treatment from a control group	It is unethical not to perform research that will establish how effective your care really is
Chiropractic works! Our patients prove it every day!	I agree! Unfortunately, we do know how much is due to placebo, spontaneous remission, and how often it works or fails for a great majority of applications; and what are those limitations of matter we learned of in philosophy class?
We may not be able to prove that chiropractic works	Ultimately, only adjustments that are more effective than placebo or "suggestion" for given applications should be used
Chiropractic involves the use of "Innate" forces that cannot be measured	Maybe so. However, so does a neck hug, a smile, a comforting grasp of the hand, or a compliment; only legitimate research can determine if there is more to chiropractic than these psychosomatic responses
You cannot create a true sham or placebo adjustment	This is an older question which has now been put to rest; not only have chiropractic researchers used placebo controls, in some trials when asked, patients indicate they believed they received actual treatment

[a]From Leach RA. Chiropractic research: attitudes that hinder. Chiropractic 1988;1:14–17. (With permission.)

mation on how to practice (25–29, 31). *Until a concerted profession-wide effort is made to orient practitioners toward receiving their clinical information from peer-reviewed science journals such as the* Journal of Manipulative and Physiological Therapeutics, *among others, it seems unlikely that a new generation of S/Ps can be either trained or sustained* (7, 25, 29). Hopefully, this was the goal of the American Chiropractic Association when it began free distribution to all ACA member doctors of the newest chiropractic science journal, the *Journal of Neuromusculoskeletal System* (JNMS), in 1993.

While osteopathic medicine has long combined research with teaching and patient care to optimize interaction between students, residents, and faculty (32), similar chiropractic programs apparently have failed to produce opportunities for faculty to integrate their potential skills as teachers, clinicians, and researchers (33). As a consequence, chiropractic students often lack the adequate role-models of faculty advisors who are actively engaged in serious research, including publishing in peer-reviewed chiropractic science journals; it seems only logical that this in turn results in a lack of graduates oriented toward being S/Ps (33). Further, it is commonly known that when students complete research projects as a requirement for graduation, they are not expected to publish or even submit their findings to a journal.

Leach (34) believes that perhaps the only way colleges can truly produce excellent clinicians is for them to produce clinicians who are consumers and producers of legitimate research. When faculty are freed and funded to interact with students and residents to produce research, multiple educational and clinical benefits can be expected (32, 34). Some of these may benefit the chiropractic profession for decades (34).

Movement of chiropractors toward the S/P model may also be promoted by creation of a postgraduate chiropractic school (35). Haldeman (35) proposed that such a school could produce graduates who would help produce the volume of research necessary to establish chiropractors as most scientifically advanced with regard to use of the adjustment. Revisitation of B. J. Palmer's Ph.C. degree or some other adaptation of Haldeman's (35) suggestion appears worthwhile for further study.

Issues in Standards of Care

Development of standards of care is proceeding rapidly in the profession, and the chiropractic S/P can be instrumental in this process (3–6). Standards of care form a legal basis for protecting chiropractors who successfully follow them and incriminating chiropractors who fail to adhere to them (36). Obviously intended to protect the patient, standards promote "standardization" of analytical, diagnostic, treatment, and adjustive procedures across the profession (37).

Ultimately, documents produced by the Mercy Conference (5) by RAND (4) researchers, and by similar meetings in the future will play a powerful role in shaping chiropractic practice. As federal regulation of health care increases, cost containment will become a primary consideration in applying chiropractic standards of care to patient populations (38). Algorithms will be used increasingly for rational clinical decision making, and hopefully, S/Ps will help develop as well as promote the use of these diagnostic and treatment "flow charts" (39). Finally, rational consensus-building will make liberal use of input from S/Ps, both in terms of analytic and diagnostic methodologies (Table 16.3), as well as in treatment/therapeutic procedures (Table 16.4) which will continue to be refined as the research data base in chiropractic swells from single-subject case studies and small-scale research projects that can effectively be contributed by these clinicians (3, 6, 40, 41).

Discussion

Despite overwhelming evidence that chiropractic is more effective than medical intervention for lower back pain (see Chapter 9), when researchers find patients more sat-

Table 16.3.
Seattle 1990 Consensus Conference Conclusions on Process for Validation of Chiropractic Analytic/Diagnostic Methods.[a]

A.	1.	Dissemination of new information should be by means of a referred journal, preferably an indexed journal.
	2.	All chiropractic research publications, from leading journals to private technique publications, should now adopt a common format or style.
	3.	Appropriate ethical guidelines should be established for all dissemination of new knowledge.
B.	1.	The validation process should combine consensus methods, using broad-based representation from the profession, and continuing scientific research and investigation.
	2.	Development of research should involve all constituencies within the profession, including technique developers, colleges, and the field. Everyone has rights and responsibilities in this process.
	3.	Scientific research must include replication of initial results by an independent investigator.
	4.	The complete validation process should be conducted according to generally accepted scientific methods.

[a]From White LB, Chapman-Smith D. Summary of roundtable III. Report from roundtable I (analytic/diagnostic methods). Chiro Technique 1990;2:157. With permission.

Table 16.4.
Seattle 1990 Consensus Conference Conclusions on Process for Validation of Chiropractic Treatment and Therapeutic Procedures[a]

A.	1.	There should be an established process for validation of chiropractic therapeutic techniques which, as in the Kaminski model, should combine consensus methods and scientific study.
	2.	The efficacy of each chiropractic procedure must be subjected to scientific investigation.
	3.	There should be guidelines on what therapeutic claims may be published or alleged pending validation of a technique by scientific methods.
	4.	Validation is a team responsibility involving the developers of a technique, other practitioners, chiropractic research foundations, colleges, and scientists outside the profession.
B.		Outcomes that are difficult to research, as in the areas of prevention and wellness, should not be discredited or neglected.

[a]From White LB, Chapman-Smith D. Summary of roundtable III. Report from roundtable II (treatment/therapeutic procedures). Chiro Technique 1990;2:157. With permission.

isfied with chiropractic than medical care (66% vs. 22%, respectively), they continue to attribute the result more to the effectiveness of the patient/chiropractor interaction than to the effectiveness of chiropractic treatment itself (42). Establishing the superiority of chiropractic adjustment for anything other than lower back pain, thus, will be a monumental task. The only conditions the public currently perceives chiropractic as having a role in treating are back and neck pain (43).

We chiropractors are challenged to debate our philosophy, create testable hypotheses, and pursue those we perceive as most important through clinical investigations, despite limited resources (3, 6, 8, 9). Will we choose the model of the limited musculoskeletal specialist and gain a greater number of sufferers, but only those with low back pain (43)? Or, will we develop a research base establishing the effectiveness of chiropractic for improving a variety of conditions, and hammer away at public acceptance with legitimate investigations that delineate our strengths and weaknesses as health care givers? Or, will we demonstrate more wellness or less dis-ease after adjustments in blinded clinical trials?

These are all questions that chiropractic S/Ps can address, using study designs and methodologies such as those reported in more detail in the next chapter and in other sources (3, 6, 41). *To bring about a sweeping change in our profession that would lead to improved and more scientific applications of chiropractic as well as increased use of chiropractic services, bold action is needed to develop an attitude of excellence in all that we do* (Table 16.5).

Conversely, by our inaction as a profession and/or by choosing to reject a role for ourselves as scientist/practitioners or at least as scientific practitioners, we may doom ourselves to the role of limited musculoskeletal providers, or worse yet, inferior providers of manipulative services (if we allow physical therapists or others to take the lead in advancing the science of spinal adjustment).

Is chiropractic's effectiveness merely due to use of effective root metaphors? ("Mrs. Smith, I have found the cause of your problem. You have a bone out of place (or alternatively, a joint fixation) here, pinching on this nerve here! We will restore the alignment, thereby relieving pressure on your nerve.) Some within and outside the profession acknowledge the power of our patient communication skills (44, 45). Only time will tell if we will use the S/P model, establish small-scale clinical research centers, and otherwise establish a research tradition that matches the purported power of our root metaphors in the 21st century (46, 47).

Summary

There are many compelling reasons why chiropractic should develop the scientist/practitioner (S/P) model for growth and expansion of scientific knowledge and practice within the profession (3, 6, 29, 41). The need for practitioner input into future standards of practice, the responsibility for development of the science of chiropractic, limited funding for chiropractic research priorities, a lack of practical applications of chiropractic theories due to a lack of clinical research, an antiscience attitude among some in chiropractic, and differences between patients presenting to chiropractic college outpatient clinics and those presenting to private chiropractic offices, point to the need for scientist/practitioners who adopt the principles and practices of science into their practices and who contribute to the advancement of science in their profession (2, 4, 5, 6–14).

Critical to the development of S/Ps, and perhaps to the elimination of some attitudes that discourage scientific research in chiropractic, is the debate over whether to allow theosophical beliefs into chiropractic philosophy (7, 16, 22, 26, 27). Some argue that such metaphysical concepts should be allowed, but that they should be debatable and not adhered to dogmatically as if chiropractic philosophy was unchangeable (20, 21, 23, 24). Others hold that theosophy holds no place in the philosophy of a health science and that such a philosophy discourages rather than guides the scientific process of critical rationalism (7, 16, 25–29).

The training of chiropractors as S/Ps has apparently not been a primary focus of chiropractic colleges, which have been underfunded and engaged in a battle with organized medicine for their very survival (9, 31). Chiropractors in the field do not appear to understand the relative power of various research designs in providing clinically useful data (31), and students, residents, and faculty in chiropractic colleges typically lack the research interactions experienced by their counterparts in osteopathy (32–34). Such interaction may be critical to the creation of S/Ps in the future (34).

Finally, the role of S/Ps in guiding the development of standards of care and indeed in defining who we are and what we do is reviewed in this chapter. Only time will tell if the profession will use the S/P model to develop a broad research base, establish small-scale clinical research centers, and otherwise establish a research tradition that will guide and enhance our patient care and that matches the purported power of our root metaphors in the 21st century (44–47).

Table 16.5.
Developing an Attitude of Excellence for the Profession: Bold Steps Necessary to Foster Increased
Use of Chiropractic[a]

I. Profession-wide steps

    A. *Develop and maintain high academic standards* in all chiropractic institutions

    B. *Develop high goals and expectations for research* production in the average chiropractors, who will in turn demand excellence in research from their chiropractic associations and academic institutions

    C. *Disseminate information gained by research* (as published in peer-review science journals and not based on information from trade journals) to the average chiropractor, thereby developing a scientific base for patient care

    D. *Market the new and improved 21st-century chiropractic practice to the media and academics,* who ultimately control public attitudes

II. Individual practitioner steps

    A. *Talk frequently about chiropractic science:* leaders of the profession including association directors, presidents, academics, postgraduate instructors and researchers must persistently take every opportunity to publicly support the need for a more scientific chiropractic, and consistently read and discuss new chiropractic research findings (as published in peer-reviewed science journals); discuss positive and negative findings, flaws in research, and ways to improve research in chiropractic

    B. *Increase research visibility:* At the colleges, researcher-of-the-year awards, bonuses, and other perks to researchers who are truly productive and innovative could be implemented. Since colleges complain of limited funding for research, researchers who produce innovative trials with limited funding should receive special recognition. In each state or province, clinician-of-the-year awards should be a high honor bestowed upon practitioners who have published case studies or research while in practice. In the past, we have made "chiropractor of the year" an honor to those who were politically active. Now we must honor those in our profession who would advance the fledgling science of chiropractic. These are the new chiropractic pioneers.

    C. *Dispel the myths regarding research:* Some in our profession still feel threatened by research. We simply must use every means available through articles, media presentations, and one-on-one contacts to persuade our colleagues that research is the only viable guarantee that our profession will grow and prosper. For example, when a practitioner states that if we publish research then physiotherapists will see how effective chiropractic is and begin to practice it, point out that 18% of all physiotherapists are already in private practice. Moreover, 21 U.S. states have enacted legislation that permits direct patient access to physical therapists. These therapists are already dabbling in manipulation. Indeed, perhaps the only way chiropractic can survive the competition of physical therapy is by doing excellent research so often that one must be a full-time chiropractor to keep up with advances in chiropractic science and practice.

    D. *Be a smart consumer of products:* Ask questions. Expect whoever is selling a chiropractic technique or instrument to be able to show you case studies, anecdotal evidence, and controlled trials establishing the reliability and validity of the product. If they can't produce, don't buy! Dr. James Cox and Dr. Arlan Fuhr are examples of chiropractors who are seriously interested in establishing the validity of their techniques. We should demand no less from others who attempt to sell us their products.

---

[a]From Leach RA. Demanding excellence in the 21st century. J Can Chiro Assoc 1990;34:189–193. With permission.

REFERENCES

1. Dunn M, Slaughter RL, Edington KG. Is there a chiropractic science? J Manipulative Physiol Ther 1990;13:412–417.

2. McMichael RA, Poortinga G, Powell J, Sheely RB, Poteete RD, Sherman RP. Reliable standards of care are determined by consensus of those who provide that care. J Manipulative Physiol Ther 1991;14:217–221.

3. Barlow DH, Hayes SC, Nelson RO. The scientist practitioner: research and accountability in clinical and educational settings. New York: Pergamon, 1984:6,7.

4. Shekelle PG, Adams AH, Chassin MR, et al. The appropriateness of spinal manipulation for low-back pain: indications and ratings by a multidisciplinary expert panel. Santa Monica, Calif.: RAND, 1991.

5. Haldeman S, Chapman-Smith D, Peterson DM, eds. Guidelines for chiropractic quality assurance and practice parameters. Gaithersburg, Md.: Aspen, 1993.

6. Keating JC Jr. A buddy system for chiropractic research. J Can Chiro Assoc 1987;31:9–10.

7. Leach RA. Chiropractic research: attitudes that hinder. Chiropractic 1988;1:14–17.

8. Sorg RJ, Shaw HA. Osteopathic research priorities. J Am Osteopath Assoc 1985;85:736–738.

9. Keating JC Jr, Mootz RD. The influence of political medicine on chiropractic dogma: implications for scientific development. J Manipulative Physiol Ther 1989;12:393–398.

10. Wilk et al. v. AMA et al. U.S. no. 76 C 3777, 25 Sept. 1987.

11. Keating JC Jr, Young MA. Who is the chiropractic scientific community? J Aust Chiro Assoc 1987;17:84–86.

12. Nardini M. There is nothing more practical than a good theory. Ann Swiss Chiro Assoc 1989;9:43–48.

13. Lädermann JP. Chiropractic theories confronted with their practical applications: a missing link. Ann Swiss Chiro Assoc 1989;9:31–42.

14. Nyiendo J. A comparison of low back pain profiles of chiropractic teaching clinic patients with patients attending private clinicians. J Manipulative Physiol Ther 1990;13:437–447.

15. Keating JC Jr. The embryology of chiropractic thought. Eur J Chiro (submitted).

16. Keating JC Jr. Commentary: beyond the theosophy of chiropractic. J Manipulative Physiol Ther 1989;12:147–150.

17. Coulter I. Speakers' corner: the philosophy of chiropractic into the 21st century. Can Mem Chiro Coll Newslett 1990;12(2):9.

18. Kreisberg J. Letter to the, editor. J Manipulative Physiol Ther 1989;12:496.

19. Harris JH. Guest opinion: exorcising metaphysics. Chiro J Feb 1990:7,18.

20. Charlton KH. Hit and myth. Chiro J Aust 1991;21:58–62.

21. Albury WR. Questioning chiropractic philosophy. Chiro J Aust 1991;21:56–57.

22. Barge FH. Letter to the, editor. J Can Chiro Assoc 1990;34:68.

23. Richards DM. The Palmer philosophy of chiropractic—an historical perspective. Chiro J Aust 1991;21:63–68.

24. Strang V. Essential principles of chiropractic. Davenport, Ia.: Palmer College of Chiropractic, 1988:13–14,103.

25. Donahue JH. A proposal for the development of a contemporary philosophy of chiropractic. Am J Chiro Med 1989;2:51–53.

26. Keating JC Jr. To the editor in reply. J Can Chiro Assoc 1990;34:68.

27. Donahue JH. Guest editorial: why the average chiropractor doesn't support research. (In submission).

28. Keating JC Jr. Common misconceptions about research in chiropractic. Minn Chiro J Nov 1986:14–17.

29. Leach RA. Demanding excellence in the 21st century. J Can Chiro Assoc 1990;34:189–193.

30. Biggs L. Chiropractic, education: a struggle for survival. J Manipulative Physiol Ther 1991;14:22–28.

31. Jamison JR. Science in chiropractic clinical practice: identifying a need. J Manipulative Physiol Ther 1991;14:298–304.

32. D'Alonzo GE. Clinical research in osteopathic medicine. J Am Osteopath Assoc 1987;87:440–445.

33. Bergmann TF, Keating JC Jr, Sawyer CE. The need for innovation in clinical training: fac-

ulty practice plans in chiropractic education. J Manipulative Physiol Ther 1989;12:491–495.

34. Leach RA. Research: a clinician/researcher replies. MPI's Dynamic Chiropractic, 1 Sept 1989:32–33.

35. Haldeman S. Why chiropractic needs a postgraduate school. J Can Chiro Assoc 1975;19:14–15,37.

36. Gledhill SJ. Expert opinion and legal basis of standards of care determination. Chiro Technique 1990;2:94–97.

37. Hansen DT. Searching for the common authority in validation and standardization of chiropractic methods. Chiro Technique 1990; 2:72–73.

38. Nyiendo J. Economic measures used in determining effectiveness and efficiency of chiropractic methods. Chiro Technique 1990; 2:143–150.

39. Hansen DT. Commentary: development and use of clinical algorithms in chiropractic. J Manipulative Physiol Ther 1991;14:478–482.

40. White LB, Chapman-Smith D. Summary of roundtable III. Chiro Technique 1990;2:157–159.

41. Center DB, Leach RA. The multiple baseline across subjects design: proposed use in research. J Manipulative Physiol Ther 1984;7:231–236.

42. Cherkin DC, MacCornack FA. Patient evaluations of low back pain care from family physicians and chiropractors. West J Med 1989;150:351–355.

43. DeBoer K, Waagen G. Commentary: the future role of the chiropractor in the health care system. J Manipulative Physiol Ther 1986;9:225–227.

44. Coulehan JL. The treatment act: an analysis of the clinical art in chiropractic. J Manipulative Physiol Ther 1991;14:5–13.

45. Robert J. Influence of the health professional-patient relationship. Ann Swiss Chiro Assoc 1989;9:233–244.

46. Charlton KH. The nature and environment of knowledge production, chiropractic theory and future progress. J Aust Chiro Assoc 1986;16:95–98.

47. Keating JC Jr, Smallie DD. Commentary: viability of small-scale clinical research centers. J Manipulative Physiol Ther 1989;12:54–55.

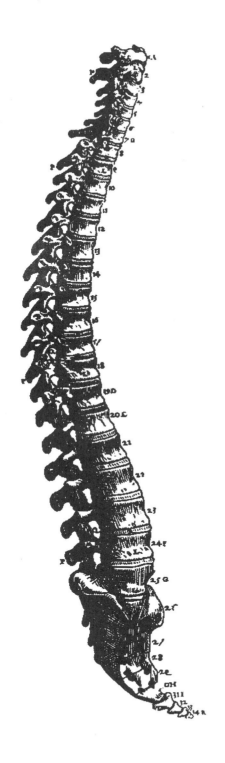

Approaches to Researching Chiropractic

Our belief in any particular natural law
cannot have a safer basis than our
unsuccessful critical attempts to refute it.

Sir Karl Raimund Popper

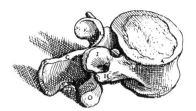

Chapter 17

Researching Chiropractic

*F*ew searches in the history of mankind have been conducted without controversy, setbacks, and frustrations. Late in the 1960s, following a personal investigation, Suh (1) concluded that the chiropractic profession needed not only broad clinical studies but also basic research. This University of Colorado professor came under pressure from colleagues, government officials, and health professionals to abandon the idea of initiating basic chiropractic research before he had even begun. Yet Suh went on to organize and develop a program of study in chiropractic in areas of biomechanics, neurophysiology, and neurochemistry (2–7).

Meanwhile, due at least in part to the medical boycott (8), similar pressures were felt by scientists who were asked to join the faculties of chiropractic colleges or to participate in research and education ventures, which had the obvious effect of limiting contact between chiropractic students and researcher/educators (9). Paradoxically, even as organized medicine complained of the lack of appropriate science and education in chiropractic, it was singularly effective in impeding improvements in these areas of the profession (9).

Nevertheless, even as the boycott began to wane toward the late 1970s—after the federal mandate to research chiropractic was made by Congress in 1974, and at least partly as a result of the legal challenge

mounted by Wilk et al. in 1977 (8)—interdisciplinary conferences in the 1970s heralded the beginning of a virtual renaissance of research for the chiropractic profession (10–13). Haldeman formed the International Society for the Advancement of Clinical Chiropractic and Spinal Research (18672 Dodge Ave, Santa Ana, CA 92705). An ACA-sponsored organization, the *Foundation for Chiropractic Education and Research* (FCER; 1916 Wilson Blvd, Arlington, VA 22201), and an ICA-sponsored organization, the *Foundation for the Advancement of Chiropractic Tenets and Science* (FACTS; 1901 L St NW, Suite 800, Washington, DC 20036), represent the largest national associations. Even the third largest chiropractic research funding agency, founded by Arlan Fuhr, D.C., the *National Institute for Chiropractic Research* (NICR; 4900 Leesburg Pike, Suite 310, Alexandria VA 22302) has already funded more than $100,000 worth of clinical chiropractic investigations, while FCER, the largest, funds upwards of $1 million annually (see Chapter 16).

An interdisciplinary chiropractic research journal, the *Journal of Manipulative and Physiological Therapeutics* (JMPT), was indexed by *Index Medicus* as well as by several other scientific indexing services (including *Excerpta Medica, Biosis*, and the *Soviet Academy of Science*), making it available to chiropractors, physicians, and scientists worldwide through the *Medline* computer retrieval system, operated by the National Library of Medicine in Bethesda, Maryland, and through software distributed by the National Technical Information Service in Washington, D.C.

Literature retrieval and blinded peer-reviewed science journals are critical for establishing a science in a modern health care profession. Blinded peer review generally improves publication quality, assuring the reader that at least minimal standards are applied to the information presented. (A list of some current science journals in chiropractic appears in Table 16.1.)

Literature retrieval and indexing are critical, since it would be exhaustively time consuming and nearly impossible to manually search all the peer-reviewed science journal articles relevant to various hypotheses and to patient care in chiropractic (the necessary first step in research)(14). However, of the chiropractic science journals now available, only *JMPT* is available through *Medline*. So with the proliferation of chiropractic science journals in the 1980s and 1990s, *ChiroLars*, an indexing and computer-based literature retrieval system, was developed by a field practitioner (and the *Index to Chiropractic Literature* was developed by the *Chiropractic Library Consortium* (CLIBCON)). Hence, through *Medline*, the chiropractic clinician and scientist/practitioner (S/P) can search medical and science sources (more than 3000 journals are indexed), while through *ChiroLars*, chiropractic journal information can be retrieved (14).

The proliferation of chiropractic science journals has provided a platform for some important chiropractic clinical research from various chiropractic college research departments and from the field (15). Another recent platform has been the FCER-sponsored *International Conference on Spinal Manipulation (ICSM)*, where S/Ps and researchers have gathered and presented abstracts of their current research, even before publication. Since conducting and publishing scientific research can be a lengthy process (a typical, even small-scale, investiga-

tion may take months to design and implement, more months to statistically evaluate and prepare for submission to a chiropractic science journal, months more for blinded peer review, and a year or more between acceptance and publication), scientific symposia like the ICSM provide a means for disseminating important *preliminary* data to peers prior to full acceptance and publication.

Many of these research projects have involved the use of blinds as well as controls, which overcomes flaws in earlier chiropractic research efforts. Central to at least some of this scientific research is the concept that chiropractic can alter the natural or "normal" course of a given disease, "dis-ease," or dysfunction by correction of the intervertebral subluxation or vertebral subluxation complex (VSC)(16). To demonstrate this concept, the design of chiropractic studies must be objective (i.e., incorporate such fundamental procedures as multiple, double, or single blinds and use statistically sound analyses) (17).

A concept that is new to chiropractic research but familiar to researchers in psychology and physical therapy is the use of single-subject and time-series research designs, which eliminate the need for more complicated research settings (18). Use of such methods assures elimination, or at least control, of the psychosomatic factor; use of statistics appropriate to the design is necessary before the data can be correctly interpreted and before conclusions can be drawn from analysis of the research.

This chapter briefly explores five key elements of quality chiropractic scientific inquiry: *design, literature review, methods, statistics* (data, results), and *conclusions*. If any of these are missing or are inappropriately applied, the research is flawed, and conclusions drawn from such a study would be suspect. It is imperative —for the appropriate and expeditious development of the science of chiropractic in the 21st century— that every chiropractor and student (and of course S/Ps and researchers) know these concepts.

Approaches to Researching Chiropractic

Several major topics need intensive investigation if chiropractic tenets are to be substantiated. McDowell (16) believes that chiropractic research should be directed to three primary areas: evaluation of chiropractic therapy, diagnostic technique, and relative basic science. This approach requires further division into laboratory, field, and clinical studies.

CHIROPRACTIC BASIC SCIENCE RESEARCH

Much of the research needed to validate or invalidate chiropractic hypotheses will require laboratory investigations and will involve chiropractic college or university settings. Experimental studies of nerve compression or irritation and animal models of subluxation are two examples of this type of research.

Nerve Compression

Laboratory investigations could be used to follow up on the work of Sharpless (6) and Luttges et al. (3). Such investigations are needed to determine the correlation between spinal nerve or root compression or irritation and protein and degenerative changes both proximal (spinal cord proper) and distal to the compression (see Chapter 11). Other basic science studies involving animals could be initiated to follow up on the work of Triano and Luttges (19). These studies are needed to determine the relationship between chronic, moderate nerve root compression or irritation (mimicking the supposed effects of subluxation) and subsequent physiological, functional, or pathological changes, if any, in the extremities and in the viscera.

Subluxation Model

The novel approach to development of an animal model for subluxation used by DeBoer and McKnight (20) at the Palmer College of Chiropractic certainly requires further research (see also Chapter 12) if chiropractic is to connect biological and clinical events; perhaps we will not discover a route to the operational definition of VSC or segmental dysfunction (SDF) in humans until we can experimentally induce and remove the lesions in animals (much as experimental genetic research has led to greater understanding and clinical progress in the treatment of a variety of disorders).

CHIROPRACTIC CLINICAL INVESTIGATIONS

Clinical research is needed for validation of all chiropractic hypotheses presented in this text. Clinical analogue investigations to determine the biological events associated with adjustments, research to elucidate the role of SDF and facilitation in initiating somatovisceral disorders thought to be amenable to CMT, studies of reliability of SDF and VSC diagnoses, chiropractic technique effectiveness, and clinical outcomes assessments are examples of research priorities for the profession.

Neurodystrophy

Certainly, a theoretical basis for chiropractic effects on the neuroendocrine system would be enhanced by demonstrating immunomodulation after adjustments in patients with pain, not merely in pain-free students, as a natural follow-up to the landmark work of Brennan and co-workers (21) at the National College of Chiropractic. Longer-lasting immune effects of adjusting in pain patients is suggested by a chiropractic investigation in Australia (22). While the conclusion of Brennan and co-workers (21) that a temporary boost in natural killer cells (cytotoxic T cells) after adjustments but not after placebo may be useful to distinguish sham from true manipulation, their findings based upon upper dorsal CMT may not apply—or may apply even more so—to other spinal regions. Perhaps upper cervical adjustments (applied closer to the hypothalamic centers known for autonomic modulation of immunity; see Chapter 14) might evoke longer-lasting immune effects in asymptomatic students with motion restrictions in the cervical spine. Such speculation awaits further study.

Similarly, clinical analogue experimentation to better understand the biological events associated with chiropractic adjustment should follow the work of Terrett and Vernon (23) at the Canadian Memorial Chiropractic College, who investigated paraspinal pressure pain thresholds; Wagnon and co-workers (24), who investigated circulating aldosterone; and Briggs and Boone (25) at the Sherman College of Straight Chiropractic, who investigated pupillary diameter as a measure of the postadjustment sympathetic response. While subsequent investigations failed to confirm the initial findings of Vernon and co-workers (26) of a plasma β-endorphin response after adjustments but not placebo, further work might consider a central release mechanism for β-endorphins or other opioids after CMT (27).

SDF and Facilitation: Somatoautonomic Influences and Clinical Outcome Assessments

Somatoautonomic phenomena and the *segmental dysfunction* (SDF) and *facilitation* hypotheses (see Chapters 5–8) definitely require further investigation. These theories may comprise the most logical justification for the use of chiropractic adjustment in the correction of conditions other than pain syndromes (28). Electromyography should be an objective indicator of muscle activity in such studies, which could be performed in the solo-practitioner clinical setting (see Chapter 7). Electromyographic determination of the effects of chiropractic adjustment on muscle spasm in the paraspinal muscles related segmentally to the viscera or function to be tested (e.g., renal secretions) could be correlated with laboratory findings to verify the relationship between the somatic and the visceral functions involved.

More complicated trials could be attempted also, but the profession must determine what systemic effects, if any, result from such phenomena as SDF and facilita-

tion. Although initial controlled trials of clinical outcomes and quasi-experimental research efforts on the effect of CMT for some somatovisceral disorders (type O) has been important (e.g., research on essential hypertension, hyperactive children, and babies with colic: see also Chapter 9), much more research is essential if chiropractic is to develop a role for management of these disorders.

Indeed, Keating (29) argues that chiropractic is in danger of losing altogether the broad treatment scope envisioned by the founder, D. D. Palmer, and by other early pioneers (see also Chapter 4), which generally included psychiatry, obstetrics, a broad range of conditions we now consider autonomically mediated and stress-related, a variety of "functional" conditions (viz., unknown etiology, without apparent pathology), and a wide array of health problems:

> Most of the traditional spectrum of chiropractic clinical interests has never been tested, let alone disproved. The necessary compromise, I believe, is to persevere in the practice of those methods which have received some scientific and social legitimacy (i.e., type M problems), and simultaneously to develop a significant research enterprise for the balance of health problems and methods for which we suspect there may be clinical value. Here is an area of professional development where a practitioner-scientist model of training and practice can be most helpful (29).

Research on the Chiropractic Lesion

Research on the chiropractic lesion(s) (regional dysfunction (RDF), SDF, VSC phases I, II, and III) is critical to all hypotheses presented in this text. As stated in Chapter 10, some college-based researchers appear to have lost hope that an operational definition of VSC (regardless of the terms used to describe it) can be agreed upon, which will stand up to the rigors of inter- and intraexaminer reliability studies. The *ACA Council on Technique*, hopeful that better definitions will help researchers more specifically compare notes, has agreed on a new terminology that may enhance both interprofessional as well as intraprofessional dialogue regarding chiropractic research (M. Gatterman, personal communication: see Chapter 3).

In addition to studies of algometry, thermography, electromyography, static and motion radiography, and active range of motion by various investigators, efforts by Dale Nansel and co-workers (30) at the Palmer West Chiropractic College to identify the manipulable lesion by the response of specific motion restrictions to adjustments delivered to different sides and at different levels stands as a classic example of innovative research (see also Chapters 6, 7, and 9). *Such studies are directed at the core of all chiropractic hypotheses: the belief that chiropractic lesions exist and can be identified and, often, corrected. We should either conduct this research with vigor or eschew these SDF- and VSC-based arguments altogether and adopt instead models suggesting that CMT merely invokes stimulatory/inhibitory neuroendocrine responses, if it is nothing more than a placebo effect.*

Research on Chiropractic Techniques/Diagnostic Methods

At Western States Chiropractic College, Kaminski (31) developed a model for the evaluation of chiropractic technique and diagnostic methods (Fig. 17.1). The model has received widespread recognition in chiropractic science literature and provides a basis for developing research priorities in these key areas of chiropractic practice.

Clinical algorithms can provide a step-by-step procedure allowing clinicians to follow appropriate guidelines easily and quickly, to arrive at a diagnosis or determine an appropriate course of care. Like the algorithm found in Figure 17.1, these delineate the steps that the clinician must follow sequentially, in a carefully thought out plan. Algorithm development has been advocated as a necessary component to the appropriate scientific advancement of chiropractic practice, and researchers have been encouraged to focus on conditions: (*a*) with a high prevalence, (*b*) commonly managed by chiropractic, (*c*) with a high morbidity, and (*d*) that are manageable/treatable (32).

There are a variety of technique systems for application of chiropractic adjustments (see Chapter 1, Table 1.1). Of the modern technique system pioneers in chiropractic, probably fewer than a dozen are involved in some clinical research to validate their procedures; however, Dr. Arlan Fuhr (Activator method) and Dr. James Cox (Cox technique—flexion-distraction) are fine examples of scientist/practitioners who have dedicated themselves fully to using scientific methods and publishing their research in peer-reviewed science journals (see citations, especially in Section III).

Ongoing research includes but is not limited to Gonstead technique, (Dr. Greg Plaugher, director), Sacro-Occipital technique (most peer-reviewed journal citations appear in osteopathic literature), and some upper cervical technique systems. Unfortunately, with the exception of but a handful of these, most are not even close to the validation envisioned by the Kaminski model. Despite the fact that we know little about which techniques perform best under which set of circumstances for which conditions, SDF or VSC, chiropractors have often adopted the attitude described by Bergmann (33) with regard to their own technique(s):

> My technique procedure is a chiropractic technique; My technique has not helped the patient; therefore chiropractic can not help the patient.

Rather than dismissing the effectiveness of some systems over others, the chiropractic clinician would be well advised to critically appraise claims and assertions made by technique innovators (33). In addition, technique innovators should be challenged to vigorously pursue the validation process by publishing research on their methods in peer-reviewed, chiropractic science journals.

Much of the initial research necessary for chiropractic methods and diagnosis concerns establishing both inter- and intraexaminer reliability. If procedures are not replicable both between and within examiners, questions of discriminability, sensitivity, and specificity are moot (34, 35).

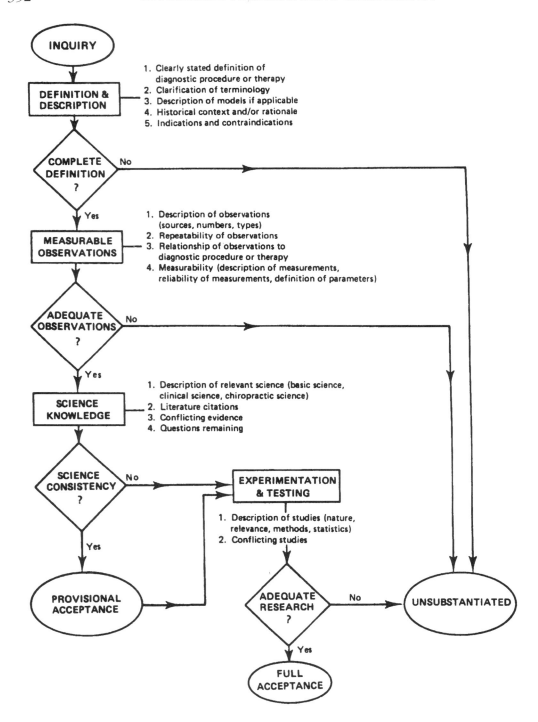

Figure 17.1.   Steps required for chiropractic diagnostic and technique validation in the so-called Kaminski model. *Ovals* represent inputs and outputs, *rectangles* indicate data entry steps, *diamonds* indicate that a decision must be made, and *arrows* direct the S/P or researcher to the next step. (From Kaminski M. Evaluation of chiropractic methods. Chiro Technique 1990;2:107–113. With permission.)

Vertebrobasilar Syndrome and Contraindications to CMT

Another area deserving in-depth research involves the role of subluxation in alteration of vertebral artery blood supply to the brainstem (see Chapter 13). Some investigators have determined that this phenomenon represents a contraindication for adjustment (36, 37). The role of correction of vertebrobasilar arterial insufficiency by manipulation, if there is such a role, and the role of chiropractic adjustment in causing stroke by this mechanism certainly merit further investigation.

Comparative Studies

Finally, human clinical studies could be devised to compare chiropractic with medical or other care in the treatment of various disorders. Such studies could also be used to compare the efficacy of the various chiropractic techniques. These studies must involve specific, measurable criteria in both initial and final patient examinations, for the data to be believable. In addition, use of a statistical method appropriate to the research design is critical to proper evaluation of the data (38).

Key Elements of Scientific Inquiry

The key elements of scientific inquiry are those that should be present in a report of the investigation. They include (*a*) an appropriate *study design* for the questions being investigated; (*b*) a thorough *literature search*, including primarily references published in peer-reviewed science journals; (*c*) description of *methods* used, including the use of appropriate *statistics* for analyzing the data, matched to the design of the study; (*d*) discussion of *results* and how they compare with prior research; and finally, (*e*) *conclusions* based upon the findings.

We briefly explored the necessity of the clinician and S/P using peer reviewed literature in Chapter 16. With the *Medline* and *ChiroLars* computerized literature retrieval systems, a good thorough literature search

is now possible even for geographically isolated practitioners. A thorough literature search is critical for the success of most inquiry. Prior literature can steer the S/P away from the practices and methods that have failed in the past, while providing up-to-date information about the question under investigation.

Other elements of scientific inquiry are not as easy to master as the literature search, but are equally important. We next briefly explore study designs and some statistical concepts associated with chiropractic research.

STUDY DESIGNS FOR CHIROPRACTIC RESEARCH

Since the first edition of this textbook, a number of chiropractic research efforts have involved the use of "placebo" or "sham" adjustments or other controls for the psychosomatic factor in research (see Chapter 9). A study design well-suited to the questions being asked and controlling for threats to validity must demonstrate improvement beyond placebo. It must be demonstrated that correction of intervertebral subluxation, VSC, or SDF by use of adjustments can alter the normal course of the disease, "dis-ease," or disorder, or at least that adjustments in some other way affect health.

Variables

Theoretically, a sham manipulation would have no substantial effect on the disease or symptom (*dependent variable*–mediating or clinical outcome variable that depends upon the patient's response to intervention) but would appear to be of value to the patient, while chiropractic adjustment (*independent variable*–procedure, something that the S/P controls) would have a substantial curative influence. The use of questionnaires, to address patient satisfaction with care, and self-reports of pain and disability (see Chapter 6) are examples of *clinical outcome variables*; *mediating variables* are those that link the independent variable (what the doctor does) with the clinical outcome (29).

Sham Procedure

The patient should be unable to differentiate between a corrective adjustment and a sham procedure or treatment (i.e., between the fake treatment and the proposed corrective treatment), and some studies have demonstrated successful sham procedures, based on poststudy questioning of the subjects (i.e., when asked if they thought they received adjustments or sham procedures, both adjusted and sham-treated groups believed they had received actual treatment)(39). Others, such as Brennan and coworkers (21), believe that certain biological markers can be used to distinguish sham-treated from manipulated subjects.

While a true "sham" manipulation may be impossible to devise (with the characteristic audible release of gasses from the joint) (40), a number of alternatives may be available. For example, mobilizing procedures such as motion palpation can be compared with specific chiropractic adjustment (41). Sham manipulations in chiropractic research have included gentle prodding at the trapezius ridge along the cervicobrachial junction (in studying the effect of thoracolumbar manipulation on arterial flow in the lower extremity), nonspecific contact of the adjuster's fingertip with the gluteal area (in researching the effect of "basic technique" adjusting for an antihypertensive response), and nonspecific detuned Activator instrument adjusting across the back and neck (in evaluating chiropractic adjustment effectiveness for children with hyperactive behaviors) (42–44).

The use of blinds and controls in research is not new, but it is a true challenge to chiropractic researchers faced with an enormous number of unknowns and variables. Before research can be initiated, the problem being investigated has to be defined, and defining VSC in a meaningful way has been the enigma of chiropractic clinical research methodology. Hence, efforts to quantify suspected components of VSC and SDF have been made instead, such as muscle spasm or hypertonicity by use of electromyography (45), passive gross motion re-

strictions (30), and tenderness, as assessed by algometry (23) and a variety of other measures (see Chapters 6, 7, and 9).

Control Group Trials

Classical medical research methodology advocates designs involving multiple, double, or single blinds (46, 47) as well as comparative treatment or sham manipulation (48–50). Criteria are established so that each patient included in the study has the same problem (51). Various degrees of impairment or dysfunction are measured before and after adjustment, by independent observers using objective reproducible means (51).

When neither the doctor nor the subject knows whether the treatment is purported to be ameliorative or sham, the study is said to be double-blind (Fig. 17.2). Chiropractic investigators have successfully used double blinds in their research using adjustments, including the novel work by Nansel and coworkers (30), whose subjects had no idea whether they were being adjusted correctly or incorrectly—they were blinded as to passive gross motion assessments—and whose treating chiropractors were told which side of the neck and at which level to adjust, similarly unaware of the results of the gross motion palpation tests.

Finally, chiropractic adjustment may be compared with physiotherapy, analgesics and bed rest, exercise and "back school" (advice concerning proper lifting, etc.), and sham physiotherapy (e.g., detuned diathermy) (Fig. 17.3).

Time-Series Experiments

Center and Leach (18) have offered an alternative research approach involving use of a single-subject research design, one of the *time series designs*. With this design, patients are their own controls for the efficacy of the treatment and are monitored continuously, both clinically and physiologically (e.g., electrodermal activity, EMG studies), before, during, and after intervention with the independent variable (Fig. 17.4). Repeated measures allow visual observation of level, trend, and variability, permitting control of

Clinical controlled study design

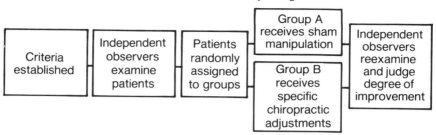

Figure 17.2. In the clinical controlled study design, as few as two chiropractors and one medical doctor could comprise the independent observer panel. These observers do not know which patients were assigned to the control (A) or adjustment (B) groups; they are, therefore, blinded. The patients are not told whether they would receive specific chiropractic care or simulated care, which would constitute the other blind. One chiropractor provides adjustments for both groups (giving appropriate adjustment and/or sham adjustment to patients in each group). (Adapted from Buerger AA. Clinical trials of manipulation therapy. In: Buerger AA, Tobis JS, eds. Approaches to the validation of manipulation therapy. Springfield, Ill.: Charles C Thomas, 1977:313–320.)

Clinical controlled study Design (large scale)

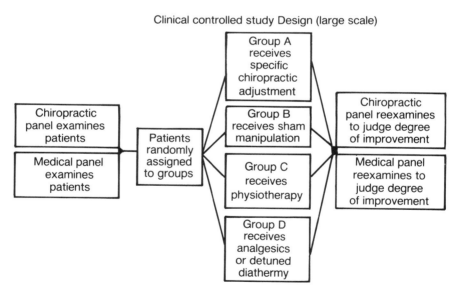

Figure 17.3. A large-scale study design for clinical chiropractic research that allows chiropractors and medical doctors to examine and evaluate subjective and objective improvement separately and independently. In this study, some patients could receive either effective or sham manipulation, and others, either effective or sham physiotherapy (detuned diathermy with no current flowing). Obviously, other therapies could be substituted for groups C and D. (Adapted from Buerger AA. Clinical trials of manipulation therapy. In: Buerger AA, Tobis JS, eds. Approaches to the validation of manipulation therapy. Springfield, Ill.: Charles C Thomas, 1977:313–320.)

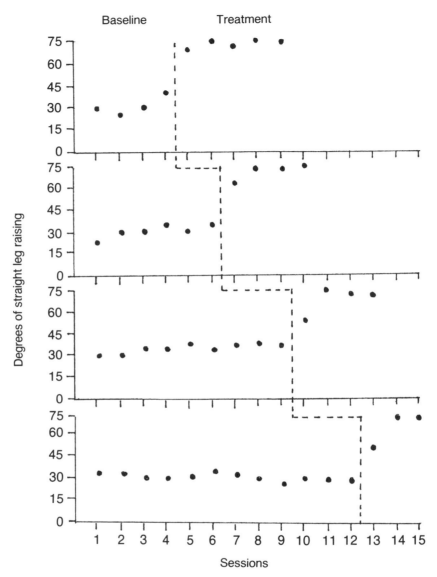

Figure 17.4.   The multiple baseline design across subjects, which has been advocated by Center and Leach, is an alternative to the use of blinds and sham manipulation. Patients are their own controls and are monitored objectively before, during, and after intervention. Once a steady state for the dependent variables has been established for the first patient, the intervention treatment is introduced. After the treatment effect on the first patient is established, the intervention treatment is applied to the second patient, etc. This study design has been used extensively by clinical psychologists and educators and, to a lesser extent, by psychiatrists and physical therapists. Here the patients are being monitored for improvement in straight leg raising during pretreatment (baseline) and treatment sessions. (Adapted from Center D, Leach RA. Multiple baseline design across subjects. J Manipulative Physiol Ther 1984;7:231–236.)

some of the threats to *internal validity* (such as measurement error or variability; Table 17.1). Advantages to the use of the multiple baseline design across subjects include its elimination of the need for a sham manipulation and its applicability in small research settings.

Keating and co-workers (29, 52) have more completely described the use of other *quasi-experimental research designs* in chiropractic settings, as well as use of appropriate statistics to interpret data collected by these and other designs. These designs have helped S/Ps in psychology establish a research base (see Chapter 16), and they have been used occasionally in physiotherapy research settings; now they have been introduced to chiropractic as well (16, 29, 44, 52, 53).

Descriptive Designs

Descriptive designs include case reports—primarily of assessment, diagnosis, or intervention—and clinical series. These offer the S/P an invaluable tool for contribution to the chiropractic scientific literature, as these designs are well within the grasp of field practitioners. A single case can be reported using a methodology or procedure that remains untested or is even controversial and otherwise might not be investigated by college-based researchers, who must justify the expenditure of large sums of money and time and so must necessarily pursue research efforts most likely to yield results.

Moreover, *clinical series* include studies in which the S/P evaluates the effect of a certain adjustment or treatment on a given dependent variable in consecutive cases, in two or more groups of subjects. When the S/P uses descriptive statistics to illustrate average scores and variability in a clinical series (e.g., standard deviation of the mean, SD), the study is termed a *quantitative clinical series.*

Such studies are termed *prospective* and are planned in advance; they are preferred because there is more control over selection

Table 17.1.
Examples of Threats to Internal Validity of Clinical Experiments[a]

History: although patient's improvement appears to have resulted from adjustments, it was actually caused by a concurrent event (e.g., analgesics taken without the chiropractor's awareness)

Maturation: improvement in patient not due to adjustments, but instead resulting from aging, fatigue, or other naturally occurring processes which may exert a clinical effect (hence, enuresis resolves because child's nervous system has matured, rather than due to adjustments)

Reactivity of measurement: due to increased involvement with parents, clinicians or other interested persons, the enuretic child focuses his attention on the problem and so is sensitized to it (viz., Hawthorne effect); meanwhile, clinician and parent may note improvement in number of "wet" nights and conclude adjustments caused the change

Interaction among methods: in some cases a combination of doctor/patient reactivity, maturation, adjustments, etc. may result in clinical improvement that could not have occurred with any one of these

Instrumentation: unreliable equipment, (e.g., weak batteries) or poorly trained operators result in unreliable data that appears to reveal improvement in the patient's condition

Selection: doctors argue that their records "prove" that a certain physiotherapy procedure decreases muscular pain; however, they fail to randomly sample their files and provide only cases that seem to support their hypotheses.

Natural history: the patient's condition is naturally variable (e.g., multiple sclerosis); the chiropractor applies adjustments when the problem is at its worst and as symptoms subside assumes adjustments effected the improvement when instead the condition was spontaneously resolving or was already in a cycle toward improvement

[a]From Keating Jr JC. Toward a philosophy of the science of chiropractic: a primer for clinicians. Stockton, Calif.: Stockton Foundation for Chiropractic Research, 1992:195.

of patients and choice of variables to monitor. However, occasionally the practitioner has an opportunity to present meaningful data after it has been collected—all the more reason for employing scientifically based outcome measures in private practice—these investigations are termed *retrospective*. A more thorough review of these types of research has been presented by Keating (29).

STATISTICAL CONCEPTS FOR RESEARCH

Feinstein (54) discussed the concept of "hardness" of clinical variables and outcome measures in some detail. He argues that some clinicians may judge a variable to be too soft and neglect to include it in the analysis of data; however, he states that even these variables can be coded, statistically analyzed, and reviewed for the relevancy of their impact on clinical judgment. While not speaking directly to the chiropractic profession in his paper, he might as well have been discussing leg length checks, algometry, self-report questionnaires, range of motion tests, and other similar chiropractic variables (see Chapters 6 and 7).

Feinstein defines *hard* (as opposed to *soft*) data as including (*a*) information acquired objectively rather than subjectively, (*b*) an observed entity that can be preserved so it can be checked and rechecked, and (*c*) measurement occurring on a scale that is *dimensional* (e.g., height, weight, serum cholesterol, and blood pressure), rather than *ordinal* (e.g., deep tendon reflexes graded 1+, 2+, etc., or none, mild, moderate, severe) or nominal (e.g., anaplastic versus epidermoid cancer).

He states that the most important attribute of hardness is reliability. For example, passive end-range assessments of cervical joints for restricted "end feel" is nonpreservable, subjective, and nondimensional; however, the data might be accepted as hard if three chiropractors—examining independently—agreed on what was found.

Indeed, his thesis is that so-called hard data are often not so hard after all; unreliability, distortion, and inflation of sample size to achieve statistical outcomes that may be irrelevant to improvement in quality of life are problems that this medical epidemiologist from Yale asserts arise out of the quest for analysis of harder clinical variables (54).

The use of statistics in chiropractic research came of age in the past decade, as scientists began to debate the relative value of concordance statistics (i.e., kappa and interclass correlation) for intra- and interexaminer reliability evaluations (34, 35, 55) and even argued the value of the Walsh test (a nonparametric test) in single-subject research designs (56, 57). For a more detailed review of statistical and nonstatistical analysis of data collected using designs reviewed in this chapter, the work of Keating (29), and Barlow, Hayes, and Nelson (53) should be consulted.

Discussion

Chiropractic research has made great strides in the past two decades. This trend needs to continue if chiropractic research is to lead the profession in the 21st century. The modern patient seeks care that has been tested against all other forms of treatment in rigorous and objective clinical trials. The federal government expects such research even more, now that chiropractic is part of a larger national health care system, and certainly if that role is to be expanded. The media demand that objectivity be the principle of any study. With interdisciplinary and intradisciplinary comparative studies, such demands can be met.

Reliability and reproducibility are critical factors in both clinical chiropractic research and in medical research. Reliability diminishes as the volume and range of data increase (58). Hence, measurement and treatment procedures should be kept simple.

Another important concept with regard to chiropractic research methodology concerns selection of patients. Patients might be selected who will classically not respond well to suggestion (as evidenced by Minnesota Multiphasic Personality Inventory), to ensure that the adjustment itself physically corrected the problem (59, 60). Obviously, such patients are excellent candidates for studies in which the dependent variable is well defined and easily measured; pain-rating scales and disability questionnaires (see Chapter 6) are also of help and may be used as predictors of candidates likely to respond to treatment in future studies (61).

Since a firm diagnosis is not possible in most patients with back pain, all aspects of the condition should be researched (62, 63). For example, initial and follow-up disability questionnaires may be used to predict outcome (patients tend to respond to treatments in proportion to their scores on certain disability questionnaires); indeed, chiropractic studies using disability questionnaires have already yielded much new knowledge and have set a new standard for outcome assessment (see Chapters 6 and 9).

Evaluation of the chiropractic lesion(s) remains perhaps the greatest frustration and challenge facing researchers and S/Ps alike. Quantitative and qualitative definition of the phases of VSC, SDF, and RDF are needed, and no operational definition of even a most generic "manipulable lesion" is available at this time. Research on this phenomenon should be a primary concern of college-based researchers and S/Ps alike, or perhaps we should eschew the concept altogether and adopt instead the belief that all we do is psychosomatic or the result of some biological response, or both.

Evaluation of chiropractic techniques will help determine which are most efficient in correcting the various phases of VSC, including SDF and RDF (once they have been operationally defined), and conditions in various individuals. These studies will assist the profession in determining the validity of certain clinical tools as well (e.g., the heat-reading instrumentation shown in Fig. 17.5). Evaluation of chiropractic analysis and diagnosis will aid in all other areas of chiropractic research and treatment. Studies in which chiropractic is compared with medical and other treatments will be more complicated to design, staff, and finance than studies of chiropractic alone; these studies are, nevertheless, a top priority, in this author's opinion.

Perhaps the most encouraging new development is the use of quasi-experimental and descriptive case studies in the 1980s in chiropractic research; such designs offer chiropractic S/Ps the opportunity to become valuable players in the research arena, and indeed, field practitioners apparently contributed heavily to chiropractic research in the last decade (15). What role S/Ps will play in guiding a new, more scientific practice of chiropractic into the next century remains to be seen, but based on their initial contributions, the future appears bright indeed.

Summary

Chiropractic research efforts at the University of Colorado (2–7) and elsewhere initially were hampered by opposition from organized medicine (8, 9). Chiropractic studies have been performed in several areas of clinical investigation, and in these studies, modern research methodology and sham manipulation and controls have been used (20–30). Key elements of scientific inquiry are briefly reviewed, including appropriate literature review, methodologies based on a design that answers questions (hypotheses) posed by the research, statistical methods appropriate to the design, and conclusions that are based upon the findings. Use of time series designs (e.g., multiple baseline design across subjects) and others are briefly reviewed, along with their advantages for the small clinic research setting (18, 29, 44, 52). Finally, the use of personality and disability questionnaires, pain-rating scales, and various chiropractic research possibilities is discussed (34–38).

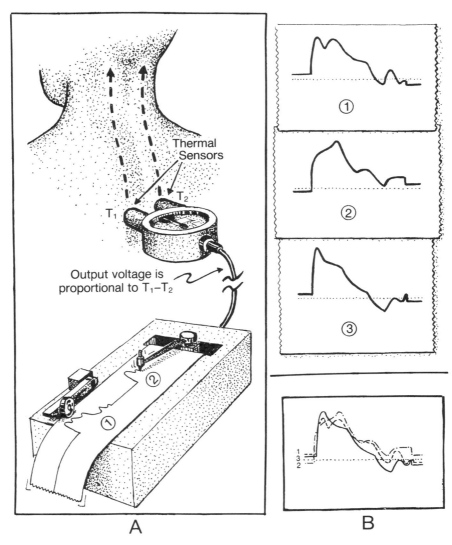

Figure 17.5. A device for determination of temperature differential along the spine. The hand-held device is moved vertically over the vertebral bodies, and a graph records the difference in temperature from both sides of the spine (A). Each graph (B) represents 6–7 seconds of vertical travel; these graphs were recorded at 5-second intervals. The examination was begun at the first dorsal level and ended with a split-second pressure contact at the base of the occiput. The graphs are shown diagrammatically; the readings were taken by the author after only 1 month of experience with this apparatus. The collage of the graphs shows the reproducibility that even an "amateur" can demonstrate. Use of this technique by chiropractors to determine neuromuscular activity, however, is being replaced somewhat by infrared thermography, owing partly to better reliability (see Chapter 7).

REFERENCES

1. Suh CH. Lecture presented at the Life Chiropractic College on 6 April 1978.

2. Kelly PT, Luttges MW. Electrophoretic separation of nervous system proteins on exponential gradient polyacrylamide gels. J Neurochem 1975;24:1077–1079.

3. Luttges MW, Kelly PT, Gerren RA. Degenerative changes in mouse sciatic nerves: electrophoretic and electrophysiological characterizations. Exp Neurol 1976;50:706–733.

4. MacGregor RJ, Oliver RM. A general-purpose electronic model for arbitrary configurations of neurons. J Theor Biol 1973;38:527–538.

5. MacGregor RJ, Sharpless SK, Luttges MW. A pressure vessel model for nerve compression. J Neurol Sci 1975;24:299–304.

6. Sharpless SK. Susceptibility of spinal roots to compression block. In Goldstein M, ed. The research status of spinal manipulative therapy. Washington, D.C.: Government Printing Office, 1975:155–161.

7. Suh CH. The fundamentals of computer aided x-ray analysis of the spine. J Biomech 1974;7:161–169.

8. Wilk et al. v. AMA et al. U.S. no. 76 C 3777, 25 Sept 1987.

9. Keating JC, Mootz RD. The influence of political medicine on chiropractic dogma: implications for scientific development. J Manipulative Physiol Ther 1989;12:393–398.

10. Goldstein M, ed. The research status of spinal manipulative therapy. Washington, D.C.: Government Printing Office, 1975.

11. Buerger AA, Tobis JS, eds. Approaches to the validation of manipulation therapy. Springfield, Ill.: Charles C Thomas, 1977.

12. Korr IM, ed. Neurobiological mechanisms in manipulative therapy. New York: Plenum, 1978.

13. Haldeman S, ed. Modern developments in the principles and practice of chiropractic. New York: Appleton-Century-Crofts, 1980.

14. Curl D, Shapiro C. Literature searching by a field doctor: a comparison of manual versus computerized methods. Chiro Technique 1993;5:15–22.

15. Keating JC, Young MA. Who is the chiropractic scientific community? J Aust Chiro Assoc 1987;17:84–86.

16. McDowell FH. Clinical research areas requiring further study. In Goldstein M, ed. The research status of spinal manipulative therapy. Washington, D.C.: Government Printing Office, 1975:309–310.

17. Haldeman S. Basic principles in establishing a chiropractic clinical trial. ACA J Chiro 1978;23:S33-S37.

18. Center D, Leach RA. Multiple baseline design across subjects. J Manipulative Physiol Ther 1984;7:231–236.

19. Triano JJ, Luttges MW: Nerve irritation: a possible model of sciatic neuritis. Spine 1982;7:129–136.

20. DeBoer KF, McKnight ME. A surgical model of a chronic subluxation in rabbits. J Manipulative Physiol Ther 1988;11:366–372.

21. Brennan PC, Triano JJ, McGregor M, Kokjohn K, Hondras MA, Brennan DC. Enhanced neutrophil respiratory burst as a biological marker for manipulation forces: duration of the effect and association with substance P and tumor necrosis factor. J Manipulative Physiol Ther 1992;15:83–89.

22. Alcorn SM. Antibodies and antigens—their definition, source and relevant function. J Aust Chiro Assoc 1978;11:18–37.

23. Terrett AGJ, Vernon H. Manipulation and pain tolerance: a controlled study of the effect of spinal manipulation on paraspinal cutaneous pain tolerance levels. Am J Phys Med 1984;63:217–225.

24. Wagnon RJ, Sandefur RM, Ratliff CR. Serum aldosterone changes after specific chiropractic manipulation. Am J Chiro Med 1988;1:66–70.

25. Briggs L, Boone WR. Effects of a chiropractic adjustment on changes in pupillary diameter: a model for evaluating somatovisceral response. J Manipulative Physiol Ther 1988;11:181–189.

26. Vernon HT, Dhami MSI, Howley TP, Annett R. Spinal manipulation and beta-endorphin: a controlled study of the effect of a spinal manipulation on plasma beta-endorphin levels in normal males. J Manipulative Physiol Ther 1986;9:115–123.

27. Christian GF, Stanton GJ, Sissons D, et al. Immunoreactive ACTH, β-endorphin and cortisol levels in plasma following spinal manipulative therapy. Spine 1988;13:1411–17.

28. Haldeman S. The clinical basis for discussion of mechanisms of manipulative therapy. In: Korr IM, ed. The neurobiologic mechanisms in manipulative therapy. New York: Plenum, 1978:53–75.

29. Keating JC Jr. Toward a philosophy of the science of chiropractic: a primer for clinicians. Stockton, Calif.: Stockton Foundation for Chiropractic Research, 1992:74–110, 139–184,195.

30. Nansel DD, Peneff A, Quitoriano J. Effectiveness of upper versus lower cervical adjustments with respect to the amelioration of passive rotational versus lateral-flexion endrange asymmetries in otherwise asymptomatic subjects. J Manipulative Physiol Ther 1992;15:99–105.

31. Kaminski M. Evaluation of chiropractic methods. Chiro Technique 1990;2:107–113.

32. Hansen DT. Development and use of clinical algorithms in chiropractic. J Manipulative Physiol Ther 1991;14:478–482.

33. Bergmann TF. Closing commentary. Chiro Technique 1990;3:140–141.

34. Haas M. The reliability of reliability. J Manipulative Physiol Ther 1991;14:199–208.

35. Jansen RD, Nansel DD. Diagnostic illusions: the reliability of random chance. J Manipulative Physiol Ther 1988;11:355–365.

36. Giles LGF. Vertebral-basilar artery insufficiency. J Can Chiro Assoc 1977;22:112–117.

37. Kleynhans AM. Complications of and contraindications to spinal manipulative therapy. In Haldeman S, ed. Modern developments in the principles and practice of chiropractic. New York: Appleton-Century-Crofts, 1980:359–384.

38. Cambell RC. Statistics for biologists. Cambridge: Cambridge University Press, 1974: 6–7.

39. Waagen GN, Haldeman S, Cook G, Lopez D, DeBoer KF. Short-term trial of chiropractic adjustments for the relief of chronic low back pain. Manual Med 1986;2:63–67.

40. Greenman P. Discussion of clinical observations and emerging questions. In: Korr IM, ed. The neurobiologic mechanisms in manipulative therapy. New York: Plenum, 1978: 77–89.

41. Wiles MR. Observations on the effects of upper cervical manipulations on the electrogastrogram: a preliminary report. J Manipulative Physiol Ther 1980;3:226–229.

42. Wickes D. Effects of thoracolumbar spinal manipulation on arterial flow in the lower extremity. J Manipulative Physiol Ther 1980; 3:3–6.

43. Dulgar G, Hill D, Sirucek A, Davis B. Evidence for a possible anti-hypertensive effect of basic technique apex contact adjusting. ACA J Chiro 1980;14:S97-S102.

44. Giesen JM, Center DB, Leach RA. An evaluation of chiropractic manipulation as a treatment of hyperactivity in children. J Manipulative Physiol Ther 1989;12:353–363.

45. Leach RA, Owens EF Jr, Giesen JM. Correlates of myoelectric asymmetry detected in low back pain patients using hand-held post-style surface electromyography. J Manipulative Physiol Ther 1993;16:140–149.

46. Berqquist-Ullman M, Larsson U. Acute low back pain in industry. Acta Orthop Scand [Suppl] 1977;170:1–117.

47. Wymore AB. Chairman's summary: comments on therapeutic studies. In: Goldstein M, ed. The research status of spinal manipulative therapy. Washington, D.C.: Government Printing Office, 1975:307–308.

48. Kane RL, Fischer FD, Leymaster C. Manipulating the patient: a comparison of the effectiveness of physician and chiropractic care. Lancet 1974;1:1333–1336.

49. Buerger AA. Clinical trials of manipulation therapy. In: Buerger AA, Tobis JS, eds. Approaches to the validation of manipulation therapy. Springfield, Ill.: Charles C Thomas, 1977:313–320.

50. Glover JR, Morris JG, Khosla T. Back pain; a randomized clinical trial of rotational manipulation of the trunk. Br J Ind Med 1974;31: 59–64.

51. Doran DML, Newell DJ. Manipulation in the treatment of low back pain: a multicenter study. Br Med J 1975;2:161–164.

52. Keating JC Jr, Giljum K, Menke JM, Lonczak RS, Meeker WC. Toward an experimental

chiropractic: time-series designs. J Manipulative Physiol Ther 1985;8:185–189.

53. Barlow DH, Hayes SC, Nelson RO. The scientist practitioner: research and accountability in clinical and educational settings. New York: Pergamon, 1984.

54. Feinstein AR. Clinical biostatistics: XLI. Hard science, soft data, and the challenges of choosing clinical variables in research. Clin Pharmacol Ther 1977;22:485–498.

55. Haas M. Statistical methodology for reliability studies. J Manipulative Physiol Ther 1991; 14:119–132.

56. Shiel RC. To the editor. J Manipulative Physiol Ther 1986;9:150–151.

57. Center DB, Leach RA. In reply. J Manipulative Physiol Ther 1986;9:151.

58. Nelson MA, Allen P, Clamp SE, DeDombal FT. Reliability and reproducibility of clinical findings in low back pain. Spine 1979;4: 97–101, 1979.

59. Dennis MD, Greene RL, Farr SP, Hartman JT. The Minnesota Multiphasic Personality Inventory. Clin Orthop 1980;9:125–130.

60. Lawlis GF, Mooney V, Selby DK, McCoy CE. A motivational scoring system for outcome prediction with spinal pain rehabilitation patients. Spine 1982;7:163–167.

61. Lehman TR, Brand RA, Gorman TWO. A low back rating scale. Spine 1983;8:308–315.

62. Roland M, Morris R: A study of the natural history of back pain part 1: development of a reliable and sensitive measure of disability in low back pain. Spine 1983;8:141–144.

63. Roland M, Morris R. A study of the natural history of low back pain part 2: development of guidelines for trials of treatment in primary care. Spine 1983;8:145–150.

Appendix A: Social Theory of Chiropractic

Let us propose an additional theory regarding the relationship between health and dysfunction and the effectiveness of chiropractic care. We will name it the *social theory*. This theory is not intended to supplant those already in existence; rather, it augments and supports the need and justification for chiropractic care.

In abstract, this theory contends that dysfunction or less than optimum health can be the result of social factors, some of which are amenable to chiropractic care. We explain this rationale below and review literature that supports this theory. A model is presented defining the practical application of this theory. The direction additional research must take to further substantiate this theory is also addressed.

Foundations

To properly develop a theory, it is imperative that terms be defined to avoid confusion and misperceptions. The following terms may have many meanings; thus, the need for precise definitions.

HEALTH

Health is a state of complete physical, mental, and social well-being and not merely the absence of disease or infirmity (1). Definitions incorporate values that bear on ethical considerations. Health as a state of well-being describes individuals in relation to a concept of normality. Normality, in a pathological sense, is the absence of disorder, impairment, or disease. Statistically, normality for a specified condition is defined from its modal distribution in a population. In a social sense, normality is defined by values relating to how things ought to be (2). Parsons defined health, in a social sense, "as the state of optimum capacity of an individual for the effective performance of the roles and tasks for which he has been socialized" (3). The three concepts are not mutually exclusive; they are strongly interrelated.

Health also appears to be a matter of degree, and standards of health seem to be relative to persons and to the time of life. A middle-aged person may be "healthy" but experience more aches, pains, and limitations than a person in the early twenties. Thus health and "unhealth," i.e., health and falling short of health, are true opposites, not health and disease.

DISEASE

Disease, as the generic name for the cluster of symptoms and identifiable pathological conditions of the body, is not a notion symmetrical with, or opposite to, health. The concept of disease is a general scheme for explaining, predicting, and controlling dimensions of the human condition. There is *one* "health"; there is a family of diseases.

The concept of disease not only describes and explains but also enjoins an action. It states what ought to be and thereby incorporates criteria for evaluation. It delineates roles, such as patient and physician, and interconnects these roles with a network of duties and expectations.

Paracelsus taught the "ontological" view of disease. Diseases are regarded as entities in themselves, distinguishable by specific changes and causes (4). This view suggests that diseases have specific causes and characters and respond to specific therapies. The "ontological" concept of disease as an entity unto itself has given rise to modern pathology that studies the specific character of the "diseased" structure and bacteriology that studies the specific cause of the "disease." Within this concept, it is possible to experience "disease" without necessarily being "sick." A classic example is an individual identified as being HIV positive but still able to play professional basketball.

In contrast to the "ontological" perspective is the "physiological" perspective. Disease is a general, not a specific, notion and thereby is related to physiological function. Thus, disease is related more to context than to substance, more the result of individual constitutions, the laws of physiology, and the effects of the environment. The emphasis is on the individual rather than the disease entity.

Modern medicine has incorporated both concepts in its management of "disease" through diagnosis, prognosis, and therapy or through the process of evaluating, predicting, and controlling "reality." Diseases are multifactorial and multidimensional, involving genetic, physiological, psychological, and sociological components. The emphasis placed on the cause of the disease entity in a multidimensional condition is often related to the orientation of the evaluator. If all you have is a hammer, than everything you see looks like a nail.

Disease, as it exists for those who both experience illness and explain it, is bound by the circumstances of that experience. Explanatory accounts are not things; things are what explanatory accounts explain and disease is a mode for explaining things, in particular, ill humans (4). The concept of disease thus becomes a method for explaining, predicting, and treating ill humans.

ILLNESS

The term "illness" is a necessary element in the discussion of health and disease. Parsons (3) describes illness in terms of incapacity for relevant task performance. Fabrega (5) discusses illness as:

> a set of behaviors, judged as undesirable and unwanted in a culture . . . Illnesses are in many respects a natural outcome of the processes of individual coping and adaptation and are to be expected in any society as a matter of course. Moreover, an increasingly bureaucratic and technological society is likely to 'produce' illness by altering physical and social environmental factors which impinge on human adaptation, just as the application of biomedical knowledge of illness can be expected to lead to the inadvertent outbreak of new (iatrogenic) illnesses. And as social values and the level of technology change, ways of defining illness (i.e., vs. nonillness) will also change. All of this means that illnesses are likely to persist as human problems.

Herzlich and Pierret (6) speak of illness as a social condition that restructures our relations with society. This relationship takes on special significance as it relates to work and the legal framework associated with wage labor in an industrialized society. Totman's (7) discussion of the illness experience is closely tied to emotions. He speaks of deep-seated frustrations and feelings of dissatisfaction with life's achievements and with one's work in a sample of diverse illnesses. He reported that feelings of resentment, frustration, depression, anxiety, and helplessness commonly preceded the onset of symptoms.

When an allopathic physician speaks of illness, a cluster of symptoms and signs are described. Sackett et al. (8) incorporate the social, psychological, and economic aspects of illness under the concept of a predicament. In a holistic paradigm, practitioners speak of illness as dis-ease, indicating various degrees of discomfort. Lowenberg (9) speaks of illness as a learned behavior in response to stress and secondary gain. This implies that a responsibility resides with the individual who makes the decision to assume illness behavior.

The patient's healing is facilitated by the practitioner, whether through providing information or applying healing interventions. The practitioner succeeds as a healer by mobilizing the innate recuperative powers within the patient. Touching and physical contact between the practitioner and patient are seen as essential components in mobilizing this internal healing power (Lowenberg, page 41).

Assumptions

To establish a social theoretical framework of chiropractic, a few assumptions must be made.

1. The chiropractic physician is an accepted entity in society in the legitimization of illness in a fashion similar to other health care providers.
2. As acceptable entities in society, chiropractic physicians are responsible for providing appropriate care that they determine will lead to improved health.
3. Appropriate care is based on a rational and critical approach to understanding the presentations of patients and the management of their predicaments within one's scope of practice and training.

Theoretical Models

DISEASE MODEL

It is not uncommon for patients to present to chiropractic physicians with distinctly defined pathophysiological abnormalities. Whatever the etiology and whatever the management may involve, chiropractic physicians take care of patients with abnormal conditions that may improve and absolve.

SYMPTOM MODEL

Most patients come to a physician because their health is less than optimum. Or, they may present with disease symptoms, dysfunction, or the inability to perform normal tasks, evidenced by the symptoms present even when identification and categorization of a disease entity may not be possible. Whatever the reason, there is justification for the patient to seek to enter into a relationship with a "healer."

SOCIAL MODEL

Whether the patient has symptoms and/or disease or not, the action of seeking care and becoming a patient is illness behavior, implying the adoption of an altered social role and function. Thus, the social model may be incurred in conjunction with the disease model and the symptom model or it may stand alone in the absence of disease or symptoms (Fig. A.1). A physician who accepts patients and legitimizes their illnesses assumes the role of a social change agent, and the social model is invoked. That is, the physician accepts the responsibility to assist the patient to return to a normal role in society, given the patient's willingness to comply with instructions.

The "hands on" physical contact provided in the patient-doctor encounter is a social as well as a physical experience. Allowing encroachment into one's personal space through physical contact creates a form of nonverbal communication. Generally, a message of care and concern is communicated from doctor to patient. Emotions spoken of by Totman (7) begin to take on a new perspective.

Verbal communication is also somewhat characteristic of the chiropractic physician, as attempts are made to help patients understand that their predicaments are the result of the inability of the body to maintain a healthy state of being. The chiropractic physician helps patients to realize that healing is the result of healthful living, a part of which includes chiropractic manipulation for the stim-

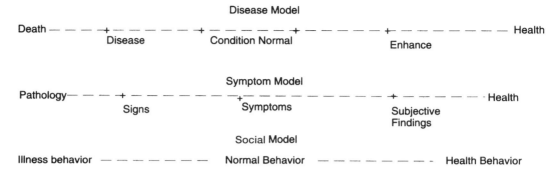

Figure A.1. Three models of behavior: disease, symptom, and social models. Although the three models appear to overlap, such correlation is not assured. Illness behavior can occur in the absence of disease or symptoms. Pathological changes herald the presence of disease but may not manifest symptoms or initiate illness behavior.

ulation of the recuperative processes within the body. Through this interactive communication, patients gain confidence in their own ability to remove themselves from the illness behavior they have assumed.

The *social change agent* role of the chiropractic physician is seldom appreciated by the practitioner. As physical signs and symptoms are reduced and removed, patients reassume their roles as members in society with the attendant contributions. The practitioner becomes the facilitator to this process.

From the holistic and naturalistic perspective espoused by the chiropractic profession, the patient–chiropractic physician encounter is consistent with the role of a social change agent. Other health care providers, marginal or otherwise, provide similar experiences. The touching component coupled with the specific manipulation makes the chiropractic encounter somewhat unique.

Chiropractic's Role in Society

The role of a social change agent for the chiropractic physician is not a unique health care encounter. Any person who affects change can be loosely referred to as a change agent. It can be argued that a specific chiropractic adjustment and its attendant effects on the neurophysiological and biomechanical functions of the patient provide a positive benefit to the patient directly and to society indirectly. However, use of manipulative procedures and even specific adjustments are not limited to chiropractic physicians.

Some believe that chiropractic's philosophical tenets make a unique contribution to society by establishing an alternative health care approach to allopathic medicine. The holistic approach to health care, however, is not unique to chiropractic phenomena. In fact, chiropractic's more recent emphasis on musculoskeletal back pain is believed to be a movement toward the role of a limited practitioner and away from the role of an alternative health care provider.

The chiropractic physician, functioning as a social change agent and facilitator of the innate healing processes, does provide an alternative approach to those seeking to improve health. With an emphasis on health enhancement and disease prevention, the chiropractic physician focuses primarily upon the neuromusculoskeletal system, through which one's health status is monitored and managed.

The evidence of successful chiropractic care is becoming ever more abundant in the scientific literature. The mechanisms underlying the success of chiropractic care are not adequately described. As part of this social theory, stress-related illness and dysfunction contribute to the manifestation of symptoms and illness behavior, and chiropractic's approach to patient care provides a significant element in the management of stress-related illness and improving the health of society.

FUNCTIONAL AND STRESS-RELATED ILLNESSES

By touching and by communicating concepts of health (as opposed to disease), the chiropractic physician provides a service unmet by allopathic medicine and inadequately dealt with by folk medicine. In the pathological model, touching (manipulating or adjusting) and communicating have limited curative value and unmeasured palliative value. In the symptom model, functional and stress-related disorders are often manifested with minimal distinct clinical signs and symptoms and are common entities in our industrialized society. Back pain and the common cold are examples of two common illnesses with large social impact, minimal clinical veracity, and even less distinctive clinical management.

In a large health insurance experiment by the RAND Corporation, health status and health utilization were closely monitored for several years in a large population. From this study, medical effectiveness was categorized (10). Four groups were identified: 1) highly effective treatment by medical care, 2) quite effective treatment by medical care, 3) less effective treatment by medical care, and 4) medical care rarely effective but self-care and over-the-counter remedies thought to be effective (Table A.1).

The first group, where "highly effective care" occurred, was characterized by disease entities with highly distinctive pathological findings and well-defined treatment protocols, such as pneumonia, fractures, anemia, and malignancies. The second group, with "quite effective treatments," included conditions usually considered amenable to treatment with medications, such as colitis, diarrhea, thrombophlebitis, and tonsillitis. The "less effective" medical treatment group included such things as musculoskeletal disease, mental retardation, prostatic hypertrophy, and varicosities. The group that was "rarely treated effectively" by medical care included such conditions as colds, chest pain, fatigue, headaches, irritable colon, low back pain, acute sprains and strains, and obesity.

The general pattern of this categorization scheme is a movement from distinct pathophysiological alteration with well-prescribed treatment regimes to the absence of a distinct pathophysiological alteration and no prescribed treatment protocols. Furthermore, less effective medical treatment is found to correlate with the absence of a distinct pathophysiological alteration. Interestingly, the further down the scale toward decreased pathology and decreased medical effectiveness, the more likely the condition would fall into a functionally (or stress) related treatment classification. The conditions listed in this last group represent ailments that could be cared for by a chiropractic physician.

CHIROPRACTIC ROLE IN THE SOCIAL MODEL

Chiropractic can provide an alternative to medicine in those areas related to functional and stress-related disorders not amenable to medical care. There is a curative value to high-touch, low-tech chiropractic care in fulfilling this unique niche left vacant by high-tech, low-touch medical care, which can benefit patients and society.

Chiropractic physicians function as social change agents affecting the health and wellness of their patients. But is the role of the chiropractic physician limited to the management of symptoms manifested by disease and dysfunction? As social change agents oriented toward "wellness" as opposed to "illness," chiropractic doctors are

Table A.1
Medical Effectiveness Groupings[a]

Group 1: Highly effective treatment by medical
  care system
 a. Medical care highly effective: acute conditions
        Eyes—conjunctivitis
        Otitis media, acute
        Acute sinusitis
        Strep throat
        Acute lower respiratory infections (acute
          bronchitis)
        Pneumonia
        Vaginitis and cervicitis
        Nonfungal skin infections
        Trauma—fractures
        Trauma—lacerations, contusions, abrasions
 b. Medical care highly effective: acute or chronic
        conditions
        Sexually transmitted disease or pelvic
          inflammatory disease
        Malignant neoplasm, including skin
        Gout
        Anemias
        Enuresis
        Seizure disorders
        Eyes—Strabismus, glaucoma, cataracts
        Otitis media, not otherwise specified
        Chronic sinusitis
        Peptic and nonpeptic ulcer disease
        Hernia
        Urinary tract infection
        Skin—dermatophytoses
 c. Medical care highly effective: chronic conditions
        Thyroid disease
        Diabetes
        Otitis media, chronic
        Hypertension and abnormal blood pressure
        Cardiac arrythmias
        Congestive heart failure
        Chronic bronchitis, chronic obstructive
          pulmonary disease
        Rheumatic disease (rheumatoid arthritis)
Group 2: Quite effective treatment by medical care
  system
        Diarrhea and gastroenteritis (infectious)
        Benign and unspecified neoplasm
        Thrombophlebitis
        Hemorrhoids
        Hay fever (chronic rhinitis)
        Acute pharyngitis and tonsillitis
        Acute middle respiratory infections (tracheitis,
          laryngitis)
        Asthma
        Chronic enteritis, colitis

(Group 2, continued)
        Perirectal conditions
        Menstrual and menopausal disorders
        Acne
        Adverse effects of medicinal agents
        Other abnormal findings
Group 3: Less effective treatment by medical
  care system
        Hypercholesterolemia, hyperlipidemia
        Mental retardation
        Peripheral neuopathy, neuritis, and sciatica
        Ears—deafness
        Vertiginous syndromes
        Other heart disease
        Edema
        Cerebrovascular disease
        Varicose veins of lower extremities
        Prostatic hypertrophy, prostatitis
        Other cervical disease
        Other musculoskeletal disease
        Lymphadenopathy
        Vehicular accidents
        Other injuries and adverse effects
Group 4: Medical care rarely effective or self-
  care effective
        Medical care rarely effective
            Viral exanthems
            Hypoglycemia
            Obesity
            Chest pain
            Shortness of breath
            Hypertrophy of tonsils or adenoids
            Chronic cystic breast disease
            Other breast disease (nonmalignant)
            Debility and fatigue (malaise)
        Over-the-counter or self-care effective
            Influenza (viral)
            Fever
            Headaches
            Cough
            Acute URI
            Throat pain
            Irritable colon
            Abdominal pain
            Nausea or vomiting
            Constipation
            Other rashes and skin conditions
            Degenerative joint disease
            Low back pain diseases and syndromes
            Bursitis or synovitis and fibrositis or
              myalgia
            Acute sprains and strains
            Muscle problems

[a] From Lohr KN, Brook RH, Kamberg CJ, Goldberg GA, Leibowitz A, et al. Use of medical care in the
RAND health insurance experiment. Medical Care [suppl] 1986;24(9):533, with permission.

poised to serve as primary contact physicians. Armed with competent diagnostic skills, thus garnering the confidence of society, the chiropractic physician has the opportunity to become the triage agent in the management of health care. Equipped with therapeutic skills focused on the treatment of functional and stress-related disorders, the chiropractic physician is capable of effectively treating a large majority of symptom-related disorders and perhaps reducing the frequency with which these symptoms progress on to disabling and pathological disorders. Finally, equipped with the concepts of health and wellness, chiropractic physicians are ready to lead their patients and society in general through the necessary life style changes to improve health status and quality of life.

As a social change agent working through the social model of health care, the chiropractic physician has a vital and integral role in the future delivery of health care.

Summary

The *social theory* of chiropractic posits that the chiropractic physician functions as a social change agent in the role of healer or doctor in society. Furthermore, emphasizing health care rather than disease places chiropractic in the position of providing an alternative approach to health that traditionally was not offered by allopathic care. The two health care delivery systems are not mutually exclusive but mutually beneficial, and they often overlap.

Chiropractic care focuses on the neuro-musculoskeletal system as the vehicle through which the body manifests its health status and through which many functional and stress-related disorders can be managed. Chiropractic care provides a low-tech approach to health enhancement and disease prevention through the holistic concept of "wellness." The chiropractic physician represents the "wellness practitioner" of the future.

REFERENCES

1. Adopted by the International Health Conference in New York, 22 July 1946, Official Record World Health Organization 2,100.

2. Susser M. Ethical components in the definition of health. Ch. 1.7. In: Caplan AL, Engelhardt HT, McCartney JJ, eds. Concepts of health and disease. Reading, MA: Addison-Wesley, 1981:95.

3. Parsons T. Definitions of health, and illness in the light of American values and social structure. Ch 1.4. In: Caplan AL, Engelhardt HT, McCartney JJ, eds. Concepts of health and disease. Reading, MA: Addison-Wesley, 1981:69.

4. Engelhardt, HT. The concepts of health and disease. Ch 1.2. In: Caplan AL, Engelhardt HT, McCartney JJ, eds. Concepts of health and disease. Reading, MA: Addison-Wesley, 1981:34, 40.

5. Fabrega H. The scientific usefulness of the idea of illness. Ch 1.10. In: Caplan AL, Engelhardt HT, McCartney JJ, eds. Concepts of health and disease. Reading, MA: Addison-Wesley, 1981:134,141.

6. Herzlich C, Pierret J. Illness and self in society. Forster E, transl. Baltimore: Johns Hopkins University Press, 1987:238.

7. Totman R. Social causes of illness. New York, Pantheon, 1979:139.

8. Sackett DL, Haynes RB, Tugwell P. Clinical epidemiology: a basic science for clinical medicine. Toronto: Little, Brown & Co., 1985:4.

9. Lowenberg JS. Caring & responsibility. Philadelphia: University of Pennsylvania Press, 1989:35.

10. Lohr KN, Brook RH, Kamberg CJ, Goldberg GA, Leibowitz A, et al. Use of medical care in the RAND health insurance experiment. Ch 5, Table 5.1. Medical Care [Suppl] 1986;24(9):S33.

Appendix B: Integrated Physiological Model for VSC

Common to all concepts of subluxation are some form of kinesiological dysfunction (kinesiopathology) and some form of neurological involvement (neuropathology). The vertebral subluxation complex (VSC) is a model that describes the common and essential elements of these components in an attempt to make their relationship more understandable in the context of chiropractic adjustive procedures. It is a descriptive model of changes in nerve, muscle, connective, and vascular tissues which accompany the kinesiological aberrations of spinal articulations. The major hypotheses presented in this text related to the concept of subluxation are thus given an organizational structure through which to interpret the clinical outcomes and basic physiological processes related to subluxation degeneration and its reversal by chiropractic adjustments. The model thereby fulfills the criteria for a scientific theory as presented in Chapter 2.

The term *complex* reflects the subtle and intricate interrelationships that exist between the different components and between components at different segmental levels of the spine, and by extension, the relationship between changes at the spinal level and the tissues and organs supplied by the associated nerves. The model thus addresses the basic sciences aspect referred to in Chapter 17, but is of necessity relevant to and consistent with chiropractic clinical experience. The primary form of kinesiopathology which is addressed in chiropractic clinical practice is hypomobility or fixation. Complete or partial immobilization leads to a consistent pattern of degeneration in all tissues associated with the immobilized joint and is referred to here as immobilization degeneration (ID) (1).

In its original formulation, the VSC consisted of five components: kinesiopathology, neuropathology, myopathology, histopathology, and biochemical abnormalities. While this selection of headings encompassed most of the acknowledged aspects of the chiropractic subluxation, it needed a more refined development. For example, all components of the five-component model were given equal status, with no indication of the degrees or types of interrelatedness of the various components.

The first attempt at documenting the model was by Dishman (2, 3), who described the original 5-component model in which histopathology was reserved exclusively for a description of cartilage degeneration. Faye, too, has published a brief overview of the model (4) in which he reserves the histopathology component exclusively for a description of the inflammatory process. A more extensive and substantial formulation of the model (Fig. B.1) included three additional components: connective tissue pathology, vascular abnormalities, and inflammatory response (5). Since that time, the model has been further refined; pathoanatomy has been substituted for histopathology, and pathophysiology has been included as a basic component.

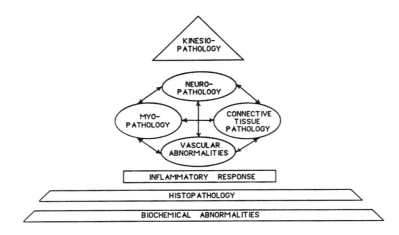

Figure B.1.

Overview of the Model

Figure B.1 illustrates the relationship of each component of the VSC to all others. Since motion disorders are the most fundamental aspect of chiropractic clinical practice, kinesiopathology assumes its place of prominence. Movement is supported and permitted by muscle and connective tissue, it is controlled by the nervous system, and all tissues are nourished and cleansed by the vascular system. These comprise the tissue-level components, and each works in coordination with the others to allow proper movement. Interfering with any single component will affect all others (6).

To characterize the degenerative changes associated with subluxation pathology, each tissue-level component must be described with regard to its pathoanatomy, pathophysiology, and pathobiochemistry. The inflammatory response is presented here as a distinctly separate component since it derives elements from all tissues and represents aspects of all fundamental processes but can be assigned to none exclusively. The term *subluxation* is taken throughout this text to mean a constellation of signs and symptoms which is identified and managed by chiropractors clinically. The VSC represents the underlying physiological and biochemical processes and related anatomical structures

involved directly or indirectly in the clinical picture.

Kinesiopathology

The basic unit of spinal mobility is the motion segment (7), which consists of two adjacent vertebrae joined by an intervertebral disc (IVD), two posterior articulations, and a number of ligaments (8), including capsules. Parke (6) includes the muscles and segmental contents of the spinal canal and the intervertebral canal (IVC). Functionally, the motion segment is viewed as a three-joint complex (9), but it may be considered to be a single, compound joint with three articulations (10), analogous to the wrist.

Sandoz (11) developed a model of spinal joint function in chiropractic theory (see Chapter 3, Fig. 3.1). In this idealized schematic, a joint has an active range of motion (ROM) that is under voluntary control. An additional ROM is possible, which requires assistance, as by an examiner. The ranges of active plus assisted motion constitute the passive physiological ROM. At the end of this range, one encounters the elastic barrier of resistance. According to Sandoz, the chiropractic adjustment takes the joint beyond this barrier into the paraphysiological space, thereby extending the range of physiological motion. At the end of the paraphysiological space, one encounters the limit to anatomical integrity, beyond which motion would result in sprain and true luxation.

Joint movement is complicated, more so in the spine than in any other organ system (12). In addition to the three planes of physiological movement, flexion/extension, lateral flexion, and rotation, there is also long-axis traction. Joint play, a springiness in the joint when it is taken to tension, represents the elastic barrier of resistance to joint motion (see Fig. 3.1).

It is difficult to discuss kinesiology of joints without discussing ligaments, capsules, and muscle/tendon systems. In addition, in the spine, the dural sac and its contents must be considered in the kinetics of movement (13, 14). The spine is further complicated in its kinesiology in that it responds as an integral unit in which restrictions of movement at one level can lead to compensatory changes in other areas (15, 16). No disorder of a single major component of a motion segment can exist without affecting first the functions of the other components of the same segment and then the functions of other levels of the spine (6).

IMMOBILIZATION DEGENERATION

All situations that lead to immobilization cause some degenerative change in the musculoskeletal system, and early mobilization, traction, and continuous passive motion overcome these harmful effects (17). Lack of movement in a joint leads initially to stiffness (18) and associated pain (19). This is followed by degeneration of the joint (1, 20), and ultimately the joint is fused by bony ankylosis. The idea that joint restriction or "fixation" is an integral component of subluxations was first proposed by Smith et al. (21). More recently, the basic concepts of the diagnosis of spinal fixations by motion palpation of the spine were formalized by Gillet (22) and organized by Faye (4) into a system of spinal joint palpation.

In a study of the effect of internal fixation on the zygapophyseal joints in dogs, degeneration occurred within two months of immobilization (23). Human patients with tuberculosis of the spine underwent ventral fusion by discectomy, thereby effectively eliminating movement between the two vertebrae (24). After six months, fusion of the zygapophyseal joints had also occurred in these patients. The lumbar spines of adult cadavers all showed intraarticular adhesions, ranging from thin thread-like filaments to dense mats that preclude any articular movement (25).

ADJUSTIVE PROCEDURES

Chiropractors use adjustive procedures to restore normal kinematics to joints. Restoring motion to a previously immobilized joint leads to normal joint function and physiology. While the degenerative effects of immobilization may be completely reversed upon remobilization (26–28), the extent of, and time for, maximum recovery depend upon the duration of immobilization (29). In extreme cases of immobilization to the point of fibrofatty consolidation of the synovial fluid, remobilization will result in the formation of a new joint cleft and articular cartilage with normal histological architecture (26). This constitutes some of the strongest evidence available supporting a physiological basis for the effectiveness of chiropractic adjustive procedures. Early mobilization is gaining a foot-hold in medical programs for treatment of whiplash (30) and following knee surgery (31). Forced motion causes physical disruption of adhesions between gross structures, such as capsule to cartilage, and leads to disruption of the intermolecular cross-bridging of collagen (32).

Neuropathology

The neurological component of the VSC is, for many, the cornerstone of chiropractic theory (33). For those who see beyond the application of chiropractic and other manipulative procedures to merely relieve headache and low back pain, the nervous system mediates vitality and health to the individual organs and tissues (34). Today, more than ever before, basic scientific and medical research supports this fundamental concept of chiropractic (35–38).

Every aspect of the nervous system's organization and function is relevant to the theory and practice of chiropractic, and many levels of neurological involvement are reflected in subluxation degeneration. This section explores some of the more pertinent aspects of this relationship (39). Pain is by far the most significant factor in a patient's seeking chiropractic care. In the diagnostic evaluation, motor function, reflexes, altered sensation, and pain responses are primary indicators in the physical examination (40). The interested reader is referred to several excellent reviews on the neurological component of the VSC (3, 41–43).

The segmental nerve is an integral component of each vertebral joint, and degeneration of the spinal articulations should have an effect on the associated spinal nerves. This is commonly recognized in the case of herniated discs that impinge on the segmental nerve roots (44, 45) as well as spurs and osteophytes around the joints of Lushka (46). Nerve impingement due to hypertrophy of the zygapophyseal joints has also been well documented (46). Chiropractic has begun to establish itself as caring for such cases (47, 48). Not all patients who benefit from chiropractic, however, suffer from herniated discs, nor do all patients with herniated discs display clinical symptoms (10, 49, 50). While cases of herniated discs may provide dramatic evidence of the effectiveness of chiropractic management programs, we must search for more general mechanisms to explain the positive results obtained by chiropractic care for the typical clinical case.

DORSAL ROOT GANGLIA

The integral relationship between the spinal joints and the dorsal root ganglia (DRG) necessitates evaluation of the role that these structures play in the VSC (51). With the exception of the first two spinal nerves, all DRG lie within the IVC in intimate association with the articular capsule (52, 53). DRG contain the cell bodies of all sensory neurons, except those found in the cranial nerves. Their strategic location between adjacent pairs of vertebrae make them prime suspects in the etiology of subluxations, and the focus of chiropractic adjustive procedures.

DRG are far more sensitive to mechanical stimulation than peripheral nerves. When inflamed, the ganglia become hyperexcitable and give rise to spontaneous discharges (54, 55). Minimal acute compression or chronic irritation lead to long periods of repetitive firing, which last longer than the stimulus itself; acute compression of peripheral nerves or nerve roots, on the other hand, does not. Aberrant impulses could lead to clinical and pathological signs and symptoms.

The ganglia are richly vascularized (56) but appear to have no blood-nerve barrier. Ganglionic capillaries are far more permeable than those of the CNS or peripheral nerve (57), and they have been implicated as a route of infection by virus and bacteria (58–61), as a site for the development of chemical irritation and inflammation by blood-borne agents (62), and as an entry portal for anesthetics injected into the epidural space (63). Any compression or sclerosis that might compromise the arterial supply to, or venous drainage from, the ganglia is likely to promote irritability as described for peripheral nerves (64).

ARTICULAR NEUROLOGY

Articular neurology is germane to the theory of chiropractic. Wyke (65) has classified the spinal joint receptors into three types of mechanoreceptors and the nociceptor (pain receptor) system. The role that each of these plays in degenerative processes and particularly in pain (66) is the subject of intensive research. Gillette (41) has proposed that coactivation of the articular receptor system and other somatic receptors is a major component of the chiropractic adjustment. The zygapophyseal joints are involved in the mechanism of referred pain (somatosomatic reflex), but the neurological mechanisms are not well understood (10, 67).

The afferent discharges derived from articular mechanoreceptors have a threefold impact when they enter the neuroaxis (66, 68): (*a*) reflexogenic effects; (*b*) perceptual effects; and (*c*) pain suppression. There is a significant correlation between proprioceptive input from the cervical spine and coordination of the extremities (68). There is a discharge of afferent fibers of the knee joint following passive movements of the leg (69). Joint inflammation sensitizes articular nociceptors to fire at rest and during normally nonnoxious joint movements (70). The proportion of neurons displaying resting discharges was higher and the receptive fields were larger in the inflamed joints. In humans (71), distension of the joint capsule of the knee led to reflex weakening of the quadriceps muscles. Injection of saline into the lumbar facets resulted in pain and significant increases in the myoelectric activity of the quadriceps (10) or the hamstrings (72), depending on the levels injected. These responses were abolished by injection of local anesthetic.

PAIN

The most common clinical characteristic of patients entering chiropractic offices is pain (39). Pain is a significant aspect of cervical spinal degeneration (58) as well as lumbar and pelvic degeneration (66). The mechanism for such pain is unquestionably related to mechanical or chemical irritation of the spinal nerves or their roots (58), or specific articular nerves (49, 66). Due to the largely subjective nature of pain, its evaluation by clinical methods and objective measures is a challenge to clinicians of all professions (66, 73). For the patient, the pain is real, whether or not there are objective clinical findings and, as in the case of phantom pain (74), whether or not the body part is present.

Numerous theories have been proposed to explain pain (75). One of the more widely discussed is the gate theory of pain (76), in which specific internuncial neurons of the spinal cord control the perception of pain. The transmission of pain sensation through the gate depends upon the relative input of large (A-beta) and small (A-delta and C) fibers converging on the gate (75). This is one of the major mechanisms evoked in modern theories of manipulative therapies to explain how adjustive procedures relieve pain (41, 77, 78).

VISCEROSOMATIC RELATIONSHIPS

Viscerosomatic relationships are widely recognized as patterns of referred pain (79). For example, pain associated with heart attack is often felt in the left shoulder and radiating down the left arm. Kidney degeneration refers pain to the low back, while pancreatic degeneration refers pain to the right shoulder. Skilled examiners can palpate spinal soft tissue changes associated with ischemic heart disease and differentiate those associated with other heart conditions (79).

SOMATOAUTONOMIC RELATIONSHIPS

Somatovisceral relationships are perhaps the key concept of chiropractic theory. The central issues can be divided into two complementary aspects: (*a*) Can spinal or paraspinal neurological dysfunction lead to visceral degeneration in the organs supplied by the involved nerves? (*b*) Can chiropractic intervention prevent degeneration and restore vitality to degenerating tissues? This is, perhaps, the most controversial issue in chiropractic theory. The evidence, however, tends to support such a concept. Responses in the nerves to the kidneys and adrenals were recorded after lateral flexion of a motion segment (36); the sympathetic response observed was correlated with alterations in heart rate and blood pressure.

Clinical studies tend to support these observations. A randomized, controlled trial (38) showed that chiropractic adjustments reduced blood pressure in humans. Another human study (80) showed that chiropractic adjustments exert a definite influence on pupillary diameter (see also Chapter 9).

NEURODYSTROPHIC HYPOTHESIS

As presented in Chapter 14, the neurodystrophic hypothesis proposes that neural dysfunction is stressful to the viscera and other body structures and leads to "lowered tissue resistance" that can modify the nonspecific and specific immune responses and alter the trophic function of the involved nerves. This has often been evoked by chiropractors to explain the positive results obtained in patients suffering from conditions of a more general nature than musculoskeletal pain, such as COPD (81), bronchial asthma, dysmenorrhea, and hypertension (82).

Current research provides growing evidence for a dynamic interaction between nervous and immune systems. Histological studies have shown that mast cells are innervated directly by sympathetic nerve fibers and that this relationship appears to serve a regulatory role in immunological response (83). These observations are consistent with those showing a reduction of norepinephrine in lymphoid tissue following an immunological challenge (84). The evidence supports the hypothesis that sympathetic innervation exerts an inhibitory effect on the immune system and that changes in tissue levels of norepinephrine can affect immunological responsiveness. In animals, sympathectomy of one side of the body leads to increased development of tumors on that side (85). This suggests that interference with the sympathetic nervous system can compromise the body's immune system (86, 87).

NEUROTRANSMITTERS

Nerves release from their termini chemicals called neurotransmitters, which elicit immediate and dramatic effects in the end organs. Release of acetylcholine in muscles, for example, causes contraction; norepinephrine in arterioles causes vasoconstriction or vasodilation, depending upon the type of receptor present; release of serotonin in the uterus leads to uterine contraction (88). Release of the same neurotransmitters in other tissues can result in inhibition: acetylcholine in the heart suppresses the intrinsic rate of discharge of the heart's pacemaker, and noradrenaline in the lungs leads to bronchodilation following relaxation of the bronchial smooth muscle. Chemical transmitters are involved in the perception of pain as well as light and sound. The chemical nature of the nervous system forms the basis of our understanding of neurological function and represents aspects of the biochemical component of the VSC.

TROPHIC INFLUENCES

It is unclear whether trophic influences are due to the release of some chemical substances, to the rates of electrical discharge of axons, or to some other aspect of nerve function (89–91). Chemicals that perform such functions are called trophic substances. Several compounds are implicated as mediators of trophic influences (92, 93), with acetylcholine being most often cited (94, 95). Trophic influences stimulate more subtle responses in tissues than do neurotransmitters, such as altered growth rate (96).

It is suggested that proper vitality, morphology, and function of the target tissues depend on adequate trophic stimulation. In muscle, for example, exchanging nerves between "white" and "red" muscle led to white muscle transforming to red and vice versa (97). This line of research gave considerable impetus to the compression models of subluxation (see Chapter 11).

Trophic substances are synthesized in the cell body and transported to the synapse by axoplasmic transport (98). Compressing the nerve and shutting off the flow of these vital supportive substances might cause the tissues to degenerate for lack of the chemical stimulation, but the force required to cut off axoplasmic flow would lead to serious neurological deficits that would far overshadow any subtle trophic changes predicted by subluxation models. It remains to be seen, however, whether chronic irritation might lead to excessive trophic stimulation that could lead to tissue hypertrophy or even pathological degeneration (see Chapter 15).

Myopathology

Joint immobilization leads to disuse atrophy (99–101). The precise role this plays in joint degeneration is not well understood. While the changes in muscle function are often completely reversible (102–104), the time required for complete restoration of muscle function depends upon the duration of immobilization (102, 103). These findings are complicated by the different responses to immobilization by different muscle types (102, 105–107) as well as by differences in degenerative response related to the position of the joint and so the length of the muscle in the immobilized state (103, 108–110).

In some cases, the muscle changes are secondary to immobilization but in turn contribute to joint degeneration (111). In other instances, such as trauma, congenital anomalies, or diseases that affect muscles (such as polio and muscular dystrophy), muscle degeneration or pathology can be primary and might also contribute to joint degeneration. It is not always possible to discern the role of muscle in joint pathology, especially that of the spine.

In particular, scoliosis poses an enigma. While muscles tend to differ on the concave and convex sides of the scoliotic curve, their contribution to the development of the curve is not understood in the vast majority of cases (112). Current trends in scoliosis theory lean toward the idea that there is a loss of unilateral regional control of muscle tone or loss of coordination of the righting (postural) response in the spinal musculature (113, 114). Virtually every significant as-

pect of muscle structure and function has been evaluated in the context of degenerative changes following immobilization.

Studies of immobilization of the knee showed that in the early stages of joint degeneration, restricted joint mobility was due almost exclusively to the muscle/tendon unit (26); cutting the muscle away restored movement to normal ranges. In later stages, mobility appears to be restricted by capsular and ligamentous stricture (115, 116) followed by intraarticular adhesions (109). Muscle tension might lead to excessive degeneration of cartilage by compressing the joint surfaces together (111), thereby contributing to the development of osteoarthritis. A vicious cycle has been described (72) in which muscle spasticity leads to joint contracture, which leads to more spasticity and muscular contracture. The specified treatment for this condition is to return the joints to their full ROM and maintain that range through the healing stages.

Muscle spindles are adversely affected by immobilization, showing significant morphological, physiological, and biochemical changes including shortening and thickening, degeneration of the primary spindle endings, swollen capsules, and loss of cross-striations (117, 118). Physiological alterations include increased sensitivity to stretch and elevation of resting rate of discharge (117, 119). One consequence of such an increase in spindle activity would be to feed excessive stimuli into the central reflex pathways, resulting in altered efferent output. This could lead to overstimulation of muscle groups that respond to the stretch reflex, leading finally to muscle spasm and tender trigger points. Alternatively, such input could lead to reflex inhibition or failure of joint musculature upon challenge (120).

When a joint is immobilized, the effect on muscles depends upon their length in the immobilized state (110, 121) or the angle at which a joint is fixed (99). Such changes have been reported for gross morphologic appearance (122) as well as biochemical (123–125) and ultrastructural (99) characteristics. Shortened muscles show a reduction in tension-producing capacity, while those chronically stretched retain their ability to generate force in direct proportion to changes in cross-sectional area.

Alteration of the distractive forces applied to the Achilles tendon induces extensive cellular and extracellular changes in the musculotendinous junction (125). The distribution of cell types and architecture of the extracellular matrix depend to a large degree on the type of force applied to the tissue (compressive vs. distractive) (126). Early mobilization of previously immobilized limbs increased the rate of healing in lacerated flexor tendons (127), whereas adhesions form in immobilized limbs between the tendon and its sheath (117).

Connective Tissue Pathology

The major impact of connective tissue (CT) changes in the VSC model involves changes following immobilization. The most remarkable effect of immobilization is joint stiffness (128), or contracture (129, 130), which also increases with age. This phenomenon has been the subject of intensive research due to the use of casting in orthopaedic procedures (130).

Every CT component is affected by immobilization, and each expresses its own unique pattern of change (1, 130). Synovial fluid undergoes fibrofatty consolidation that progresses to more adherent fibrous tissue, ultimately providing a matrix for the deposition of bone salts (26). Articular cartilage, on the other hand, shrinks due to the loss of proteoglycans (131), exhibits a reorganization of cellular components (111), develops ulcerations that connect the synovial space with the subchondral bone, and ultimately becomes ossified itself (132). Softening of articular cartilage following immobilization renders it more susceptible to damage by minor trauma (133). Adhesions form between adjacent articular structures (26, 111), and forced motion causes a physical disruption of adhesions as well as a disruption of intermolecular cross-linkages (32). It is also important to note that adhesions may form between the nerve root sleeve and the adjacent osseous and capsular structures in the IVC (134).

The effect of immobilization on articular CT, as with muscle, depends upon the position of the joint when it is immobilized (20, 135). This reflects the forces placed upon the respective tissues (133, 136). The age of the CT is also important in determining the response to altered forces (137, 138). In a young growing bone, excessive pressure inhibits bone growth, while a reduction of pressure may accelerate bone growth (139). In mature skeletons, abnormal distribution of stresses leads to altered mineral deposition and osteophyte formation (140). Weight-bearing and motion appear to exert separate influences on the maintenance of CT (133).

Ligamentous contracture is widely discussed as a mechanism for joint stiffness (32). This may well apply to later stages of immobilization, but in the earlier stages of ID, ligaments become more pliable and compliant, a condition referred to as ligamentous laxity (129, 141–143). Alterations of the point of attachment of ligament to bone following immobilization are also well described (129, 144), and this is a significant factor in the ligament's response to stress.

The vast majority of research on joint immobilization has been performed on extremities, especially knees and elbows (1), and on experimental animals such as rats (111), rabbits (145), and dogs (137). Studies with humans have suggested that the animal findings are applicable to human spinal degeneration (24, 115, 146, 147). Very little research has been done on the effects of immobilization on the spine in either animals or humans. Most of the studies that have been done are related to scoliosis (140) or lumbar discectomy (24). In scoliotic spines, changes on the concave side of the curve differed from those on the convex side (148), the former resembling ligamentous changes in immobilized joints, the latter resembling changes in hypermobile joints. If the discs are analyzed as a unit, the two effects cancel, giving the appearance of no change in the IVD.

Vascular Abnormalities

Vascular abnormalities have been widely discussed as contributing or complicating factors in a range of clinical symptomatologies from thoracic outlet syndrome (149) to trigeminal neuralgia (150) and vertigo (151). Several vascular anomalies are widely discussed as being significant to subluxations. First and foremost is the vertebral artery (VA).

Vertebrobasilar insufficiency is a major contraindication to cervical rotatory adjustments (152). Paralysis, hemiparesis, Wallenberg's syndrome, or death have resulted from extreme rotation and extension of the cervical spine, whether chiropractically through adjustments (152) or voluntarily on the part of the patient (153). Often these situations are thought to be caused by a dislodged thrombus from the VA, but structural anomalies must be considered as well (154, 155). The VAs are known to occasionally develop asymmetrically in size, with one side making an insignificant contribution to cranial blood flow (156). In addition, the VA is known to buckle, or form loops within the transverse canal (155), and this is believed to lead to signs and symptoms of cerebral ischemia (see Chapter 13).

The segmental arteries that supply the spinal nerves divide into the dorsal and ventral radicular arteries (157). Occasionally, one of these carries most of the blood for that segment (56), and such asymmetries may contribute to radicular-type symptoms. Experimental arterial or venous occlusion leads to joint stiffness (128). Finally, compression within the IVC by disc protrusion, osteophytes, tumors, or hypertrophied bone would potentially affect the vascular component before affecting the neurological structures directly (158). Diminished venous return leads to alterations in capillary distribution around joints (159), and a similar mechanism has been suggested in immobilized joints (160, 161).

The vertebral column is drained by a system of veins that form an intricate plexus (Batson's plexus) around the vertebral column and spinal cord (162). The plexus lacks valves, as in the systemic veins, to control the direction of venous flow (158). This unique anatomical arrangement allows retrograde flow (venous reflux), which contributes to the effect of posture on venous drainage in the spine. Batson's plexus is also believed to account for metastatic dissemination to the spine (162).

Toxins or inflammatory agents from one area of the spine (e.g., the vertebral bodies or spinal articular capsule) could influence areas of the spine remote from the origin of these substances, such as the dorsal root ganglia, through this same route. The role of intersegmental mobility in such a process is unknown, although movement in other parts of the body is critical to proper venous circulation (163). Blood flow increases upon resisted rhythmic contraction of the calf and thigh muscles (161). Immobilization would likely lead to localized venous stasis, which would effectively create a negative relative pressure at the area of immobilization. Venous reflux would then potentially bring toxins into the area of immobilization. Venous stasis reduces the rate of removal of metabolic toxins, which, in turn, leads to inflammation and accelerating degeneration.

Inflammatory Response

Inflammation leads to pain, which is the major presenting complaint in chiropractic offices (39). The inflammatory response is a composite of cellular and biochemical processes, largely mediated via the vascular system (164), but initiated and supported by local events within the tissues themselves. Fibrous CT does not manifest an inflammatory response in the same way as skin, muscles, or viscera (165). Lacerated tendons can repair themselves intrinsically by recruitment of tissue macrophages and proliferation of fibroblasts (127), more representative of a chronic inflammatory response (165, 166). Chronic inflammation also leads to an alteration of collagen types in CT (167, 168), fibrosis, and long-term exposure to the destructive actions of macrophages (165). There is clearly an inflammatory response associated with immobilization of joints (160), and ossification is considered the end product of inflammation (169). Inflammatory spill-over into surrounding tissue is a critical parameter to monitor (170) as implied in the concept of chemical radiculitis (171). It represents one way in which the degeneration of spinal joints may affect the neurological components.

ARTHRITIS

Arthritis means simply inflammation of a joint, and it can affect any joint of the body, including the spine (142, 146). Although osteoarthritis, or degenerative joint disease (DJD), is classically considered a noninflammatory condition (172), as many as 75% of cases of osteoarthritis show evidence of inflammation (173). All forms of arthritis are associated with pain and decreased movement of the involved joints. Joint immobilization is the most widely used tool for the study of arthritis in experimental animals (174–177). All situations that lead to the immobilization can cause osteoarthritis (178), which is also closely related to scoliosis (146). The restoration of movement can decrease the rate of degeneration or even restore the joint to normal functional capacity (179), as evidenced clinically (180, 181) and shown by basic animal studies (17, 182). Arthritis is intricately interwoven with the inflammatory, kinesiological and CT components. Molecular fragments of collagen (183, 184) and proteoglycans (185–187) are inflammatory stimuli and have been associated with rheumatoid arthritis (188–190), as well as polyarthritis in mice (191) and humans (192), osteoarthritis, (193) and other arthritic conditions (194).

INFLAMMATION OF
NERVES AND NERVE ROOTS

Inflamed nerves are hyperexcitable (54) and exhibit behavior different from that of

normal nerves. The dorsal root ganglia (DRG) of normal nerves respond to mechanical stimulation by a discharge of action potentials that stops upon cessation of the stimulus. Inflamed ganglia, however, continue to fire long after the mechanical stimulus has ceased. The ganglia themselves are more susceptible to blood-borne agents such as small molecular weight inflammatory agents. Such a process has been proposed, under the name *chemical radiculitis*, to explain radicular symptoms following discal herniation (171). It is proposed here that such a mechanism is a frequent mediator of neurological involvement in subluxations.

Fundamental Aspects

To completely characterize the VSC as a clinical entity, all involved tissues must be described in terms of their pathoanatomy, pathophysiology, and pathobiochemistry. These fundamental aspects of the VSC represent the foundation of knowledge upon which is formed the details of the model.

PATHOANATOMY

The 5-component model of the VSC included histopathology, a subset of pathoanatomy. The broader category allows anatomical variations, such as asymmetrical development or other vertebral arteries, and congenital anomalies, such as agenesis of the dens, to be formally included as aspects of the VSC. Variations in anatomical structures are well recognized as contributing to abnormal spinal biomechanics and symptomatic clinical presentations. Facet trophism is a case in point, as are wedged and blocked vertebrae. While not exhibiting abnormal histological characteristics, they cause or contribute to the development of the VSC.

For each tissue there is a histological description of degenerative processes that occur in various pathological conditions, and there may be several different histopathological processes for each tissue (e.g., changes in muscle tissue with muscular dystrophy compared with those from polio). Degeneration of muscle tissue following joint immobilization consists of a loss of mass (atrophy) succeeded by fibrofatty replacement. Muscle spindles show a pattern of degeneration which differs from that of the extrafusal muscle fibers (195, 196). Within the spindle, nuclear bag and nuclear chain fibers show different patterns of response to immobilization and exercise (196).

The histopathology of CT degeneration has been well described (1). With regard to ID, the first observable sign of tissue change is a loss of metachromatic staining of cartilage, which indicates a loss of proteoglycan (27). This is observed after the first day of immobilization, but changes in cellular activity have been demonstrated within four hours of immobilization (131). Histological changes in cartilage are more pronounced in areas apposed by other cartilage (111, 135).

Fibroblasts initially become rounded, then disappear. Chondrocytes similarly disappear and begin to form clusters, the "brood capsules," at the edges of the areas of apposition (111). These become very active metabolically but ultimately become necrotic and create ulcerations in the articular surface (111). The synovial fluid undergoes fibrofatty consolidation with the invasion of inflammatory cells and the formation of a CT matrix (115). Substantial regeneration of cellular and extracellular components of the joints is seen following remobilization of previously immobilized joints (26).

In the dorsal root ganglia, one can distinguish six distinctive cell types (197), which presumably correspond to different classes of peripheral receptors (53). It is believed that the larger A-type cell bodies, localized in the proximal poles of the ganglia, are associated with muscle spindle receptors or proprioception in general, while the small C-type cell bodies, concentrated at the distal poles, are associated with the unmyelinated C-fibers believed to be involved in nociception (198). With degeneration or trauma at

the proximal pole of the ganglion, the first functions affected would be movement and coordination; pain perception would only be affected by more extensive involvement of the ganglion. Pathological changes occurring in the ganglia in association with cystic invasion were reported by Smith (199) to include pyknosis, hyperchromatism, and chromatolysis of the perikarya.

PATHOPHYSIOLOGY

Changes in physiological responses are characteristic of all degenerative processes. The kinesiopathological component, including biomechanical considerations, consists almost exclusively of pathophysiological processes. In the VSC, this would include alterations of biomechanical characteristics of CT components such as tendons (37) and the IVD (200), including changes in the extensibility and load characteristics of ligaments following immobilization (126, 141, 175). Alterations of neuronal response patterns (52) and reflex adaptations to increased neuronal input and neurophysiological changes in the DRG as a result of inflammation (54) are good examples of pathophysiology. Each tissue level component will manifest a number of pathophysiological changes in association with subluxation degeneration.

PATHOBIOCHEMISTRY

The aspects of biochemistry relevant to the VSC range from neurotransmitters to proteoglycans. Biochemistry is the common language of all biological sciences, and a knowledge of its principles is essential for understanding areas as diverse as histopathology, digestion, axoplasmic flow, muscle contraction, and endocrinology. Although chiropractic is rarely thought of as having a basis in biochemistry, certain alterations in metabolism are necessarily involved in the degenerative processes of the VSC. An exhaustive treatment of this topic would require establishing fundamental principles, molecular structure, a detailed description of metabolism, etc. This section highlights some of the more important aspects of biochemistry as they relate to chiropractic.

Connective Tissue

Mechanical failure of ligaments, discs, capsules, or other CTs can result from local variations in chemical composition (200). In addition, alterations of the biomechanical forces that stress CT lead to local changes in the biochemical composition of the tissue (1). We thus have a clearly delineated link between biomechanics and biochemistry as it relates to CT structure and function.

Collagen forms chemical cross-linkages that hold adjacent collagen molecules together and stabilize its overall structure (32). The number of cross-linkages increases with advancing age (201) and in states of degeneration (202). This is involved in the formation of CT adhesions as are known to form between the nerve root sheath and the articular capsule (26, 111). The sulfated glycosaminoglycans draw water into the spaces between individual collagen fibrils. The water contributes to the space-filling properties of the proteoglycans but also provides lubrication between adjacent collagen fibrils (32, 203), especially in fibrous CT.

Upon immobilization of a joint, the first measurable biochemical change is a decrease in proteoglycan; a change that occurs in all CT components of the joint (131). This allows the collagen fibers to approximate each other more closely and facilitates formation of more collagen cross-linkages (201). The longer a joint is immobilized, the more collagen cross-linkages are formed. This would appear to be a mechanism for stabilizing the joint in its new ROM. Remobilization of a previously immobilized joint leads to a disruption of collagen cross-linkages (202, 203), as by the high-velocity, low-amplitude thrust that is characteristic of the chiropractic adjustment.

Inflammation

Another significant aspect of CT biochemistry are the antigenic and inflammatory properties of fragments of collagen (183, 184) and proteoglycans (204). Fragments of hyaluronic acid are potent angiogenic agents; that is, they stimulate the development of new capillaries (205). It has long been believed that rheumatoid arthritis is an autoimmune disease, with the organism producing antibodies to its own collagen (183). Collagen plays a significant role not only in rheumatoid arthritis (206) but in osteoarthritis and other joint diseases as well (193, 194); antibodies to collagen are frequently found in patients suffering from nonrheumatoid arthritis. Antibodies to proteoglycans exist in rheumatic diseases such as polychondritis, osteoarthritis, and rheumatoid arthritis (191).

CT releases specific chemical mediators of the inflammatory response called autocoids (186), including a group called CT-activating peptides. There is an inflammatory response to tissue injury, such as ligamentous or capsular tear (162), but the inflammatory response to simple immobilization is less well understood. Evidence of such a response includes the development of pain (19) and the marked alterations of joint morphology seen on immobilization (26, 111). The products of CT degradation could stimulate an inflammatory process as an initial step in tissue remodeling and adaptation to new dynamic joint function, such as limited motion.

The role of histamines in inflammation must be understood, as well as the events that control their release from the mast cells and other immunological components (207, 208). Similar consideration must also be given to the role of prostaglandins in the pain response (209, 210).

Endocrinology

Serum aldosterone levels decrease following chiropractic adjustments in patients with hypertension (211). Spinal mobilization resulted in specific sympathetic input into the adrenal gland (36). Although adrenal hormonal output was not monitored, one would expect a change in circulating medullary hormones, based on neurophysiological observations and observed changes in heart rate and blood pressure. Cortisol levels increase following spinal manipulation, but this is a generalized stress response, not a specific effect of chiropractic adjustive procedures (212). Muscle disuse following immobilization leads to insulin resistance, altering glucose metabolism (213). No doubt other hormonal effects on neuromusculoskeletal tissues have a significant impact on biomechanical function or response, such as the effect of pregnancy in softening the ligaments of the female pelvis to facilitate delivery.

Pharmacological Considerations

Given the widespread use of drugs by the medical profession to treat a variety of diseases and conditions, including musculoskeletal disorders, the effects of drug usage on the course of chiropractic management programs must be considered. In addition, there is a growing movement in the chiropractic profession toward the use of proprietary and nonproprietary drugs (214). While it is not our purpose to debate the use of drugs in chiropractic, the effects of drugs on human physiology and function cannot be ignored. As an example, the regular use of muscle relaxants might well alter the outcome of a chiropractic adjustment program. Conversely, narcotic use leads to a type of muscular rigidity (215), which could have a dramatic impact on the patient's response to care. The use of injectable and topical steroids to treat inflammatory conditions can lead to adverse effects (216, 217) that could interfere with effective chiropractic care.

SUMMARY

This chapter attempts to provide a comprehensive and inclusive conceptual basis for the chiropractic lesion or subluxation. This has evolved into a component-based model of spinal dysfunction and degeneration that has implications for all manual, somatic approaches to patient care. Accomplishing this required including all relevant tissues: nerve, muscle, vascular, and connective, as well as the clinically relevant aspects of kinesiopathology and the inflammatory response. Each of these tissue level components can be subdivided into their anatomically identifiable elements for more precise diagnostic descriptions. Emphasis is placed on the organization and interaction of the components and their specific elements. Each component must be described in terms of its pathoanatomy, pathophysiology, and pathobiochemistry to fully characterize the changes that take place during subluxation degeneration and subsequent reversal following adjustive/manipulative procedures. Perturbations of a single element may have an impact on the entire system.

Kinesiological considerations are of primary importance to the model, and the relationship of the various components to motion is a major theme. Central to the conceptual basis of the model is immobilization degeneration; once an articulation is immobilized, it will undergo degeneration that will affect all aspects of the joint's structure and function. The neuromusculoskeletal aspects of this process are the immediate focus of the model.

There are three levels of application of the model in a clinical setting: the basic scientific knowledge, the diagnostic/evaluative applications of technology to the individual components, and finally the mechanisms of therapeutic intervention. The model has practical application as a means of organizing the vast amount of information that is to be assimilated and used by clinical practitioners; it stimulates inquiry into the physiological processes involved in spinal degeneration and dysfunction; it offers a conceptual framework in which to develop basic and clinical research; it allows ready exchange of information between basic scientists and clinical practitioners; and it can serve as a basis for organizing educational curricula. The model is internally self-validating and is consistent with all currently accepted knowledge within the basic and clinical sciences, but it is flexible enough to allow virtually unlimited growth as our understanding of spinal structure and function expands.

It is hoped that this model can become a focus for discussion among clinicians and basic scientists. To that end, it is possible to map each component onto specific diagnostic modalities (e.g., myopathology onto EMG, kinesiopathology onto range of motion) and adjustive/manipulative intervention procedures (the effect of a high-velocity thrust on the articular capsule or IVD in question). In this way the VSC model can stimulate communication among all members of the profession.

REFERENCES

1. Lantz CA. Immobilization degeneration and the fixation hypothesis of chiropractic subluxation. Chiro Res J 1988;1:21–46.

2. Dishman RW. Static and dynamic components of the chiropractic subluxation complex. A literature review. J Manipulative Physiol Ther 1988;11(2):98–107.

3. Dishman R. Review of the literature supporting a scientific basis for the chiropractic subluxation complex. J Manipulative Physiol Ther 1985;8:163–174.

4. Schafer RC, Faye J. Motion palpation and chiropractic technique. Huntington Beach, Calif.: Motion Palpation Institute, 1983.

5. Lantz CA. The vertebral subluxation complex. ICA Rev 1989;45:37–61.

6. Parke WW. Applied anatomy of the spine. In: Rothman RH, Simeone FA, eds. The spine. Ch 2. Philadelphia: WB Saunders, 1982.

7. Nachemson AF, Schultz AB, Berkson MH. Mechanical properties of human lumbar spine motion segments. Influences of age, sex, disc level and degeneration. Spine 1979;4(1):1–8.

8. Roaf R. A study of the mechanics of spinal injuries. J Bone Joint Surg 1960;42B:810–823.

9. Farfan HJ. Biomechanics of the lumbar spine. In: Kirkaldy-Willis WH, ed. Managing low back pain. New York: Churchill Livingstone, 1988:9–21.

10. Mooney V, Robertson J. The facet syndrome. Clin Orthop 1976;115:149–156.

11. Sandoz R. Some physical mechanisms and effects of spinal adjustments. Ann Swiss Chiro Assoc 1976;6:91–141.

12. Vanderby R, Daniele M, Pattwardhan A, Bunch W. A method for the identification of in-vivo segmental stiffness properties of the spine. J Biomech Eng 1986;108:312–316.

13. Lance J, Anthony M. Neck-tongue syndrome on sudden turning of the head. J Neurol Neurosurg Psychiatry 1980;43:97–101.

14. Breig A. Adverse mechanical tension in the central nervous System. New York: John Wiley & Sons, 1978.

15. Jirout J. Studies in the dynamics of the spine. Acta Radiol 1956;46:55–60.

16. Stokes I, Wilder D, Frymoyer J, Pope M. Assessment of patients with low-back pain by biplanar radiographic measurement of intervertebral motion. Spine 1981;6:233–240.

17. Videman T. Connective tissue and immobilization. Clin Orthop 1987;221:26–32.

18. Akeson WH. An experimental study of joint stiffness. J Bone Joint Surg 1961;43A:1022–1034.

19. Hills W, Byrd R. Effects of immobilization in the human forearm. Arch Phys Med Rehabil 1973;54:87–90.

20. Jackson R. The cervical syndrome. Springfield, Ill.: Charles C Thomas, 1977.

21. Smith OG, Langworthy SM, Paxson MC. Modernized chiropractic. Cedar Rapids, Mo.: Laurence Press, 1906.

22. Gillet H, Liekens M. Belgian chiropractic research notes. Huntington Beach, Calif.:Motion Palpation Institute, 1989

23. Kahanovitz N, Arnoczky S, Levine D, Otis J. The effects of internal fixation on the articular cartilage of unfused canine facet joint cartilage. Spine 1984;9(3):268–273.

24. Tarlov IM. Cyst (perineural) of the spinal roots. Another cause (removable) of sciatic pain. JAMA 1948;138:740–744.

25. Harris RJ, MacNab I. Structural changes in the lumbar intervertebral discs. Their relationship to low back pain and sciatica. J Bone Joint Surg 1954;36B(2):304–322.

26. Evans EB, Eggers GWN, Butler JK, Blumel J. Experimental immobilization and remobilization of rat knee joints. J Bone Joint Surg 1960;42A:737–758.

27 Palmoski M, Pericone E, Brandt KD. Development & reversal of a proteoglycan aggregation defect in normal canine knee cartilage after immobilization. Arthritis Rheum 1979;22:508-517.

28. St. Pierre D, Gardiner PF. The effect of immobilization and exercise on muscle function. A review. Physiother Can 1987;39:24–36.

29. Krusen FH. Handbook of physical medicine and rehabilitation. Philadelphia: WB Saunders, 1971.

30. Mealy K, Brennan H, Fenelon GCC. Early mobilization of acute whiplash injuries. Br Med J 1986;292:656–657.

31. Marwah V, Gadegone WM, Magarker DS. The treatment of fractures of the tibial plateau by skeletal traction and early mobilization. Int Orthop 1985;9:217–221.

32. Woo SL-Y, Matthews JV, Akeson WH, Amiel D, Covery FR. Connective tissue response to immobility. Correlative study of biomechanical and biochemical measurements of normal and immobilized rabbit knees. Arthritis Rheum 1975;18:257.

33. Palmer DD. The science, art and philosophy of chiropractic. Portland, Ore.: Portland Printing House, 1910.

34. Janse J, Hildebrandt RW. Principles and practice of chiropractic. Lombard, Ill.: National College of Chiropractic, 1976.

35. Vernon HT, Dhami MS, Howley TP, Annett R. Spinal manipulation and betaendorphin. A controlled study of the effect of spinal manipulation on plasma betaendorphin levels in normal males. J Manipulative Physiol Ther 1986;9(2):115–123.

36. Sato A, Swenson R. Sympathetic nervous system response to mechanical stress of the spinal column in rats. J Manipulative Physiol Ther 1984;7(3):141–147.

37. Korr IM. The collected papers of IM Korr. Colorado Springs, Colo.: American Academy of Osteopathy, 1979.

38. Yates G, Lamping D, Abram N, Wright C. Effects of chiropractic treatment on blood pressure and anxiety. A randomized, controlled trial. J Manipulative Physiol Ther 1988;11(6):484–488.

39. Phllips R, Butler R. Survey of chiropractic in Dade County Florida. J Manipulative Physiol Ther 1982;5(2):83–89.

41. Gillette R. A speculative argument for the coactivation of diverse somatic receptor populations by forceful chiropractic adjustments. Manual Med 1987;3:1–14.

42. Slosberg M. Effects of altered afferent articular input on sensation, proprioception, muscle tone and sympathetic reflex responses. J Manipulative Physiol Ther 1988;11(5):400–408.

43. Gunn C, Milbrandt W. Early and subtle signs in low-back sprain. Spine 1978;3(3):267–281.

44. Tay E, Chacha P. Midline prolapse of a lumbar intervertebral disc with compression of the cauda equina. J Bone Joint Surg 1979;61B(1):43–46.

45. Lindblom K, Rexed B. Spinal nerve injury in dorsolateral protrusions of lumbar discs. J Neurosurg 1948;5:413–432.

46. Lyon E. Uncovertebral osteophytes and osteochondrosis of the cervical spine. J Bone Joint Surg 1945;27(2):248–253.

47. Bronfort G. Chiropractic treatment of low back pain. A prospective survey. J Manipulative Physiol Ther 1986;9(2):99–113.

48. Mierau D, Cassidy J, McGregor M, Kirkaldy-Willis W. A Comparison of the effectiveness of spinal manipulative therapy for low back pain patients with and without spondylolisthesis. J Manipulative Physiol Ther 1987;10(2):49–55.

49. Shealy C. Facet Denervation in the management of back and sciatic pain. Clin Orthop 1976;115:157–164.

50. DeVilliers, P Booysen E. Fibrous spinal stenosis. Clin Orthop 1976;115:140–144.

51. Lantz C. The role of dorsal root ganglia in the development of chiropractic subluxations. A chiropractic theory. Proceedings of the 3rd Annual Current Topics in Chiropractic. 1981;C2:1–12.

52. Svaetichin G. Electrophysiological investigations on single ganglion cells. Acta Physiol Scand 1951;24(86):5–57.

53. Lieberman A. Sensory ganglia. In: D Landon, ed. The peripheral nerve. New York: John Daily Sons, 1976:188–278.

54. Howe JF, Loeser JD, Calvin WH. Mechano-sensitivity of dorsal root ganglia and chronically injured axons. A physiological basis for the radicular pain of nerve root compression. Pain 1977;3:25–41.

55. Kirk EJ. Impulses in dorsal spinal nerve rootlets in cats and rabbits arising from dorsal root ganglia isolated from the periphery. J Comp Neurol 1975;115:165–175.

56. Bergman L Alexander L. Vascular supply of the spinal ganglia. Arch Neurol Psychiatry 1941;46:761–782.

57. McCabe JS, Low EN. The subarachnoid angle. An area of transition in peripheral nerve. Anat Rec 1969;164:15–3.

58. Wakesman BH. Experimental study of diptheric polyneuritis in the rabbit and guinea-pig. III. The blood nerve barrier in the rabbit. J Neuropathol Exp Neurol 1961; 20:35–77.

59. Clements GB, Subak-Sharpe JH. Recovery of herpes simplex virus 1 ts mutants from the dorsal root ganglia of mice. Brain Res 1983;59:203–207.

60. Sato A, Schaible H, Schmidt R. Types of afferents from the knee joint evoking sympathetic reflexes in cat inferior cardiac nerves. Neurosci Lett 1983;39:71–75.

61. Brierley JB. The sensory ganglia. Recent anatomical, physiological and pathological contributions. Acta Psychiatr Neurol Scand 1955;30:553–576.

62. Chang LW, Yip RK. Corn oil-induced changes in dorsal root ganglia of rats. Envir Res 1983;30:50–57.

63. Cousins MJ, Bridenbaugh PO. Neural blockade in clinical anesthesia and management of pain. 2nd ed. Philadelphia: JB Lippincott, 1989.

64. Porter EL, Wharton PIS. Irritability of mammalian nerve following ischemia. J Neurophysiol 1948;12:109–116.

65. Wyke B. The neurology of joints. A review of general principles. Clin Rheum Dis 1981;7(1):223–239.

66. Wyke B. The neurology of low back pain. In: M Jayson, ed. The lumbar spine and low back pain. 2nd ed. New York: Pitman Medical, 1980.

67. Lippitt A. The facet joint and its role in spine pain. Management with facet joint injections. Spine 1984;9(7):746–750.

68. deJong PTVM, deJong JMB, Cohen B, Jogkees LBW. Ataxia and nystagmus induced by injection of local anesthetics in the neck. Ann Neurol 1977;1:240–246.

69. Schaible H, Schmidt R. Responses of fine medial articular nerve afferents to passive movements of knee joint. J Neurophysiol 1983;49(5):1118–1126.

70. Coggeshall R, Hong K, Langford L, Schaible H, Schmidt R. Discharge characteristics of fine medial articular nerve afferents at rest and during passive movements of inflamed knee joints. Brain Res 1983;272:185–188.

71. DeAndrade J, Grant C, Dixon A. Joint distension and reflex muscle inhibition in the knee. J Bone Joint Surg 1965;47A(2):313–322.

72. Stauffer ES. Rehabilitation of the spinal cord-injured patient. Ch 19. 1982.In: Rothman RH, Simeone FA, eds. The spine. Philadelphia: WB Saunders, 1982.

73. Mooney V. Where is the pain coming from? Spine 1987;12(8):754-759.

74. Howe J. Phantom limb pain. A re-afferentation syndrome. Pain 1983;15:101–107.

75. Melzak R, Wall PD. The challenge of pain. New York: Basic Books, 1982.

76. Melzak R, Wall PD. Pain mechanisms. A new theory. Science 1965;150:971.

77. Zusman M. A theoretical basis for the short-term relief of some types of spinal pain with manipulative therapy. Manual Med 1987;3: 54–56.

78. Irving R. Pain and the protective reflex generators. Relevance to the chiropractic concept of spinal subluxation. J Manipulative Physiol Ther 1981;4/2:69–71.

79. Nicholas A, DeBias D, Ehrenfeucther W, England K, England R, et al. A somatic component to myocardial infarction. J Am Osteopath Assoc 1987;87(2):123–129.

80. Briggs L, Boone W. Effects of a chiropractic adjustment on changes in pupillary diameter. A model for evaluating somatovisceral response. J Manipulative Physiol Ther 1988;11(3):181–189.

81. Deal MC, Morlock JW. Somatic dysfunction associated with pulmonary disease. J Am Osteopath Assoc 1984;84:179–183.

82. Wiles M, Diakow P. Chiropractic and visceral disease. A brief survey. J Can Chiro Assoc 1982;26(2):65–68.

83. Bienenstock J, Tomioka M, Matsuda H, Stead R, Quinonez G, et al. The role of mast cells in inflammatory processes. Evidence of nerve/mast cell interactions. Int Arch Allergy Appl Immunol 1987;82:238–243.

84. DelRey A, Besedovsky H, Sorkin E, DaPrada M, Arrenbrecht S. Immunoregulation mediated by the sympathetic nervous system II. Mol Immunol 1981;63–329–344.

85. Coujard R, Heitz F. Cancerologie. Production de tumeurs malignes consecutives a des lesions des fibres sympathiques du nerf sciatique chez le Cobaye. C R Acad Sci 1957;244:409–411.

86. Besedovsky H, DelRey A, Sorkin E, DaPrada M, Keller H. Immunoregulation mediated by the sympathetic nervous system. Cell Immunol 1979;48:346–355.

87. Stein-Werblowsky R. The sympathetic nervous system and cancer. Exp Neurol 1974;42:97–100.

88. Goodman LS, Gilman A. The pharmacological basis of therapeutics. 4th ed. London: MacMillan, 1970.

89. Salmons S, Sreter FA. Significance of impulse activity in the transformation of skeletal muscle type. Nature 1976;263:30–34.

90. Drachman D. Trophic actions of the neuron. An introduction. Ann NY Acad Sci 1974;228:3–5.

91. Davis HL. Trophic action of nerve extract on denervated skeletal muscle. "In vivo": dose dependency, species specificity, and timing of treatment. Exp Neurol 1983;80:383–394.

92. Davis HL, Heinicke EA. Prevention of denervation atrophy in muscle. Mammalian neurotrophic factor is not transferring. Brain Res 1984;309:293–298.

93. Davis HL, Kiernan JA. Neurotrophic effects of sciatic nerve extract on denervated extensor digitorum longus muscle in the rat. Exp Neurol 1980;69:124–134.

94. Drachman DB. Is acetylcholine the trophic neuromuscular transmitter? Arch Neurol 1967;17:206–218.

95. Guth L. "Trophic" influences of nerve on muscle. Physiol Rev 1968;48:645–687.

96. Close R. The effects of cross-union of motor nerves to fast and slow skeletal muscles. J Physiol 1964;173:831–832.

97. Close R. Dynamic properties of fast and slow skeletal muscles of the rat after nerve cross-union. J Physiol 1969;204:331–346.

98. Fernandez H, Inestrosa N. Role of axoplasmic transport in neurothropic regulation of muscle end-plate acetylcholin-esterase. Nature 1976;262:55–56.

99. Tomanek RJ, Lund DD. Degeneration of different types of skeletal muscle fibers. II. Immobilization. J Anat 1974;118:531-541.

100. Fuglsang-Frederiksen A, Scheel W. Transient decrease in number of motor units after immobilization in man. J Neurol 1978;41:924–929.

101. Fudema J, Fizzell J, Nelson E. Electromyography of experimentally immobilized skeletal muscles in cats. Am J Physiol 1961;200:963–967.

102. Witzmann FA, Kim DH, Fitts RH. Recovery time course in contractile function of fast and slow skeletal muscle after hindlimb immobilization. J Appl Physiol Respir Environ Exercise Physiol 1982;52(3):677–682.

103. Tabary JD, Tabary C, Taridieu C, Tardieu G, Goldspink G. Physiological and structural changes in the cat soleus muscle due to immobilization at different lengths by plaster casts. J Physiol 1972;224:231–244.

104. Booth FW, Seider MJ. Recovery of skeletal muscle after 3 months of hindlimb immobilization in rats. J Appl Physiol Respir Environ Exercise Physiol 1979;47(2):435–439.

105. Witzmann FA, Kim DH, Fitts RH. Hindlimb immobilization. Length-tension and contractile properties of skeletal muscle. J Appl Physiol Respir Environ Exercise Physiol 1982;53(2):335–345.

106. Kovanen V, Suominen H, Heikkinen E. Mechanical properties of fast and slow skeletal muscle with special reference to collagen and endurance training. J Biomech 1984;17:725–735.

107. Edgerton VR, Barnard RJ, Peter JB, Maier A, Simpson DR. Properties of immobilized hindlimb muscles of the "Galago Senegalensis." Exp Neurol 1975;46:115–131.

108. Tardieu C, Tabary JC, Tabary C, Tardieu G. Adaptation of connective tissue length to immobilization in the lengthened and short-

ened positions in cat soleus muscle. J Physiol Paris 1982;78:214–220.

109. Spector SA, Simard CP, Fournier M, Sternlight E, Edgerton VR. Architectural alterations of rat hindlimb skeletal muscles immobilized at different lengths. Exp Neurol 1982;76:94–110.

110. Fournier M, Roy R, Perham H, Simard C, Edgerton V. Is limb immobilization a model of muscle disuse? Exp Neurol 1983;80:147–156.

111. Thaxter TH, Mann RA, Anderson CE. Degeneration of immobilized knee joints in rats. J Bone Joint Surg 1965;47A:568.

112. Cassidy JD, Brandell BR, Nykolation JW, Wedge J. The role of paraspinal muscles in the pathogenesis of idiopathic scoliosis. A preliminary EMG study. J Can Chiro Assoc 1987;31:179–184.

113. Herman R, Mixon J, Fisher A, Maulucci T, Stuyk J. Idiopathic scoliosis and the central nervous system. A motor control problem. Spine 1985;10:1–14.

114. Shalstrand T, Ortengren R, Nachemson A. Postural equilibrium in adolescent idiopathic scoliosis. Acta Orthop Scand 1978;49:354.

115. Enneking WF, Horowitz M. The intraarticular effects of immobilization on the human knee. J Bone Joint Surg 1972;54A:973–985.

116. Videman T, Michelsson JE, Rauhamaki R, Langenskiold A. Changes in 35 S sulphate uptake in different tissues in the knee and hip regions of rabbits during immobilization, remobilization and the development of osteoarthritis. Acta Orthop Scand 1976;47:290–298.

117. Yellin H, Eldred E. Spindle activity of the tenotomized gastrocnemius muscle in the cat. Exp Neurol 1970;29:513–533.

118. Esaki K. Morphological study of muscle spindle in atrophic muscle induced by immobilization. Nagoya Med J 1966;12:185–201.

119. Maier A, Eldred E, Edgerton V. The effects on spindles of muscle atrophy and hypertrophy. Exp Neurol 1972;37:100–123.

120. Ferrell W, Nade S, Newbold P. The interrelation of neural discharge, intra-articular pressure and joint angle in the knee of the dog. J Physiol 1986;373:353–365.

121. Simard C, Spector S, Edgerton V. Contractile properties of rat hind limb muscles immobi-

122. Ralston HJ, Feinstein B, Inman VT. Rate of atrophy in muscles immobilized at different lengths. Fed Proc 1952;11:127.

123. Kurakami K. Studies on changes of rabbit skeletal muscle components induced by immobilization with plaster cast. Nagoya Med J 1966;12:165–184.

124. Maier A, Crockett J, Simpson D, Saubert C, Edgerton V. Properties of immobilized guinea pig hindlimb muscles. Am J Physiol 1976;231(5):1520–1526.

125. Flint M. Interrelationships of mucopolysaccharide and collagen in connective tissue remodeling. J Embryol Exp Morphol 1972;27(2):481–495.

126. Merriless MJ, Flint MH. Ultrastructural study of tension and pressure zones in a rabbit flexor tendon. Am J Anat 1980;157:87–106.

127. Gelberman R, Manske P, Akeson W, Woo S, Lundborg G, Amiel D. Flexor Tendon Repair. J Orthop Res 1986;4:119–128.

128. Wright V, Johns JJ. Physical factors concerned with the stiffness of normal and diseased joints. Bull Johns Hopkins Hosp 1960;106:216–231.

129. Noyes FR. Functional properties of knee ligaments and alterations induced by immobilization. A correlative biomechanical and histological study in primates. Clin Orthop 1977;123:210–228.

130. Akeson WH, Amiel D, LaViolette D. The connective tissue response to immobility. A study of the chondroitin-4 and 6-sulfate and dermatan sulfate changes in periarticular connective tissue of control and immobilized knees of dogs. Clin Orthop 1967;51:183–198.

131. Troyer H. The effect of short-term immobilization on the rabbit knee in joint cartilage. Clin Orthop 1975;107:249–257.

132. Bowness J. Present concepts of the role of ground substance in calcification. Clin Orthop 1968;59:233–247.

133. Palmoski MJ, Colyer RA, Brandt KD. Joint motion in the absence of normal loading does not maintain normal articular cartilage. Arthritis Rheum 1980;23:325–334.

134. Bobechko W, Hirsch C. Auto-immune response to nucleus pulposus in the rabbit. J Bone Joint Surg 1965;47B(3):574–580.

135. Salter R, Field P. The effects of continuous compression on living articular cartilage. J Bone Joint Surg 1960;42A(1):31–49.

136. Ginsberg J, Eyring E, Curtiss P. Continuous compression of rabbit articular cartilage producing loss of hydroxyproline before loss of hexosamine. J Bone Joint Surg 1969;51A(3):467–474.

137. Akeson WH, Amiel D, LaViolette D, Secrist D. The connective tissue response to immobility. An accelerated aging response? Exp Gerontol 1968;3:289–301.

138. Adams P, Muir H. Qualitative changes with age of proteoglycans of human lumbar discs. Ann Rheum Dis 1976;35:289.

139. Arkin A, Katz J. The effects of pressure on epiphyseal growth. J Bone Joint Dis 1956;38A(5):1056–1076.

140. Rothman RH, Simeone FA, Bernini PM. Lumbar disc disease. The spine. Ch 9. In: Rothman RH, Simeone FA, eds. Philadelphia: WB Saunders, 1982.

141. Binkley JM, Peat M. The effects of immobilization on the ultrastructure and mechanical properties of the medial collateral ligament of rats. Clin Orthop 1982;203:301–308.

142. Resnick D, Niwayama G. Degenerative disease of the spine. In: Resnick D, Niwayama G, eds. Diagnosis of bone and joint disorders. Philadelphia: WB Saunders, 1981.

143. Boyle AC. Color atlas of rheumatology. Chicago: Year Book, 1980.

144. Laros GS, Tipton CH, Cooper RR. Influence of physical activity on ligament insertions in the knees of dogs. J Bone Joint Surg 1971;53A:275–286.

145. Finstrebush A, Friedman B. Early changes in immobilized rabbit knee joints. A light and electron microscopic study. Clin Orthop 1973;92:305–319.

146. Lewis T. Osteoarthritis in lumbar synovial joints. A morphological study. Acta Orthop Scand 1964;[suppl]73:1–112.

147. Lipson SJ, Muir H. Experimental intervertebral disc degeneration. Arthritis Rheum 1981;24:12–21.

148. Taylor TKF, Ghosh P, Bushnell GR. The contribution of the intervertebral disc to the scoliotic deformity. Clin Orthop 1981;156:79–90.

149. Leibenson C. Thoracic outlet syndrome. Diagnosis and conservative management. J Manipulative Physiol Ther 1988;11(6):493–499.

150. Kanoff R. Microvascular decompression for trigeminal neuralgia. J Am Osteopath Assoc 1985;85–7:458–461.

151. Calbucci F, Tognetti F, Bollini C, Cuscini A, Michelucci R, Tassinari C. Intracranial microvascular decompression for 'cryptogenic' hemifacial spasm, trigeminal and glossopharyngeal neuralgia, paroxysmal vertigo and tinnitus. I. Surgical technique and results. Ital J Neurol Sci 1986;7:359–366.

152. Schellhas K, Latchaw R, Wendling L, Gold L. Vertebrobasilar injuries following cervical manipulation. JAMA 1980;24413:1450–1453.

153. Okawara S, Nibbelink D. Vertebral artery occlusion following hyperextension and rotation of the neck. Stroke 1974;5:640–642.

154. Barton J, Margolis M. Rotational obstruction of the vertebral artery at the atlantoaxial joint. Neuroradiology 1975;9:117–120.

155. Pierron D, Lopez-Ibor L, Halimi P, Doyon D, Hurth M. Boucle de l'artere vertebrale et cervicalgies. J Radiol 1985;66(6–7):447–449.

156. Pasztor E. Decompression of vertebral artery in cases of cervical spondylosis. Surg Neurol 1978;9:371–377.

157. Williams R, Warwick PL, eds. Grey's anatomy. 36th ed. Philadelphia: WB Saunders, 1980:896.

158. Theron J, Moret J. Spinal phlebography. New York: Springer-Verlag, 1978.

159. Cuthbertson EM, Siris E, Gilfillan RS. The femoral diaphyseal medullary venous system as a venous collateral channel in the dog. J Bone Joint Surg 1965;47A:965.

160. Davis D. Respiratory manifestations of dorsal spine radiculitis simulating cardiac asthma. Ann Intern Med 1950;32:954–959.

161. Liew M, Dick W. The anatomy and physiology of blood flow in a diarthrodial joint. Clin Rheum Dis 1981;7(1):131–148.

162. Bullough PG, Vigorita VJ. Atlas of orthopaedic pathology with clinical and radiological correlations. New York: Gower Medical, 1984.

163. Guyton A. Venous circulation. Textbook of medical physiology. 6th ed. Philadelphia: WB Saunders, 1981.

164. Ruddy S. Process and principles of inflammation. Vol 1. In: Kelly WN, Harris DE Jr.,

Ruddy S, et al. Textbook of rheumatology. Philadelphia: WB Saunders, 1981:3–7.

165. Heymer B. Causative agents, mediators and histomorphology of inflammation. Pathol Res Prac 1985;180:143–150.

166. Mecklenburg G, Czarnetzki B. In vitro and in vivo migratory response of connective tissue mast cells to inflammatory mediators. Agents Action 1986;19(5/6):344–345.

167. Narayanan A, Engel L, Page R. The effect of chronic inflammation on the composition of collagen types in human connective tissue. Collagen 1983;3:323–334.

168. Nimi M, Deshmukh H. Differences in collagen metabolism between normal and osteoarthritic human articular cartilage. Science 1973;181:751–752.

169. Lussier A, DeMedicis R. Correlation between ossification and inflammation using a rat experimental model. J Rheum 1983;11:114–117.

170. McNicol D, Pace S. Cell receptors to sulphated polysaccharides in the acute and chronically inflamed synovial joint. Clin Orthop 1987;224:105–109.

171. Marshall LL, Trethewie ER, Curtain CC. Chemical radiculitis. A clinical, physiological and immunological study. Clin Orthop 1977;129:61–67.

172. Rodman G, ed. Degenerative joint disease. Primer on rheumatic diseases. 7th ed. Atlanta, Ga.: Arthritis Foundation, 1973.

173. Howell DS. Etiopathogensis of osteoarthritis. In: McCarty DJ. Arthritis and allied conditions. A textbook of rheumatology. Philadelphia: Lea & Febiger, 1985:1400–1407.

174. Peacock EE. Some biochemical and biophysical aspects of joint stiffness. Role of collagen synthesis as opposed to altered molecular bonding. Ann Surg 1966;164:1–12.

175. Moskowitz R. Experimental models of degenerative joint disease. Semin Arthritis Rheum 1971;1:95–116.

176. Pita JC, Manicourt DH, Muller FJ, Howell DS. Studies on the Potential reversibility of osteoarthritis in some experimental animal models. In: Kuettner K, et al., eds. Articular cartilage biochemistry. New York: Raven Press, 1986:349–363.

177. Langenskiold A, Michelsson J, Videman T. Osteoarthritis of the knee in the rabbit produced by immobilization. Acta Orthop Scand 1979;50:1–14.

178. Videman T. Experimental osteoarthritis in the rabbit. Acta Orthop Scand 1982;53:339–347.

179. Jayson M. Intra-articular pressure. Clin Rheum Dis 1981;7(1):149.

180. Valias AC, Tipton CM, Batthes RD, Gart M. Physical activity and its influence on the repair process of medial collateral ligaments. Conn Tissue Res 1981;9:25–31.

181. Burks R, Daniel D, Losse G. The effect of continuous passive motion on anterior cruciate ligament reconstruction stability. Am J Sports Med 1984;12:323–327.

182. Salter R, Simmonds D, Malcolm B, Rumble E, MacMichael D, Clements N. The biological effect of continuous passive motion on the healing of full-thickness defects on articular cartilage. J Bone Joint Surg 1980;62(A)8:1232–1251.

183. Andriopoulos N, Mestecky J, Wright G, Miller E. Characterization of antibodies to the native human collagens and to their component alpha chains in the sera and the joint fluids of patients with rheumatoid arthritis. Immunochemistry 1976;13:709–712.

184. Hahn E, Timpl R, Miller E. The production of specific antibodies to native collagens with the chain compositions. J Immunol 1974;113/1:421–423.

185. Liauw L, Lewis L. Editorial: Mast cells in inflammation and allergy. Agents Actions 1985;17:77–79.

186. Castor C. Regulation of connective tissue metabolism by autocoid mediators. J Rheum 1983;11:55–60.

187. Sandson J, Rosenberg L, White D. The antigenic determinants of the protein-polysaccharides of cartilage. Exp Med 1966;9:817-828.

188. Andriopoulos NA, Mestecky J, Miller EJ, Bradley EL. Antibodies to native and denatured collagens in sera of patients with rheumatoid arthritis. Arthritis Rheum 1976;19: 613–617.

189. Michaeli D Fudenberg HH. The incidence and antigenic specificity of antibodies against denatured human collagen in rheumatoid arthritis. Clin Immunol Immunopathol 1974;2:153–159.

190. Trentham DE, Dynesius RA, Rocklin RE, David JR. Cellular sensitivity to collagen in

rheumatoid arthritis. N Engl J Med 1978; 299(7):327–332.

191. Mikecz K, Glant T, Poole R. Immunity to cartilage proteoglycans in BALB/c mice with progressive polyarthritis and ankylosing spondylitis induced by injection of human cartilage proteoglycan. Arthritis Rheum 1987;30(3):306–318.

192. Golds EE, Stephen IBM, Esdaile JM, Strawczynski H, Poole AR. Lymphocyte transformation to connective tissue antigens in adult and juvenile rheumatoid arthritis, osteoarthritis, ankylosing spondylitis, systemic lupus erythematosus and a nonarthritic control population. Cell Immunol 1983; 82:196–209.

193. Nifbauer G, Wolf B, Bashey R, Newton C. Antibodies to canine collagen types I and II in dogs with spontaneous cruciate ligament rupture and osteoarthritis. Arthritis Rheum 1989;30(3):319–327.

194. Trentham D, Townes A, Kang A, David J. Humoral and cellular sensitivity to collagen in type II collagen-induced arthritis in Rats. J Clin Invest 1978;61:89–96.

195. Tower S. Atrophy and degeneration in the muscle spindle. Brain 1932;55:77–90.

196. Maynard J, Tipton C. The effects of exercise training and denervation on the morphology of intrafusal muscle fibers. Int Z Angew Physiol Einschl Arbeitsphysiol 1971;30:1–9.

197. Ranbourg A, Clermont Y, Beandet A. Ultrastructural features of six types of neurons in rat dorsal root ganglia. J Neurocytol 1983; 12:47–66.

198. Carmel PW, Stein BM. Cell changes in sensory ganglia following proximal and distal nerve section in the monkey. J Comp Neurol 1969;135:145–166.

199. Smith D. Cyst formations associated with human spinal nerve roots. J Neurosurg 1961; 18:654–660.

200. Adams P, Eyre DR, Muir H. Biochemical aspects of development and aging of human lumbar intervertebral discs. Rheum Rehabil 1977;16:22–29.

201. Akeson WH, Amiel D, Mechanic GL, Woo SL-Y, Harwood FL, Hamer ML. Collagen linking alterations in joint contractures. changes in the reducible cross-links in periarticular connective tissue Collagen after nine weeks of immobilization. Conn Tissue Res 1977;5: 15–19.

202. Vater C, Harris E, Siegel R. Native cross-links in collagen fibrils induce resistance to human synovial collagenase. Biochem J 1979; 181:639–645.

203. Amiel D, Wood SL-Y, Harwood FL, Akeson WH. The effect of immobilization on collagen turnover in connective tissue. A biomechanical correlation. Acta Orthop Scand 1982;53:525–332.

204. Glant T, Csongor J, Szucs T. Immunopathologic role of proteoglycan antigens in rheumatoid joint disease. Scand J Immunol 1980;11:247–252.

205. West DC, Hampson IN, Arnold S, Kumar S. Angiogenesis induced by degradation products of hyaluronic acid. Science 1985;228: 1324–1326.

206. Bennett J. The etiology of rheumatoid arthritis. In: Kelly WN, Harris ED Jr., Ruddy S, et al., eds. Textbook of rheumatology. Philadelphia, WB Saunders, 1981:887–895.

207. Chakravart N. Histamine release from mast cell granules. Agents Actions 1982;12(1/2): 94–110.

208. Sorgenfrei J, Danerau B, Vogt W. Role of histamine in the spasmogenic effect of the complement peptides C3a and C5a-desArg (classic anaphylotoxin). Agents Action 1982;12(1/2):118–212.

209. Ehrlic HP, Wyler DJ. Fibroblast contraction of collagen lattices in vitro inhibition by chronic inflammatory cell mediators. J Cell Physiol 1983;116:345–351.

210. Willis A, Cornelsen M. Repeated injection of prostaglandin E2 in rat paws induces chronic swelling and a marked decrease in pain threshold. Prostaglandins 1973;3(3):353–357.

211. McKnight ME, DeBoer KF. Preliminary study of blood pressure changes in normotensive subjects undergoing chiropractic care. J Manipulative Physiol Ther 1988;11:261–266.

212. Vernon H, Seggie J, Engel G, Brown G. The effect of upper cervical spinal manipulation in sheep on circulating levels of melatonin and cortisol. In: Wolk S, ed. Proceedings International Conference on Spinal Manipulation. Washington D.C.: FCER, 1989.

213. Seider M, Nicholson W, Booth F. Insulin resistance for glucose metabolism in disused

soleus muscle of mice. Am J Physiol 1982; 242:E12-E18.

214. Williams S. Take two aspirin. Today's Chiro 1989;18:7–9.

215. Themann P, Havemann U, Kuschinsky K. On the mechanisms of the development of tolerance to the muscular rigidity produced by morphine in rats. Eur J Pharmacol 1986; 129:315–321.

216. Dougherty J, Fraser R. Complications following intraspinal injections of steroids. J Neurosurg 1978;48:1023–1025.

217. Rosner I, Malemud C, Goldberg V, Papay R, Getzy L, Moskiowitz R. Pathologic and metabolic responses of experimental osteoarthritis to estradiol and an estriol antagonist. Clin Orthop 1982;171:280–286.

Index